D1379884

THE COMPLETE HEALTH & BEAUTY BOOK

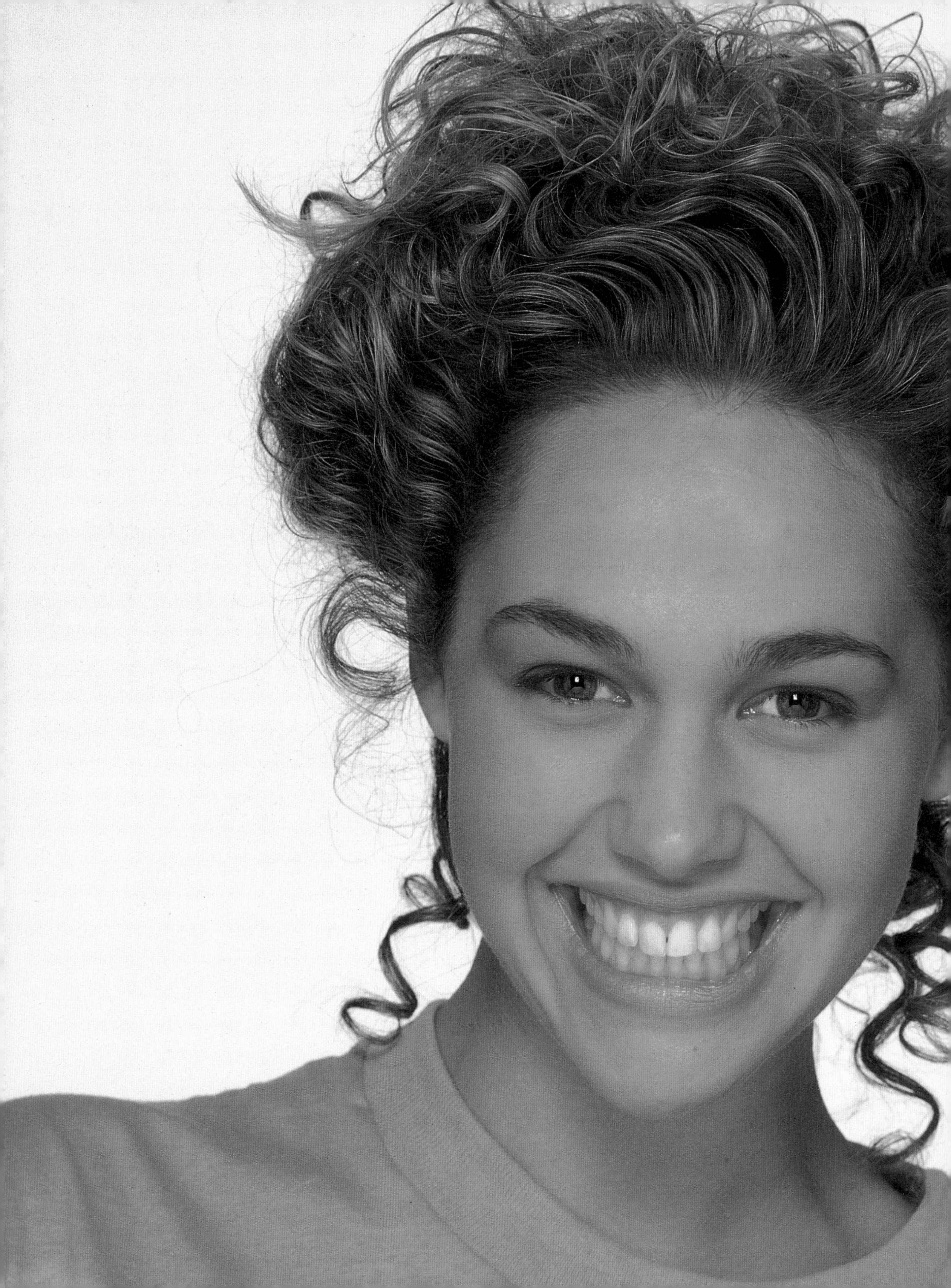

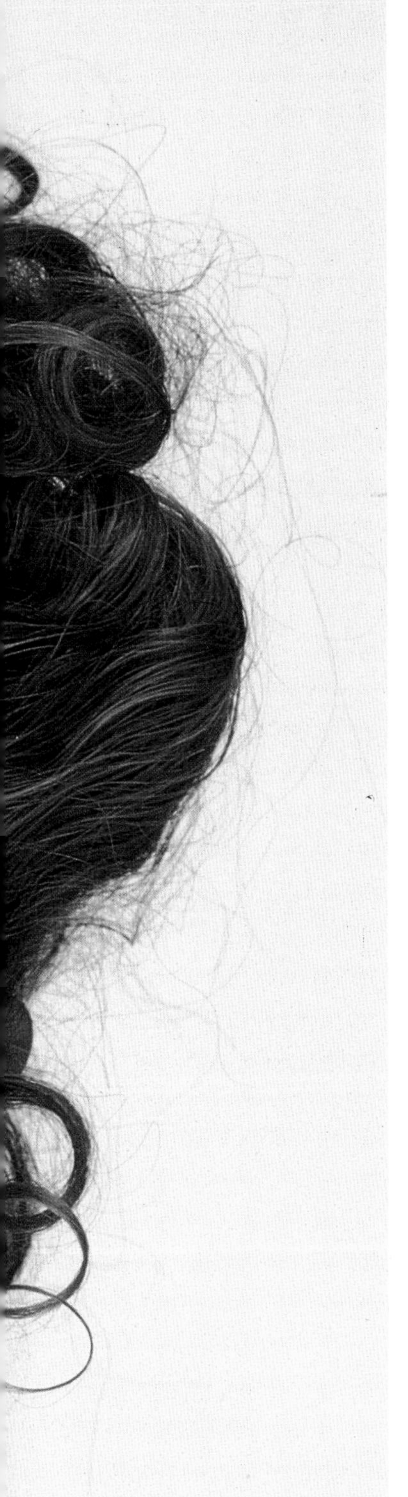

THE COMPLETE HEALTH & BEAUTY BOOK

CHANCELLOR
PRESS

First published in 1992 by
Chancellor Press, an imprint of
Reed International Books Limited,
Michelin House, 81 Fulham Road,
London SW3 6RB

ISBN 1 85152 259 X

Printed and bound in Great Britain by
BPCC Hazells Ltd
Member of BPCC Ltd

CONTENTS

You care about the way you look, what you eat and the way you live your life. **The Complete Health and Beauty Book** is a modern reference which will show you how to look good and stay healthy - and it's all step-by-step!

Stuck in a beauty rut? Bring a touch of glamour to your face or find out how to make-up the natural way. Discover the experts' beauty secrets and work with the right colours to create your personal beauty plan.

There are professional tips on top-to-toe skin care as well as the low-down on safe tanning. And you can pick up the latest salon techniques like waxing, manicure and pedicure so you can use them at home.

See how a good hair-care programme will give you bags more confidence and brush-up on style ideas, working with the right products and styling accessories.

With in-depth facts on lifestyle issues such as diet, vitamin advice and combating stress you'll have the answer to every health and beauty problem!

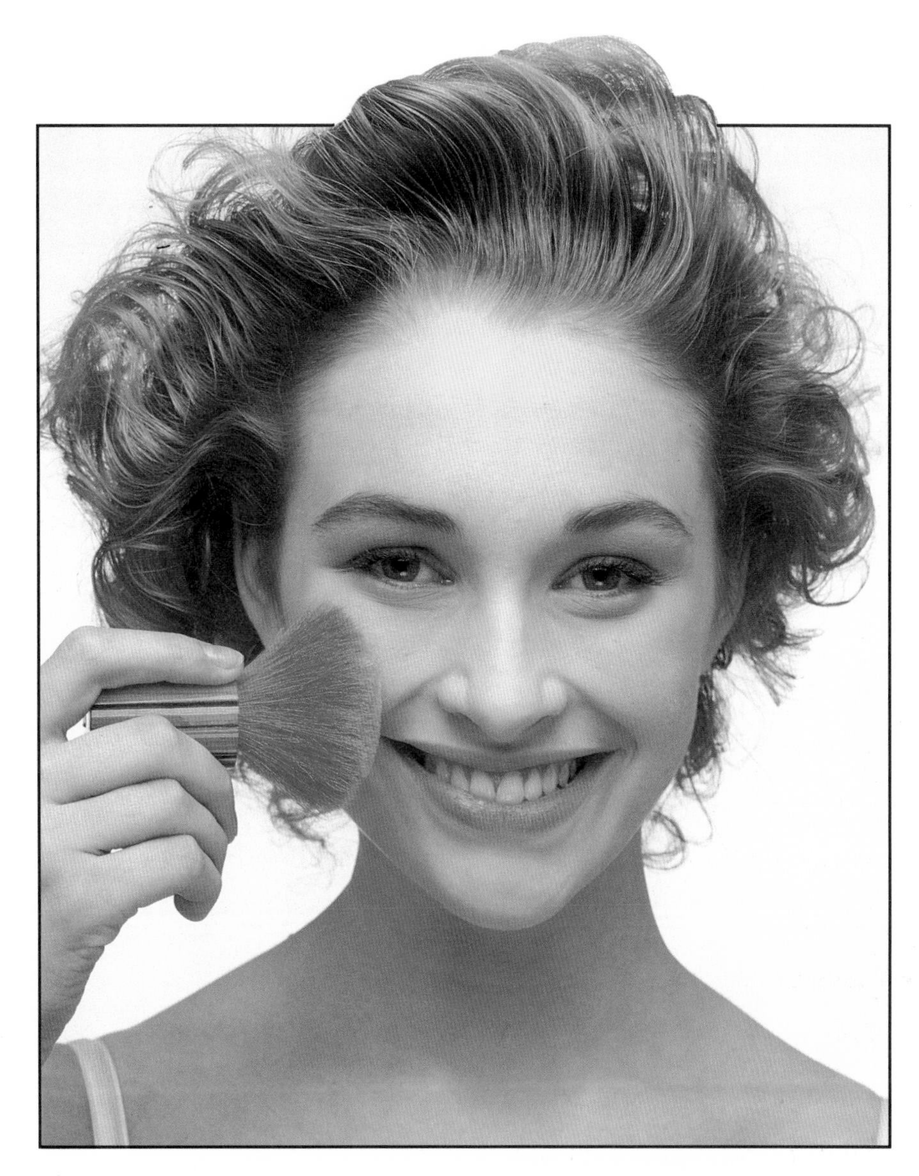

CHAPTER ONE

Beauty Basics

BACK TO BASE

◄ **For a natural finish, choose a foundation in a shade to match your skin tone.**

Foundation is the basis of good looking and long-lasting make-up. It evens out skin tone and primes your complexion for other cosmetics. Here's how to ensure a flawless finish for your face

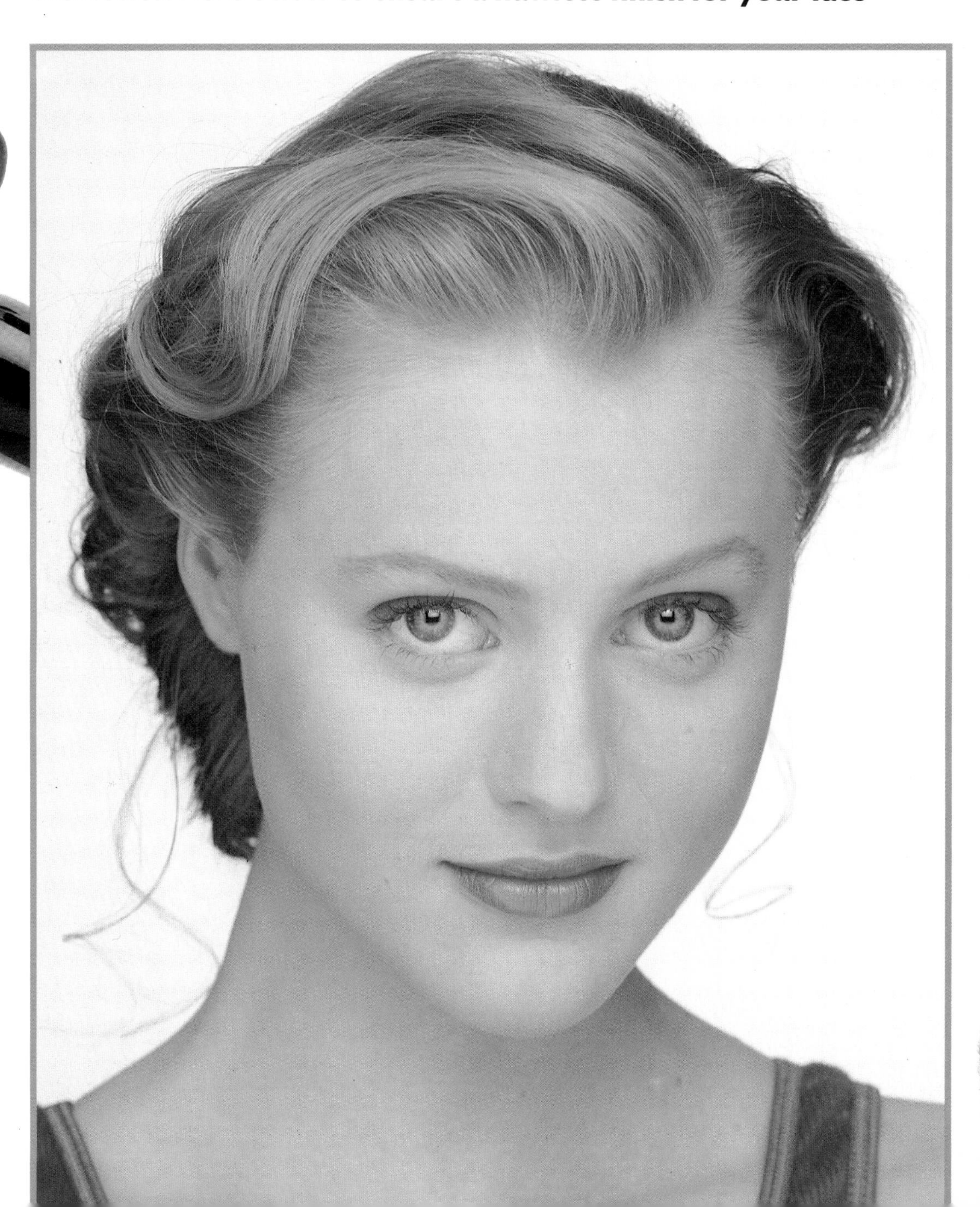

Tip

To avoid diluting the foundation or even washing it off, partly dry your sponge in a tissue before you put on the colour.

GET IT RIGHT!

- Ideally you should put on foundation in natural daylight. If this isn't possible, make sure you have light shining directly onto your face as any shadows falling across your face make it difficult to put foundation on evenly.
- Concealer is great for hiding dark circles under your eyes. But if you use it on under-eye bags it'll act as a highlighter making them look even worse.
- To freshen up foundation at the end of the day, ready for a night out, lightly spritz your face with water then re-powder any oily patches.

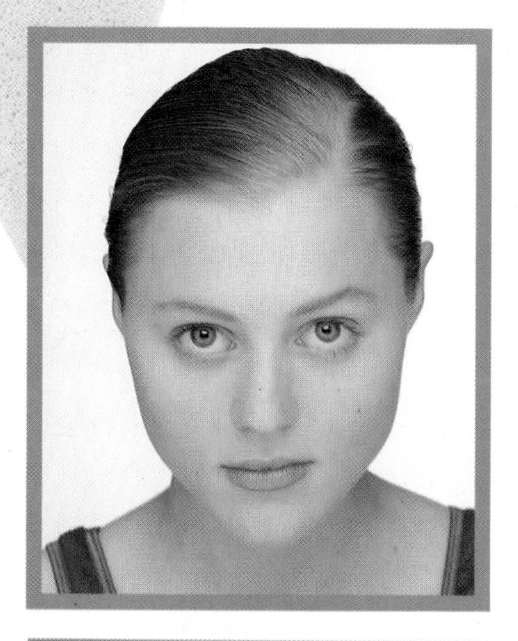

1 **Without make-up your skin may look clear, but foundation will make it look even better. After cleansing, moisturise your face and neck leaving the moisturiser to soak in thoroughly for a couple of minutes.**

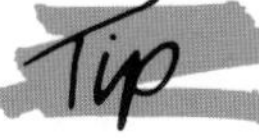

If your skin is oily, press a tissue lightly over the greasiest areas to help prevent breakthrough shine later on in the day.

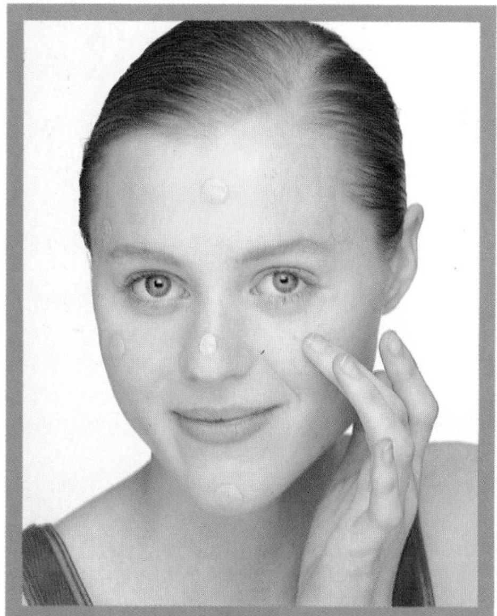

2 **Whatever type of foundation you choose, use only the smallest amount necessary to give adequate and even cover. The best way to do this is to dot on small blobs of foundation with your fingertips.**

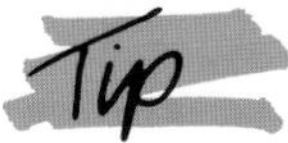

Foundation acts as the base for all other make-up, so don't forget to cover your eyelids and your lips.

3 **You can blend foundation with clean fingers, but take a tip from the professionals and use a damp sponge. Beginning at the centre of your face, gently blend the colour around your nose and under your eyes, then sweep over the rest of your face. To avoid an unsightly tidemark along your jawline, use the clean side of the sponge and blend the foundation down onto your neck.**

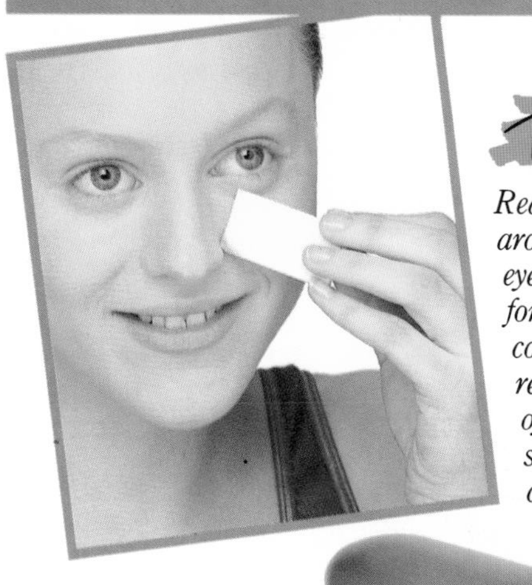

Tip

Reaching the crevices around your nose and eyes can be difficult. Opt for a wedge-shaped cosmetic sponge that can reach the awkward bits of your face. Use the straight sides for covering and blending.

► **To make sure concealer blends with your foundation, choose a shade that's slightly lighter than the base colour.**

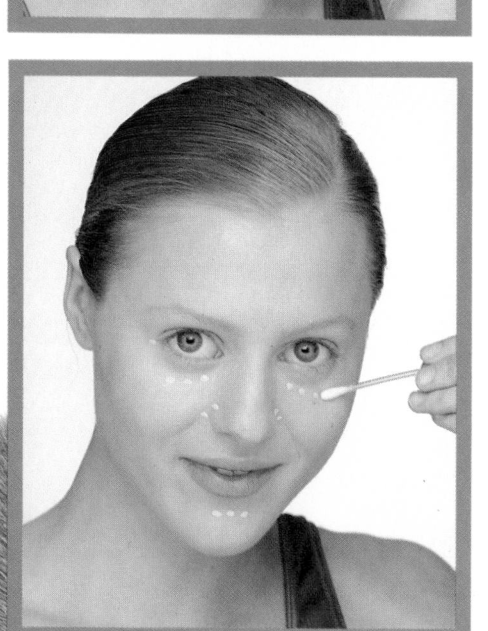

4 **Any major cover-up work that needs doing is a job for concealer and not foundation. Leave your foundation to settle for a few moments before putting it on. Dot it onto dark circles under your eyes, over red veins and small spots. Use a cotton bud to put it exactly where it's needed, then gently blend it into the skin. If you only use your finger you're more likely to rub off the concealer and the foundation with it!**

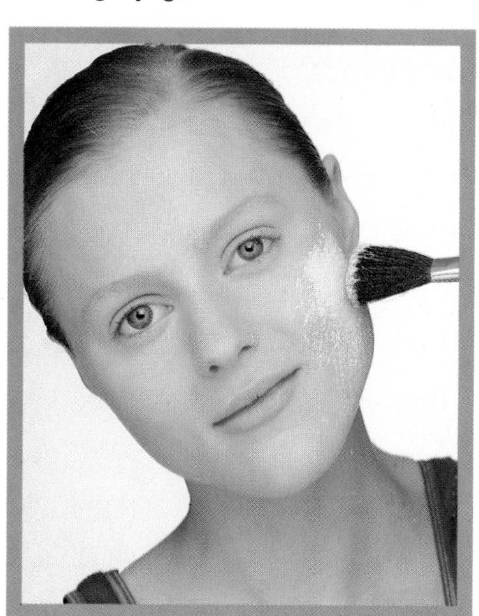

5 **Use loose, translucent powder as soon as you're happy with your foundation. Put a generous amount on a medium-sized brush and sweep over your face and neck. Put more on your nose, forehead and chin but go lightly around your eyes. Too much powder here can leave you looking dry and floury. Finish by lightly brushing off any excess powder leaving just a fine coating over your skin.**

Photographs: CHRIS LANE/Hair & make-up: KARIN DARNELL/Vest top: KNICKERBOX/Still life: ADRIAN TAYLOR

FOUNDATION

Since your foundation is the base for the rest of your make-up it's essential to choose the right one. Here's how to find the perfect formulation to suit your skin

A perfect skin is one of those things that just about everyone dreams of but most of us haven't got. That's why foundation is a girl's best friend.

If you can get your skin to look good – with a little help – then you're halfway to perfect make-up. It's well worth taking time and care over choosing and using your foundation. Get your skin right and you'll be able to skimp on the amount of other make-up you need to wear.

A good foundation is the key to long-lasting make-up as everything else sits on top of it. If your base stays looking good all day there's more chance of the rest doing the same.

You can cover almost any kind of imperfection with the right foundation – it's simply a matter of choosing the right texture for the finish you require. Foundation won't harm your skin at all even if you suffer from spots or blemishes. Cover up with the right formulation and no one will even know they exist! You'll actually be protecting your skin by wearing foundation and so long as you take care to cleanse thoroughly every night, your skin will look nearly as good without make-up as it does with it.

Powder and concealers go hand in hand with your foundation so match them carefully for a co-ordinated face.

But before you do battle at the make-up counter, sort out which cover-up is going to suit you best.

THE RIGHT STUFF

Foundations come in a bewildering variety of colours and formulations. What you're looking for is a foundation that covers all your imperfections. It should be able to minimise blemishes, dark shadows and red veins, and it should smooth out uneven skin tone. The two things you have to consider when you're choosing a foundation are texture and colour.

TEST FOR TEXTURE

Textures vary from the sheerest mousse to heavy creams that will cover just about any blemish. As a general rule, the creamier and more solid the foundation the better the cover. Test for texture on the back of your hand.

Put on water-based foundations with a damp sponge.

COVER STORY

MOUSSE is good for skins that only need very light coverage. The texture of mousse makes it extremely easy to use.

LIQUID gives a light-textured base that will cover small blemishes without looking too heavy, and can be used on all skin types.

CREAM gives more coverage so it's good for quite blemished skins. Creams usually contain a high percentage of oil which makes them ideal for dry and older complexions.

CAKE comes in a compact and is handy to carry around for quick touch-ups. It gives good coverage and is usually put on with a sponge. Cake can be either oil or water-based. Use oil for dry skin and water-based for greasy skin.

STICK is usually oil-based and better for dry skins. Can give light or heavy cover.

POWDER is best suited to oily skin as it will accentuate fine lines on dry skins. It's excellent for quick matt coverage and touch-ups during the day.

TINTED MOISTURISERS are not really foundation but will give a very light cover that's great when you've got a bit of a suntan. Don't cover with powder as you'll lose the natural looking glow.

SATIN FINISH contains tiny particles that reflect the light giving your skin a slight sheen. Only use on dry skins and even then save for evenings only.

HYPO ALLERGENIC products are made from ingredients that are less likely to cause allergies. As they don't usually contain perfume or other known irritants they are good for sensitive skins. They're available in most textures and colours.

CONCEALER could be what you need if you've spots or blemishes that won't disappear under your foundation. Try to get as close a match to your skin colour as possible. If it's lighter or darker the concealer will draw attention to, rather than away from, your spot. Don't put the concealer directly onto spots as you may spread any infection. Use a cotton bud to put it on, and your finger to blend.

Sticks are good for dry skin that needs extra cover.

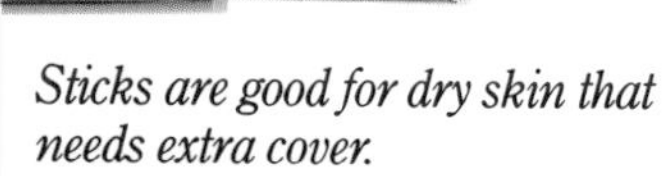

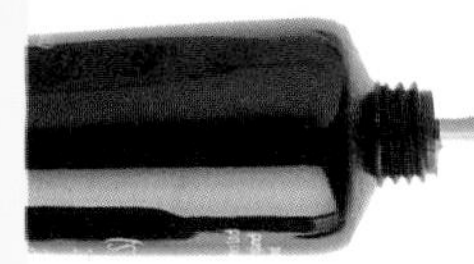

Liquid gives even cover on all skin types.

Concealers in stick, pencil or compact form hide bits you'd rather no one else sees!

Photographs: ADRIAN TAYLOR

Natural sponges have a lovely soft texture when damp.

COURSE

A large soft brush is the easiest way to put on loose powder.

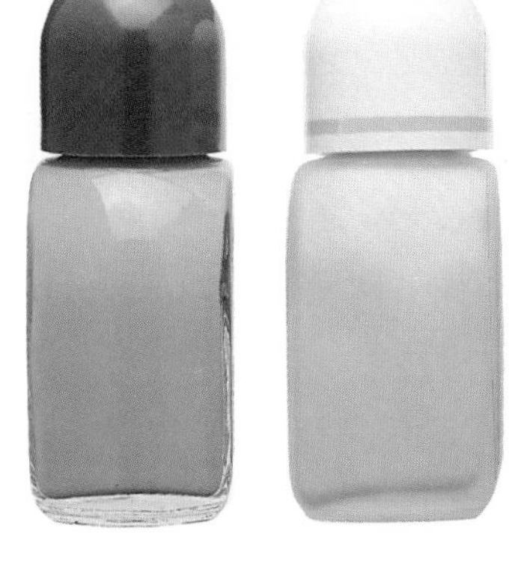

From light to dark – choose the shade that matches your skin tone.

Latex sponges help to give a well blended finish.

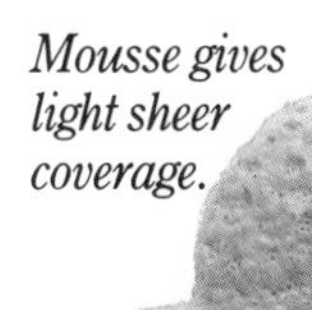

Mousse gives light sheer coverage.

Powder foundations give a matt finish to oily skins.

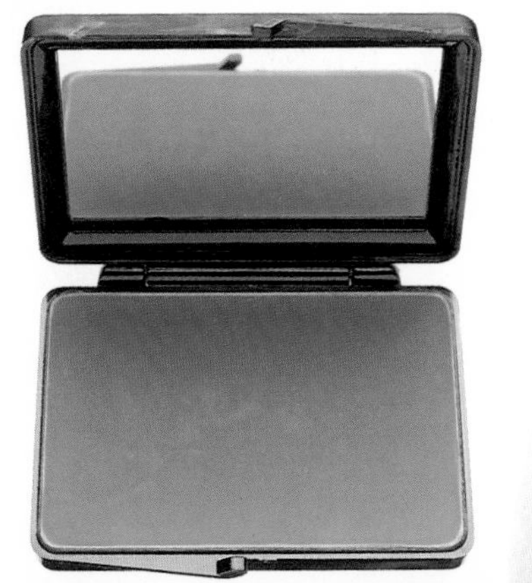

Large sponges for quick cover-ups.

CHOOSING THE COLOUR

The perfect foundation is the same shade as your skin. Never try to change the colour of your skin with your foundation – too light and it'll look like a mask and too dark will look theatrical and far too orangy.

Forget testing for colour on your hand – the only way to see if the shade's right for you is to try it on your face where you're going to wear it.

To get a good colour match, make-up artists test foundation on the neck rather than the face where skin tone is often uneven.

When shopping for a new foundation go out with a bare face so you can test it out along your jawline. Take your time and try out several – the one that almost disappears is the right shade. The colour will look different under artificial light so take a mirror along and go outside to see how they look. Don't forget that your colouring changes all through the year so you'll probably need a lighter and a darker foundation. Invest in a few extra shades and mix these with your base colour as the seasons change.

Look out for trial sizes and try out each foundation before you invest in a full-sized product.

FINGERS OR SPONGE?

It's really just a matter of personal preference whether you use clean fingertips or a cosmetic sponge to put on your foundation. Fingers are easier to get around all the awkward bits, but a sponge can give a lighter finish. Take a tip from make-up artists and apply foundation with a damp sponge for better blending. There are also sponges that are cut into wedge shapes to make it easier to work around eyes and nostrils, or flat ones to cover large areas quickly. Keep your sponges scrupulously clean by washing them out each time you use them and boiling occasionally.

YELLOW OR RED?

If choosing foundation is a real problem, it'll probably help to know more about your individual skin tone.

Whether your skin's a pale or dark shade there will be underlying tones of either red or yellow. To find out what your tone is, check a bit of skin that doesn't usually get tanned (the inside of your arm is ideal). Hold a piece of white paper next to it to exaggerate the difference. A hint of pink or blue and your tone is in the red group, slightly olive and you're definitely yellow.

Red toned skins look best with a flat beige foundation without any pink or peach in it and not too much blusher. Yellow tones are best with a foundation that's very slightly pinker than the skin to warm the face up.

MONEY SAVERS

When you're running low on foundation make the last few drops last a bit longer:

- Mix the foundation with a few drops of moisturiser on the back of your hand.
- Stand the bottle on its top overnight – you'll find a bit extra in the morning.
- Cut the foundation tube in half – it's amazing quite how much is still left inside.
- If your skin is basically good then only use foundation down the centre panel of your face to disguise those oily patches.
- If you've run out altogether – just cover blemishes with concealer and a layer of powder until you can get to a shop.

VANISHING TRICKS

If you've got dark circles or unsightly bags, focus on our eye-catching cover-ups, and watch those niggling problems simply disappear before your very eyes!

SHADOW SHIFTERS

A shadow is a dark area under the eye – like a dent or slight bruise. Permanent dark shadows can be hereditary and don't necessarily mean you've had too many late nights.

In the short term, they can be caused by poor diet, constipation, drinking too much alcohol or taking some kinds of medication.

If your lifestyle isn't to blame and the shadows won't go away, it could be a sign of a medical condition such as anaemia, so go and see your doctor at once.

BAGS EYE

Bags are raised areas that stick out above a dark shadow, and vary from a small lip to a large bulge. They're usually hereditary so there's really nothing you can do to make them disappear altogether (apart from cosmetic surgery), but with clever concealing they can look a lot less prominent.

Using too much thick night cream under and around your eyes can make them worse! The delicate skin around your eyes acts like a sponge, absorbing the oil in the cream, causing puffiness and swelling. So take care when applying cream and use it sparingly, keeping it well away from the eye area. Switching to a lighter gel formulation may also help.

An oil-free eye make-up remover will also prevent puffiness. To use, simply dip a cotton bud in eye make-up remover, then stroke it up and down your lashes and over lids. Use clean cotton wool to gently wipe off make-up and remover in one sweep. Repeat with fresh cotton wool until there's no more colour rubbing off.

You may be allergic to certain ingredients in some products. Heavy perfume can irritate the eye area, so look out for hypo-allergenic fragrance-free eye products to minimise the risks. Loose mascara filaments or particles of shadows can also flick under the eyes, so always put on a base of powder or foundation first.

Don't just think of the obvious causes. Fingers come in contact

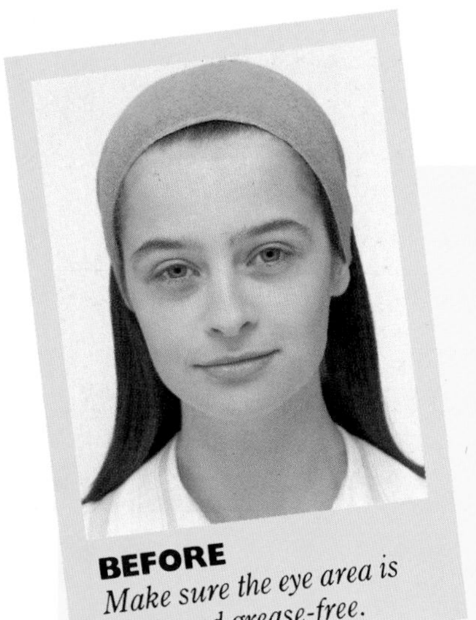

BEFORE
Make sure the eye area is clean and grease-free.

IN THE SHADOWS

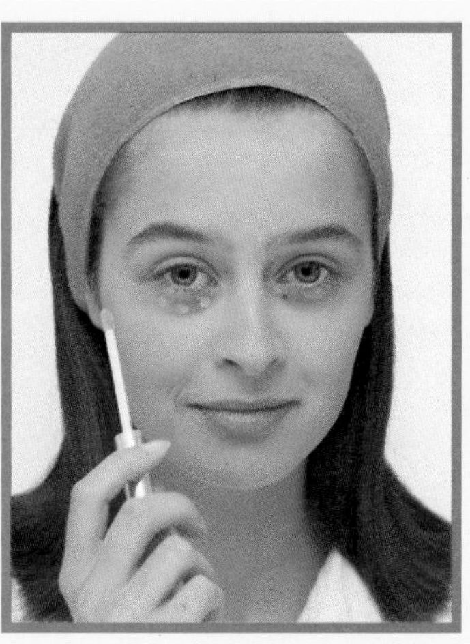

1 *Dot the concealer underneath your eyes in a shade lighter than your skin tone.*

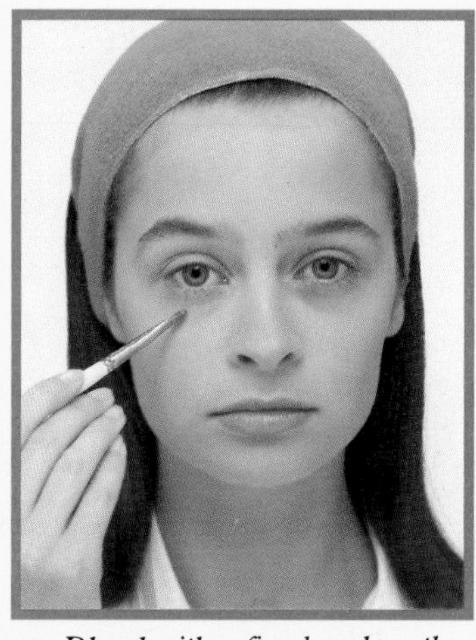

2 *Blend with a fine brush or the tip of a clean finger. Check the result in a mirror.*

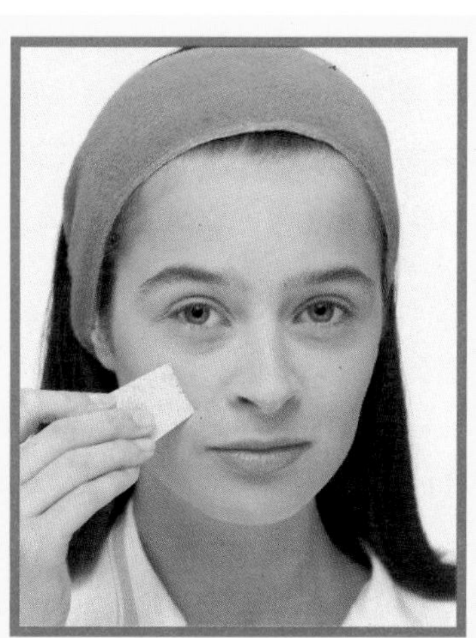

3 *Smooth on foundation with a damp sponge, using light, upward strokes. Try not to dislodge the concealer.*

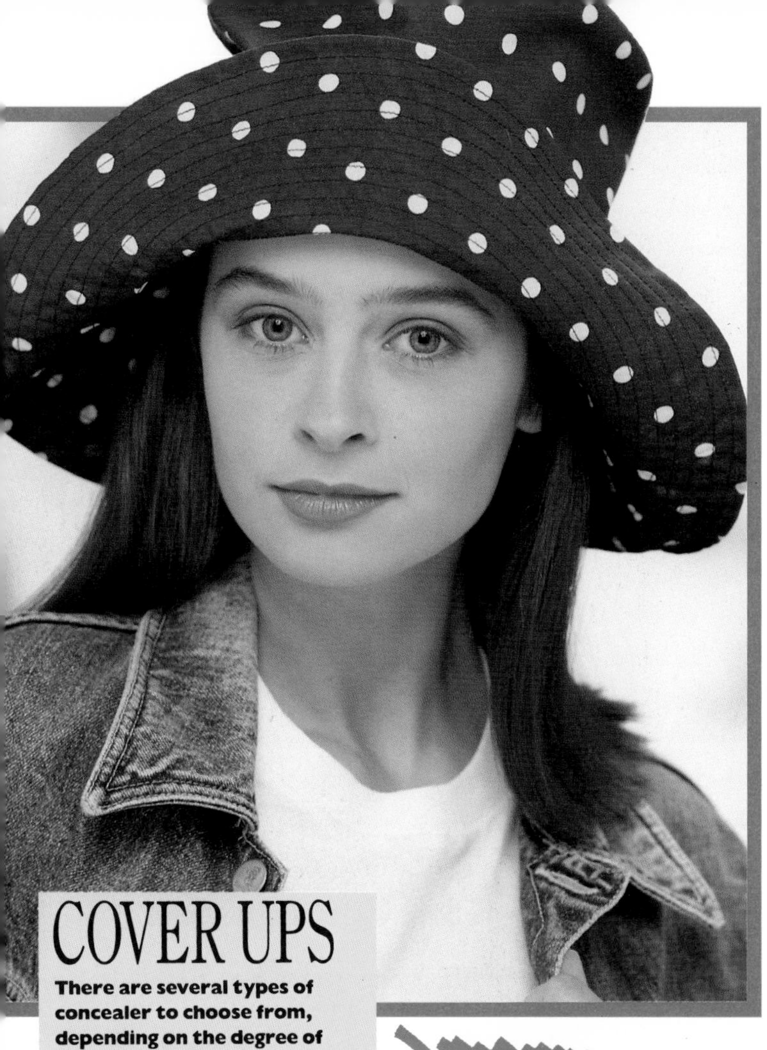

COVER UPS

There are several types of concealer to choose from, depending on the degree of coverage you want.

Younger skin can take heavier creams without looking clogged but it's a good idea to stick to lighter formulations if your skin is very dry, sensitive or lined.

You'll find that most brands come in a limited shade range – usually light, medium or dark. Use light-medium colours for shadows and darker ones for hiding bags.

Watchpoint

Never drag or pull the skin under the eyes as you risk making the bags look even bigger.

with the eyes and face, and could well be allergic to the ingredients, such as formaldehyde which is used to harden nail varnish.

Another possible cause of bags is water retention. You can end up with water being retained around your eyes. This happens to some women just before their periods. If the problem persists and is accompanied by swollen ankles or other symptoms, you should see your doctor.

4 Pat on loose powder with a velour pad, and whisk off the excess with a soft brush.

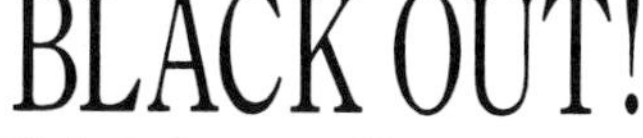

BLACK OUT!

To help improve the circulation around each eye and drain away excess fluid, try the following two to three times a day:

Press your fingers gently back and forth along the socket bone, then pat the under-eye area with the index finger.

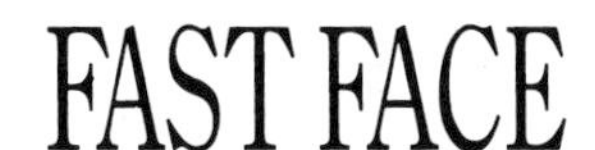

FAST FACE

Come 5.30pm, your eyes may not look so sparkling. Even up the skin tone under your eyes in next to no time.

1 Spritz skin with a water spray to refresh it and to instantly reduce any puffiness.

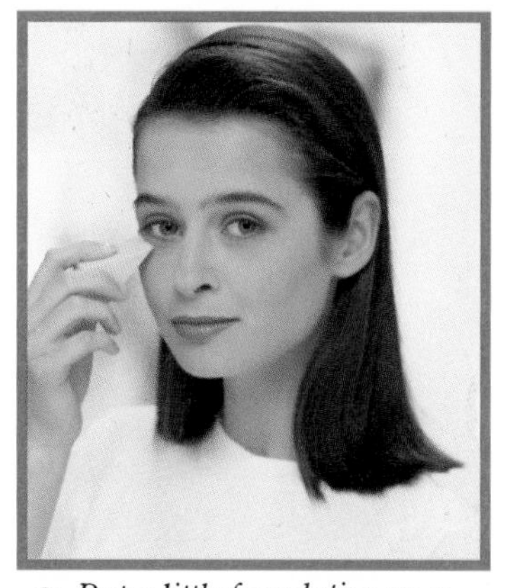

2 Put a little foundation on a damp sponge and gently blend it under the eyes.

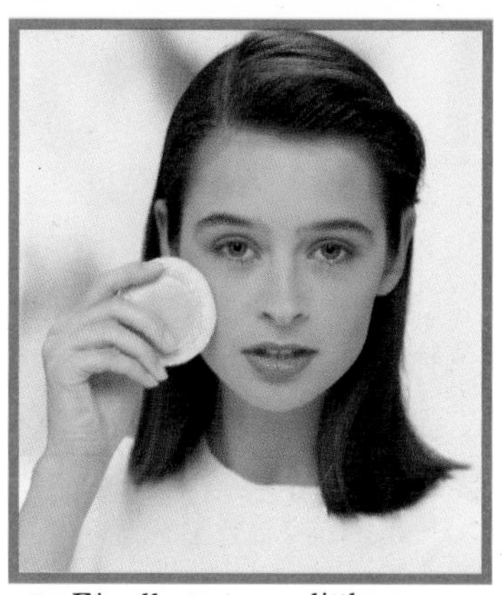

3 Finally, pat on a little loose powder for a smooth, even finish.

TOP TIPS

Try these simple solutions for perfect peepers!

- **Avoid pearlised eyeshadow if eyes are puffy or swollen as it'll highlight the problem.**
- **If you have dark shadows under your eyes, ease the problem temporarily by using a cube of ice wrapped in a handkerchief to gently massage the area. Then disguise with concealer and make-up.**
- **Look to natural remedies like witch-hazel, camomile, cucumber, cornflower and the plant eyebright found in many eye products to help soothe puffiness.**
- **Watch what eye make-up you are using and where you're putting it! Keep colours simple and avoid pinky shades or cream textures which will only draw attention to dark shadows and make eyes look even puffier. Avoid grey shades too – which can make you look hollow-eyed! Taupe and beige look best, blended with dark brown shades in the socket area.**
- **Avoid using eyeliner under the lower lid and only use mascara on the top lashes.**
- **If your eyes are very red and irritated, splash them with cold water, then relax in a bath or darkened room with slices of chilled cucumber or cold tea bags placed over each closed eye.**

BAGS AWAY!

You can't disguise bags, but it is possible to even up the skin tone around them so that they don't look quite so noticeable.

- *Use a concealer one shade darker than your skin tone.*
- *Draw a semi-circle from the inner corner of your eye, following the line of the bag but blending just outside its outer edge.*
- *Finish with a light covering of foundation.*

Photographs: ALISTAIR HUGHES/Hair and make-up: JUDITH PALLAN/Hat: THE HAT SHOP/T-shirt: THE GAP

POWDER POWER

Add the final polish to your make-up with powder! The latest ones can blot shine, shade and shape! So dust up on how to use them

If you've looked at any make-up adverts recently, it's more than likely that the product being advertised was good old face powder. Not only has it enjoyed a massive image revival but most professional make-up artists agree that it's *the* make-up essential. And luckily it's a far cry from the days of granny's sweet-smelling pressed compact in a less-than-flattering shade of Misty Dawn!

Not so long ago the pressed variety was the only sort of powder available at the cosmetic counters, but now you can buy it in spray form, in all shades, shapes (powder balls are the latest invention) and blends. Follow our guide to the powder options and make sure you get the perfect one for your skin's needs.

What's more it's actually dead trendy to own a stylish gold compact and equally swanky cosmetic brush! They're the ultimate beauty accessories.

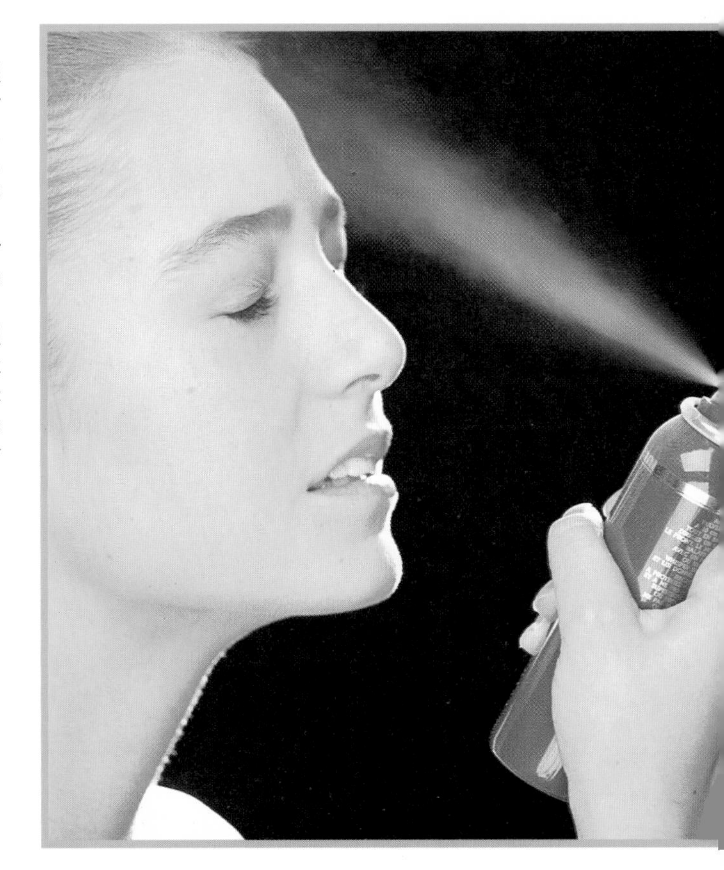

WHAT'S YOUR TYPE?

Here are the main types of powder available:

Loose powder: which comes in a tub and should be used for setting your foundation at the very beginning of the day.

Pressed powder: which comes in a compact or 'book' and is ideal for quickly retouching your make-up during the day. Since it is hard to buff pressed powder as it is quite solid, don't make the mistake of using it all over your face – it will just lift off your foundation, or make your face look patchy.

Powder pages: these work in exactly the same way as pressed powder but come as convenient, non-spillable, tear-off powdered paper pages.

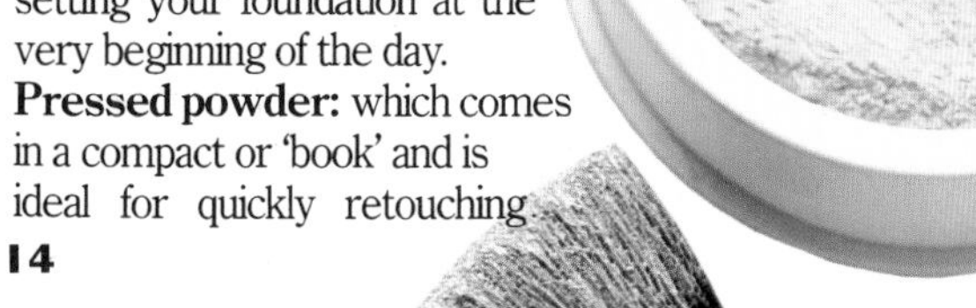

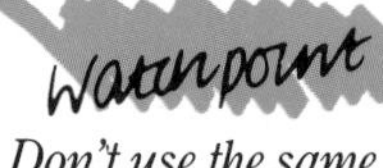

Don't use the same brush for powder and blusher – your skin will look blotchy.

COLOUR CODES

As well as skin-coloured or colourless powders, there are others designed to correct underlying skin faults. They should be applied to clean, bare skin or over foundation. You can add transparent or colourless powder over the top to help blend in the colour.

Green-tinted powder: is good for counteracting redness and hiding broken veins around nose and cheeks.

Lilac-tinted powder: helps liven up a pale sallow-looking skin.

Bronzing powder: is great for evening-up a patchy or fading tan or adding a healthy golden glow to your face, shoulders and body.

Pearlised or metallic powder: this will add a sparkly sheen to your skin. A little goes a very long way, so use it sparingly. For best results keep it for special occasions, since it can leave you looking very made-up. Sometimes called highlighting powder it can also be used to add a sparkle to your temples, browline and cleavage. Glow for it – if you really want to sparkle the night away.

PUFFING AWAY

Most of us apply powder with a big fat brush, but an innovative and time-saving idea is spray-on powder. Just hold the can about 25 cm/10 in from your face and, with your eyes shut, spray it on your forehead, nose, cheeks and chin. Then use a large brush in light, sweeping strokes over your skin to spread the powder evenly.

Another new powder concept is powder balls. All you do is run a fat brush over the surface of the pressed powder spheres to mop up colour. Even if you apply a lot of pressure, it's difficult to load the brush with too much colour, so this type of powder is great for the make-up beginner. The newest type of powder spheres don't just come in one colour either, but a kaleidoscope of pastels to give the skin a very natural luminous glow.

WHY POWDER?

- **It fixes your foundation.**
- **It helps mop up shine.**
- **It gives skin a matt finish.**
- **It adds a flattering, velvety sheen to your skin.**
- **It's quick and easy to use.**
- **It makes your pores look much smaller.**
- **It helps to improve your skin's texture.**

POWDER PLUS

There are now several clever new formulations available that do more than powder alone, and can be used as the perfect all-in-one make-up base:

Custom-blended powder: this is the latest craze at cosmetic counters. A consultant will analyse your skin and blend a face powder that matches its colour and type perfectly. It can be light-textured or heavily-pigmented, have extra moisturisers added or be based on an oil-free formula – it all depends on your skin type.

The very latest in powder technology is the use of something called Sericiate – coated microparticles used in place of talc and which help to control the amount of oil that reaches the skin's surface.

All-in-one bases: all-in-one foundations are a mixture of base and powder together. This means that you can apply your base quickly without the need to add a layer of powder on top.

THE POWDER PLOT

Follow these powder points and you'll get a flawless finish from your loose powder every time.

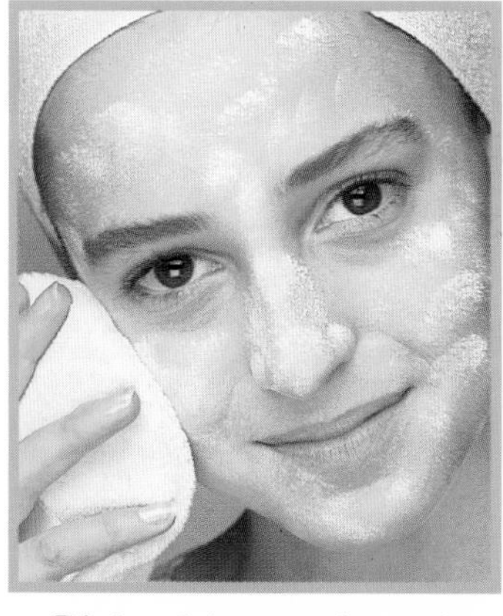

1 *Dip brush into powder, and tap off excess on the back of your hand. Mop up powder with a velour pad and put on face with a 'slap/pat' action.*

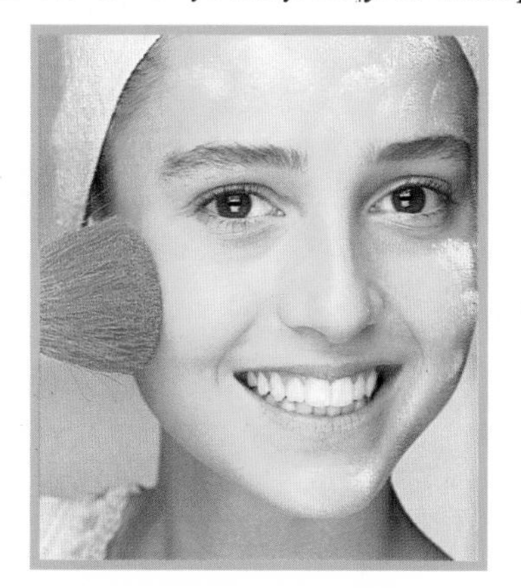

2 *Now carefully dust off the excess in downward strokes using a big, soft powder brush until your complexion is smooth and velvety-looking.*

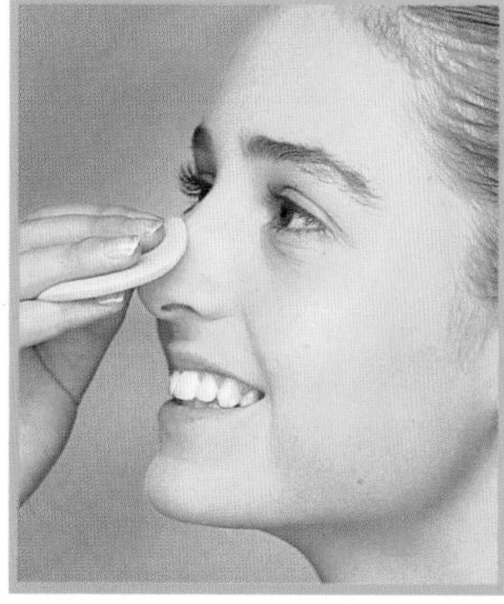

3 *Make sure you carry a pressed powder compact around with you during the day to patch up oily panels and keep your skin looking matt.*

DID YOU KNOW?

- **One of the first commercial face powders was marketed in the nineteenth-century and was made from finely-ground rice powder.**
- **In the sixteenth-century, Queen Elizabeth I used ceruse, a potentially lethal mixture of mercury and lead-based white powder to give her skin a chalky white, porcelain finish. In later life, she had to layer it on thickly to hide the holes where the lead had eaten into her skin.**

NATURALLY DOES IT

Whether you go for loose or pressed powder, there are lots of colours to choose from. But as a general rule, go for a powder with little or no colour if you want it to look as natural as possible. You can always add colour to your skin with a touch of blusher. Look out for the following naturals:

Transparent powder: which is light, matt and colourless.

Translucent powder: which lets light through and gives the skin a delicate sheen. But remember that most powders are translucent so try and choose one in a flesh-tinted shade.

Pure white: gives the skin a very white porcelain appearance. Great for party time, but avoid it if your skin is yellow-toned.

POWDER TRICKS

- **If you're going out straight from work and haven't got time to re-apply your base, just press a tissue over your face to absorb shine and then apply loose powder for a perfect, flawless finish.**
- **If under-eye shadows are a problem, simply dip a cotton bud in a little loose powder and roll it under each eye.**
- **Prevent eyeshadow particles from spoiling your foundation by dusting lots of loose powder over your cheeks. The powder will catch any loose specks and can be dusted off once your eye make-up is finished.**
- **Dust powder over your lashes to thicken them, then put mascara over the top.**
- **Make light foundation heavier and more pigmented by adding a large pinch of loose face powder to it.**

Photographs: IAN HOOTON/Hair and make-up: KIZZY HARRISON/Tops: KNICKERBOX

POWDER TRICKS

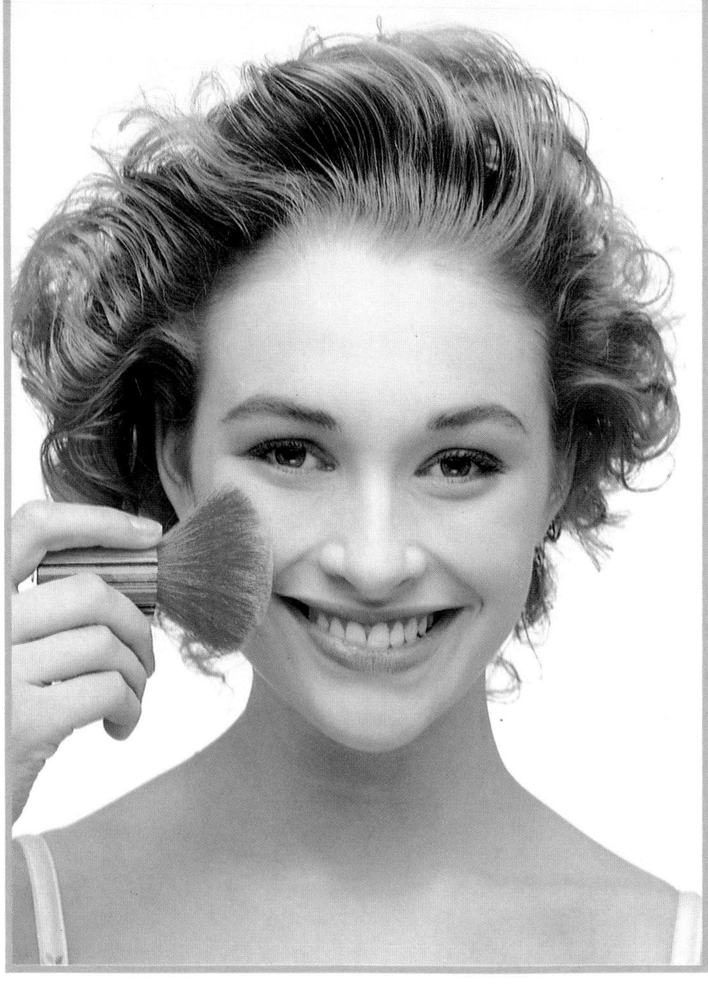

Loose powder is a make-up artist's best friend. It's versatile, easy to use, suits everyone and covers a multitude of sins! Here's your chance to learn a few tricks of the trade

If you've ever used powder, it's probably been to finish off your foundation base, or maybe you've just dabbed a bit on your nose to stop it looking shiny.

And that's what face powder is really for – stopping your skin from looking shiny. It's usually made of very finely ground talc (which could be mixed with kaolin, colour, scent and preservatives) and it comes in a range of colours to suit your skin tone – or you can use translucent powder which is probably the easiest and best to use. Because translucent powder is colourless it's hard to look as if you're wearing too much and it doesn't matter if you don't spread it completely evenly. It's also perfect to put over any coloured eyeshadows and lipsticks, and it mixes well with other kinds of powdered make-up.

You can buy compressed powder in compacts (it's the same as loose powder, but mixed with wax or oil to keep it flat in the compact) and these are especially handy for popping in your handbag. However, you get a better finish from loose powder in shakers, and the most effective way to use it is with a brush straight from the pot.

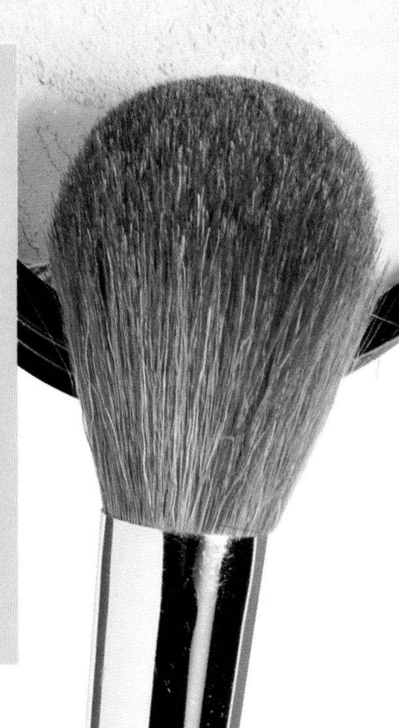

NO-SMUDGE LIPS

In the same way that powder sets foundation, it's excellent for setting lips. Brush a little over your lipstick and you'll be left with a lasting matt colour that won't come off on coffee cups.

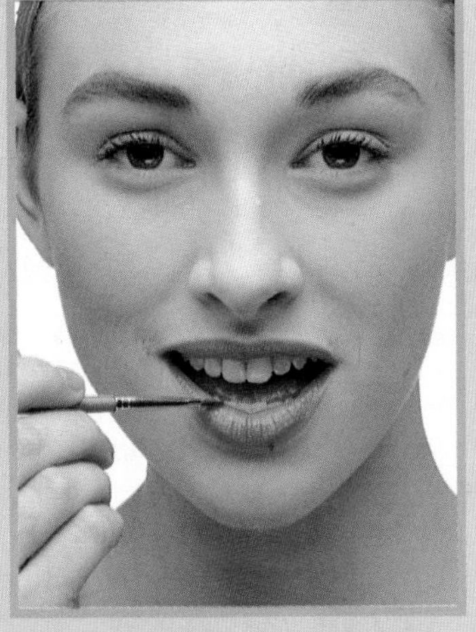

1 *Put on your lipstick as usual – preferably with a brush. Then split a tissue into individual layers.*

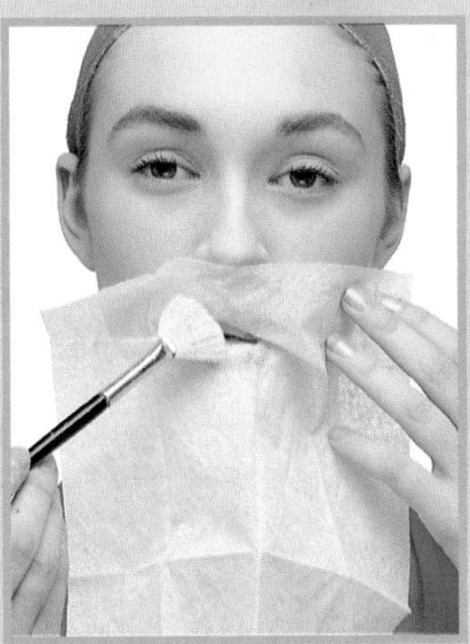

2 *Hold the tissue over your lips and use a brush to dab powder over the top for lasting lip colour.*

Photographs: PAUL MITCHELL/Hair and make-up: CHASE ASTON
Pink body: KNICKERBOX/Rose print bra: NEXT

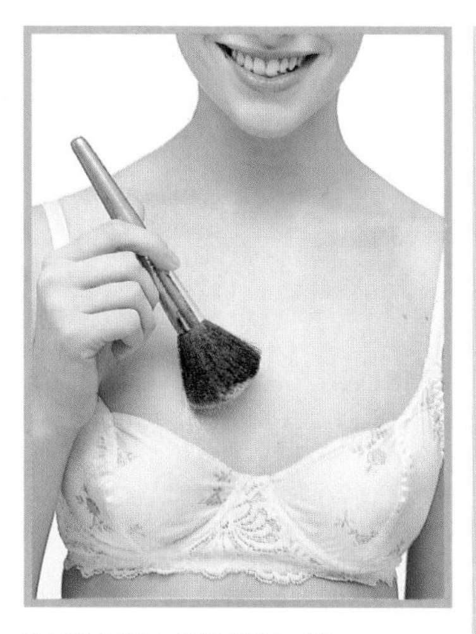

PROFESSIONAL EYES

If you wear dark or bright coloured powder eye-shadow you'll know how hard it is to stop it from smudging around your eyes while you're putting it on. For perfect results, protect the skin under your eyes by covering it in a light dusting of loose powder, then just brush it away when you've finished your make-up.

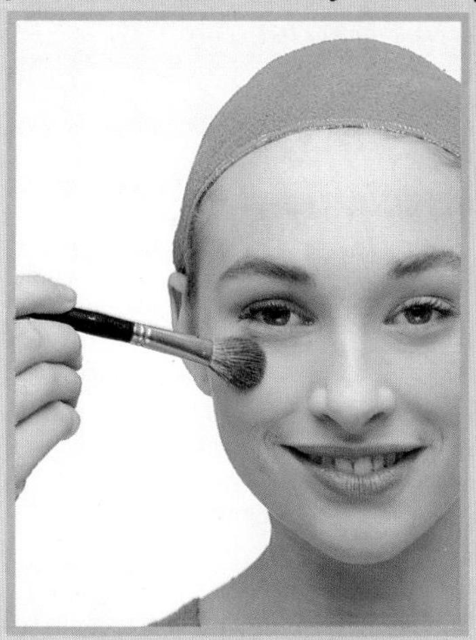

1 When you've put on your foundation and before you start making up your eyes, dab a thick covering of loose powder under each eye.

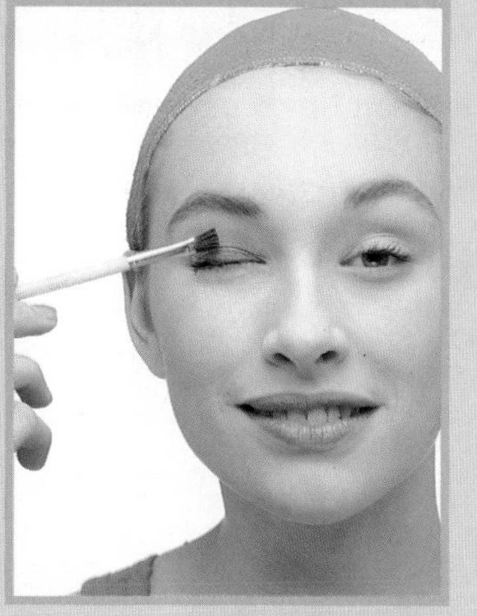

2 Leave the powder there while you make-up your eyes as usual. It'll catch falling specks of colour and stop them smudging on the skin.

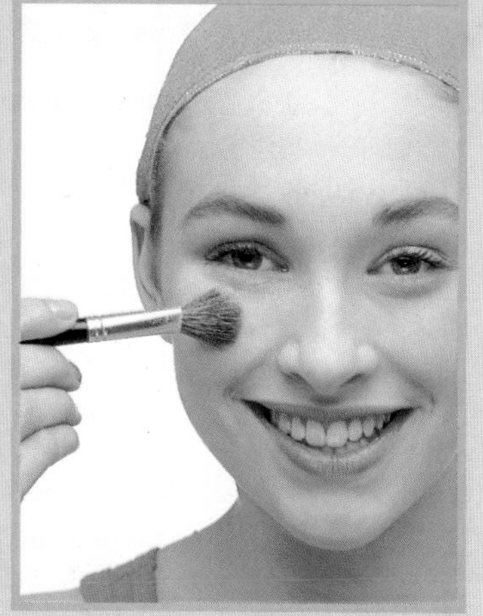

3 When you've finished working on your eyes, brush away the powder and you'll whisk away any stray shadow dust with it.

A DUSTED CLEAVAGE!

Daring necklines expose skin which should be toned to match the skin on your face – or at least powdered to stop it from shining! A light dusting of powder before you dress (don't put it on afterwards, or you'll get specks and smudges of powder on your party frock), will improve your skin texture and take care of any perspiration that may arise during an energetic evening.

Take a tip from filmstars and models and enhance (or fake!) your cleavage by lightly dusting it with a bronzing powder – it really works.

ULTRA-SUBTLE BLUSHER

The secret of natural-looking blusher is to wear very little and spread it very evenly. You can tone down your powder blusher by mixing it with your usual or a translucent face powder. Mix them together on a plate or saucer, rather than directly in their packs. This will keep the individual colours clean for future use. You only need to use a tiny amount of colour for a natural-looking complexion, so save any spare powder you have mixed and then not used in a clean jar with a tight seal.

Tip

Mix translucent powder with old powder shadows to create new subtle colours.

A PERFECT FINISH

For perfect, long lasting make-up, set your foundation with a dusting of powder all over your face – including your ears and neck! Powder absorbs any oil or perspiration that would otherwise disturb and remove your make-up. Use a big soft brush for all-over application, and don't forget to wash the brush regularly to keep it clean!

Overdone it with the blusher? Then quickly and easily tone the colour down by dusting powder over cheeks.

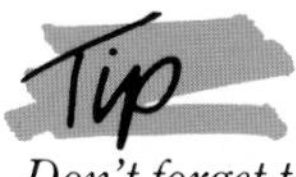

Don't forget to dust a fine layer of powder over your neck, but only use translucent powders as coloured ones can mark clothes.

NON-CREASE EYES

Guarantee crease-proof, glossy eye colour with a fix of powder! When you've put on your eyeshadow, load a small make-up brush with powder, shake off the excess, and then gently stroke the brush over your lid, working from the inside corner outwards. It'll set your eyeshadow, and should stop it from creasing. For a wide-eyed look dust powder over lashes after you've applied your first coat of mascara, and it has dried, to make lashes look thicker.

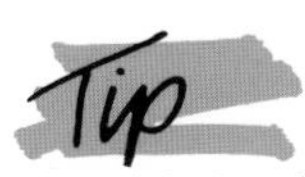

A quick dusting of powder when you put on your lipstick should keep your skin looking silky all evening long.

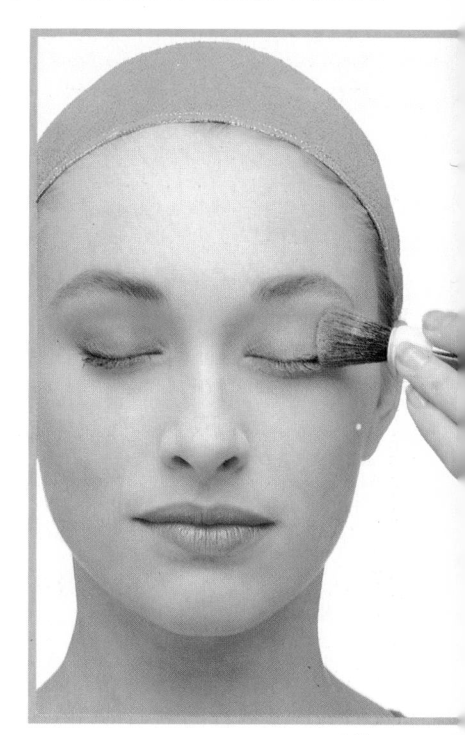

BROW BEATERS

Have you been turning a blind eye to straggly brows? If so, here's your chance to master the art of shaping up with our eye-opening info on perfect plucking

Plucking your eyebrows doesn't have to mean thin, over-arched brows that make you look permanently surprised. Careful plucking can really make a difference to the shape, not only of your brows, but your whole face.

The key to successful plucking is first to tidy up your eyebrows by removing unruly, straggly hairs. You can always pluck a few more if they look too bushy but you can't put back the hairs you've removed! It's also important to take your features into account. If they're small and delicate, you can get away with thinner, finer-shaped eyebrows. But if you have stronger features you'll probably look better with thicker, heavier brows.

1 Make sure your eyebrows are the right width for your face by measuring them first. Find out where your brow should begin by holding a pencil or fine make-up brush vertically against the side of your nose. The inner edge of your eyebrow should start where the pencil and brow meet.

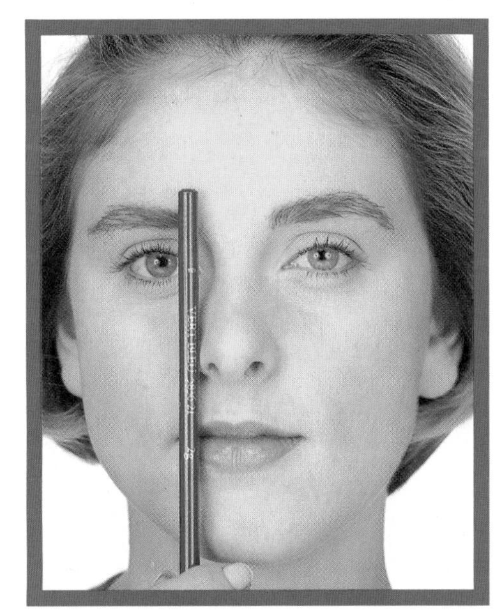

2 Using the same pencil, swing it across in a straight line from the side of your nose to the outside of your eye. Follow the line of the pencil and where it meets your eyebrow is where the outer edge of your brow should end.

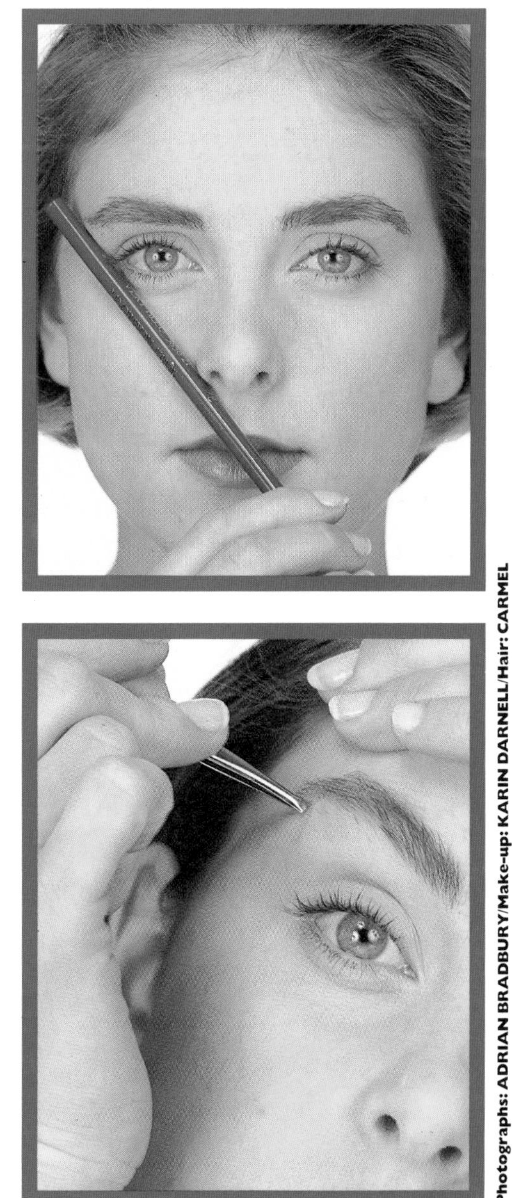

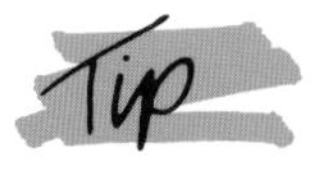

Make sure you don't overpluck by measuring with the pencil several times during plucking.

4 Hold a warm flannel over your eyebrow for a few seconds before you begin to pluck. This will help soften the skin and open your pores. Plucking isn't quite so painful when your skin is warm and it's easier to pull the hairs out too.

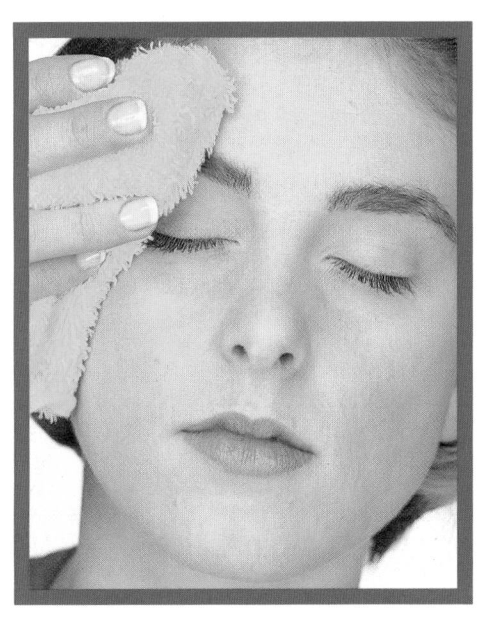

Watchpoint

Make sure the flannel isn't too hot – the skin around your eyes is very delicate.

5 Pull the skin around your brows taut and grasp the hair with the tweezers close to the root. Pull it out quickly in the direction of the hair growth. Always pluck under your eyebrow. Start with the stragglers first, then pluck more if you need to.

Watchpoint

Never pluck above your brows. It makes them look unnatural and will change the shape of your face.

Photographs: ADRIAN BRADBURY/Make-up: KARIN DARNELL/Hair: CARMEL

SHAPING UP

Give your eyebrows that special touch for a sleek natural finish

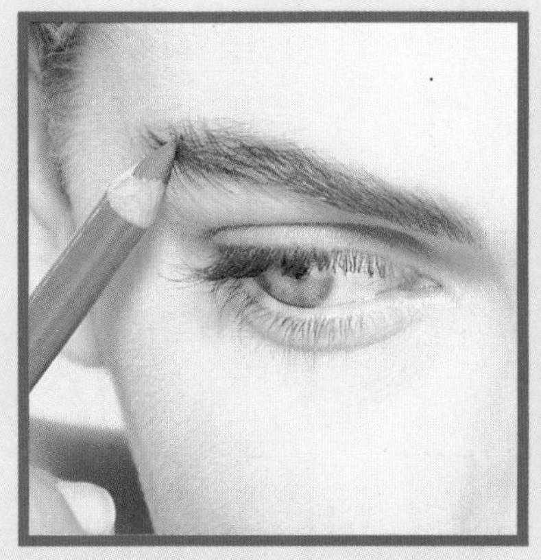

Add extra definition to your brows by using an eyebrow pencil. Use feathery strokes for a natural effect.

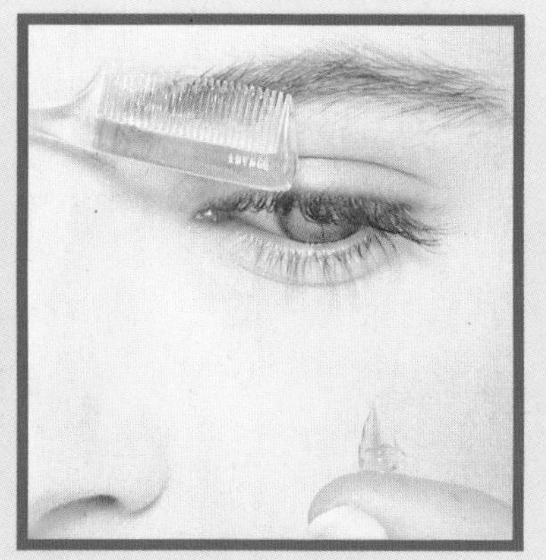

Hair gel is great for taming unruly brows. Just put a little onto an eyebrow comb and comb in the direction of the hair growth.

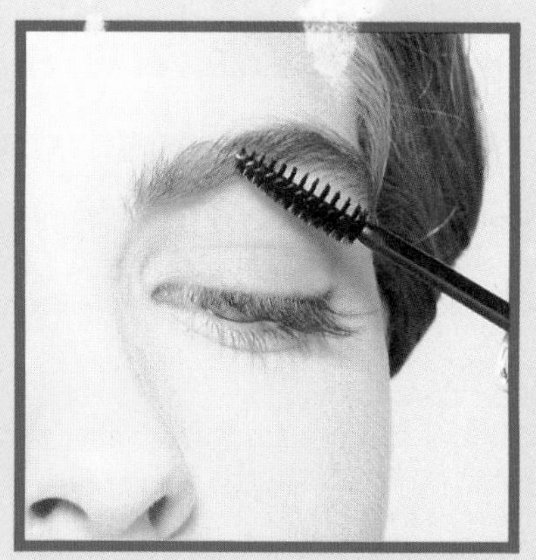

Use an old mascara wand as an eyebrow brush – but make sure it's perfectly clean first. Or you could try colourless mascara.

3 Check the area around your brows is clean and grease-free before you start plucking. Then using a brow brush or an old toothbrush, brush your eyebrows upwards. This will make straggly hairs more visible.

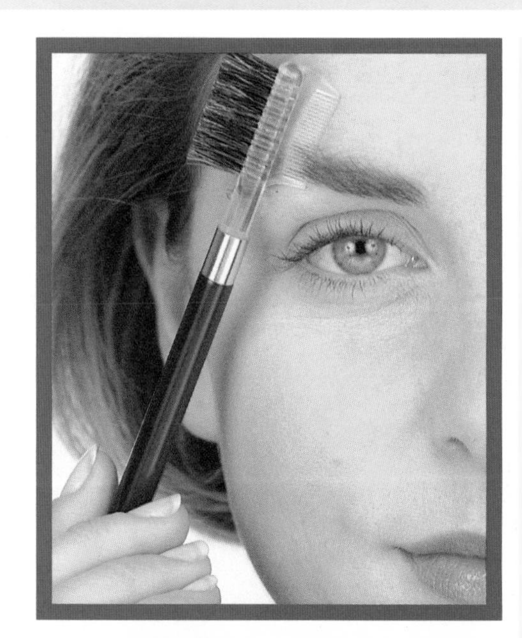

Slant-edged tweezers are best for plucking as they make it easier to grip the hair.

6 When you've finished plucking, soak a cotton wool pad in a mild antiseptic or witch hazel to tone down any redness. Squeeze the soaked cotton wool pad until it's almost dry and hold it over your eyebrow for a few seconds.

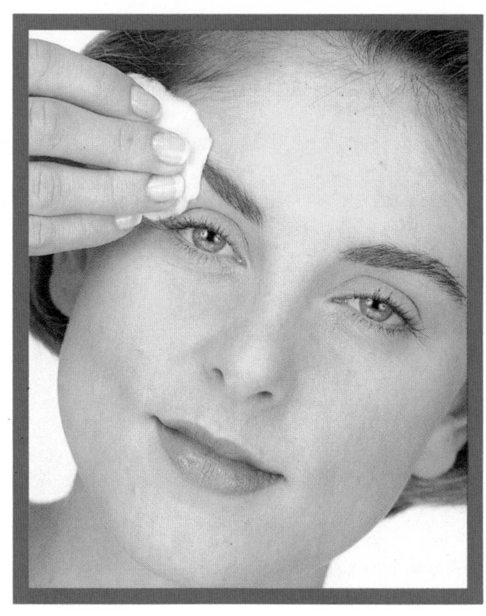

GET IT RIGHT

If you're worried about plucking your brows because you've heard horror stories in the past, check the facts first.

MYTH Plucking makes your brows grow back bushier.

FACT It doesn't. In fact, continual plucking can discourage hair growth. That's why it's so important not to overpluck.

MYTH You need to pluck your eyebrows every day.

FACT If you want to tidy up the odd straggler you can pluck daily but it's not really necessary. It's better if you don't pluck too often as it's easy to overpluck without realising it.

MYTH Plucking eyebrows will make them grow back darker.

FACT Your eyebrows, just like the hair on your head, are made up of several different colours. If your brows are fair you may notice the odd dark hair but this isn't caused by plucking.

MYTH Eyebrow pencils look obvious and unnatural.

FACT If you use an eyebrow pencil to try and fill in sparse eyebrows it will look awful. But tiny feathery strokes of a pencil in a colour that matches your brows will help define their shape. Brush with an eyebrow brush afterwards to smudge any hard lines.

ANY QUESTIONS?

Q Can I use hair removal cream to tidy my eyebrows?

A No! You need to pluck hair by hair for precision. Cream can easily remove too many of your eyebrows and is too strong for your face.

Q Can I use a permanent hair colourant to darken my eyebrows?

A It's best to keep any chemicals well clear of the delicate eye area. The safest way to darken brows is with an eyebrow pencil.

Q My brows are dark and bushy and almost meet in the middle. They're so embarrassing. What can I do?

A Electrolysis will remove unwanted hair permanently, but do remember that fashions in brow shapes change so think carefully before you invest in a course of treatment.

COLOUR COUNSEL

Are you a passionate pink or a burnished bronze? The secret of choosing the right make-up lies in understanding your skin tone. Once you know this, finding cosmetics to suit will never be a problem

There are many different colours to suit every complexion, but basically you are either a cool or warm skin type and should choose cosmetic colours accordingly. If not, your make-up will do nothing for you. But wearing shades that complement your skin tone will make your face come alive. It means, too, that your eye, cheek and lip colours are in harmony, rather than clashing.

To find your skin type, try this quiz – just tick the answers that apply to you, then check your score.

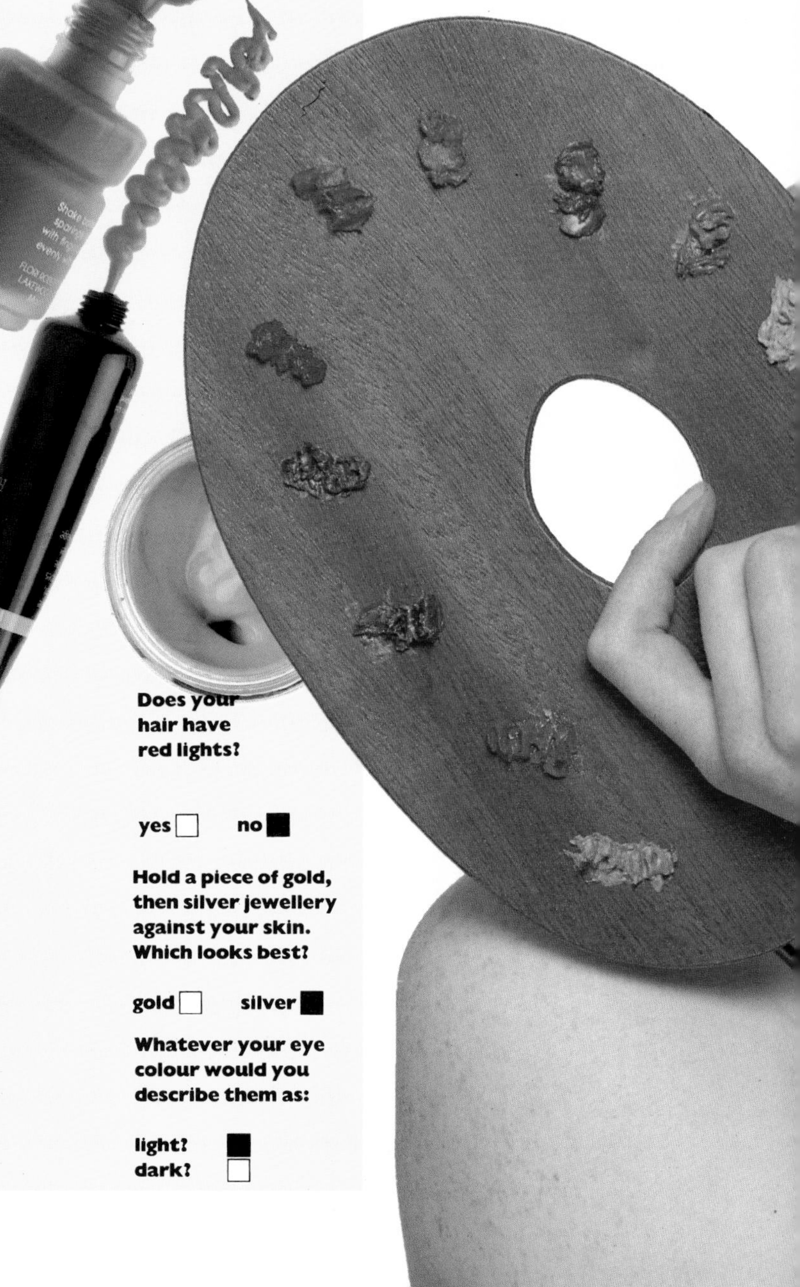

QUESTIONS

Do you have quite a few moles on your face and body?

yes □ no ■

When you wear foundation, does the colour seem to change after a few hours?

yes □ no ■

Do you get compliments when you wear:

pink? ■
emerald green? □
denim? ■

Do your lips turn blue when it's cold?

yes ■ no □

In bright sunlight, do you squint without sunglasses?

yes ■ no □

When sunbathing, do you?

burn easily? ■
freckle rather than tan? □
tan easily? □

Do you have a tendency to broken veins?

yes ■ no □

Do you have a problem with blackheads or open pores?

yes □ no ■

A few hours after cleansing is your skin:

fairly dry? ■
oily in patches? □
greasy? □

Is your skin translucent?

yes ■ no □

Is it easy to see blue veins under your skin?

yes ■ no □

Does your skin go red:

after crying? ■
after exercise? ■
very rarely? □

Does your hair have red lights?

yes □ no ■

Hold a piece of gold, then silver jewellery against your skin. Which looks best?

gold □ silver ■

Whatever your eye colour would you describe them as:

light? ■
dark? □

MOSTLY □

You have a warm skin which has mainly yellow undertones. You may be a golden blonde with honey coloured skin, or a brunette with olive or black skin. A tendency to oiliness often accompanies these skin tones. Redheads' fair skin also tends to be creamy ivory rather than pale blue-toned. Check out these warm make-up colours:

FOUNDATION

If your skin is very sallow, use a corrective mauve make-up base first. Choose a foundation with neutral beige rather than honey undertones.

Sheer formulas are also a good option for you. A tinted moisturiser, for instance, will allow your natural colouring and any freckles to show through. If you wear face powder, take care that it matches your skin tone. If it's too light, it can look floury on your skin – even some translucent powders have this effect. Similarly, avoid powders with a pink tint.

BLUSHER

Use glowing shades of coral, peach and terracotta, but don't use too brown a blusher, unless you've got a deep tan.

EYE MAKE-UP

Mix and match shades of green and metallic colours such as rust, copper and bronze. Most earthy shades of brown will suit you too. Chalky colours may make you look ashen but just a hint of gold or sandy shadow, on the centre of your eyelid or browbone, will highlight your eyes. The darker your skin, the more intense your colours can be. Stick to dark brown mascara, or black if your lashes are very dark.

LIPSTICK

Choose from a soft apricot or peach, to a bright coral or a rich orange-red to enhance the warm tones in your skin. If your skin tends to be sallow opt for colours with less yellow, such as a clear red, cranberry or wine red.

MOSTLY ■

You have a cool skin colour which means your complexion is fair with undertones of blue and red – a typical English rose! Your skin tends to be fragile, fine-textured and sensitive with a tendency to flushing and broken veins. Your hair is probably fair or light brown, but it's not unusual for raven-haired women to have cool complexions too. Here are the colours for cool skin tones:

FOUNDATION

Don't try to warm up pale skin with an orangy foundation. Make sure it matches your complexion exactly as even a shade too dark will look mask-like. Before buying, test the foundation on your lower cheek, not your hand which may be a slightly different shade to your face. Look for shades like pearl or ivory.

BLUSHER

You could look drained without this! For a subtle glow, opt for 'cool' pinks from shell-like pastel to rose.

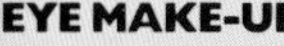

EYE MAKE-UP

The spectrum of suitable eyeshadows includes the same pinks as your blusher or lavender and lilac. Also try all shades of blue, although this can overwhelm blue eyes and will look better against grey eyes. Pale eyeshadow on its own can make you look washed out, so blend with navy or grey, in the socket or outer corner and define with eyeliner. Charcoal grey will look less harsh than black. The same goes for mascara – dark brown is a much softer choice.

LIPSTICK

Again go for pink – this may sound limiting, but it comes in a wide range of hues. The darker your hair the more vivid your lipstick can be. Fuchsia, for instance, is a cool but bright pink and can look stunning against dark hair and pale skin, but would be too intense on a fair-skinned blonde.

SEEING RED

If your skin has a red tinge, you may not need blusher. Choose lipstick in wine-coloured pinks or go for softer, peachy pinks. Foundation will even out your skin tone and a green colour corrective powder or make-up base can be used to help tone down an especially ruddy complexion.

Photographs: SARAH HUTCHINGS/Hair & make-up: KARIN DARNELL

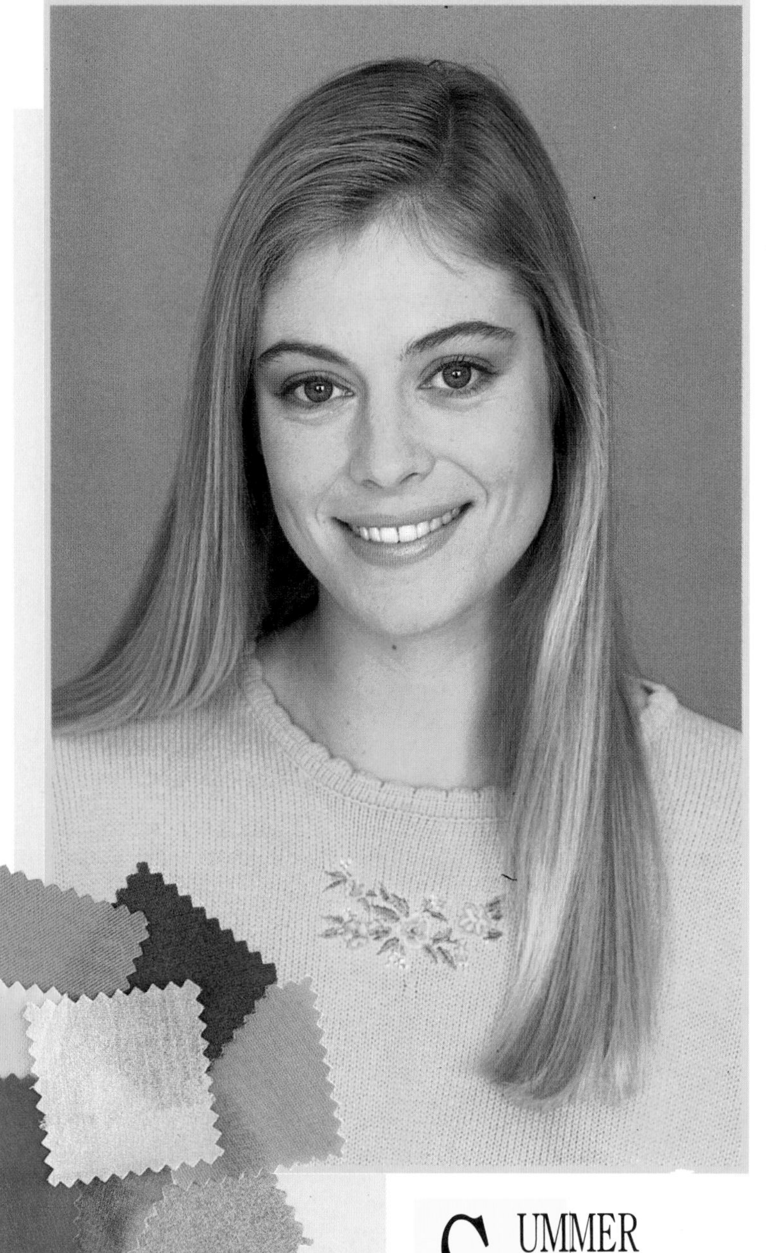

THE FOUR SEASONS

Are you a warm Spring or an icy Winter? Find out your true season with our colourfast guide and get suited to success

Why is it that some colours look wonderful on other people but on you they're a wash-out? Finding your true colours can boost your confidence by helping you look well co-ordinated and stylish. No wonder it's big business!

A professional consultation with a colour counsellor, who specialises in finding clothes and make-up in the right colours to suit you can cost a small fortune. However, with a little know-how, you too can find the shades that help you project the right image for your lifestyle.

The system that's used to find the best colours for you is quite simple: each basic colouring type is described by the characteristics of one of the four seasons – Spring, Summer, Autumn or Winter. Answer these questions and find out which season you fall into – then you can start choosing the colours to suit you.

SPRING

Skin colour: Pale ivory, peach, light to medium beige, florid or peaches and cream.

Eye colour: Hazel, green, light to dark blue or brown.

Hair colour: Flaxen blonde to golden and dark brown or grey.

Springs suit: Warm colours ranging from crisp, contrasting pastels to medium brights.

Make-up and clothes colours: Mauve, yellow, apple green, pale green, indigo, apricot, baby pink, beige and brick red.

Avoid: Dark, heavy and cool blue-toned shades.

SUMMER

Skin colour: White, rose beige or fair with pink tones.

Eye colour: Hazel, blue, grey-blue, blue-green or brown.

Hair colour: White, ash blonde, mousy brown or silver grey.

Summers suit: Soft, light to medium-toned shades.

Make-up and clothes colours: Sky blue, teal, soft grey, aqua, deep blue-green, jade, pale pink, lemon, raspberry and lilac.

Avoid: Golden tones, orange, and black and white.

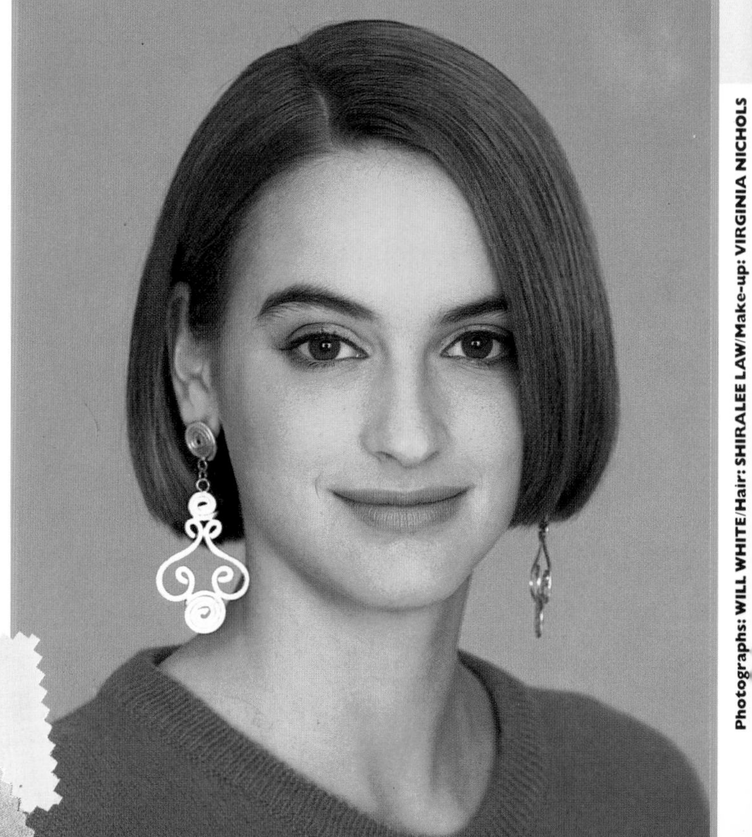

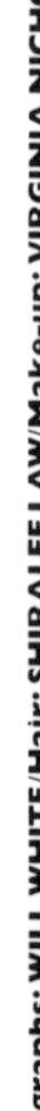

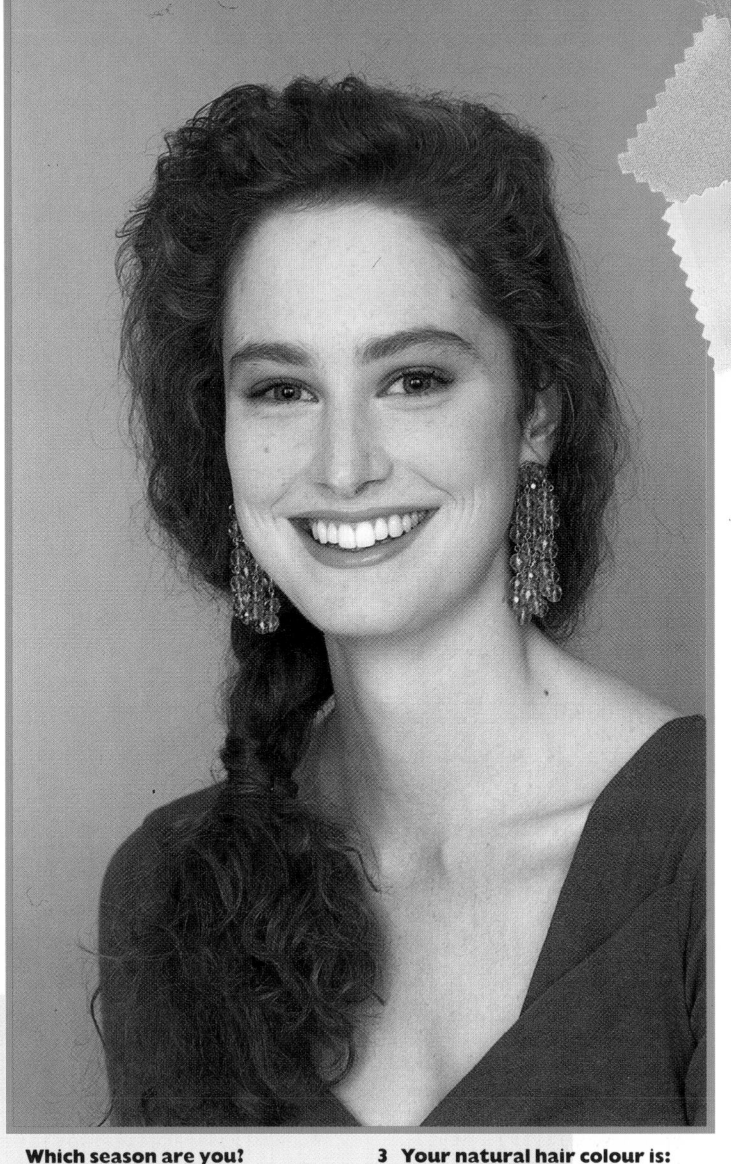

Dress: HENNES/Earrings: FLASH HARRY

AUTUMN

Skin colour: Pale cream, champagne, ivory, light to warm beige, golden brown, freckled, florid, ruddy peach.

Eye colour: Mid to dark brown, hazel, green, brown, turquoise, clear or dark blue.

Hair colour: Light auburn, golden brown, red, chestnut, copper, rust, dark brown and black.

Autumns suit: Warm earthy colours ranging from medium to dark tones. The colours should always have a rich quality even in the lighter shades.

Make-up and clothes colours: Bronze, gold, coral, aubergine, forest green, teal blue, mahogany brown, terracotta, mustard, rust, pumpkin orange, burnt orange, soft yellow and salmon pink.

Avoid: All blue-based colours, fuchsia, silver grey, as well as black and pure white.

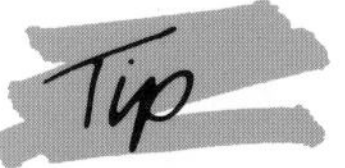

To help you decide on the shades that suit you, stand with your back against a white wall and hold different coloured scarves around your face or drape them around your shoulders.

Which season are you?

1 Your eyes are:
a. Clear blue or green, gold or turquoise
b. Grey/blue-grey or hazel
c. Greenish or golden brown
d. Dark blue or brown

2 In the sun your skin:
a. Burns easily, freckles or tans lightly but fades fast.
b. Tans with a pinky tone
c. Turns a golden brown, maybe with freckles
d. Tans easily

3 Your natural hair colour is:
a. Light to medium golden brown
b. Ash blonde or mousy brown
c. A shade of red or a warm shade of brown
d. Dark brown or black

Whichever letter you've chosen the most is the season most likely to be yours.
Mostly a – and you're likely to be a Spring person
Mostly b – Summer
Mostly c – Autumn
Mostly d – Winter

WINTER

Skin colour: Porcelain, white with pink tones, florid with deep rose tones, light olive, deep olive, brown, oriental, black.

Eye colour: Light to dark brown, hazel, blue-grey, dark blue, grey-green and dark grey.

Hair colour: Platinum blonde, medium to dark brown, black, silver grey, pure white.

Winters suit: Bright, contrasting colours especially primaries. She wears black and white well and cool icy pastels.

Make-up and clothes colours: Royal blue, deep sky blue, emerald green, blood red, deep purple, magenta, shocking pink, turquoise, navy, marble or slate grey, black and white.

Avoid: Gold, golden browns, orange, and muted shades.

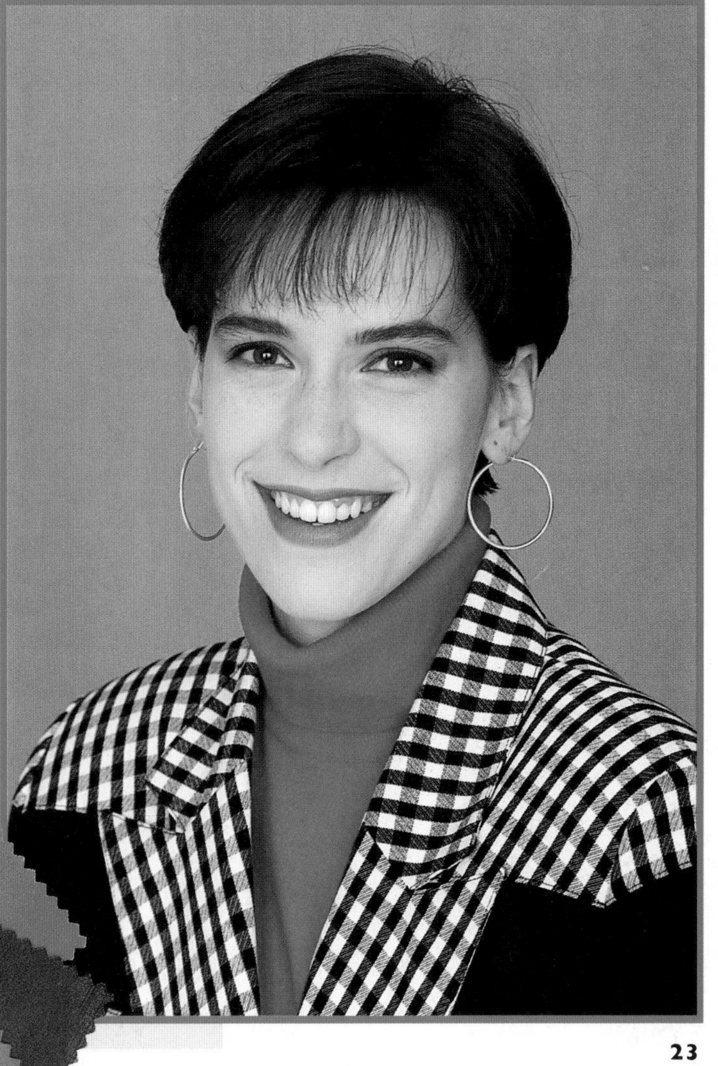

Top: DEBENHAMS/Jacket: HENNES

PLAY IT COOL

You needn't pale into insignificance because you've got light-coloured skin. Choose the coolest looking colours to complement your skin tone and make sure you're always in the pink!

Make-up is very important if you have a pale skin. Without it you can look tired and washed-out. But it's a mistake to try to warm up your complexion with colours that are strong and vibrant. Instead you should go for 'cool' colours which, like your skin tone, have a blue-pink tinge to them, in contrast to 'warm' colours which have a yellowy hue.

You probably have light-coloured eyes and blonde or mousy hair, but it is possible to have black hair and a cool skin tone. Redheads are more likely to fall into a warm skin tone category because although they have fair skin it tends to be more creamy.

Pale skins tend to be quite fine and translucent, making blue-grey under-eye shadows and thread veins show up more, so disguise with concealer in a shade lighter than your usual foundation.

FOUNDATION: Many foundations will be too dark for you and should be avoided or your make-up will look artificial. Look for shades described as ivory, fair, pearl or porcelain and go for a light, liquid type rather than a cream. Check the colour by putting a little over the back of your hand to see how it matches up. Foundation can help tone down ruddy cheeks, but steer clear of rose-tinted bases and try a green colour-corrective cream.

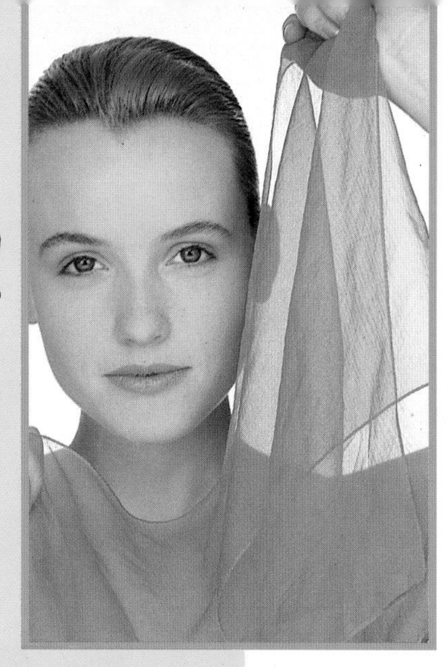

COLOUR UP!

Before choosing your make-up shades, hold different fabrics up against your face to determine which colours clash with and which ones complement your skin, hair and eyes. It helps to know this when buying clothes too, so you can co-ordinate a look.

OK CORAL?

A warm colour like this coral, which is essentially a combination of fiery red and yellow, does nothing for a cool skin tone. It simply drains the face. White or black outfits also have the same effect. White exaggerates your pale skin and black is too stark a contrast with it.

PINK 'N' SHEER

This soft pink is a lot more flattering to pale skins. It gives them subtle radiance.

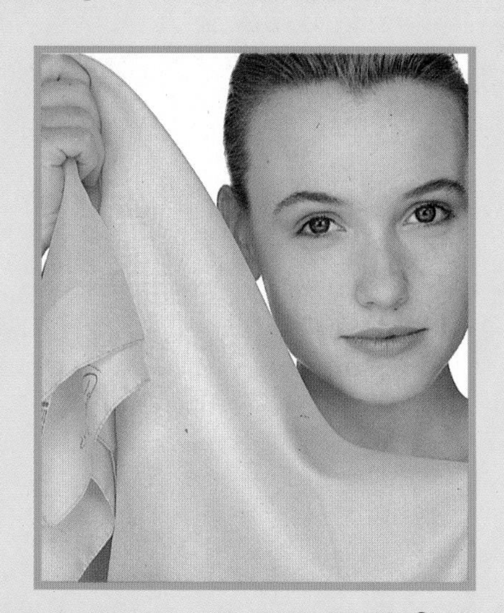

PASTEL PERFECT

Generally pastels suit you best. As you can see, the lilac fabric in the left hand contains a hint of pink and blue, and is very flattering, as is the peppermint green. You needn't wear peppermint green eyeshadow if you don't want to though! Look out for 'cool' make-up colours such as pale grey or lilac eyeshadow and pink lipstick.

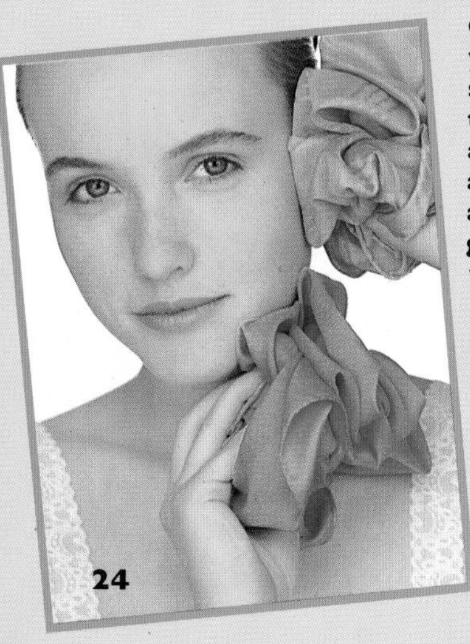

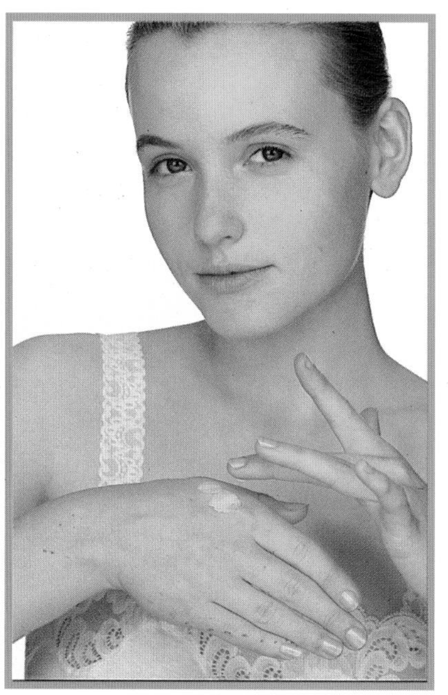

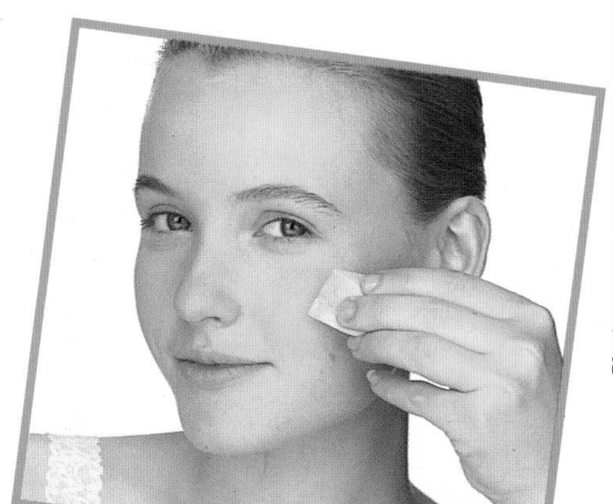

Photographs: ADRIAN BRADBURY/Hair and make-up: KIZZY HARRISON
Denim jacket: FREEMANS/T-shirt: DEBENHAMS/Underwear and jewellery: FENWICK

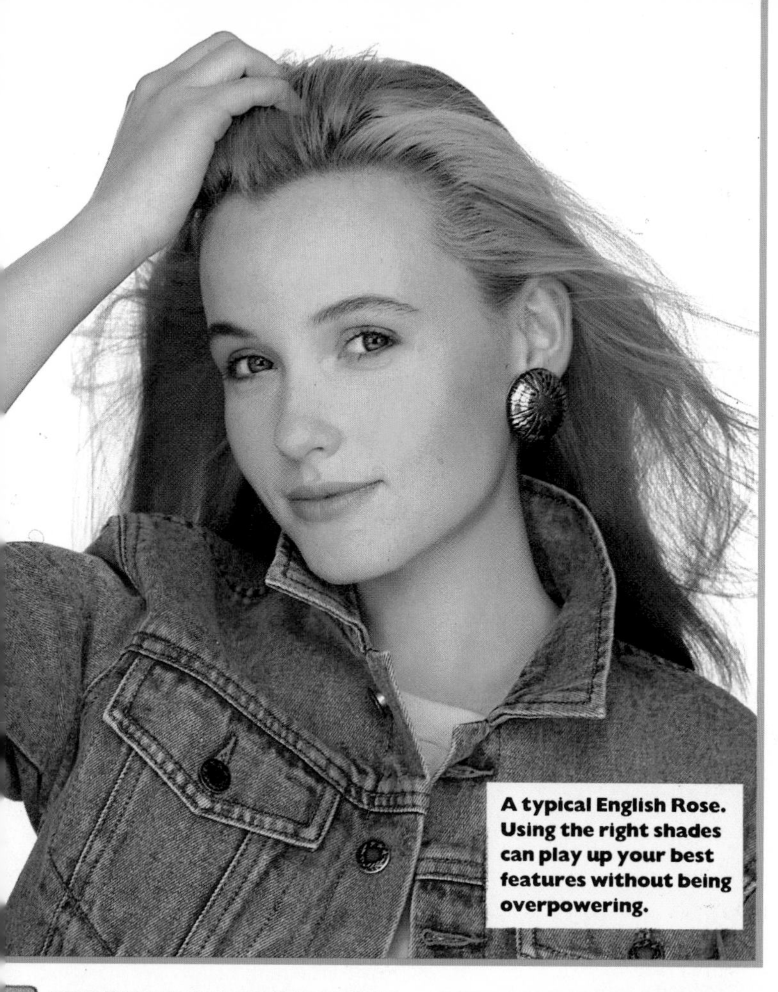

A typical English Rose. Using the right shades can play up your best features without being overpowering.

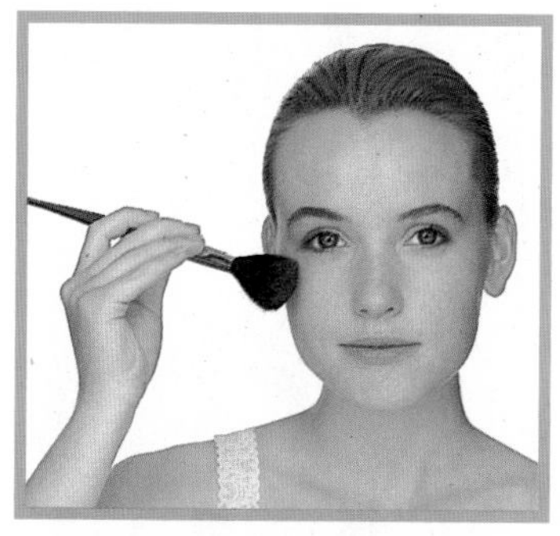

▲ **BLUSHER: again pink rather than peach tones are more likely to suit you best, but keep the effect very soft and natural by avoiding garish, fuchsia-bright pinks. Build up the intensity gradually, using a soft brush.**

▼ **LIPS: you can't go wrong with a shade of rose-pink lipstick. Understated and very feminine, it's ideal for a daytime look. Go for sheer matt lipsticks rather than pearly or extra glossy ones.**

LIP LINE-UP

(from top to bottom)

CLOVER – quite a shocking pink, but take great care clothes don't clash with it.

SHELL – very sheer, looks good with a tan.

BUBBLEGUM PINK – sugary sweet for blondes, but too light for brunettes.

RASPBERRY PINK – a shimmering option for evenings.

CLASSIC ROSE – suits most people.

CLARET – red looks great on pale-skinned brunettes, but make sure it is a bluey-red.

HEATHERY PINK – be careful to avoid purply tones if you have bluey-tinged lips.

EYES BRIGHT

Eye colours for you are purply brown, smoky grey, and pewter, plus all the blues and pinks and shades between these two such as lilac, lavender and plum, turquoise and jade green. Mix and match them in any combination, contrasting light with dark to shape your eyes. Azure blue liner tends to play down blue eyes, whereas it can enhance grey eyes; if your eyes are blue, opt instead for a flattering grey liner!

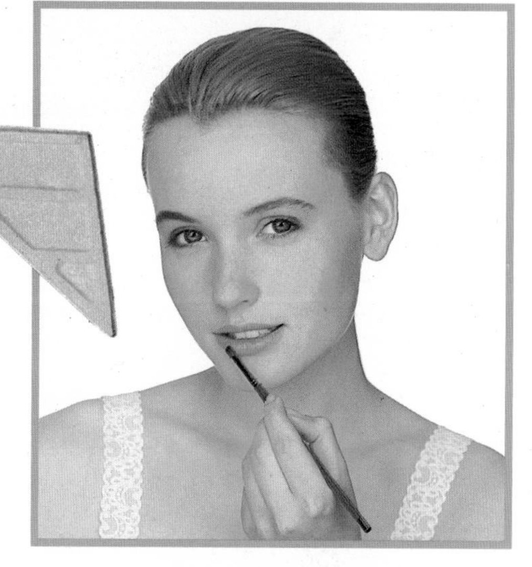

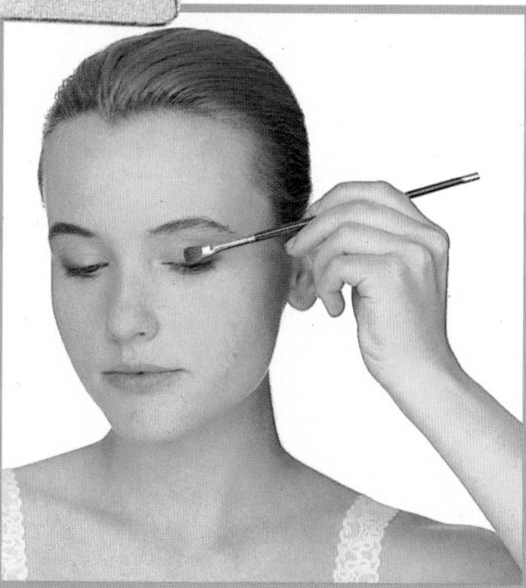

◄ **EYES: give your eyes more emphasis by blending a darker shade in the socket, or around the outer corner of your eye. Try a soft pink shade over the lid and up to the brow, with a darker smoky purple on the outer corner and underneath the lower lashes.**

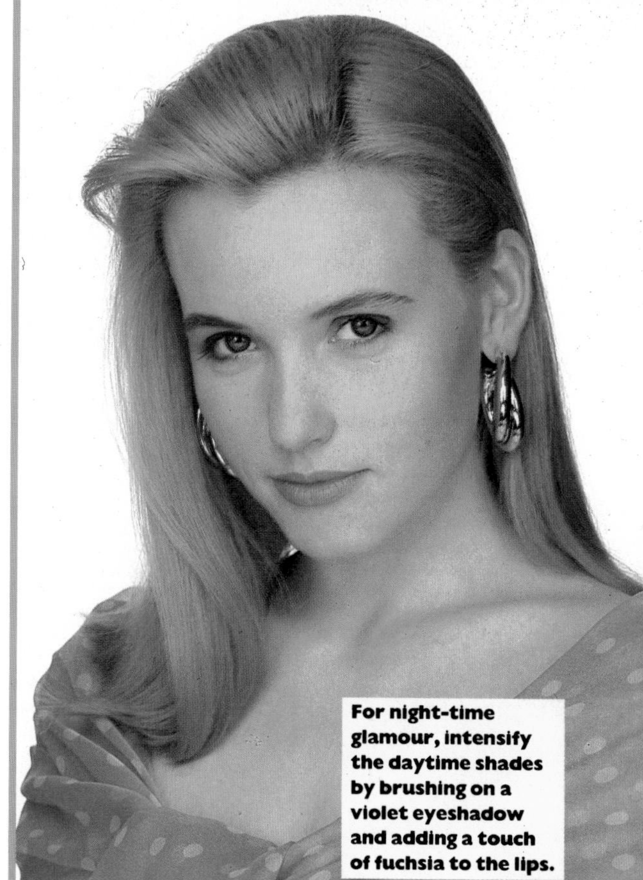

For night-time glamour, intensify the daytime shades by brushing on a violet eyeshadow and adding a touch of fuchsia to the lips.

GLOW FOR IT!

If you've got dark hair and eyes you've probably got a 'warm' golden skintone, but even if your complexion is quite pale and your hair is blonde your skin can also fall into the 'warm' category. This means that the skin has underlying tones of warm yellow and red. And these are the colours you should look for when selecting clothes and make-up.

Colours such as green and brown can be cool or warm so you have to be careful which shades you choose. It helps if you think of mixing paint. Blue and yellow make green, and the more blue, the cooler the green, while the more yellow, the warmer the green. So an olive green or a reddy-brown would suit you but not a bluey-jade or bluey-brown. Read on to see what we mean.

Choose the coolest colours for a warm complexion. Find out what you need to get glowing

FINISHED: This make-up looks great if you've got dark hair and if you're blonde or red-haired with golden skin.

EYES RIGHT

Brown eyeshadows are perfect for you. Wear metallic bronze and copper with a touch of gold. Or go for matt, earthy colours. Highlight with ivory, peach, and pearly pink shades.

COLOUR COUNSEL

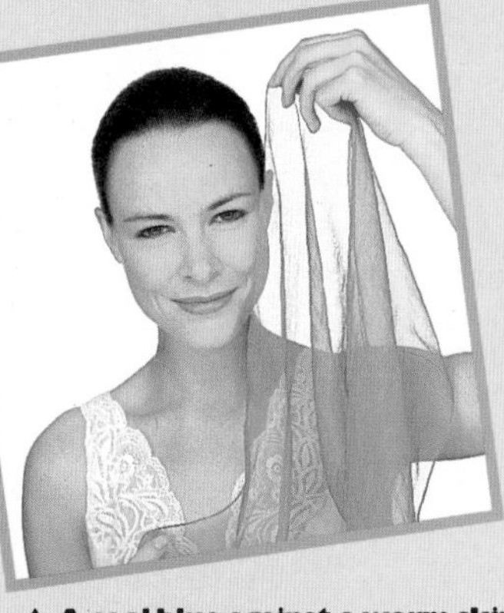

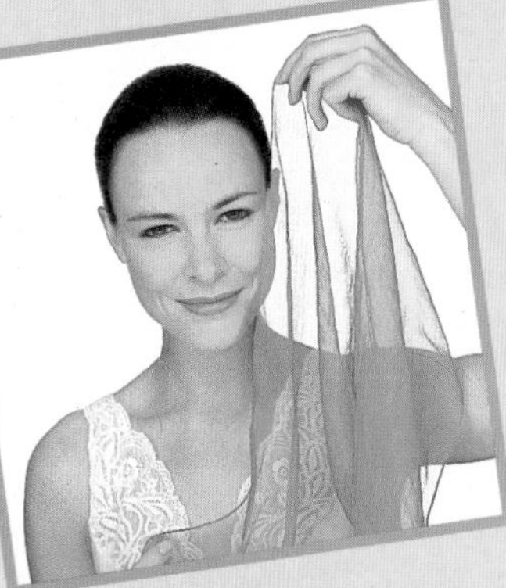

▲ A cool blue against a warm skin makes the complexion look dingy, dull and tired.

▲ A warm colour like coral seems to bring the complexion back to life, giving it an extra glow.

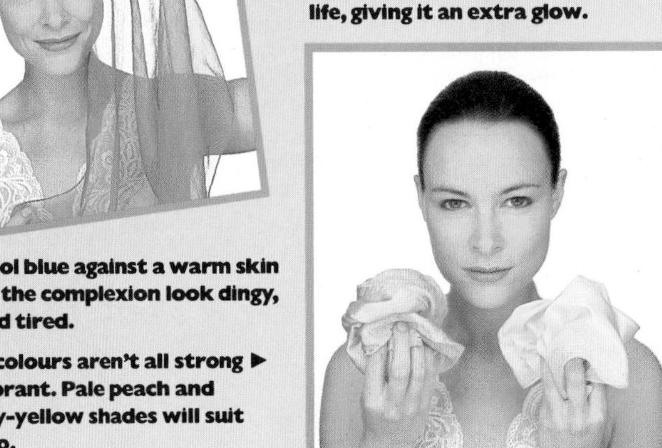

Warm colours aren't all strong ▶ and vibrant. Pale peach and creamy-yellow shades will suit you too.

HOT LIPS

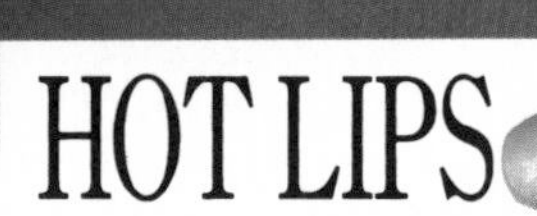

(From top to bottom)

Tangerine – an orangy-red colour. Strong and vivid for evenings. Looks good with a tan.

Coral – more subdued than the tangerine. Ideal for daytime use.

Peach melba – subtle and understated. Ideal for redheads.

Apricot – brighter than peach melba. Flatters everyone.

Chestnut – beautiful on brunettes.

Copper – softer than chestnut and ideal if you can't wear deep colours.

Melon – pearlised for a hint of colour.

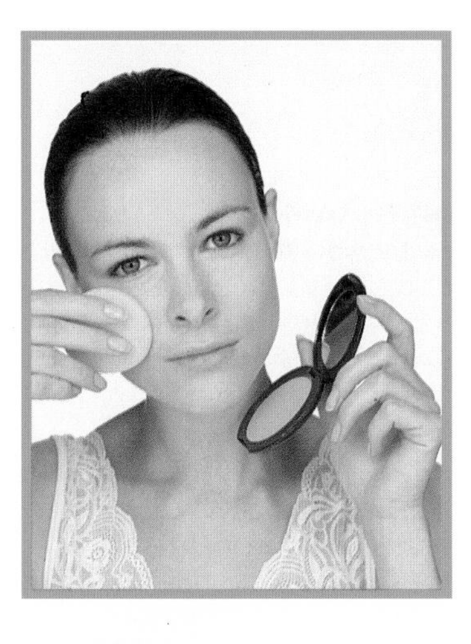

DAY BRIGHT

FOUNDATION

Look for base colours described as honey or light tan. If you have a sallow skin, tone down its yellowy tinge and go for a neutral beige foundation. Look for a face powder that matches your skin tone too. If it's too light or pinky it could leave a floury finish.

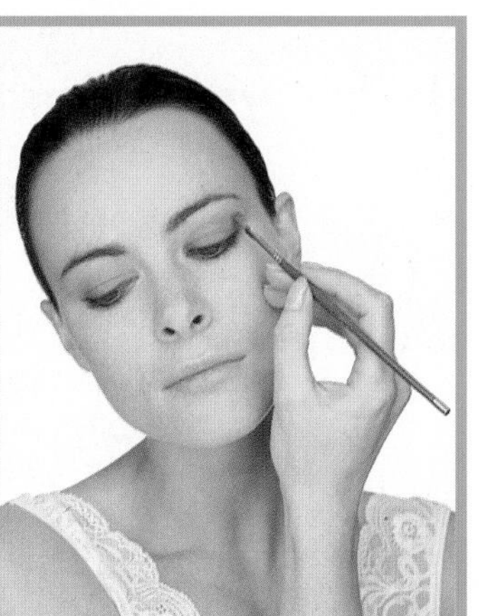

EYES

Highlight with pale matt shades such as peach or cream and add contrast with earthy colours such as russet, gold or muddy browns. Here we used a sandy shade on the brow bone, a rust colour over the rest of the lid and dark brown close to the lashes for extra definition. Add two coats of browny-black mascara to finish.

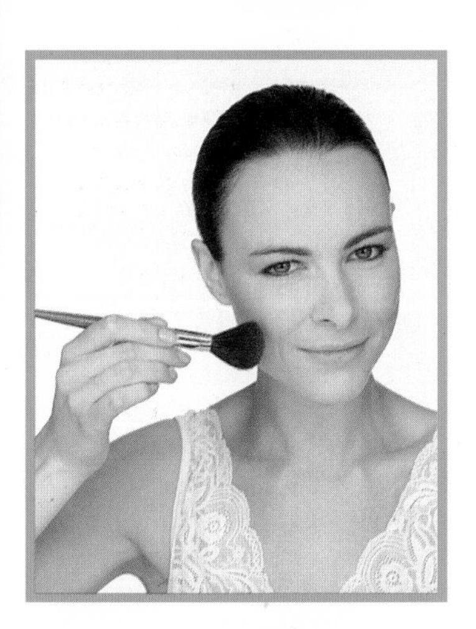

BLUSHER

Your skin often has a natural healthy glow, so just sweep on a little blusher to define your face shape and add a hint of colour. Choose gold, russet or biscuit-coloured shades but steer clear of dark brown blushers. For a barely-there blush, mop up a little colour on a cosmetic sponge and stroke it over your cheekbones.

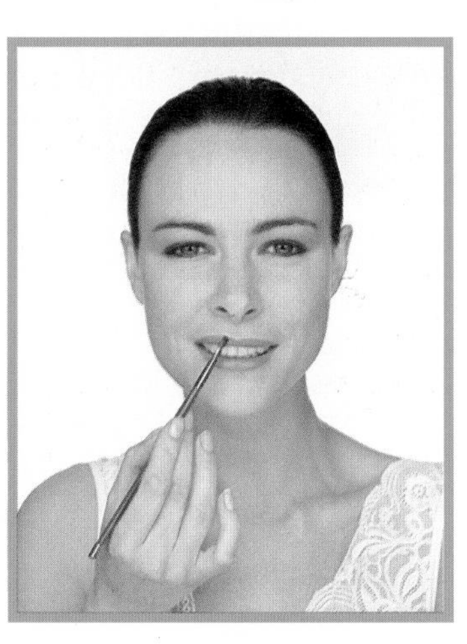

LIPS

Rich, red-browns and cinnamon shades look lovely on you, especially with autumn and winter clothes. In summer, opt for lighter, more peachy tones and save stronger lip colours for the evening. We used a cinnamon shade for this daytime look but you can spice it up for the evenings.

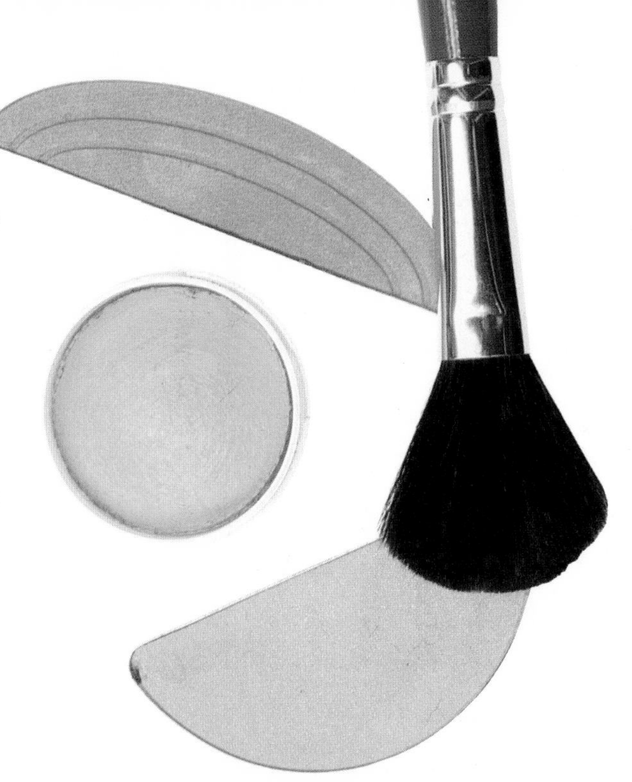

CHEEKY LOOKS

Three perfect blushers: the terracotta colour (top) suits a dark skin while the peachy pink (middle) looks great on a paler skin. If you have auburn hair, opt for a blusher with more yellow in it than red such as the golden peach shade (bottom).

Use bronzing powder instead of blusher to really glow.

Photograph: ADRIAN BRADBURY/Hair and Make-Up: KIZZY HARRISON/Jumper: DEBENHAMS
Dress: PINEAPPLE/Underwear and Jewellery: FENWICK

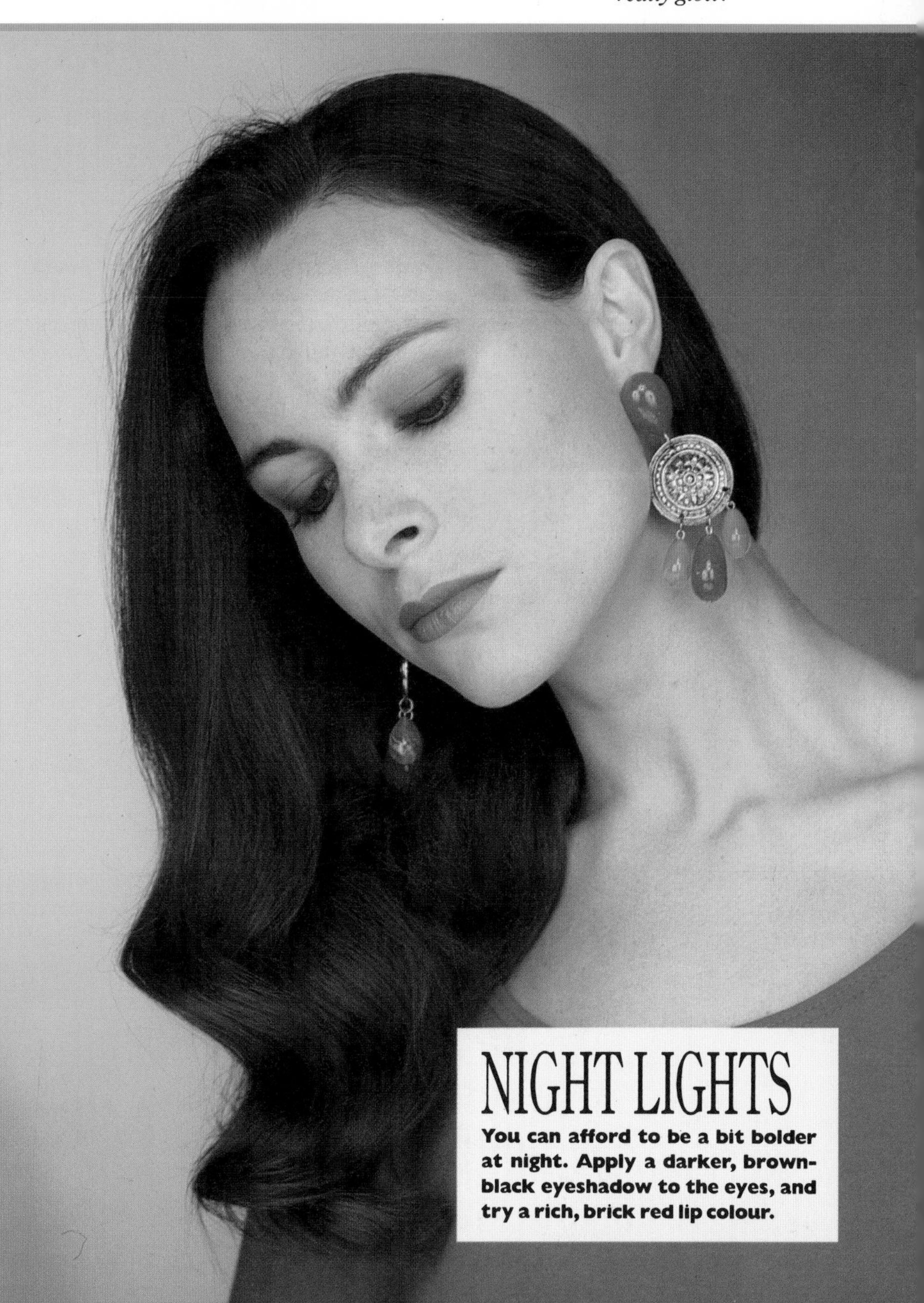

NIGHT LIGHTS

You can afford to be a bit bolder at night. Apply a darker, brown-black eyeshadow to the eyes, and try a rich, brick red lip colour.

ON YOUR MARKS

If freckles, moles and other marks bother you follow our spot-check. We can help you prevent more blemishes and cover up existing ones

Only the lucky few are blessed with skin that's completely free from blemishes. For the rest of us, freckles and other marks are all part of our body's natural make-up. They may be present at birth, appear during childhood, or even develop later in life – when they're often caused by exposure to the sun.

The majority of marks are harmless and can be concealed if necessary, though some may need special treatment and will benefit from protective care to minimise how much they show up.

FRECKLES

These are formed when melanin, the brown pigment in your skin, reacts to strong sunlight. Blondes and redheads are especially freckle-prone.

If you're not a freckle fan, you can help them to fade with lemon juice. Moisturise your skin first, then soak a cotton-wool pad in the juice. Pat it over freckles then rinse off after 15 minutes and moisturise again. To stop freckles getting darker, use a high factor sunscreen or a sun-block whenever you go out in the sun.

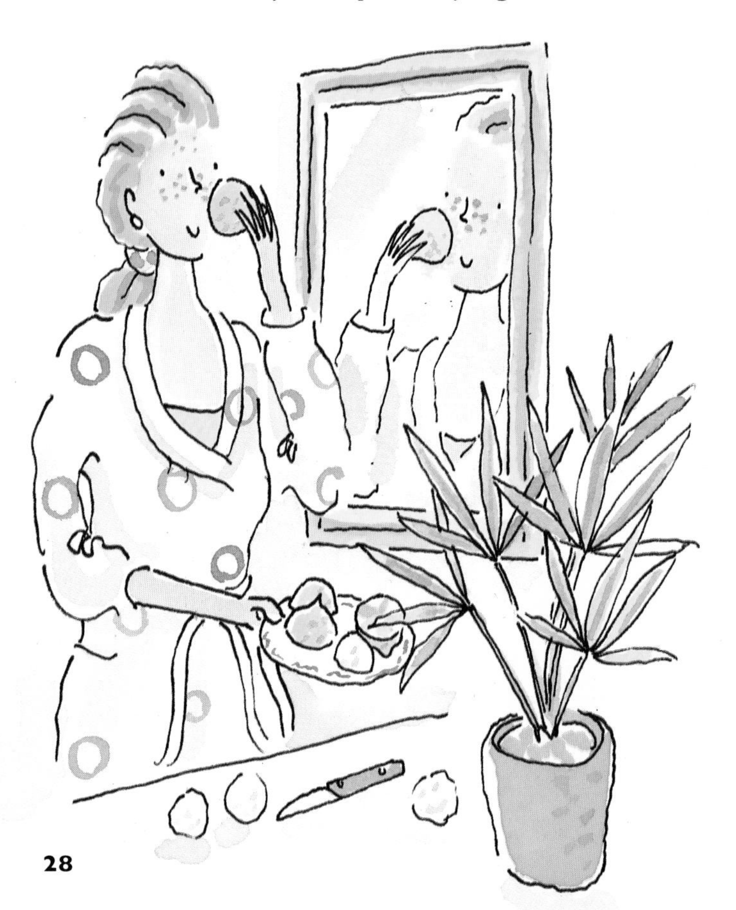

LIVER SPOTS

Liver spots are caused by long-term exposure to the sun, so they are more likely to appear from your thirties onwards. A dermatologist can freeze them off with liquid nitrogen; but the best action is to cover up with sun-block whenever you go out in the sun and use tinted creams to hide any existing marks.

MOLES

Moles, like freckles, are made up of clusters of melanin. They most frequently appear when you're young and are permanent. Large or unsightly-looking moles can be removed – ask your doctor to refer you to a dermatologist. You should also consult him if a mole bleeds or changes in size or shape – as occasionally they can become malignant. For safety's sake keep them covered when you're in strong sunlight.

Moles may sometimes sprout the odd hair – don't be tempted to pluck it, just snip it off with a sharp pair of scissors.

VITILIGO

This is a condition where the skin loses pigment, leaving patches which are paler than the rest. The cause of vitiligo is, as yet, unknown – but the condition, if severe, can cause quite a lot of distress. Special concealing creams can be skilfully applied to completely hide vitiligo, by evening out the contrasting skin tones. You should also use a sun-block on the lighter areas in strong sun, to protect them from burning.

BIRTHMARKS

Birthmarks may occur anywhere on the body and can be distressing if they appear on the face. They may be brown or reddish purple (port wine stains) – the result of a high concentration of blood vessels close to the skin's surface. In a few cases, laser therapy can fade discoloration to some degree, but this treatment – which is not yet widely available – won't help in every case. Ask your doctor to refer you to a dermatologist if you think this treatment may help.

COVER-UPS

CONCEALERS

Available in both stick and liquid form, their heavy coverage will blot out small marks like freckles. Select a shade to match your skin and dab the concealer on with a small brush, blending with your fingertips.

FOUNDATIONS

If you use a foundation as well as concealer you can choose a light liquid formula, or a good tinted moisturiser for a natural look. A heavier cream will give better coverage for concealing liver spots and vitiligo.

Apply gradually with a slightly damp sponge so that it spreads easily to build up an even colour. Take away any excess shine with a dusting of translucent powder.

If you're in doubt about which shade to choose, test a few on the skin inside your wrist, as this is the closest match to your face colour. As a general guide, opt for pale ivory or cream with a hint of pink if your skin is very fair, light beige and peachy tones for medium skins, and shades of warm beige to mahogany for olive and black skins.

COVERING CREAMS

To successfully cover birthmarks requires a specialist covering cream, heavier than most foundations. Hypo-allergenic ones are best. Try a green-tinted base cream underneath if you have an especially severe blemish.

Illustration: BILL PIGGINS

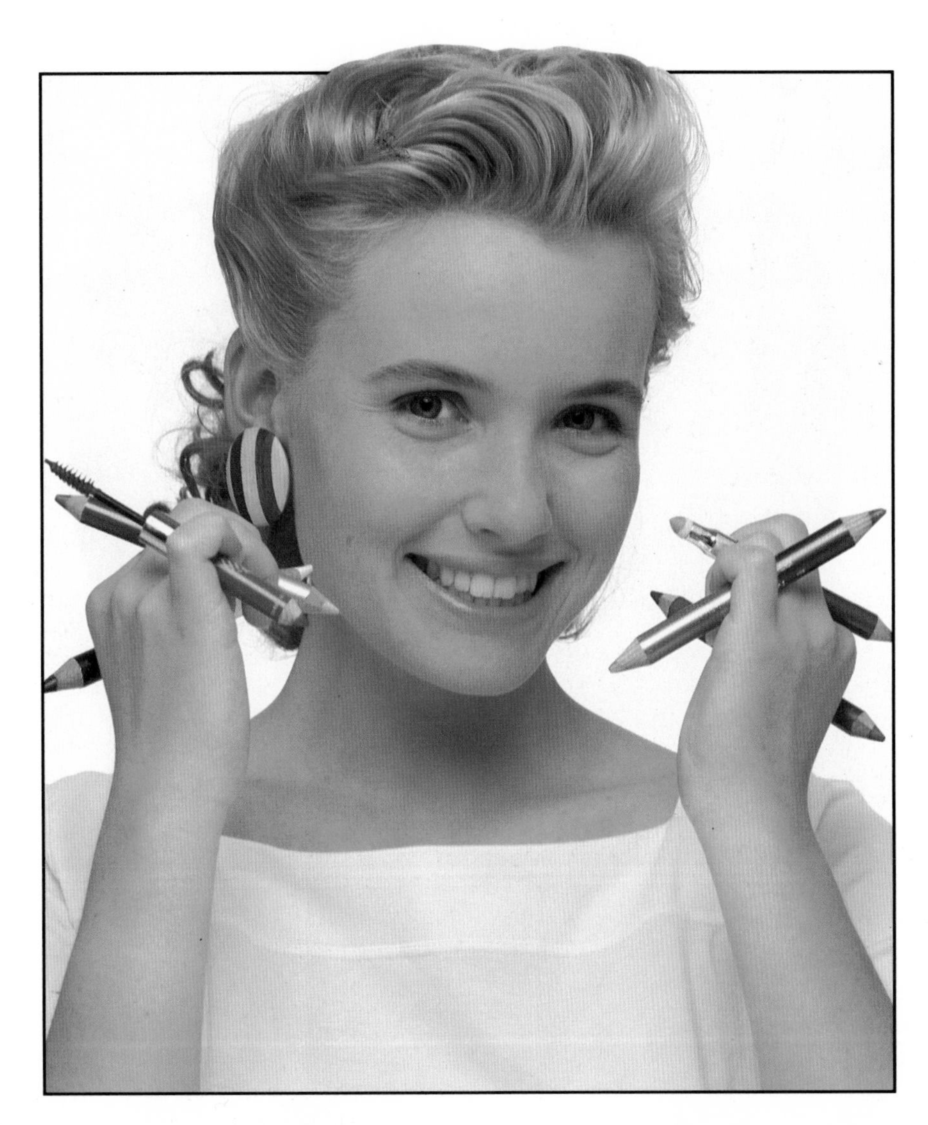

CHAPTER TWO

Making Up

FOCUS ON EYES

Here's a chance to open your eyes to our exciting make-overs! Lash on the glamour and you'll look a vision of beauty!

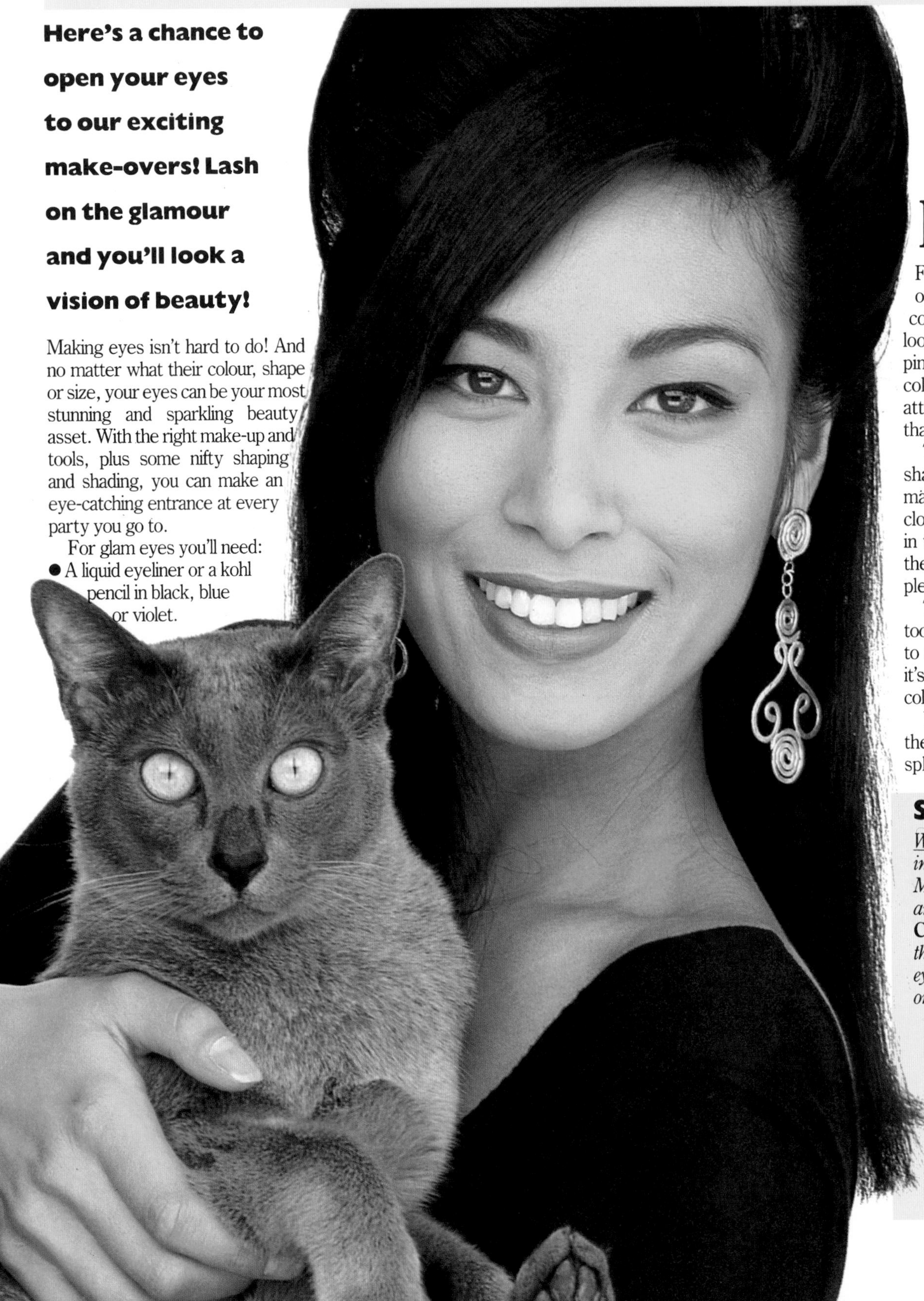

Making eyes isn't hard to do! And no matter what their colour, shape or size, your eyes can be your most stunning and sparkling beauty asset. With the right make-up and tools, plus some nifty shaping and shading, you can make an eye-catching entrance at every party you go to.

For glam eyes you'll need:

- A liquid eyeliner or a kohl pencil in black, blue or violet.
- A dark brown or brown-black eyebrow pencil.
- A selection of bright and neutral eyeshadows.
- A black lash-lengthening but fibre-free mascara.
- False eyelashes.

EYE TO EYE

For maximum impact go for one or two complementary colours that make your eyes look really dazzling. Avoid slapping on a rainbow of eyeshadow colours. This will just draw attention to your eyelids rather than enhancing your eye colour.

To find the perfect make-up shades for your eyes, look in a magnifying mirror and take a close look at the flecks of colour in the iris (the coloured bit) and then hunt for colours that'll complement them.

Take a look at your skin tone too: if it's warm and peachy, stick to shades like bronze and gold, if it's pale or pinky, go for the cool colours, such as silver or white.

You'll also need to consider the colour of your clothes before splashing out on new make-up.

SHADOW PLAY

Where you put eyeshadow is just as important as the colours you choose. Make the most of your eye shape and size by remembering:

Close-set eyes: *need emphasis at the outer corner of the eye with an eye-opening, lighter shade brushed on towards the bridge of your nose.*
Suits you: Cleopatra's eyes.

Small eyes: *make them appear larger with a pale lid colour and a dark contrasting colour in the socket.*
Suits you: doe eyes.

Very round eyes: *make them look more almond-shaped with a pale shadow on*

EYE TRICKS

● Unsteady hand? Prevent a wobbly line of eyeliner by dotting on the colour close to the lash roots. Smudge the dots into a line with a cotton bud.
● Eyeliner pencil too hard? Soften it up by holding the pointed end under the hot tap before you use it.
● When using liquid eyeliner, carefully trim the application brush with scissors so that it's very fine and won't splay out.
● Always keep a few cotton buds in your bag to mop up any smudges.
● Use an eyelash curler *before* you put on mascara.
● Hold your mascara wand vertically and use the point of the wand, rather than the thicker middle and end, to separate your eyelashes and stop the mascara clogging.
● Don't draw attention away from your eyes by wearing lots of bright blusher.
● Go for a dramatic contrast with a matt lipstick in a contrasting colour to your eyes.
● If you're going out straight from work or college then create smouldering eyes in seconds by smudging a little eyeshadow in the socket line, fading it at the outer edge – a touch of black is best for instant glamour.

FIRST BASE

● Always test out the eyeshadows on the back of your hand or smudge them on to a clean piece of white paper. Shades can look different in the palette – some even appear matt when they're actually slightly pearlised.
● Once you've decided on the eye colours you want to use, lightly smooth on foundation over each lid and dust with translucent powder. This will provide a base for the shadow and prevent it from fading or smudging.
● Next, dust your lashes lightly with loose face powder applied on a cotton wool ball. This makes the lashes look thicker and prevents your mascara smudging.
● Start with a base eyeshadow colour. Blend it with a cosmetic brush not your fingers.
● Add colour to socket crease.
● Carefully check your make-up at each stage in a mirror before moving on.

Watchpoint

Always make up in the light in which you'll be seen!

EYE-EYE

Here's the low-down on creating fabulous eyes.

SILVER LINING
To create **Cleopatra eyes:** stroke a silver shadow across the whole lid area, blending it well. Then brush on a charcoal grey colour, winging it outwards. Moisten a sponge-tipped applicator and take the same colour into the socket line and then under the lower lashes. Define the outer corner with a smudge of black kohl pencil. Finish with two coats of black mascara.

Finally, define and shape your brows using a dark pencil. This should balance the overall look.

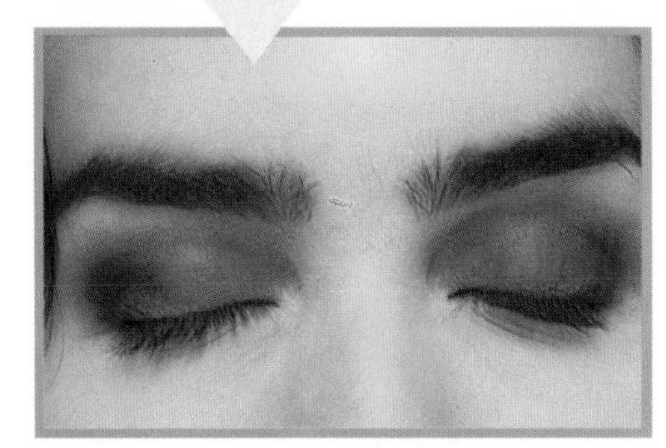

PURPLE REIGNS
To make lovely **doe eyes:** keep colours sharp and bright. Begin with a base colour, like violet and brush it over the whole lid, winging it outwards at the outer corner. Smudge a pale highlighter on to the centre of the eyelid. Blend it well. Use a chunky kohl pencil in a complementary colour to draw a soft line under the lower lashes. Move the line outwards to make a 'V' shape at the outer corner. Finish the look with two coats of mascara. Comb lashes between applications while you are waiting for the mascara to dry. For a glitzy party look substitute a bold stroke of gold for the pale highlighter powder.

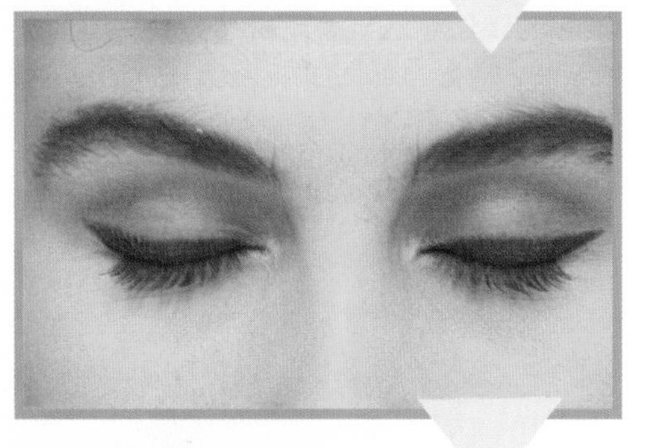

WILD THING
For purr-fect **cats' eyes:** brush a subtle base shade such as bronze over the whole lid. Use the same colour on a damp sponge-tipped applicator to define the socket line. Then draw a thin line of liquid liner across each lid close to the lash roots, winging it out at the outer corners. Rest your elbow on a table to help stop the liner going everywhere.

For dramatic drop-dead glamour stick a couple of individual false eyelashes onto your real outer lashes. And then you can have a little flutter!

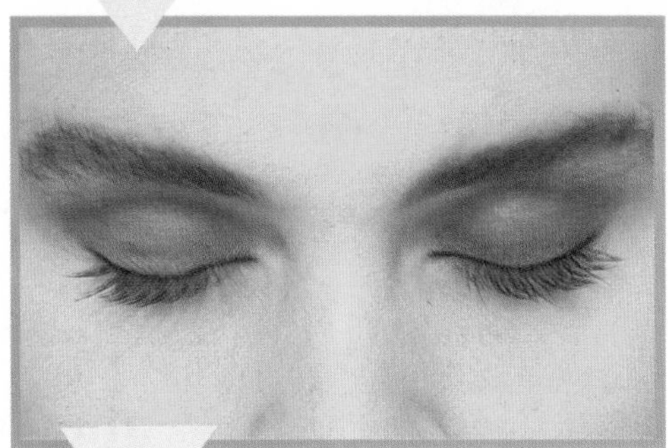

the whole lid and a strong line of black painted close to the top lashes, winging upwards and outwards.
Suits you: cats' eyes.
Protruding eyes: *need to be deepened and darkened with dark smoky colours.*
Suits you: Cleopatra's eyes.
Narrow upper lid: *widen by stroking on a light, bright shadow over the whole lid and take it just under the lower lashes to draw attention away from the upper lid.*
Suits you: doe eyes.

Now you know the shape you should be aiming for, you can follow our simple tips and create your own glamorous eyes.

BRIGHT SPARK

Even if your eyes are expertly and beautifully made-up, they won't look good if they're all pink or puffy. Follow these sparkling tricks to put a twinkle in your eye:
● *Drink plenty of water.*
● *Try to get enough sleep.*
● *Exercise your eyes regularly by rolling them in the sockets; screwing them up tightly and then opening them really wide.*
● *Avoid too much alcohol and smoky atmospheres.*
● *Remove your eye make-up gently and carefully each night to prevent irritation.*
● *Avoid putting heavy night creams on your eyes. The skin here is very absorbent and heavy creams will tend to make them puffy.*
● *Prop up your head with two pillows in bed to help drain fluid from around your eyes.*

WAKE-UP TRICKS

If you've got time before going out and your eyes look tired:
● *Place two slices of chilled cucumber or potato over the lids and relax for ten minutes.*
● *Wrap a couple of ice cubes in a hankie or clean tea-towel and put them on your eyes for about five minutes. This will help to reduce eye puffiness.*
● *Splash your eyes with a little cold water.*
● *Try shop-bought eye drops, but try not to use them every day. Natural remedies are kinder to your eyes.*

Other photographs: ADRIAN BRADBURY/Make-up: DENISE/Top: MARY QUANT/Earrings: ACCESSORI

EYE OPENERS

Your eyes are often the first things people notice about you. So make yours bigger and better than ever before with our quick and easy eye-opening tricks

LASH OUT

Your lashes are a wonderful, natural frame for your eyes. By making them look longer and thicker than ever before you'll make your eyes look much bigger and more noticeable. So even if you find you haven't time for anything else in your beauty routine, be sure you always make-up your lashes

MASCARA TRICKS

Everyone's lashes look longer and thicker with mascara, so follow our step-by-step guide with hints and tips and you'll have perfect lashes every time. Use eyelash curlers to accentuate your lashes, or build up thin lashes with a light dusting of powder before you put on your mascara. Before you start, always check that your mascara wand is free of lumps or stray hairs which could cause smudges.

Tip

Make your mascara last longer by not pumping the brush in and out. This breaks the inner seal and quickly dries out the mascara.

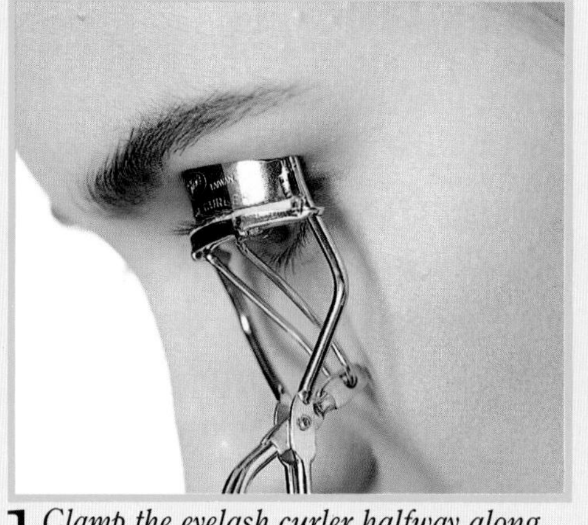

1 *Clamp the eyelash curler halfway along your lashes, hold for a couple of seconds and then release. (Remember never to use the clamp too close to your eyelid or press too hard or you'll end up pulling out your lashes and making your eyes sore.)*

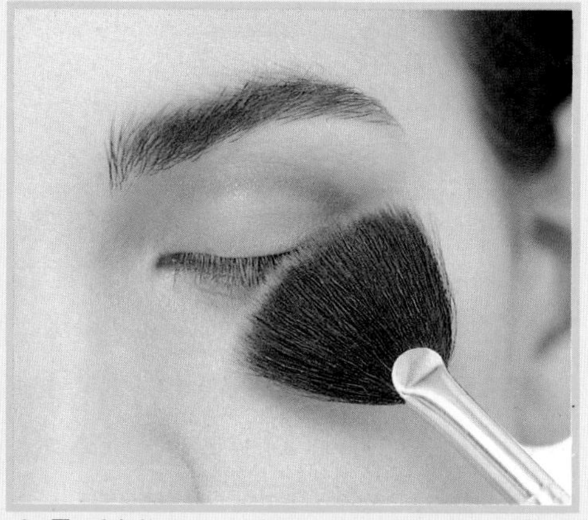

2 *To thicken your lashes, dust them with powder before you apply mascara. Load a medium-sized brush with a little loose powder (the colour doesn't matter), shut your eyes tightly then sweep the brush gently across your lashes.*

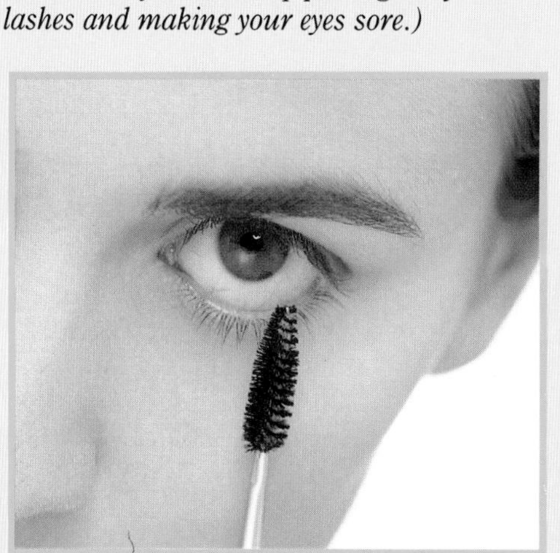

3 *Start with the bottom lashes. Hold the mascara wand upright (being careful not to poke it in your eye), then lightly sweep it across your lashes. Wait a few seconds for them to dry before you start to put the mascara on your top lashes.*

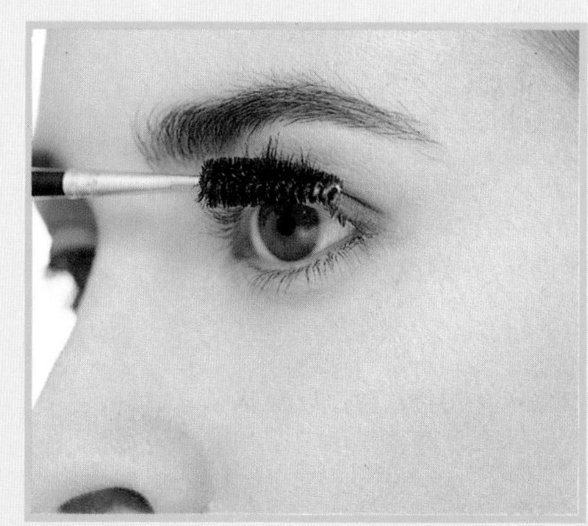

4 *Carefully reload your wand, then looking downwards stroke the wand through your lashes from underneath. Wait a couple of seconds for the first coat of mascara to dry and then apply a second coat, if you need it, for extra-thick lashes.*

BRIGHT EYES

EYE DROPS
Use a few drops every now and again if your eyes look a bit red. They work by constricting the tiny blood vessels so they disappear. Only use these once in a while rather than relying on them too often.

RELAX
Spend 10 minutes with either a cold tea bag or cotton wool pad soaked in witch hazel on each eye for a cooling effect.

BROW BEATING

Plucked to oblivion or left straggly, your brows won't do anything for you. But brushed and shaped they'll become a frame which will make the most of your eyes

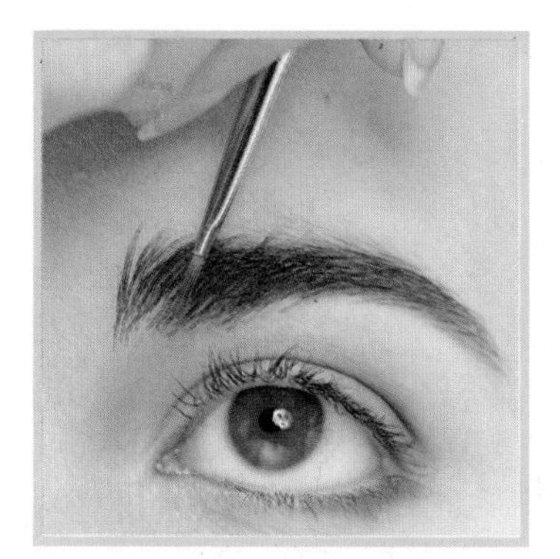

1 First, strengthen the colour of your brows. Use a small brush to fill in any gaps with matt, dark brown powder shadow. Make sure you do it lightly and evenly so you don't end up with hard lines.

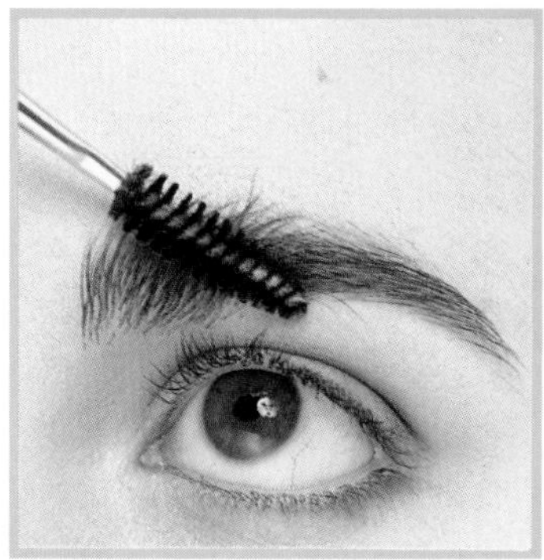

2 Now brush them into shape with a clean mascara wand, an eyebrow brush or a small toothbrush. Brush them gently upwards with a sweeping motion and outwards. This will give your eyes a lift.

SHADY DEALS

Eyeshadow plays an important part in making more of your eyes. Here's how to do a basic re-shaping job using two subtle tones of brown – a colour which works for just about everyone

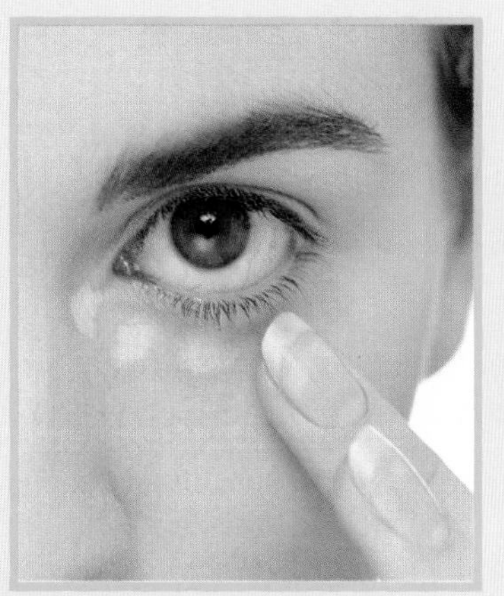

1 Disguise any dark circles under your eyes by dotting on small quantities of concealer and then gently blending it in.

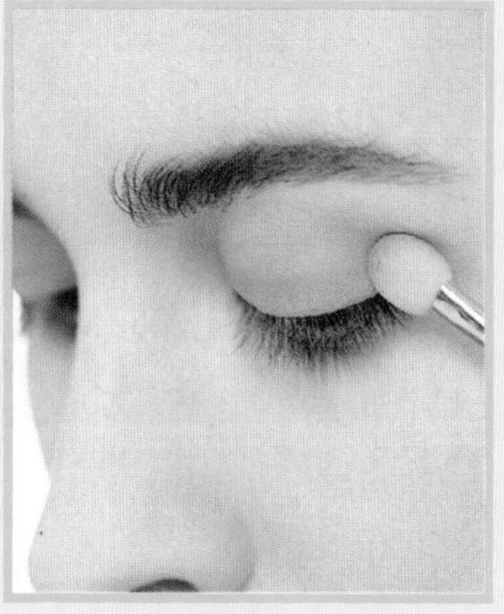

2 To highlight your eyes and create an even base to work on, brush warm brown, slightly shimmery shadow from lid to brow.

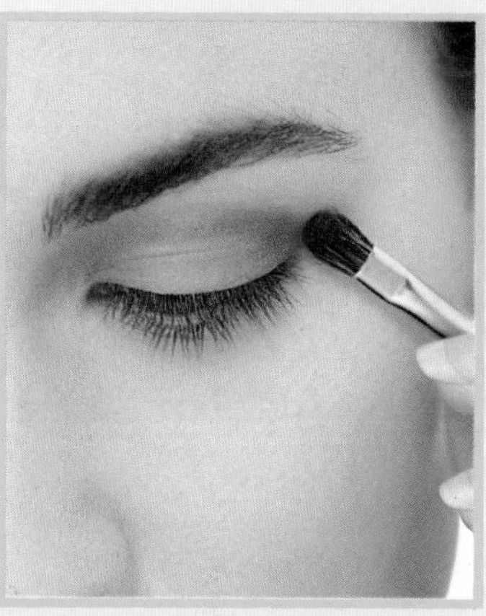

3 Brush a dark brown, matt shadow along each eye socket, carefully blending it upwards to lift and emphasise the shape.

EYE LINES

Used the right way, eyeliner can make your eyes look dramatic. Forget thick black lines which make your eyes smaller, here are two liner tricks guaranteed to make your eyes wider

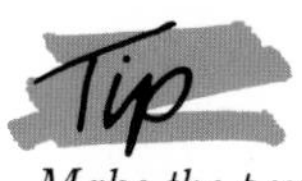

Make the pencil softer and easier to use by warming the tip in your fingers.

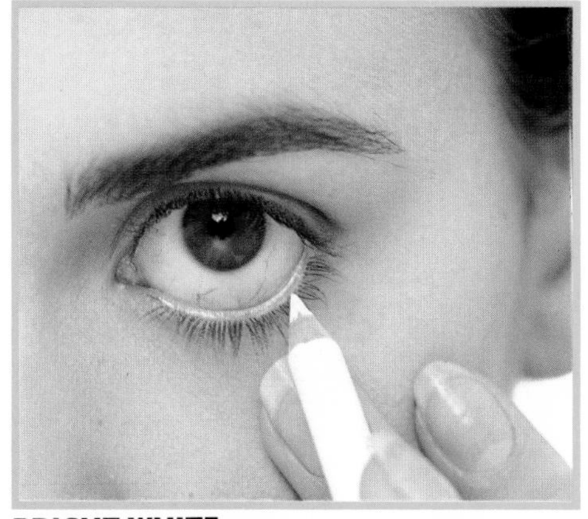

BRIGHT WHITE
This old Hollywood trick never fails to make the whites of your eyes look really bright and sparkling. All you do is use a white eyeliner pencil to draw along the bottom rim of each eye.

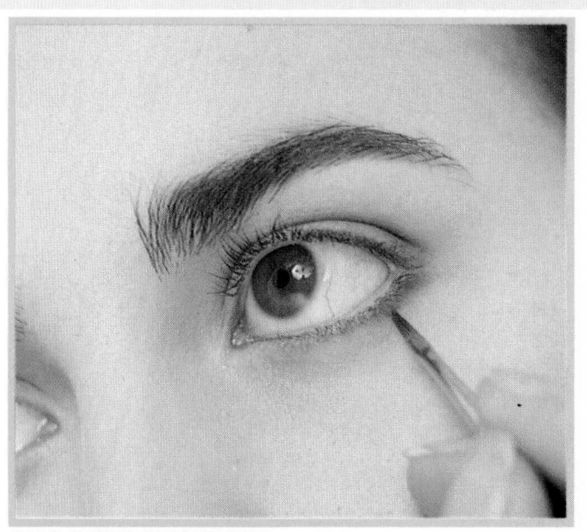

SHADOW SMUDGES
Eyeshadow is the easiest thing to use to line your eyes, it leaves you with a smudge of colour rather than a hard line. Apply before mascara, and use a fine brush to smudge it under your lower lashes.

Photographs: MATTHEW SMITH/Hair & Make-up: ELLIE WAKAMATSU

EYE-TO-EYE

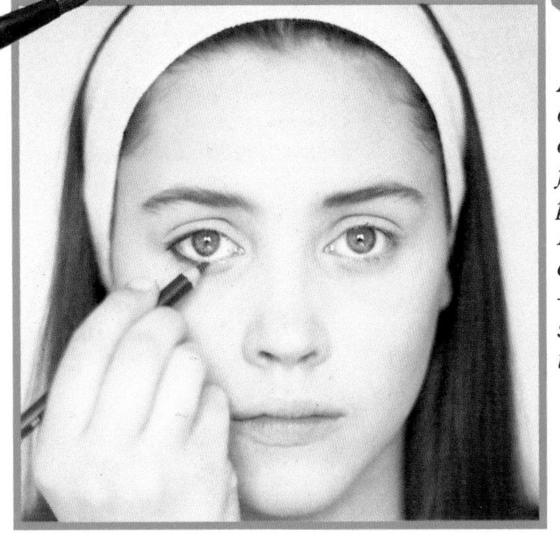

Watchpoint

Add a darker colour on your socket line to create depth – great for softening protruding eyes. But choose complementary tones – bright rainbow stripes can be difficult to blend!

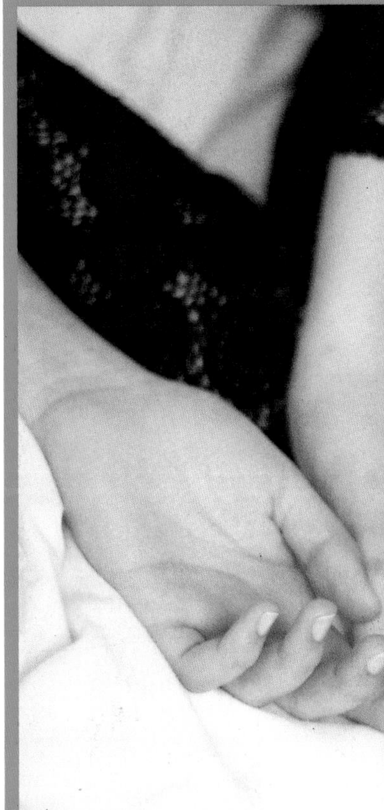

BRUSH UP

▼ On a tight budget? You don't need loads of new products to ring the changes! Your favourite *eyeshadow* and an eyeliner *brush* will do a great job.

Dip liner brush in eyeshadow, tap off the excess powder, and carefully draw along your top lash line, moving outwards and working as close to the roots as possible. For extra depth, dampen the tip of the brush first.

WIDE EYED

▲ Use an eyeliner *crayon* or *pencil* to subtly enhance the shape of your eyes. With just a little clever brushwork you can make your eyes seem wider and lashes longer and thicker. And, underneath your eye, where lashes are sparse, drawing a line can be more effective and flattering than a layer of mascara.

Opt for a matt soft brown shade so that the total effect is more obvious than the colour! Use firm, short strokes from halfway along your lower lid to the outer corner, working as close to your lash roots as possible.

Always put on mascara after eyeliner to cover any colour that you might have left on the lash roots.

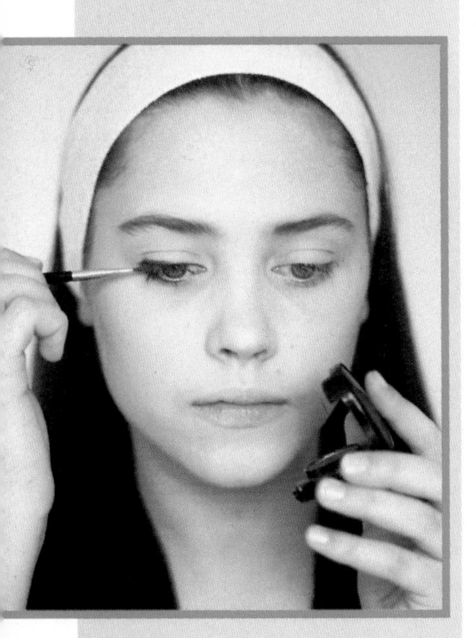

SOFT OPTION

► To create a softer look, use a *cotton bud* or a *sponge-tipped applicator* to smudge and blend eyeliner. Work the 'smudger' in all directions over your socket line and the outer curve of your eyelids.

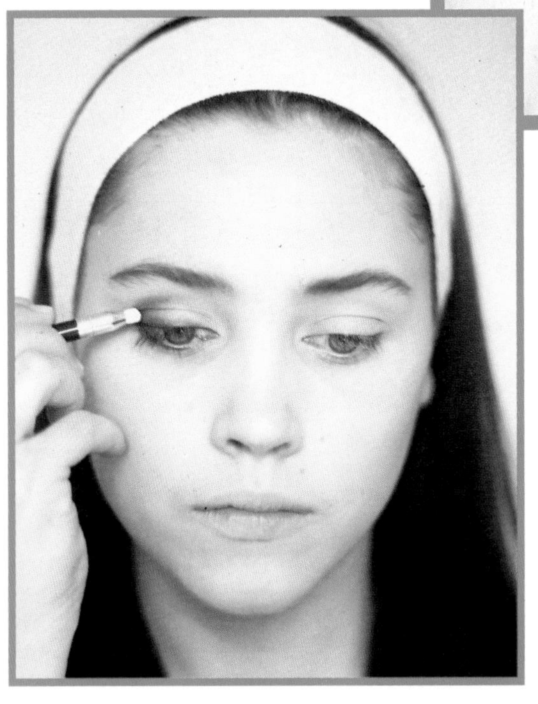

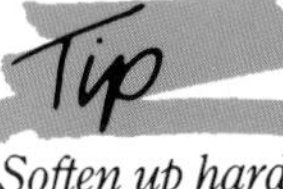

Soften up hard-tipped pencils and crayons by running them under the hot tap for a few seconds.

Keep eye pencils and crayons sharpened for accuracy.

For shaping or shading, liner makes wonderful eyes. Follow our eye-catching advice on how to use pens, pencils, liquids and crayons for the prettiest peepers

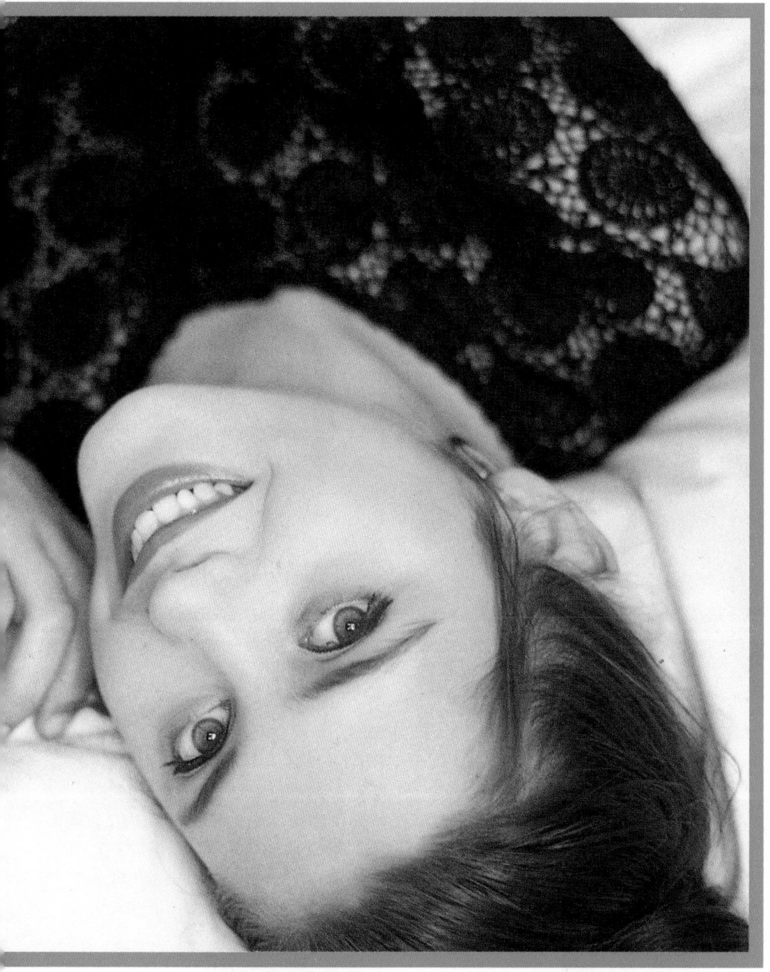

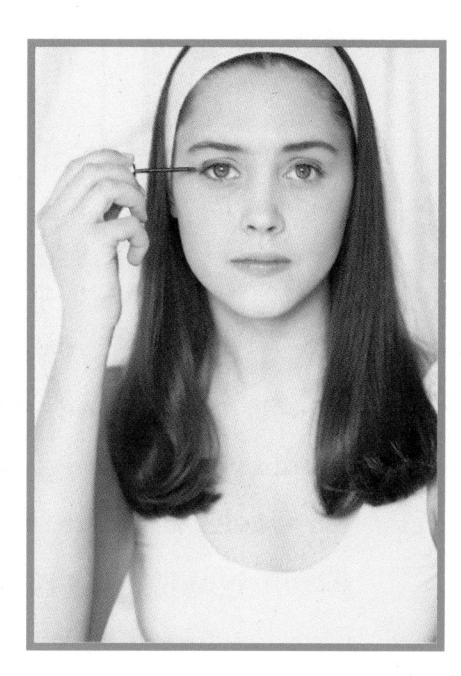

EYE LINE UP

- **Check eyes balance by following your progress in a magnifying mirror.**
- **Don't use eyebrow or eyeshadow pencils as eyeliners – they're too hard. You'll risk stretching the delicate skin around your eye.**
- **Buy a proper make-up pencil sharpener rather than clogging up the office one!**
- **Eye infections are easily passed on, so don't share liners.**
- **Use short, gentle movements rather than dragging ones which will stretch the skin.**
- **Test crayons and pencils before buying. Stroke on the inside of your wrist to make sure they're soft enough for your eyes.**

GO FOR BOLD!

▲ Liquid liner is perfect for creating dazzling looks and the fine applicator brush is ideal for drawing accurate, bold lines. For strokes of brilliance, go for the brightest colour over bare lids.

Got the wobbles? Rest your elbow on a table top to steady your hand, and put your little finger on your chin, then draw outwards along your top eyelid, following the line of your lashes. Use firm strokes.

If you accidentally smudge your eyeliner, dip a cotton bud in make-up remover and dab it over the mistake.

FELT TIP

► The doe-eyed look oozes sex appeal! Create this by using any of the methods already described, but a pen eyeliner is the most accurate applicator to use for a thicker, more dramatic line.

Black is best! Draw a line along your top lid, starting at the inside corner and sweep outwards, gradually getting thicker – imagine the shape of cats' eyes.

Keep your eye open while drawing along the inner edge so that you can draw close to the lash line. As you move outwards, partially close your eye and work slightly higher over the lid without smudging. Take the line just outside the socket crease and finish with a short upwards sweep. Then draw a sideways 'V' shape at the outer corner, taking it just under lower rim.

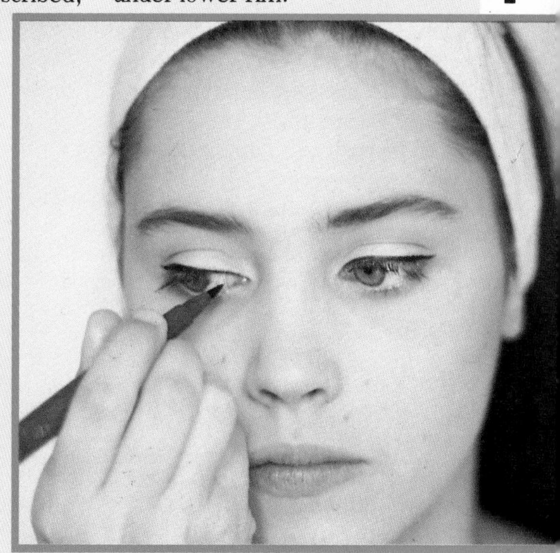

WHITE ON!

◄ Take a tip from the professionals for this eye-catching look. Draw a line inside your lower lash line using a soft white pencil to give the illusion of large, bright eyes. For instant sparkle, blend a little white eyeliner pencil at the inner corner of lids.

Watchpoint

Don't wear dark colours inside your lash line as they'll make your eyes look smaller.

Photographs: DAVID TODD/Hair and make-up: KAREN LOCKYER/Top: OASIS/Earrings: ACCESSORIZE

BLINKING GOOD LASHES

Would you like long, dark lashes that stay that way for weeks without the help of mascara? Then open your eyes to home dyeing and get ready to flash those lashes!

Eyelash dyeing is the answer to pale lashes if you want to darken them without the risk of smudges!

Home lash kits are simple to use – each contains an applicator, a tube of dye and a bottle of activating solution which you mix together in the dish provided.

Lash dye contains just two per cent peroxide while hair dye is much stronger with between 20 and 30 per cent peroxide. So for safety's sake only ever use lash dye on your eyelashes.

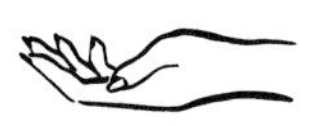

Ask a friend to help – you'll need to keep your eyes closed throughout the process so choose someone with a steady hand!

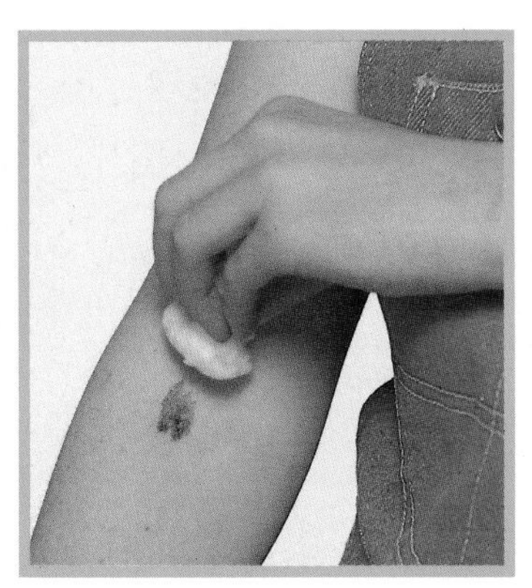

TAKE THE TEST

The day before you dye your lashes, do a patch test. Mix up a little dye and wipe it over a cleansed, grease-free patch of skin in the crook of your elbow. Leave it on for 10 minutes then rinse off. If after 24 hours there's no irritation, it's safe to continue. If you have sensitive skin, allow 48 hours for any irritation to develop.

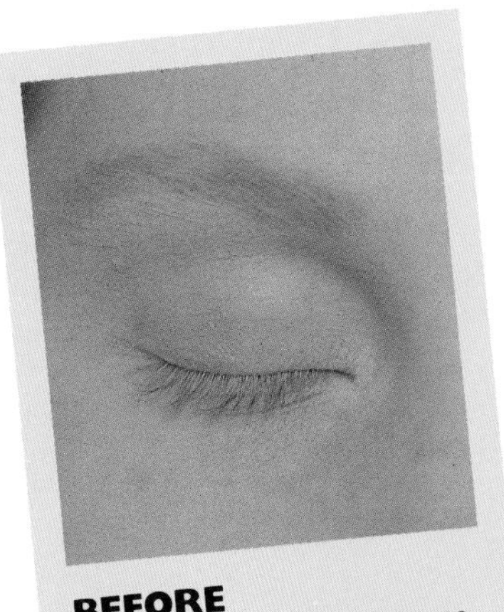

BEFORE
Do the whole dyeing process one eye at a time.

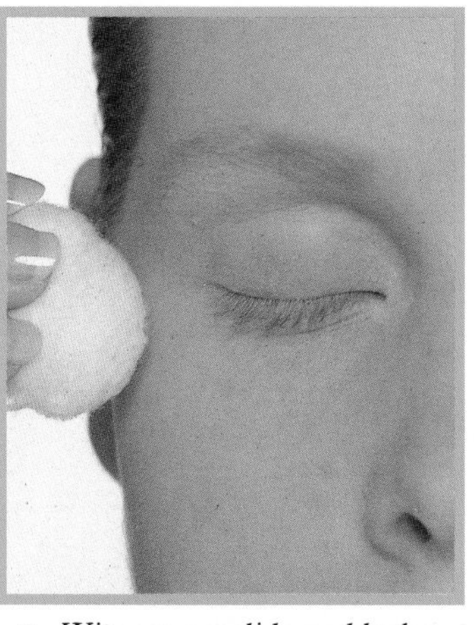

1 *Wipe your eyelids and lashes with an oil-free cleanser so that all traces of make-up and natural oils are removed.*

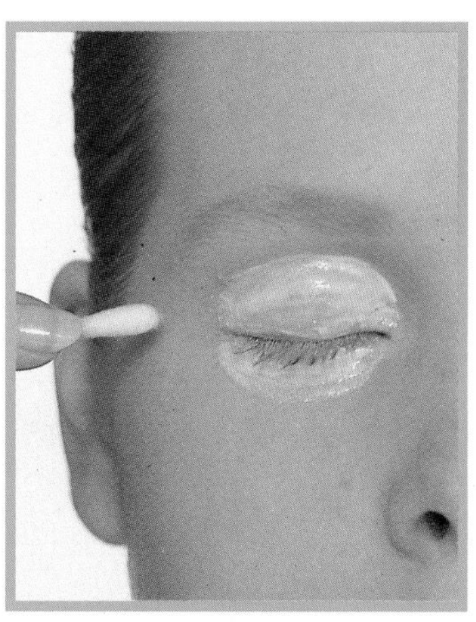

2 *Using a cottonwool bud smooth barrier cream above and below the top and lower lashes of one eye. Smooth the cream up to the roots but don't touch the lashes.*

Watchpoint

Never dye your eyelashes if you suffer from eye infections.

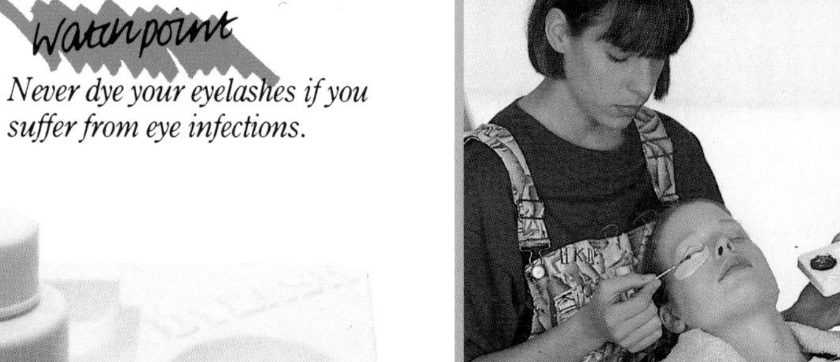

5 *Your friend should now paint your lashes from roots to ends. Keep your eyes closed so you don't smudge the colour by blinking.*

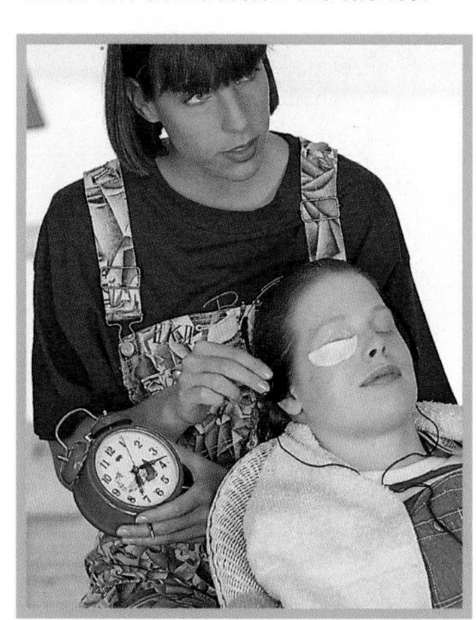

6 *Get your friend to set the clock. Leave the mixture on your lashes for 10 minutes. If any dye gets into your eyes rinse immediately with warm water.*

Photographs: SARAH HUTCHINGS/Hair and make-up: KARIN DARNELL/Floral jacket: TOP SHOP/Dungarees: C17/T-shirts: BENETTON/Earrings: ACCESSORIZE/Walkman: BOOTS

ANY QUESTIONS?

Q Only a few of my lashes are fair, should I try to dye them individually?

A It's almost impossible to single out lash hairs. Make life easier by dyeing them all!

Q Can I still wear mascara to thicken and lengthen my eyelashes even though they've been dyed?

A Yes, but try just coating the tips of your lashes to avoid a heavy look. Or opt for a contrasting colour on the eyelash tips for evening glamour. You could also use clear mascara to give extra length without colour.

Q Will make-up remover lift the dye?

A No, the lash dye will last as long as the lash itself. You will need to re-dye after six weeks or so.

Q Can I use the dye on my eyebrows too?

A Yes, but you'll get a more natural effect if you put the colour on with an eyebrow brush rather than the applicator.

WHY DYE?

- Dyeing is ideal for contact lens wearers who want to avoid wearing fibre-rich mascara. But make sure you remove your contact lenses before you start dyeing your lashes.
- Several applications of mascara can cause clogged lashes, whereas eyelash dye gives a very natural effect.
- Dyed lashes will last until the lashes themselves fall out – after about six weeks.
- There's no need to worry about smudging or runs.
- It's time-saving! You can put your mascara wand away and save time in the mornings.
- Lash dyeing can look stunning whatever your colouring, and just like mascara eyelash dye comes in various shades. You can choose from black, brown, grey and navy – whatever suits you.
- It's particularly convenient if you're a sporty type – especially if you're into water sports and don't like emerging from the water panda-eyed!
- Dyeing gets over the problem of dark roots and sun-bleached lash tips.

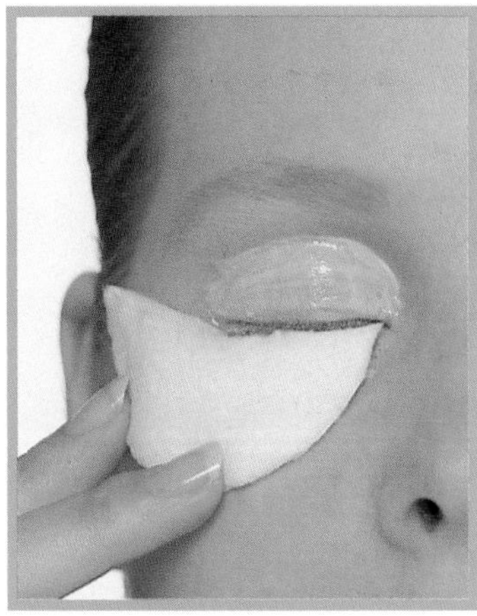

3 *For extra protection, cut a damp make-up remover pad in half and press it underneath your lower lashes on top of the barrier cream.*

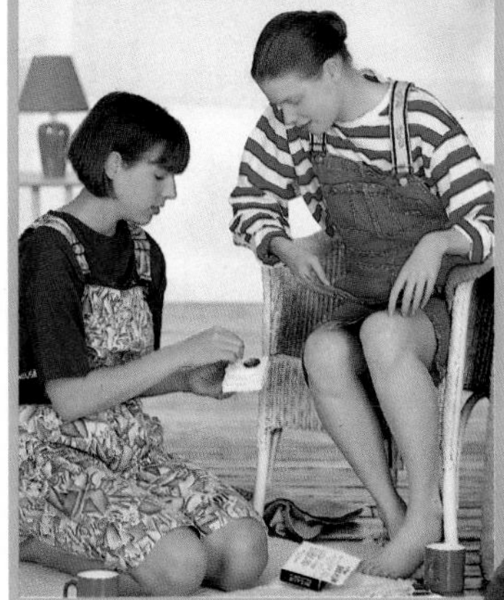

4 *In the meantime, get the friend who's helping you to mix up the dye.*

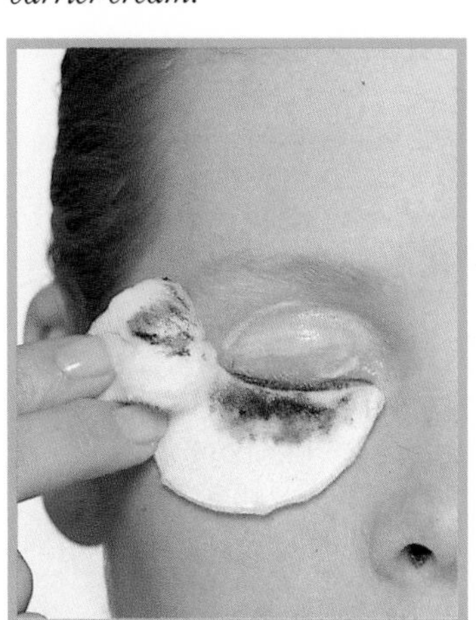

7 *Without opening your eye, use a damp cottonwool pad to wipe away excess dye. Repeat until cottonwool comes away clean, then remove the under-eye pad.*

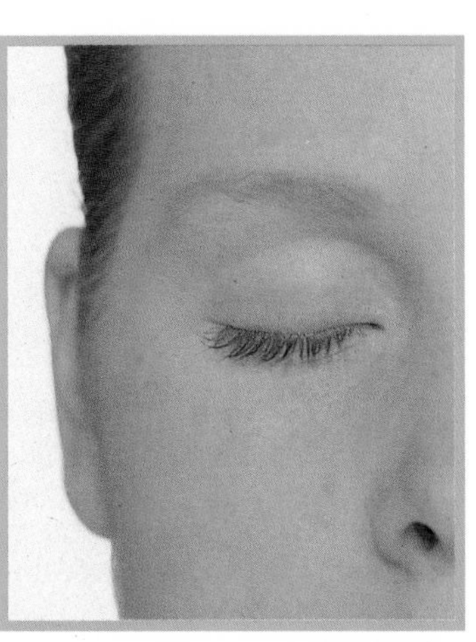

8 *Now prepare your other eye in the same way and repeat the dyeing process.*

Tip

Rinse stains away with warm water or use a cotton bud to dab on a little diluted surgical spirit.

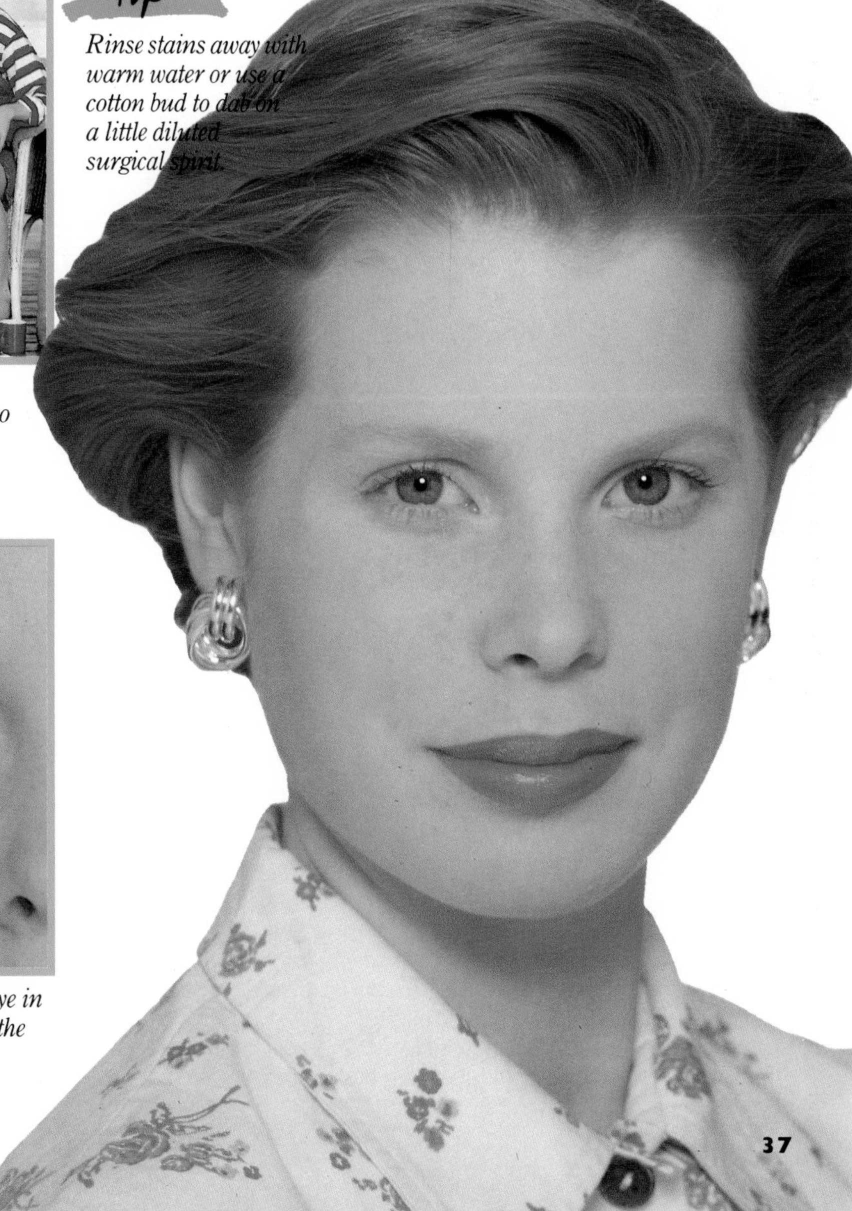

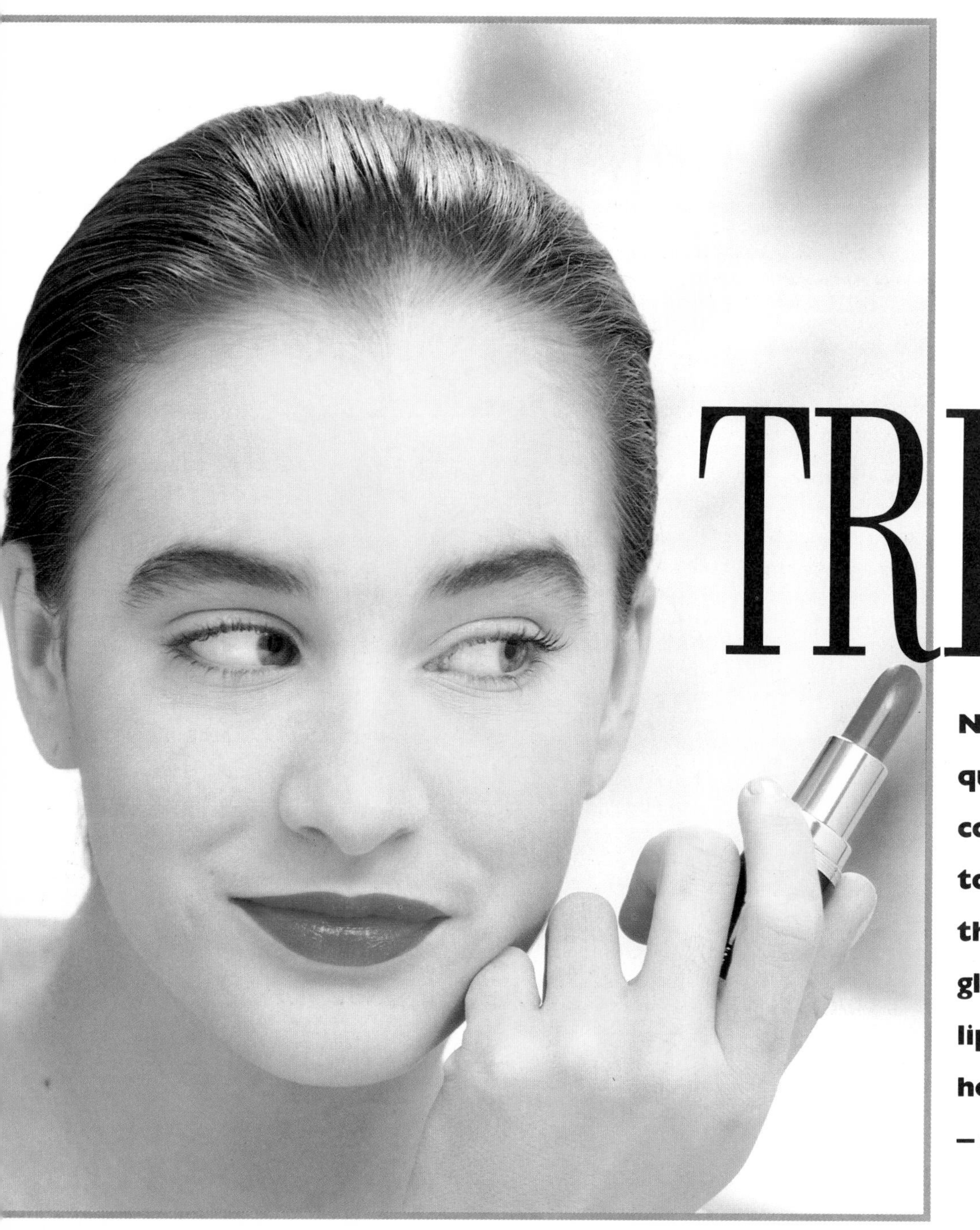

LIP TRICKS

Nothing flatters your face quite like luscious lip colour, but there's more to lip smacking good looks than a quick smudge of gloss. If you want your lips to shape up, here's how to make – and keep – a perfect pout

Lipstick is the essential finishing touch to your face, and out of all your make-up it's the one that works the hardest. If you want to come up smiling after a day's talking, eating, drinking and kissing, catch on to our lip tricks.

CHECK IT OUT

To avoid mistakes, always test lipstick before you buy – there's more to making the right choice than you might think.

- For hygiene's sake always test lipstick on your hand, not on your lips.
- Take the smell and taste into account by wiping a dot of colour onto your wrist, sniffing it and then licking it off. Some tastes can put you off and flavour and fragrance strengths vary enormously from brand to brand.
- Check the colour in daylight. Fluorescent shop lighting can distort the true shade.
- Adapt the colour to suit the season. Choose light, bright and sunny colours for the summer. Winter ones should be much richer, deeper and warmer.
- If an old favourite has been discontinued it's always worth asking whether the shade still exists – often the makers just change the name to bring it up to date.

LIP CARE

It's no use lashing out on lipstick if your lips aren't fit to be seen. The skin covering your lips is delicate – just one twentieth of a millimetre thick – so they can easily become rough. Lips are also very vulnerable to the drying effects of sun and wind as they contain neither oil-producing sebaceous glands nor melanin for sun protection. Treat them to their own special beauty routine.

SMOOTHIE

Lip moisturisers come in the form of balms or salves and are wax-based with added oils. They work by forming a film over your lips to protect them from further moisture loss and need to be re-applied several times a day to be really effective.

BRUSH UP

Regular moisturising protects your lips, but you may sometimes need to slough away loose skin. The easiest way to do this is

If you suffer from chapped lips choose lipsticks that are 'moisture rich'.

COLOUR WAYS

Lip colour is largely decided by trends, but as fashion becomes more diversified so the choice gets wider, and you can feel free to pick the most flattering shade for you. Invest in four or five colours to co-ordinate with your wardrobe, basing your choice on your skin, hair and eye colouring.

Blue-based colours **– light reds, pinks and plums – suit the English rose cool pink complexion, brunettes and ash blondes with blue or grey eyes. If you're the sort whose skin reddens in the sun then these are the shades for you.**

Yellow-based colours **– orange, peach and burgundy – suit olive skins and ruddy complexions with golden blonde or red hair and green or brown eyes.**

Vivid colours **– pillar box red, bright pink, vivid purple – suit black skins and those with dark olive skin and deep brown eyes.**

If in doubt, go for the shades recommended for your particular eye colour.

Lip colour should complement or match your blusher. Go for matt textures for a natural day look and save pearly ones to give your evening make-up a dazzling finish.

with your toothbrush! Run the brush under warm water to wet and soften the bristles then gently work it over your lips using circular movements. Blot dry with a soft tissue and moisturise.

SOAKING UP THE SUN

Lips can't protect themselves in strong sun, so protect them with a total sun block stick to keep harmful rays at bay.

PROBLEM SPOTTING

Allergies can cause dry lips. If you suffer from chapped lips despite all your best efforts to keep them smooth, you could be allergic to something in your lipstick. Unfortunately, contents aren't listed on the packaging so the only way to find them out is to write to the manufacturer. One common cause of allergy is lanolin, a natural oil from sheep's fleece used for its softening properties. Another to look out for is eosin, a red stain that's sometimes used to make lipsticks last longer. But any one of the ingredients could be the culprit.

Tip

Keep brushes and gloss applicator pads clean to avoid accidentally mixing colours. Wipe pads with a clean tissue after use, and wash sticky lip brushes in warm soapy water.

If you do suspect an allergy, stop wearing lipstick until it's better. And once the signs of reaction have gone, experiment with hypo-allergenic brands.

Lipstick bleed occurs when the colour spreads into the fine creases around your mouth, and is more of a problem for older skins. Stick to matt lipsticks which stay put better than glossy ones.

Cold sores, as the name suggests, are triggered by extremes of temperature – 'hot' sores are possible too! They are caused by a virus and can't be cured altogether. But they will clear up faster if you protect lips with a moisturiser and use a special 'cold sore' cream at the first sign of trouble. Ask your chemist to recommend one.

Yellow teeth are emphasised by bright shades and blue-based colours, while yellow-based colours make them appear whiter. Invest in peach, russet and orange shades.

BRUSH STROKES

The way you apply lipstick will give it more staying power.

- Don't put lipstick on straight from the tube – you won't be able to spread it evenly or match your lip edges. A lip brush is essential for a perfect pout so don't leave home without it!
- Lip pencils are ideal for outlining your lips or you can use them instead of lipstick. Soften any hard lines by blending in with a brush.
- Brush on the first coat of lipstick. Blot with a tissue, then apply a second coat. Dust very lightly with loose translucent powder for a matt finish.
- For a really glossy look, blot the final coat, then apply lip gloss. Keep it subtle – a light stroke over the centre of your bottom lip is quite enough.
- If you always smudge your lipstick, try lip powder instead. It looks like eye shadow and is put on with a sponge applicator. It can be tricky to apply but once on, it's hard to smear or wipe off.
- A palette of lip colours lets you mix your own shades. Or you can create the same choice by mixing colours on your hand with a lip brush.

GET IT OFF!

Lipstick removal should be gentle so that the delicate skin is not damaged.

- Use a creamy cleanser and a tissue to gently dab your lips free of colour.
- Blot your lips dry with a clean tissue.
- Slough rough skin if necessary, and condition with moisturiser.

SHAPE UP!

Improve on nature's design – you won't be able to alter the shape completely, but a bit of colour skill can even up unbalanced lips or make them look larger or smaller.

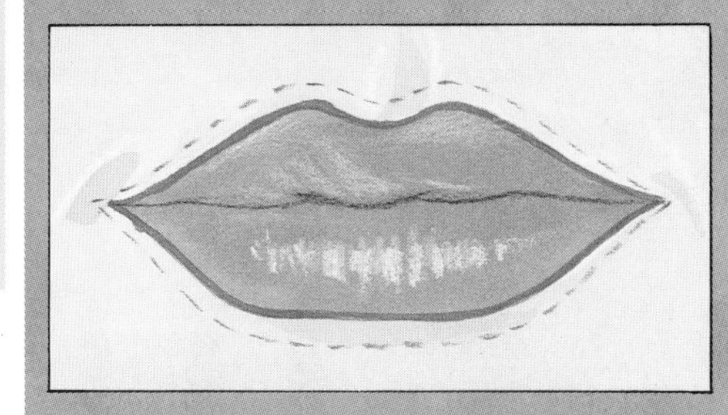

FULL LIPS can be narrowed by pencilling just inside your lip line. Fill in with a matt, subtle lipstick and avoid bright, glossy colours.

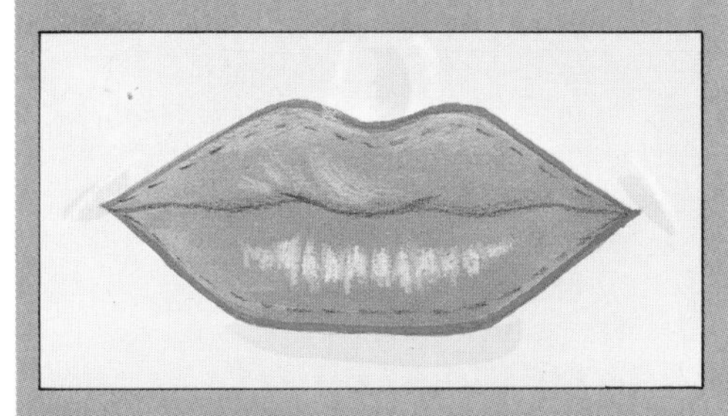

THIN LIPS can look fuller – pencil just outside the lip line and blend with a lip brush. Fill in with a clear, bright shade and dab lip gloss on the centre. Avoid matt, dark colours and primary reds.

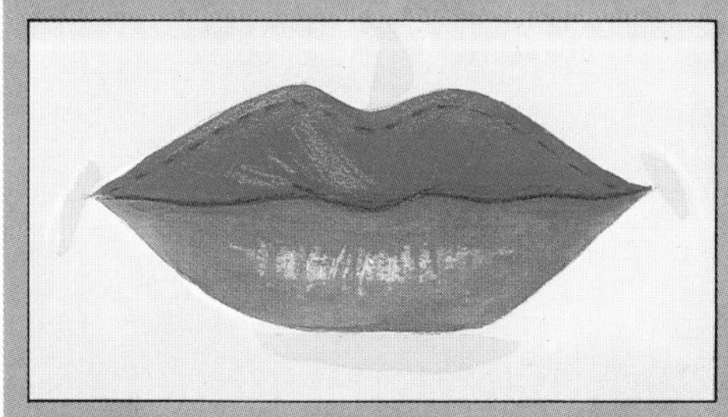

THIN UPPER LIP is balanced by pencilling just outside the top lip line and filling in. Make sure you use a slightly lighter application on the bottom lip.

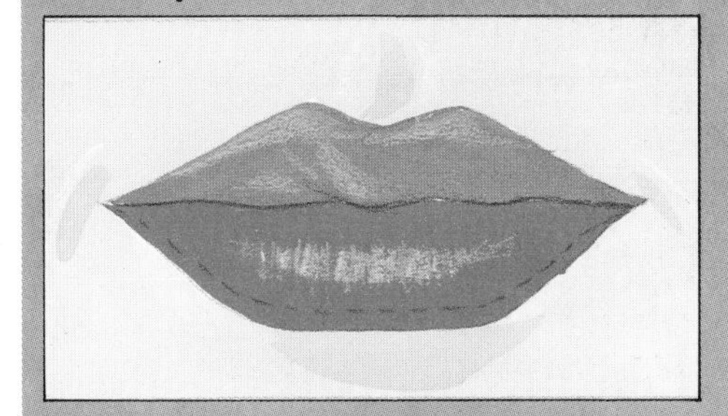

THIN BOTTOM LIP can be corrected by outlining the bottom lip only, and then using a slightly thicker coat of colour on the top lip.

Main photograph: ALISTAIR HUGHES/Still-life photographs: ADRIAN TAYLOR/Illustrations: NEIL GREER/Make-up: JACQUIE REYNOLDS

PAINT A PERFECT POUT

Make sure your lips are worth puckering up to with carefully chosen, skilfully applied lip colour. Here's a routine for lipstick that lasts!

A pair of beautiful red lips has, for a long time, been an image that's hard to beat for pure sexiness. Movie stars like Marilyn Monroe and Jean Harlow all had the perfect pout. But you don't have to be a great actress to paint your own lips. In fact if you really want to put yourself in a party mood, there's no easier way of doing it than reaching for your lipstick.

However perfectly you've applied the rest of your make-up, chances are you just won't feel dressed if you're not wearing lipstick. If you want to ooze confidence choose hot fuchsia or sizzling scarlet for your next night on the town. Opt for more muted shades during the day.

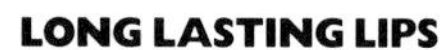

LONG LASTING LIPS

The latest way for the rich and famous to put forward a perfect pout is to have collagen injected into their lips. This puffs out the lips giving them that much sought-after 'bee-stung' look. But for ordinary folk, the quest for full lips need not involve anything so drastic. With a few professional make-up tricks you can make your lips look fuller and get your lipstick to stay fresh-looking, and on your lips rather than being left behind on cups and glasses. And remember, it's how you put your lipstick on that counts – put it on well and it'll look great for ages.

1 **Moisturise your lips before putting on the colour. This'll get rid of any dry skin that would spoil the look of your lipstick. Rub on a small amount of moisturiser and leave it to sink in for a couple of minutes.**

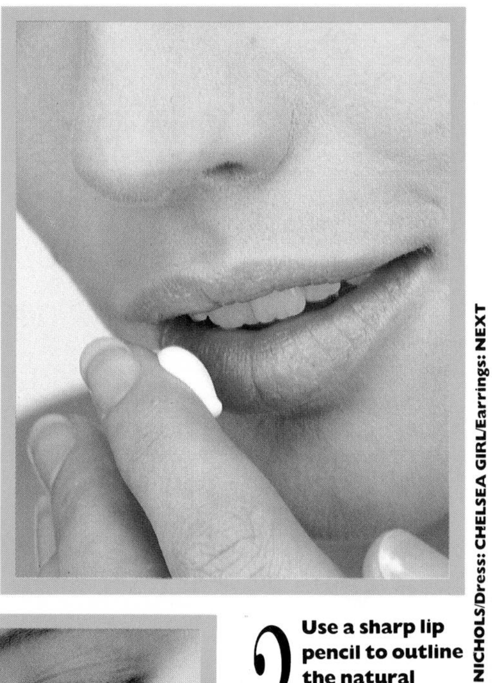

2 **Use a sharp lip pencil to outline the natural shape of your mouth. Avoid changing the shape of your lips too drastically as this will look unnatural.**

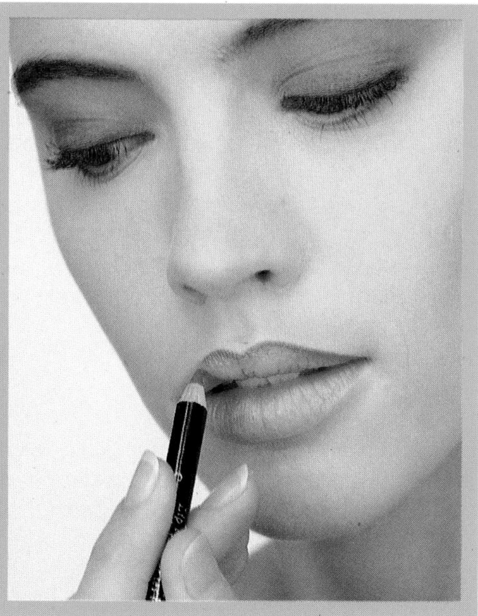

Tip

To find the perfect shade of lipstick, try mixing colours together on the back of your hand.

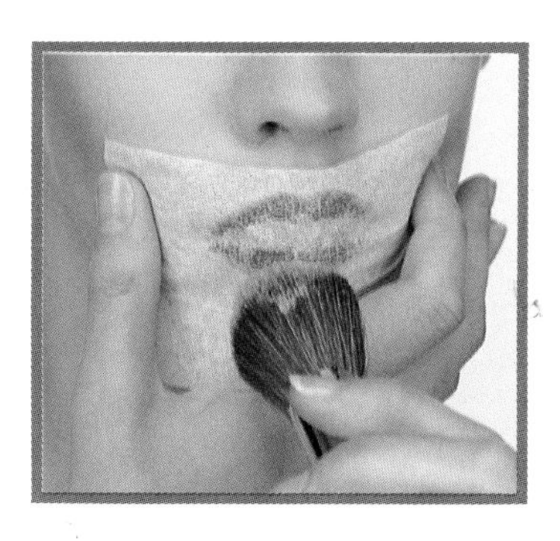

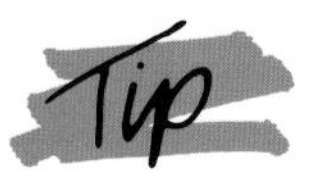

To set your lipstick without making it look dull or too matt, separate a tissue into two, fold one sheet over your mouth and dust with powder.

Use a slightly lighter-coloured pencil but in the same tone as your lipstick for a natural shape without a hard line.

Photographs: ADRIAN BRADBURY/Hair & make-up: VIRGINIA NICHOLS/Dress: CHELSEA GIRL/Earrings: NEXT

3 **Use a fine brush to fill in your lips with colour. The brush gives a more professional finish and helps you reach right into the corners.**

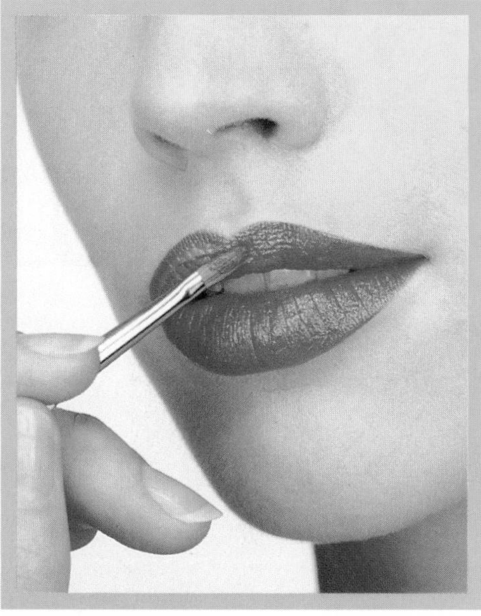

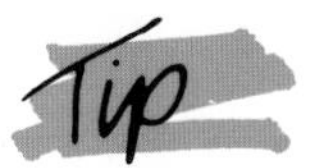

Try putting on a darker shade of colour at the corners of your mouth to make your lips look even larger.

5 **A slick trick for a perfect pout is to dot lip gloss onto the centre of your lower lip. But don't overdo it or you'll end up with greasy lips.**

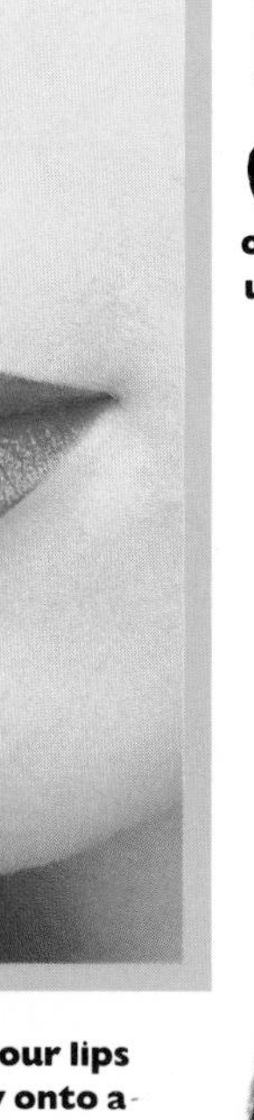

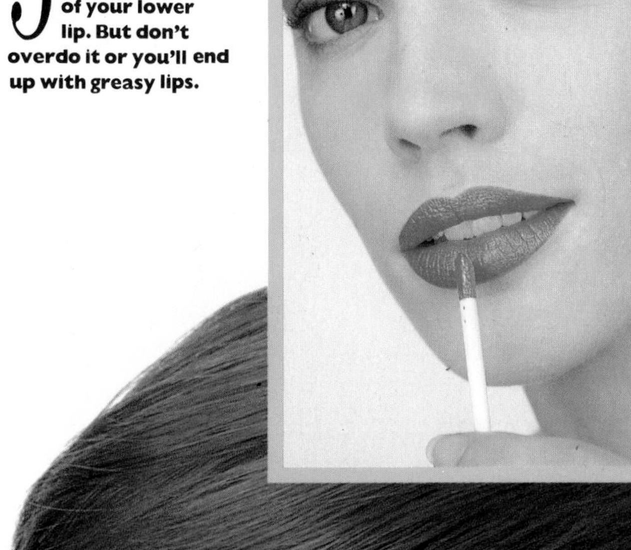

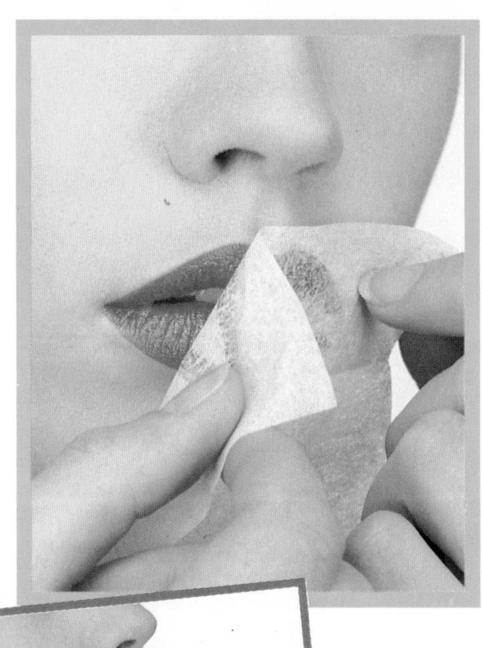

4 **Blot your lips lightly onto a tissue. Don't rub – the aim is to blot gently to remove any excess not take it all off.**

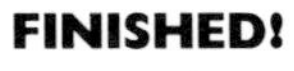

FINISHED!

The perfect pout – kissable lips that will last all night long.

To stop lipstick ending up on your teeth put your finger in your mouth and pull it out. Any excess lipstick should come off on your finger not on your teeth.

WHAT A CHEEK!

Haven't a clue what to do with blusher? Then pick up some cheeky ideas to make you glow gorgeously

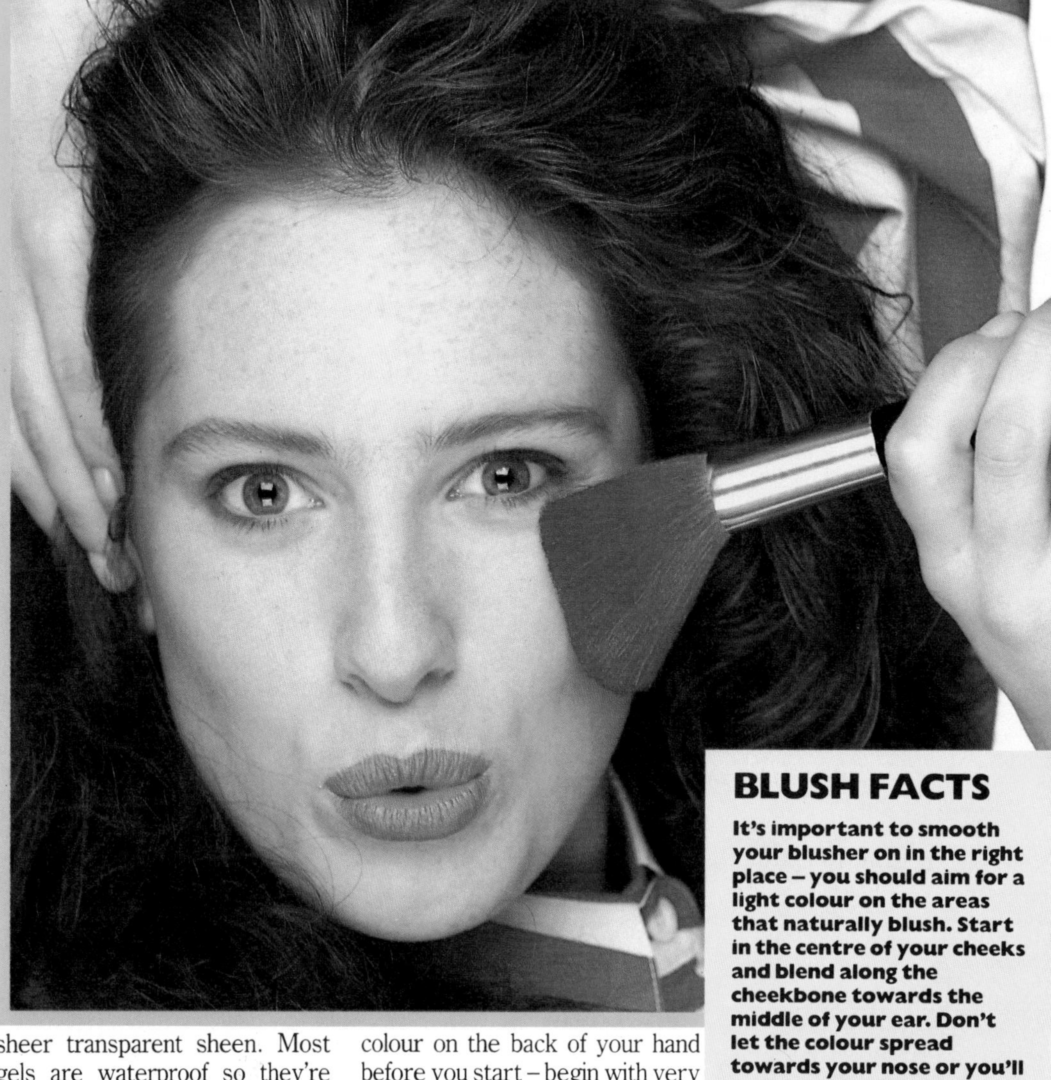

Blusher is the most versatile product in your make-up bag. Don't just use it on your cheeks though, there are plenty of ways you can lift your looks with artful brush strokes.

CHEEKY TYPES

Powder is by far the most popular type of blusher. It suits all skin types, but is especially good for oily skins as it helps preserve a good matt finish. Dust on your face with a thick brush after powdering, not straight on top of moisturiser as this tends to make it look caked and blotchy. It's also the most convenient type to use during the day as you can just brush on a little extra on top of your other make-up.

Cream is especially good for dry skin and gives it a healthy glow. Use on top of foundation but before powdering. Put on with a damp sponge for best results.

Gel helps to give your skin a sheer transparent sheen. Most gels are waterproof so they're great for swimmers and sunbathers. Use just a dab on top of moisturiser and blend well with your fingertips for soft, long-lasting colour.

OH GLOW ON!

Use a soft fluffy brush to put on powder blusher. The bigger the brush, the softer the effect. Always tap off any excess colour on the back of your hand before you start – begin with very little colour and gradually build it up – it's easier than having to wipe it off and start again if you put too much on!

Use dabbing rather than stroking movements so you don't end up with theatrical-looking stripes! Professionals often use two brushes, one to put the colour on and one for blending, to give a cover girl finish.

Wash brushes frequently, as they're good dust collectors and can harbour germs. Leave brushes to dry flat rather than standing them upright so the bristles don't splay out.

With cream or gel blusher use a dampened cosmetic sponge for a really even, natural finish (and to stop you getting it on your fingers). Put a few small dots on your cheeks and blend away!

BLUSH FACTS

It's important to smooth your blusher on in the right place – you should aim for a light colour on the areas that naturally blush. Start in the centre of your cheeks and blend along the cheekbone towards the middle of your ear. Don't let the colour spread towards your nose or you'll end up looking flushed!

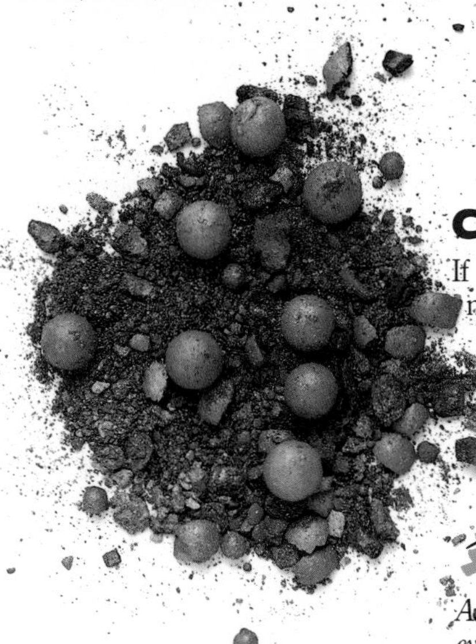

COLOUR CODES

If you're after a soft blush you need a colour that's as near to your own skin tone as possible. Pinch your cheeks slightly, make a note of the colour and try to find a shade to match.

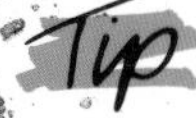

As a general rule make up your eyes first, then add blusher followed by lipstick.

CHEEKY TRICKS

Blusher isn't just for the cheeks. Give your face a touch of colour too! Put it on:

- over eyelids and browbones – but stick to soft matt shades for daytime make-up.
- across the bridge of your nose for a sunkissed look – but keep it light or you may end up looking sunburnt!
- on the tip of your chin – this helps to shorten a long face.
- around the hairline – for an all-over healthy glow.
- down the centre of your cleavage – just a light touch to emphasise your natural assets!
- on your lips as lip gloss – for a barefaced look.

AS A GUIDE

Yellow-toned skins suit peach, pale orange and apricot. Pink-toned skins look good with shades of rose and blue-pinks. Black skins need deeper shades which match their underlying tones. Bronze and copper are great for the evening.

Avoid vivid colours if you're pale and browns and russets if your skin's sallow. And steer clear of frosted shades – except after dark!

If you need an emergency blusher, try using a touch of lip pencil or soft, chunky lip crayon.

GLOWING PAINS

Q My blusher always fades away leaving me looking pale and peaky. What can I do to make it last longer?

A Try layering the colour by using a cream blusher first, then dusting a powder blusher over the top of your make-up once you've powdered your face.

Q Blusher always goes streaky on me. Am I putting it on incorrectly or am I using the wrong type?

A Streaky blusher is often caused by patchy skin. Blusher won't stay on skin that is dry or rough. If your skin is in top condition, check that you're using the colour at the right stage in your make-up routine. Powder won't sit well on top of bare skin, nor will cream over loose powder.

Q Blusher makes me look flushed – what am I doing wrong?

A It may be the shade you're using, the amount you're putting on, or where you're putting it! So follow our steps to glowing success.

Q Sometimes if I'm in a hurry, I put too much blusher on. How can I correct this without starting from scratch?

A Powder blusher can be toned down with a little light face powder. Dust it over the top with a brush. With cream or gel, smooth foundation over the top.

SHAPING UP

Use blusher in the right way and you can highlight your features or play them down.

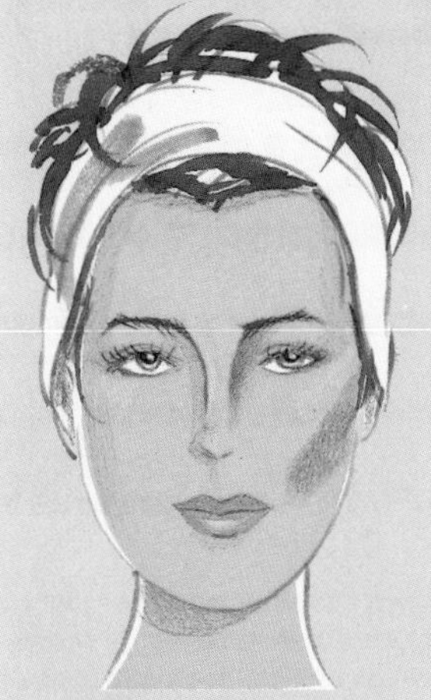

ROUND

Slim down your face with a concentration of colour on the cheekbones, fading out at the temples.

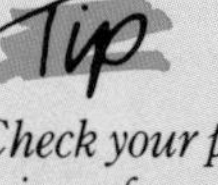
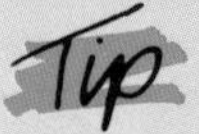

Check your profile carefully in the mirror for any hard edges on the sides of your cheeks, then blend them in with a brush.

OVAL

Add colour to the fullest part of your cheeks. Smile with your mouth closed to find the right starting point.

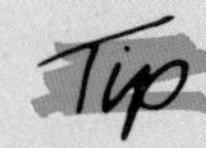

When mixing shades for your cheeks, stick to the same textures – powder with powder, gel with gel.

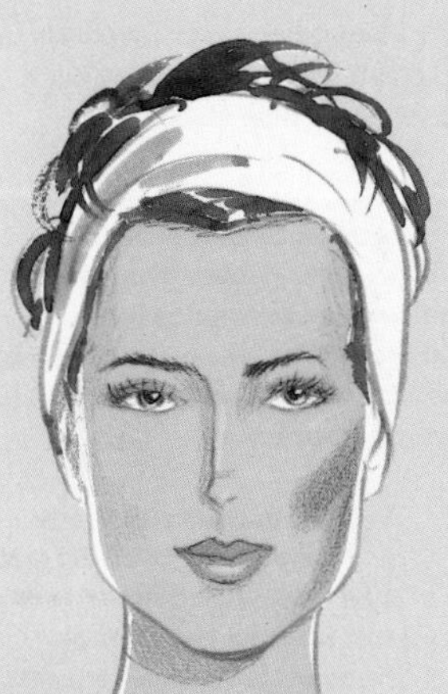

SQUARE

Add colour from just below the cheekbone and blend outwards, then stroke the same colour along your jawline to soften it.

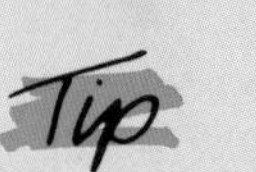

Don't forget to check the finished look with your hair styled in place. You may need to re-shade to balance the look.

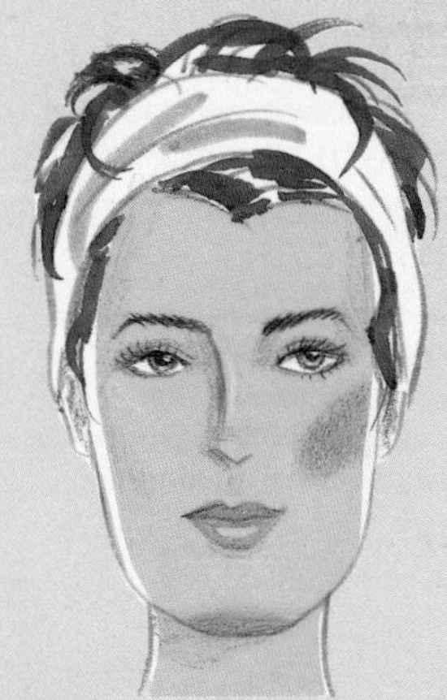

LONG

Make your chin recede with a touch of dark matt blusher on the tip. Use it on the cheekbone, fading out to a lighter shade.

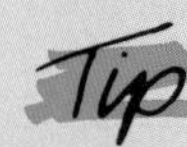

Always use the lightest touch and brush outwards and downwards to prevent any fine facial hairs from sticking up.

Photographs: IAN HOOTON/Hair: PENNY ATTWOOD/Make-up: KARIN DARNELL/Shirt: FREEMAN

50 TRADE SECRETS

Creating a flawless face takes more than a splodge of blusher and a dab of lipstick. Borrow a few artful tricks from professional make-up artists and you'll be well on the way to perfection

1 Test a foundation shade on your cheek or jawline in natural daylight, not on your wrist. If necessary, buy two shades from the same range and mix them together to get an exact match with your skin.

2 Make eyelashes appear thicker by powdering them before you apply any mascara.

3 Hide tired, pink-looking eyes by applying a flesh-toned foundation to the lids using a damp cosmetic sponge and line the inner rim of the lower lid with a beige eye pencil.

4 Using a cream blusher? Blend it in with your foundation sponge to create subtle definition without hard edges.

5 For that dewy-eyed look, paint a tiny amount of white highlighter at the inner corner of your eyes.

6 To help determine your face shape and which features to play up and down, pull your hair back from your face with an Alice band before making-up.

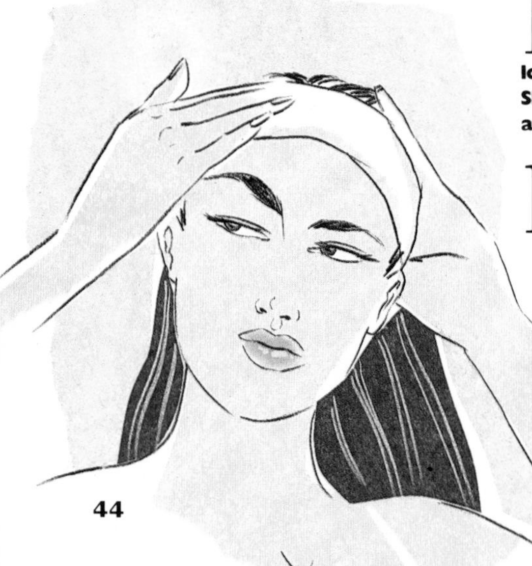
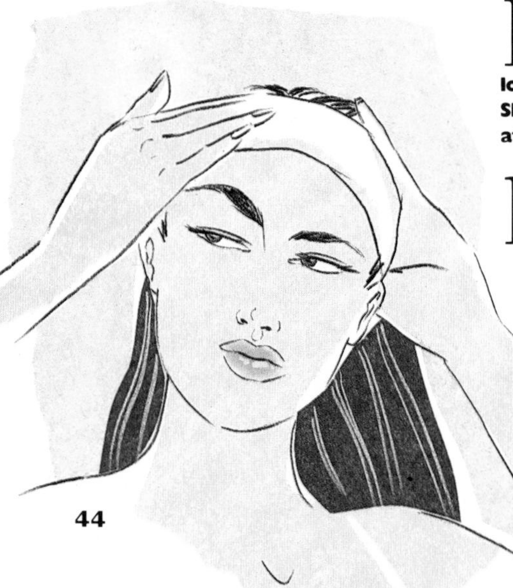
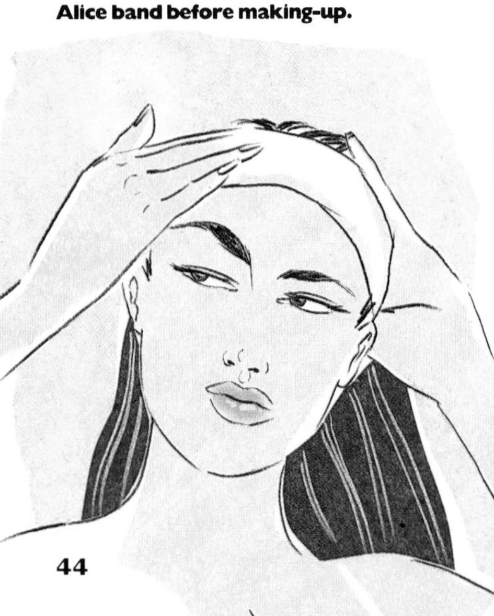

7 When choosing and using make-up, don't go entirely by shade names or how each one looks in its palette – make the most of testers in shops to avoid mistakes.

8 Set your foundation with loose translucent or transparent (colourless) face powder rather than a pinky shade. Add warmth to your skin with blusher instead.

9 Creating an O-shape with your mouth will help to stop you blinking – great for when you're stroking on mascara.

10 Mash and remix lipsticks and powder eyeshadows to create new shades.

11 Treat yourself to a set of natural bristle make-up brushes rather than using your fingers as applicators. Colours will be easier to blend and you'll be able to add definition just where you want it.

12 To apply under-eye concealer properly, tilt your head down and look up into the mirror. Shadows look their worst at this angle.

13 A terracotta-coloured eyeshadow can make blue eyes appear more vibrant.

14 To prevent looking down in the mouth, extend your lipliner slightly beyond the natural line of your upper lip, so that it slants upwards.

15 Dust off surplus face-powder with a big soft brush using light downward strokes so that your facial hairs lie flat.

16 Prevent eyeshadow particles from falling onto your foundation by pressing a clean tissue under each eye while you apply the colours.

17 Make yellow teeth look instantly pearly by wearing red or pink lipsticks rather than yellow-pigmented ones such as terracotta and peach.

18 Making up for an evening under artificial light? To prevent shadows falling across your face, use a mirror surrounded by lightbulbs.

19 Keep a supply of cotton buds – they're great for blending colours, and mopping up nail and lip colour smudges.

20 Don't let colour run riot over your features. Avoid running blusher up into the temples or hairline, creating a lip line too far outside your natural shape or taking eyeshadow up into the brows – you'll look like a clown!

21 Avoid a blue-pink blusher if your skin is already ruddy – it could make your cheeks look bruised.

22 Tame unruly brows and prevent the panda-eyed look under your lower lashes by using a colourless mascara.

23 When using a cream blusher, wear an all-in-one foundation which combines liquid and powder. Ordinary face powder can make a cream formula go blotchy on your skin.

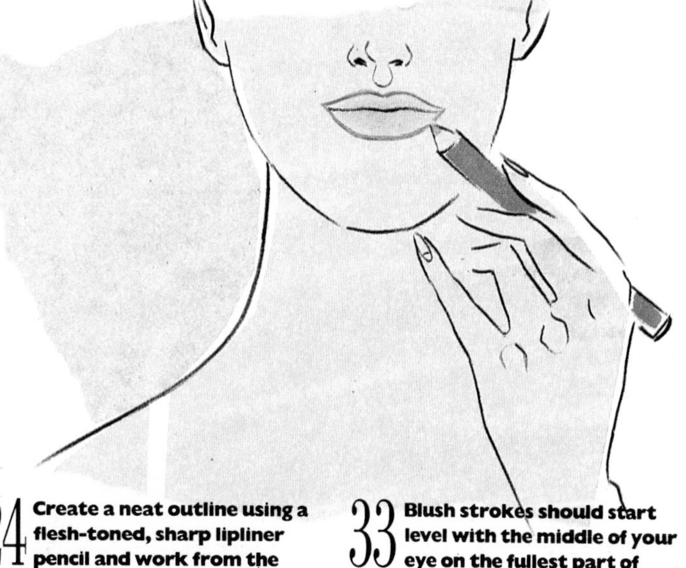

24 Create a neat outline using a flesh-toned, sharp lipliner pencil and work from the centre of each lip outwards. Hold the pencil close to the point and rest your little finger on your chin to prevent the wobbles.

25 For a flawless professional finish, always make-up using products with a similar consistency or texture.

26 Build-up the intensity of all colours gradually. Use the back of your hand as a mixing surface to gauge the shade before applying it to your face.

27 Spotty skin around your chin and mouth? Play down any redness by wearing a peach-toned lipstick.

28 Take foundation over lids and lips to help give colours depth and staying power.

29 Add depth to eyeshadows by applying them on a damp sponge-tipped applicator.

30 Create the illusion of perfectly proportioned lips by slicking on a darker lipstick on the fuller lip and a pearly one in the same shade on the thinner lip.

31 Make close-set eyes look further apart by emphasising the outer corners of each eye with a deep eyeshadow colour applied along the socket and winged upwards.

32 Prevent clogged lashes by brushing them between coats using a lash comb.

33 Blush strokes should start level with the middle of your eye on the fullest part of your cheek and extend upwards and outwards along the jawbone to the centre of your ear.

34 Don't match eyeshadow to your eye colour as it can look 'flat'. Look at the colours in the iris of your eye for inspiration.

35 Check your make-up from every angle to make sure the colours are well balanced.

36 Lining the inner rim of the lower lid with black can make your eyes look smaller.

37 Tone down overpowering blusher by pressing a little loose face powder on a velour pad and whisking off the excess with a soft brush.

38 If you wear red nail polish, stroke on a clear base coat to protect your nails from the pigment, which can stain them yellow.

39 Create a flawless complexion by blotting out your natural skin tone with an under-foundation base in lilac or white.

40 When choosing a foundation go for a shade lighter than your skin tone.

41 Got a bruise? Mix a little translucent face powder with a blob of foundation and paint it out. Set with more powder.

42 Make eyelashes thicker by dotting a fine pencil line close to the lash roots.

43 Make up in the following sequence to make sure the colours complement each other: base, eyes, lips and cheeks.

44 Get a friend to make up one side of your face so you can get a different perspective and then make up the other side yourself. Take the best from both attempts for a new stunning face.

45 Light colours enhance and emphasise features while dark ones can make them deepen and recede.

46 Got a spot? Paint on medicated cream concealer round it to hide the redness. Dab on foundation.

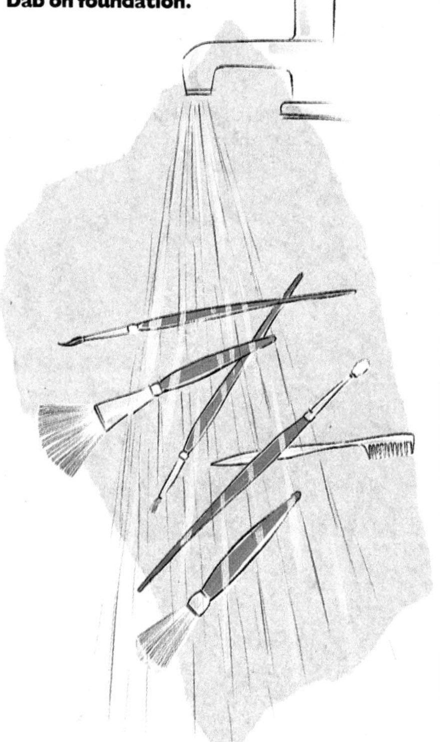

47 Wash your brushes and applicators daily so that shades will look fresh.

48 For an eye-catching mouth, paint a fine line of white highlighter along the edge of the Cupid's bow, and blend in to your foundation.

49 Matt colours are a make-up artist's best friend for creating a natural effect.

50 Avoid pinching your skin when plucking brows by choosing chisel-ended tweezers. Pull the skin taut and then pluck in the direction of hair growth.

Illustrations: JACQUELINE BISSETT

Natural make-up doesn't mean going bare-faced. Read on for some topping tips on making up with a lighter touch

BARE ESSENTIALS

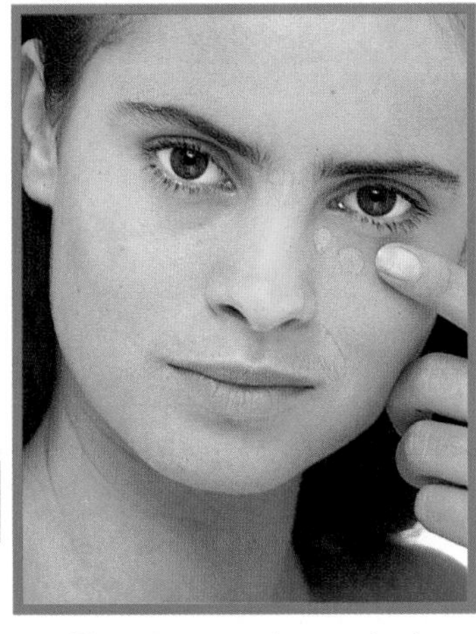

▲ *Tone down under-eye shadows and cover up minor blemishes with a few dabs of concealer. Blend in a tiny amount using a clean finger.*

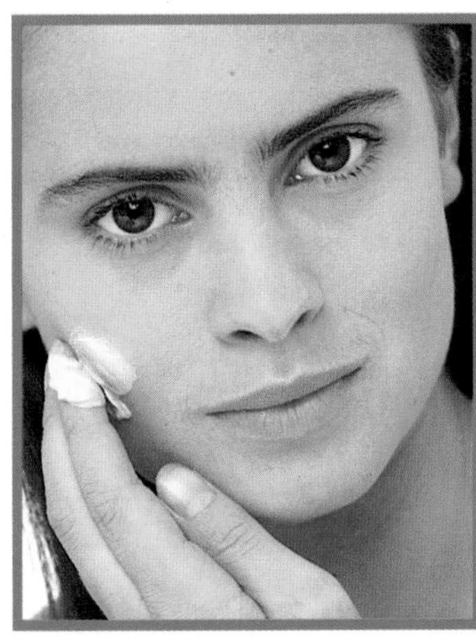

▲ *If you need to wear foundation choose one with a matt or semi-matt texture for a natural finish. Put on with your fingertips.*

▼ *If you have an oily or combination skin you'll get a longer lasting matt finish if you put on powder with a puff. Press it on using a rolling action.*

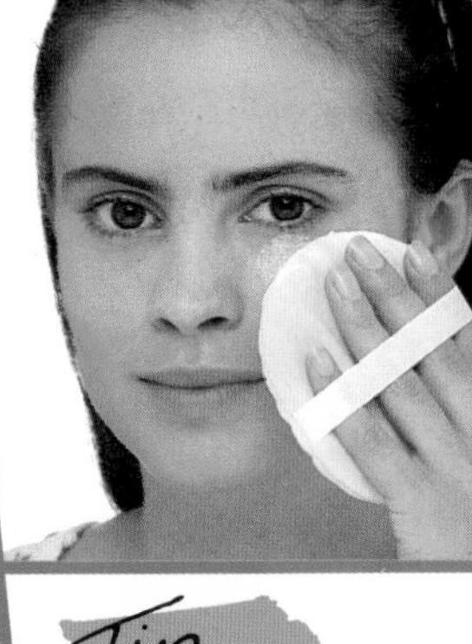

◄ *A favourite eye-opening trick of many make-up artists is to dust a little blusher lightly around the outer eye socket. It also helps make your eyes look brighter and means you don't need to bother with eyeshadow!*

NATURAL KNOW-HOW

- **If you've got very fair lashes forget mascara and have them dyed! But remember mid-brown will look better than black unless your hair is dark.**
- **Powder blushers and eyeshadows tend to look more natural than anything creamy because they're usually matt not glossy.**
- **Lift a washed-out complexion with a very light sweep of blusher over your nose. Then, to make you look instantly healthy, fake a few freckles with an eyebrow pencil!**
- **Put away your tweezers unless your brows are really unruly. Heavier eye-brows are definitely in, and make more of eyes that aren't wearing make-up.**
- **Get back to nature with your pick of the colour palettes: brown, terracotta and all the pastel shades.**
- **If you're going to be a real natural beauty then only buy products that put the environment first. Cruelty-free cosmetics, ozone-friendly aerosols and biodegradable hair care products are as good as anything else, just kinder to nature!**

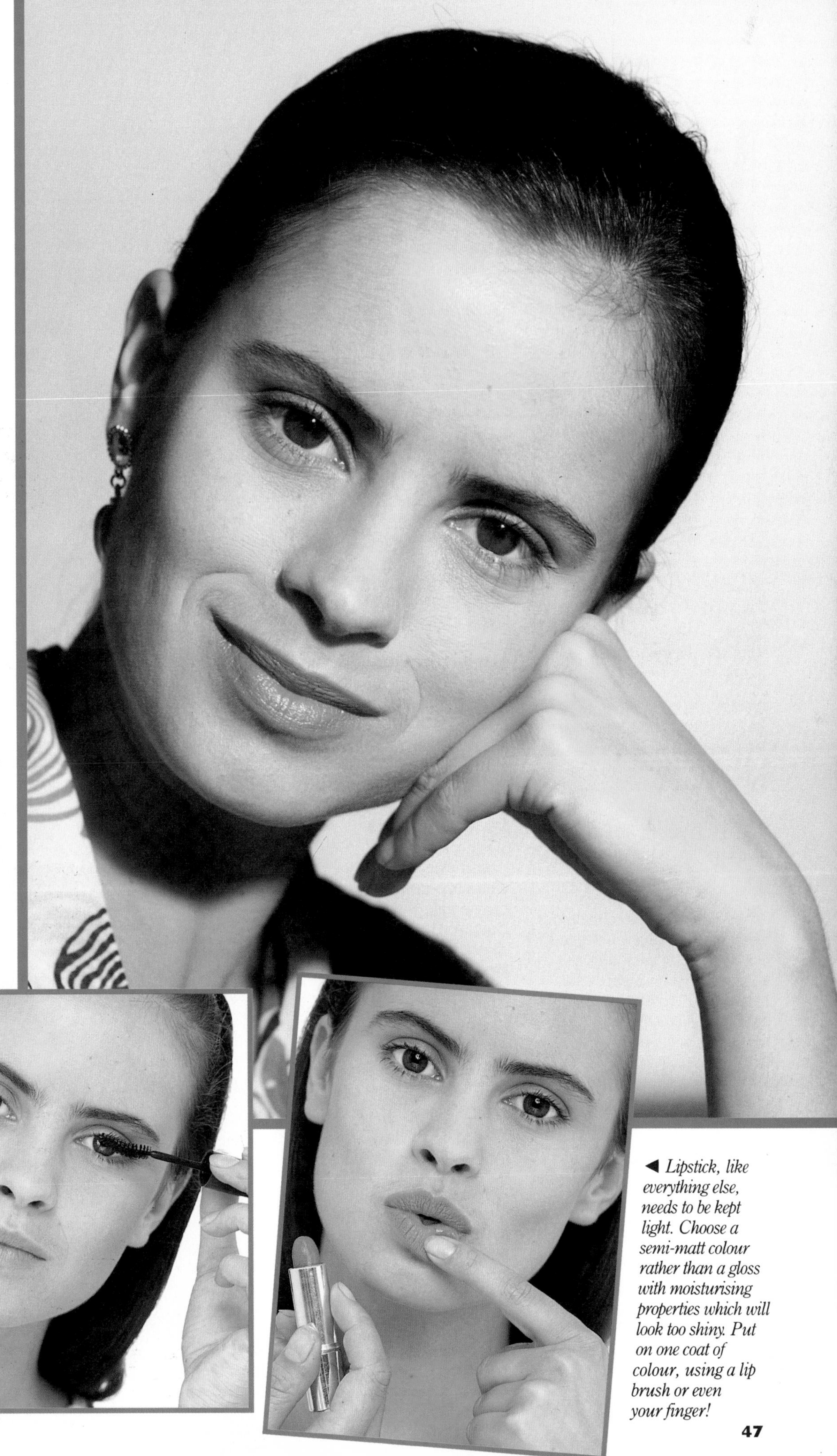

Photographs: JUTTA KLEE/Still-lifes: STEVE CABALLERO/Hair: KARIM MITHA/Make-up: VIRGINIA NICHOLS/Top and earrings: NEXT

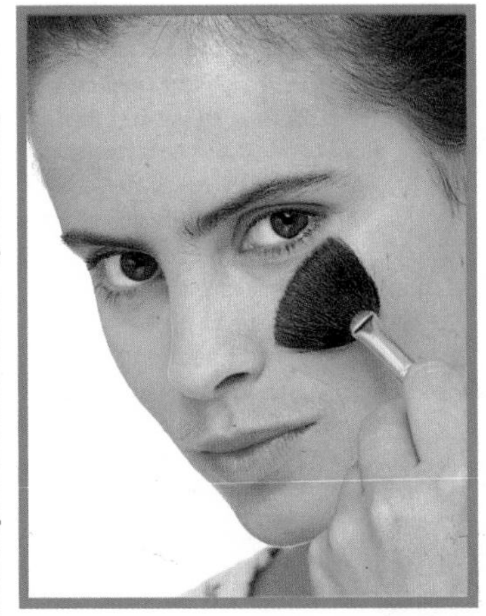

▲ *To set foundation and prevent shine, dust with loose face powder using a soft brush. Make sure you cover eyelids and lips, too!*

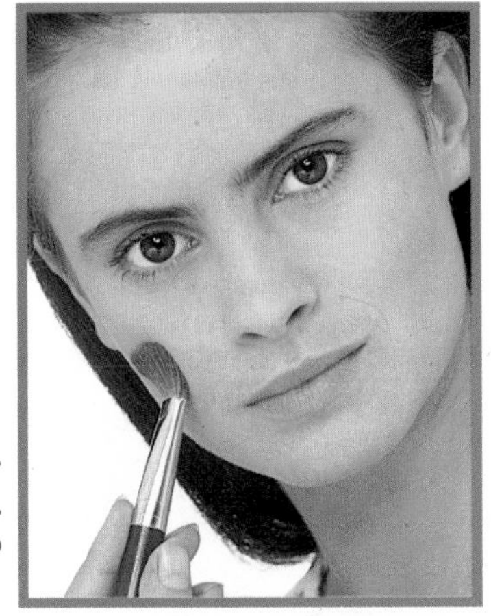

▲ *A touch of blusher, swept over cheekbones with a brush, adds a healthy glow. If you've put on too much, lightly cover with powder.*

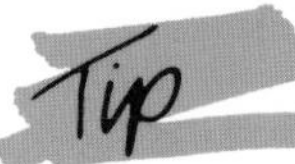

Use rose pink as the blusher shade for cool skin tones.

► *To avoid clogged lashes, which won't look natural, put on mascara in three or four individual sweeps pausing between each one to let it dry.*

Watchpoint

Avoid mascara that's 'lash building' – it's much more difficult to put on lightly.

◄ *Lipstick, like everything else, needs to be kept light. Choose a semi-matt colour rather than a gloss with moisturising properties which will look too shiny. Put on one coat of colour, using a lip brush or even your finger!*

MAKE-UP MADE EASY

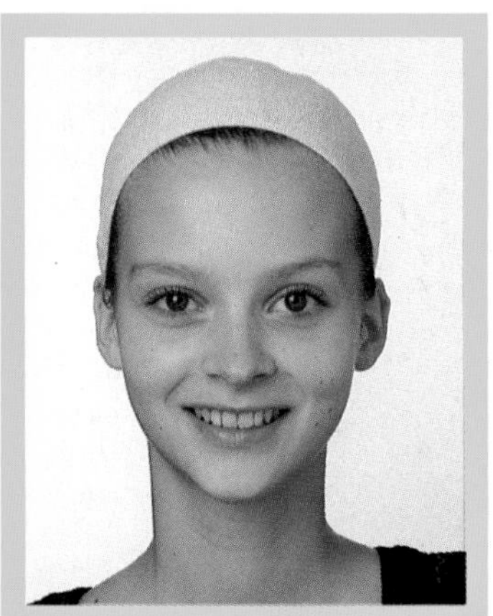

READY TO START
Give your moisturiser a few minutes to sink in then you're ready to start making up.

QUICK TIPS

- Use neutral shades on eyes – bright colours need more time to make them look good.
- Put mascara on carefully and comb your lashes through. A single coat can look much more effective than several clogged coats on top of each other.
- Mascara your lower lashes before your upper ones, to prevent the top ones from dotting or smudging.
- Your lipstick will last a lot longer if you blot your lips on a tissue before putting on a second coat.
- Try a touch of rose-pink blusher on your lids, instead of eyeshadow.
- Brush your brows with clear, colourless mascara to keep them in place.
- Tint your lashes with permanent colour. It'll make them look darker for about six weeks, then you won't have to bother with mascara at all!

You don't have to spend hours on your make-up to look good. Whittle your routine down to the basics

Sometimes the idea of putting on make-up in the morning can be one long yawn. If you're in a hurry you may think you have to choose between being late or going bare-faced. But there's another choice open to you, and that's to go for a natural look that won't take ages to apply. What you need to do is re-think your colours and how you use them. Remember that you're going for a softer look. It doesn't mean you won't look good. It just means that your make-up will flatter you in a much gentler way.

Make sure the night before that you have everything you need for the morning. Lay your things out, so that you do not have to waste time hunting for your mascara or lipstick.

Follow our step-by-step guide and you'll soon be looking great and still manage to get out of the house on time!

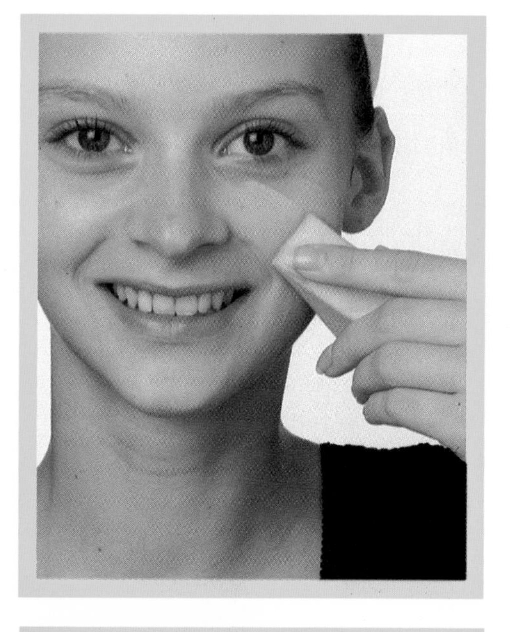

1 Forget fiddly foundation and powder. Make things easy and fast by going for a mixture of the two with a creamy powder. Use a damp sponge for even coverage. Pat on a little at a time, then use the sponge to blend it all over your face.

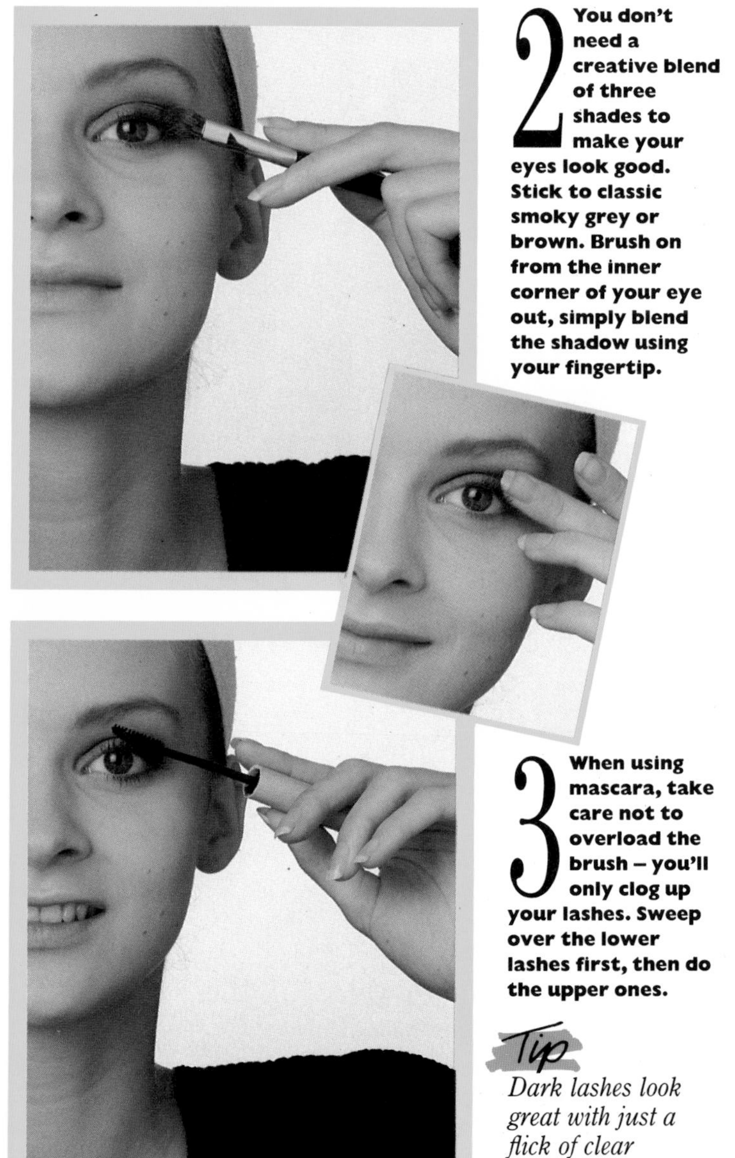

2 You don't need a creative blend of three shades to make your eyes look good. Stick to classic smoky grey or brown. Brush on from the inner corner of your eye out, simply blend the shadow using your fingertip.

3 When using mascara, take care not to overload the brush – you'll only clog up your lashes. Sweep over the lower lashes first, then do the upper ones.

Tip
Dark lashes look great with just a flick of clear mascara.

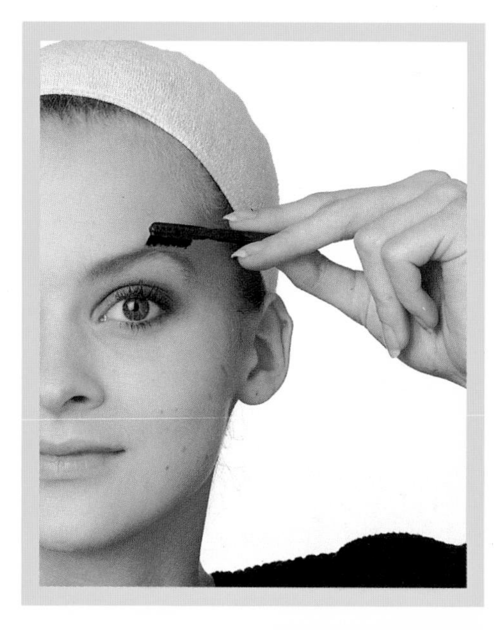

4 Improve the shape and definition of your eyebrows by brushing them with an eyebrow brush or the almost dry mascara brush and now your brows will look, and stay, neat all day long.

5 Keep blusher down to a minimum or you'll end up looking like a clown. Dust a soft peach or rose pink shade onto a big powder brush, tapping it first against the back of your hand to get rid of excess colour. Brush upwards onto the widest part of your cheeks for a soft, gentle glow.

6 You don't have to go to all the trouble of lip pencils and lip brushes to achieve a model-look make-up. Just use your fingers to put on a pinky red shade of lipstick for a soft look rather than a perfectly painted effect.

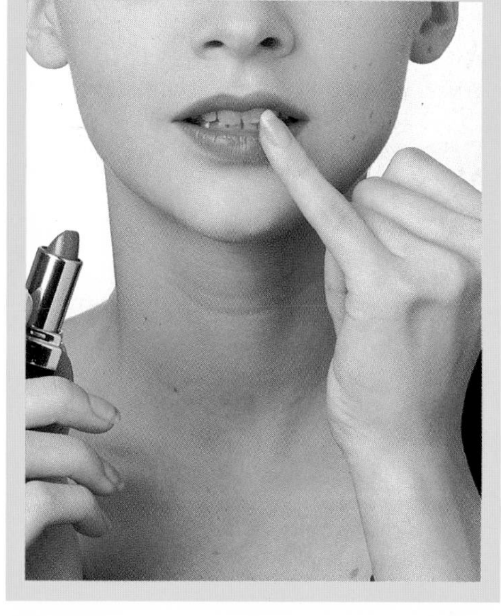

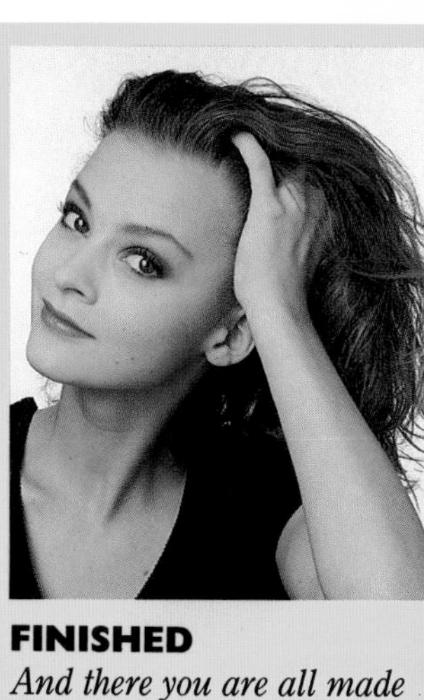

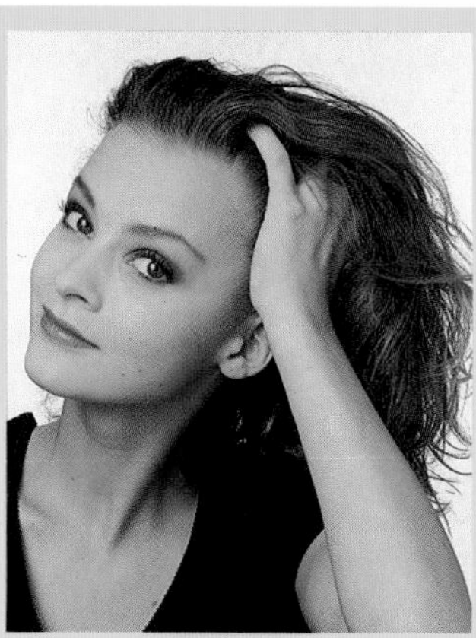

FINISHED

And there you are all made up with plenty of time left to dress, do your hair and leave the house on time.

Photographs: MATTHEW SMITH
Hair and make-up: ELLIE WAKAMATSU

COLOUR STORY: BROWNS

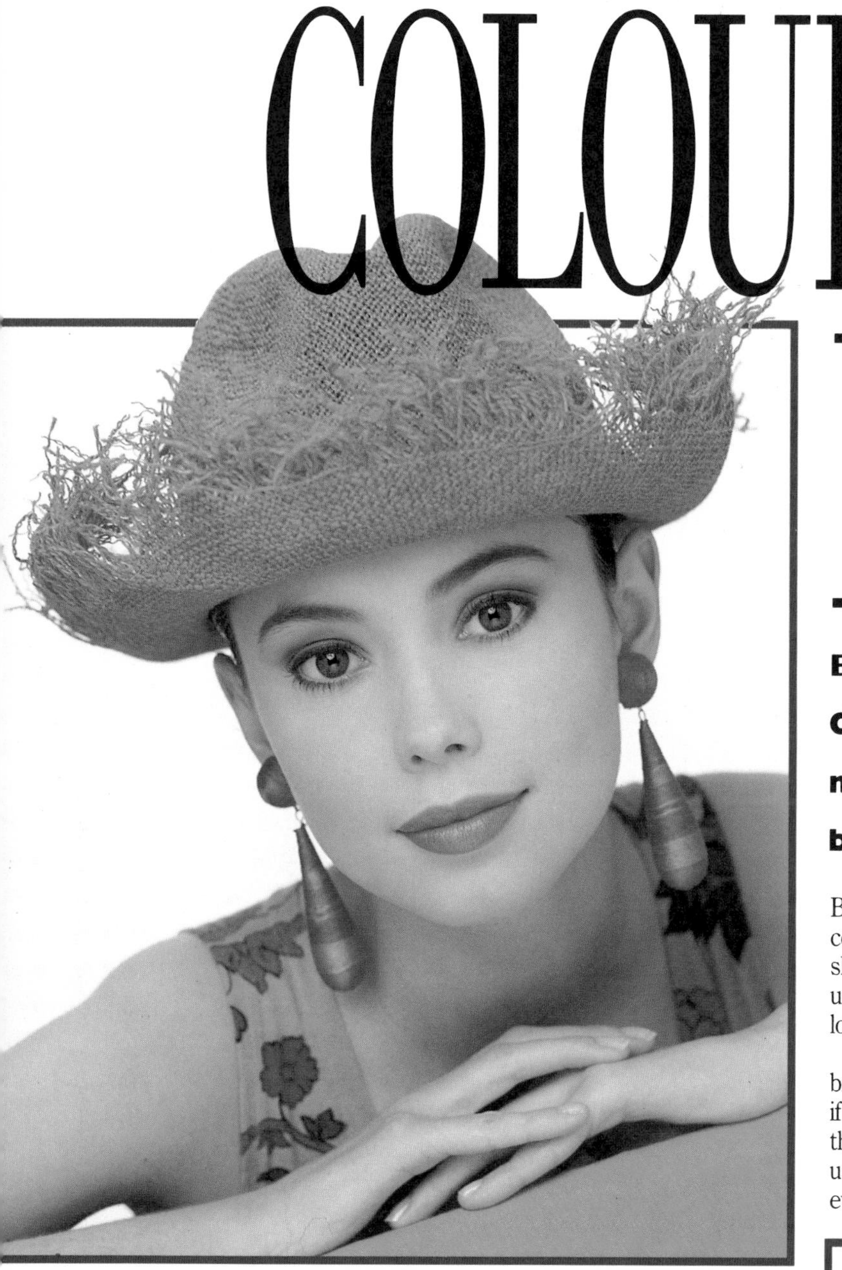

Browned off with the same old eyeshadow? Open your eyes with our guide on how to mix and match for the best effect – you'll be sure to score brownie points!

Brown is a firm favourite when it comes to eye colour. It suits most skin tones and eye colours and, if used properly, is the most natural-looking eyeshadow you can use.

However, like most colours, brown can look rather flat and dull if you just stick to one shade over the whole eye. Instead, practise using a combination of two or even three different shades of brown, such as light golden russet with rich spicy nutmeg and soft woody brown – you'll be surprised at the different effects you can achieve.

Read on and we'll show you how the experts use the light and shade in brown eye colours to gently define the eyes and give them that wonderfully subtle 'unmade-up' look.

EYE OPENERS

- **If you have oily skin, dust your lids with translucent powder before putting on shadow to help stop the colour creasing.**
- **Always put eyeshadow on with clean soft brushes and not with your fingers which tend to be too greasy.**
- **Dab, don't drag skin around the eyes as it is very delicate.**
- **If you want to test a colour against your skin tone to see whether it suits you, try it out on the back of your hand first.**
- **For a totally co-ordinated face choose a blusher and lipstick with brown rather than pink overtones.**
- **To add definition to patchy brows use a little brown powder shadow – it will always give a far more natural look than black.**
- **There's a shade of brown to suit everyone. As a general rule blondes look wonderful in camel, brunettes in chocolate and redheads in russet. Black skins suit copper and golds.**

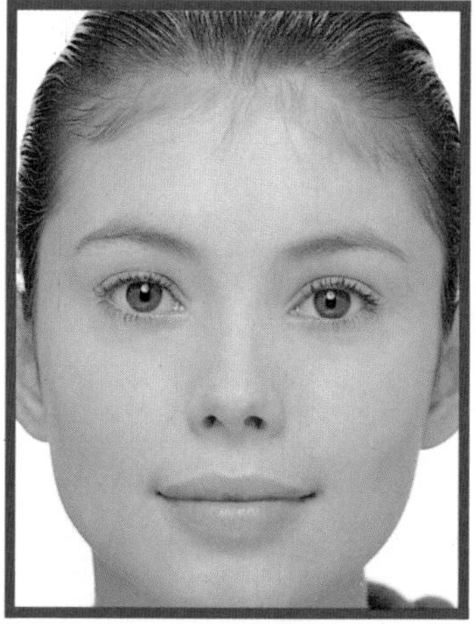

1 *Before you start make sure that your skin is thoroughly cleansed and moisturised.*

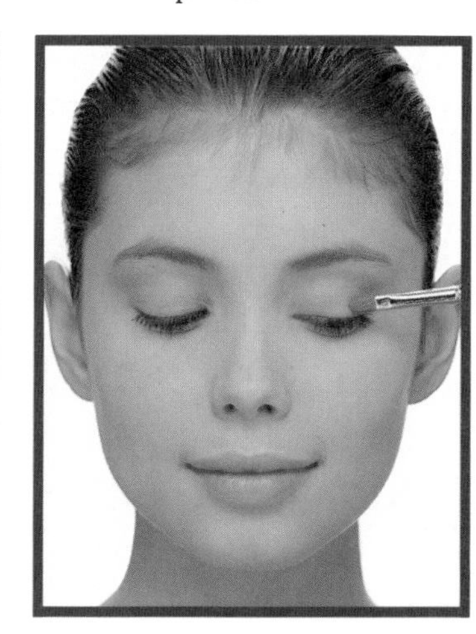

2 *Stroke a light shade such as peach or beige over both lids and up to the brows as a base colour.*

3 *Define your socket line with a mid-tone brown shadow. Dab the colour outwards from the centre of the socket, blending as you go.*

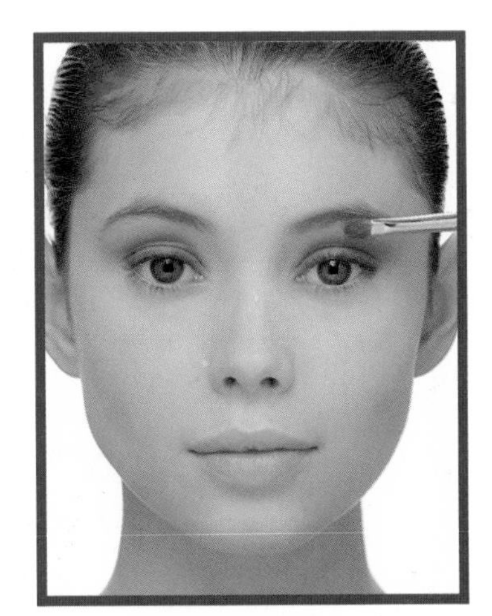

4 *Blend a darker brown shadow just above your socket line to give eyes greater definition.*

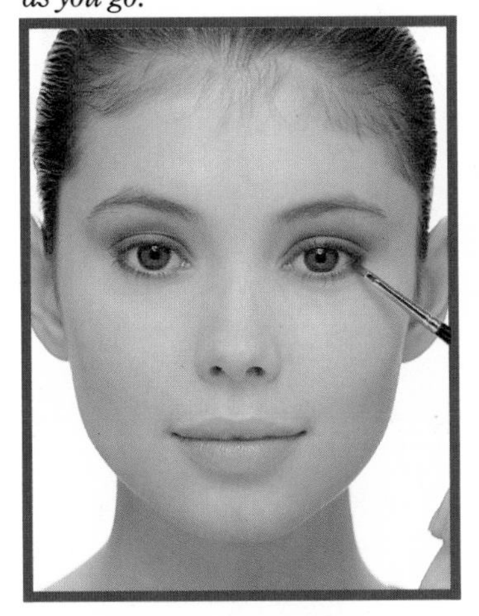

5 *Using the same shadow on a dampened brush, draw a line beneath the lower lashes, then smudge it with a dry brush.*

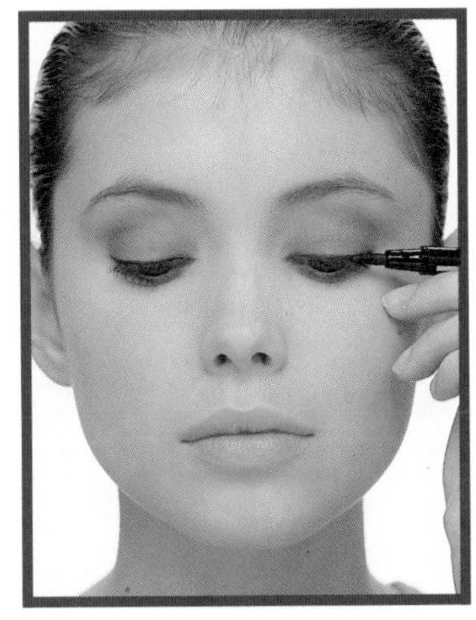

6 *Draw a fine line of dark brown eyeliner a third of the way along the top lids. This will help make your eyes look bigger.*

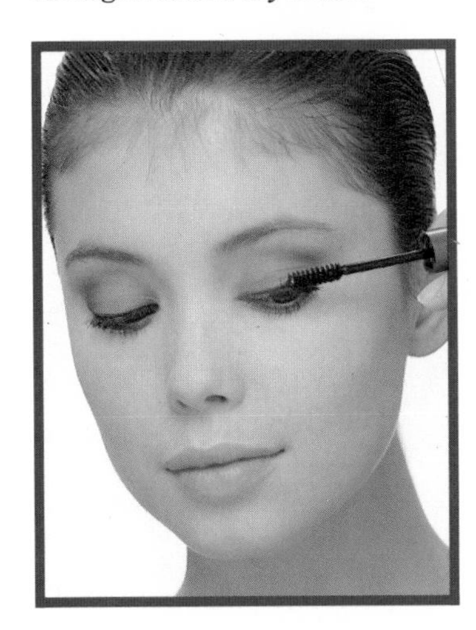

7 *Finish with a coat of soft brown mascara. When dry separate lashes with a clean mascara wand or an eyelash comb.*

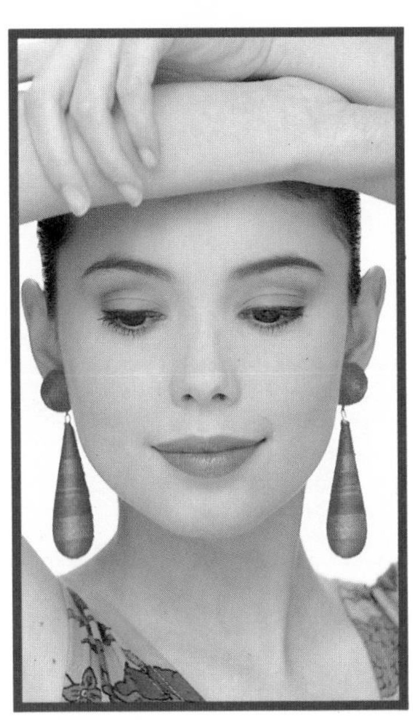

MATCHMAKERS

When it comes to choosing brown colours that go well together there are really no hard and fast rules. Most brands have testers so you can always try out a few before you go to the expense of buying.

We've put together a few suggestions to help you select lipsticks and eyeshadows that complement each other.

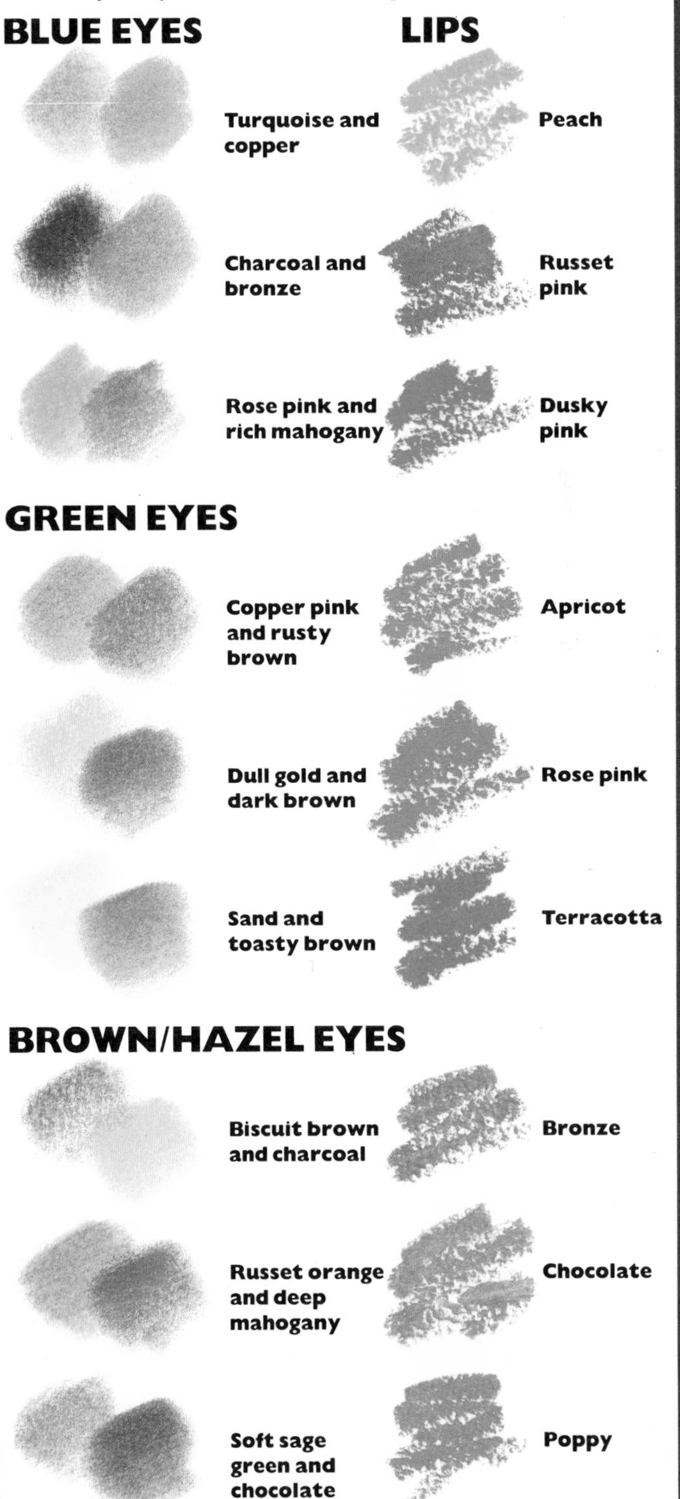

Photographs: ALISTAIR HUGHES/Hair and make-up: YA'NINA/T-shirt: NEXT/Floral top: NEXT/Earrings: NEXT/Hat: FRED BARE

GLAMOUR TRICKS

You don't have to be born beautiful to look stunning. With just a few slick tricks you can have flawless looks that say star quality!

Some people have it, some don't. And it's not natural beauty, or even how much money you spend on making yourself look good.

It's that difficult to define quality called glamour. Looking glam is all about making the most of what you've got. It's about skilfully applying make-up, not slapping it on. It's about looking polished yet making the end result seem effortless. And the greatest thing about this type of beauty is that you can have it!

BACK TO BASE

The very basis of a super smooth image is perfect skin. And if you haven't got it naturally, fake it! The queen of glamour, Joan Collins, is said to use 15 different shades of foundation to even up her skin tone. Now this may be taking it to extremes, but no skin is flawless and most can benefit from a bit of help.

For instance, if your skin is ruddy and flushes easily, try wearing a green fluid corrector under your foundation or try one of the new pale blue corrective powders which have been specially designed to counteract redness. If you've got sallow skin, try a pink or lilac corrective fluid to 'lift' and brighten your skin tone. Or try brushing on an apricot or rose powder for radiance.

WHAT'S GLAM

IN

Opaque black tights
Louis heels
Champagne, Pimms
Velvet, tafetta, suede
Chunky fake jewellery
A glimpse of a silk camisole
A curvaceous shape
Understated style, not all up front!
Not smoking

OUT

Fishnet tights
Stilettos
Cocktails, lager
Glitter-spangled lurex, leather
Gold 'rope' chains, coin rings
A glimpse of a discoloured bra strap
Looking twig-thin
A gaping cleavage
Smoking and leaving red lipstick on the butt!

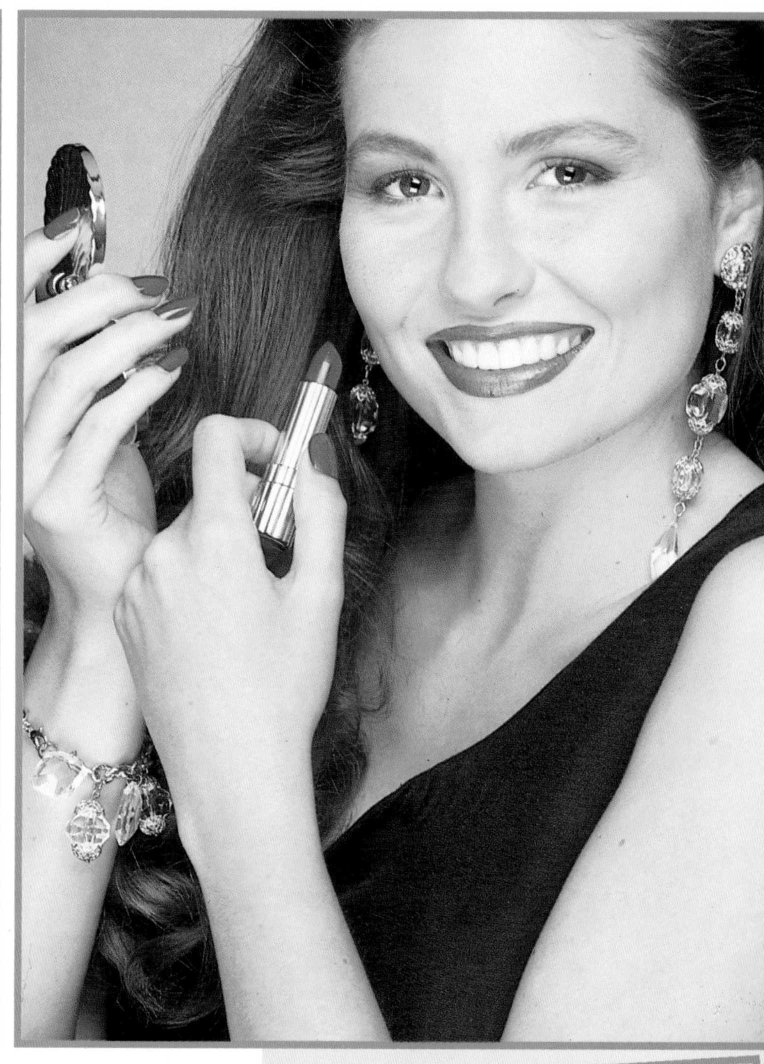

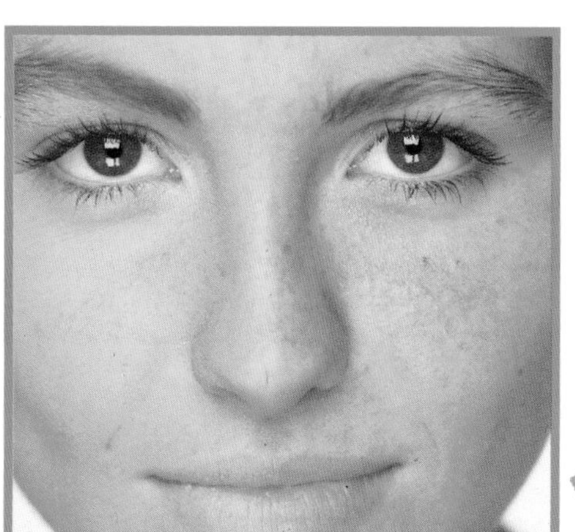

Disguise under-eye shadows and blemishes with a concealer and then dot foundation on to your face and blend it quickly in downward strokes with a slightly damp cosmetic sponge. Pat on a translucent powder with a velour pad, and dust off the excess with a big brush to 'set' your base.

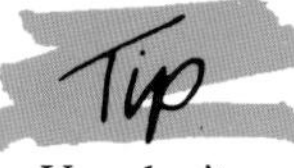

You don't want to end up with a green or purple face, so blend in colour correctives well!

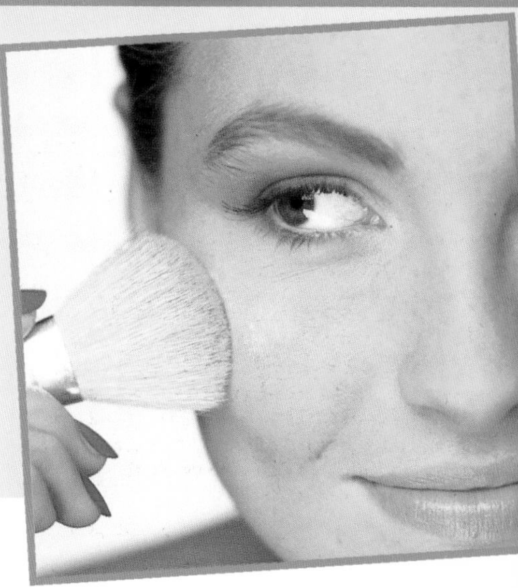

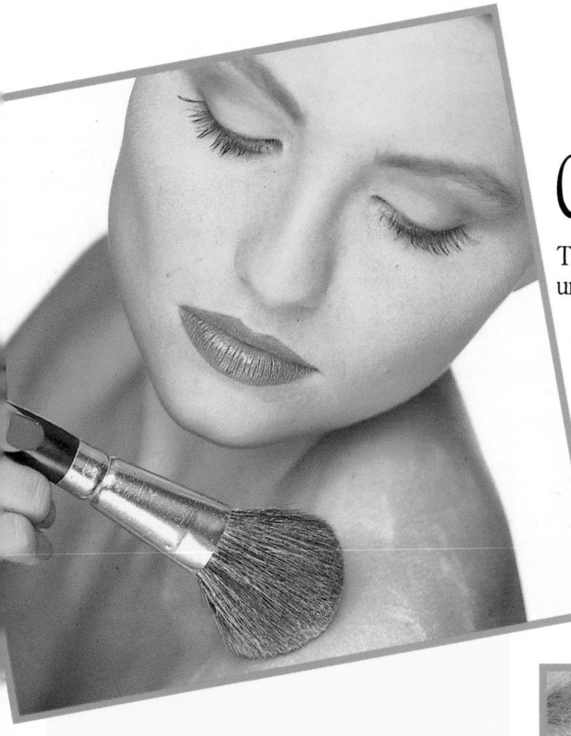

CAT'S EYES

The most gorgeous eyes are subtle and understated – not brightly coloured and loud!

To create mysterious cat's eyes – make an exaggerated 'V' shape with your shadow at the outer corner of your eye. Brush on your shadow to the socket line only in two flattering combinations. Draw a line of eyeliner close to your eyelashes and blend colour outwards and upwards into a sideways 'V' shape. For extra depth use a sponge-tipped applicator. To add that final flash, stick on individual false eyelashes at the outer corner of each eye. Gently pick a single lash up with some tweezers. Put a blob of glue on base of the lash and attach close to the lash line.

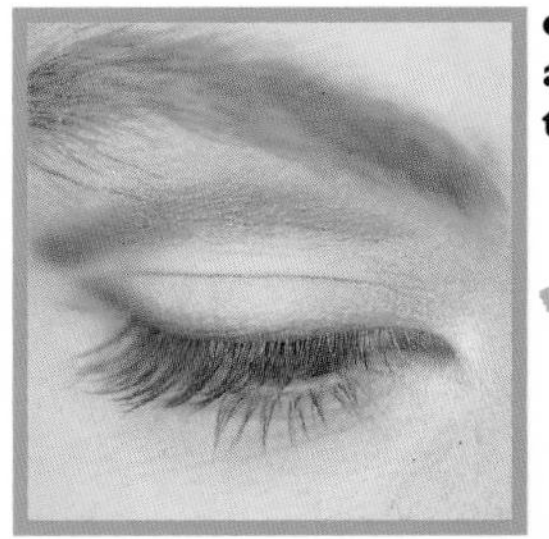

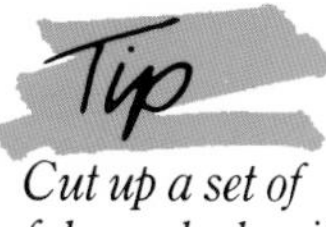

Cut up a set of false eyelashes if you can't buy single ones.

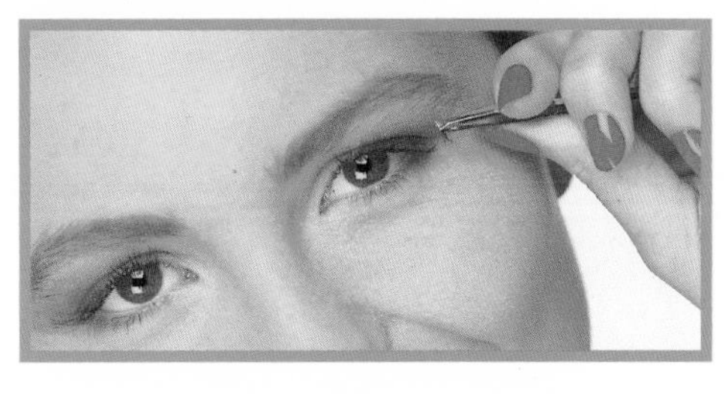

BE SOMEBODY

The most glamorous women look good all over. So don't spoil your image by spending all your time on your face and neglecting the rest of your body. Make sure the colour of your face is more or less the same as the skin on your neck, back and shoulders – especially if you wear clothes that show them off.

Dust your neck, chest and shoulders with translucent powder as you would your face. This will give you an all over flawless finish. If you've got a tan, use bronzing powder instead of a translucent one.

Tip

Exfoliate (scrub off dead skin cells using an abrasive product) once a week to keep your skin in peak condition and to make a super smooth base for your make-up.

POWDER POWER

Obvious stripes of blusher on both sides of your face is a definite no-no. Use colour on your cheeks sparingly and just dust it gently over the widest area with a soft fat brush building up the intensity gradually.

A real glamour trick is to apply a highlighter (try using a matt white eyeshadow or buy a special white cosmetic highlighter) above your cheekbones and just below your eyes. (But use the colour very sparingly – you don't want to look like a corpse.) This will highlight your cheekbones and give your skin a beautiful luminous glow.

TALON TRICKS

Chewed up nails and chipped-off nail varnish? Hands are on show just as much as your face so it's worth spending a bit of time on them.

If your nails are in a very bad state, cheat and stick on falsies! But don't just use them as they come out of the box. Cut and file them down to a reasonable length – you don't want three-inch talons, you just want your hands to look well groomed.

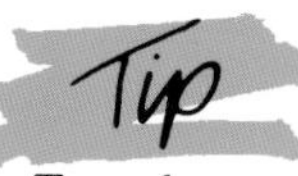

To make your own nails look longer, paint colour down the centre, leaving a small area on each side free from colour..

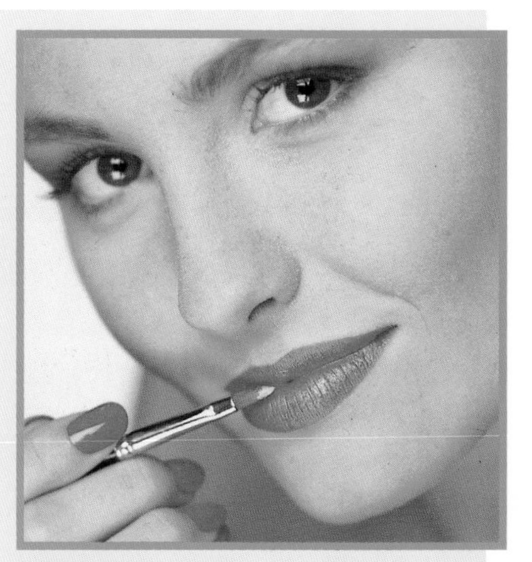

TWIST 'N' POUT

If you usually slap your lipstick on straight out of the tube when you're on the bus don't! Take time to get a good bold outline. Take the pencil line just outside your natural lip shape if lips are thin.

Use a lip brush to apply lip colour. Blot with a tissue and reapply. For true glamour, go for the richest red for a big, bold, kissable mouth.

A really quick but effective tip is to put a bit of gold lipstick onto the centre of your lower lip. This will highlight your bottom lip and make your pout particularly eye-catching! Don't be tempted to put on tons of lip gloss – it'll just make your lips greasy and increase the risk of smudging.

If you use a lipliner pencil – make sure it matches your lip colour. Nothing looks worse than a brown outline with lips filled in with pink or red lipstick.

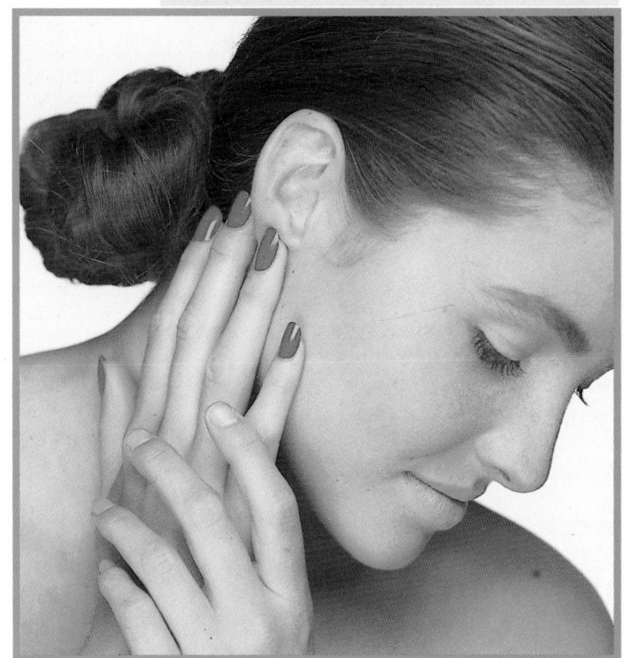

Photographs: IAN HOOTON/Hair and make-up: JO GILLINGWATER/Dress and jewellery: OASIS

IN THE PINK

From palest pastel to magnificent magenta, pink is the colour to be seen in. Mix it with your favourite shades or wear it alone. Follow our brilliant brush strokes for a fabulous day into night face

BEFORE
Cleanse, tone and moisturise, then let your skin settle.

Pink has always been a firm make-up favourite for eyes, cheeks, lips and nails. It looks great and is so versatile that many products can double-up so you don't have to carry loads of jars around!

Even if you're not a 'pink' person, a flash of pink eyeshadow or lipstick will liven up your looks.

And it's easy to build up the colour and change your daytime make-up in seconds so you'll be ready for a night out. Just add a touch more radiant raspberry or a stroke of fantastic fuchsia, and you've really got no excuse for not looking pretty in pink!

FUCHSIA PERFECT

- Find a moisturiser from the same cosmetic range as your foundation. The two are designed to work together.
- To get your foundation exactly the right shade to match your skin tone, buy two bottles – one to match winter pallor and the other to match a summer tan. Mix both shades to get the right colour for all year round.
- Pink eyeshadow tends to highlight blemishes, ruddy complexions and broken veins. The 'bluey' tints in some pinks will also emphasise bags under the eyes. If this is the case, use pink sparingly.

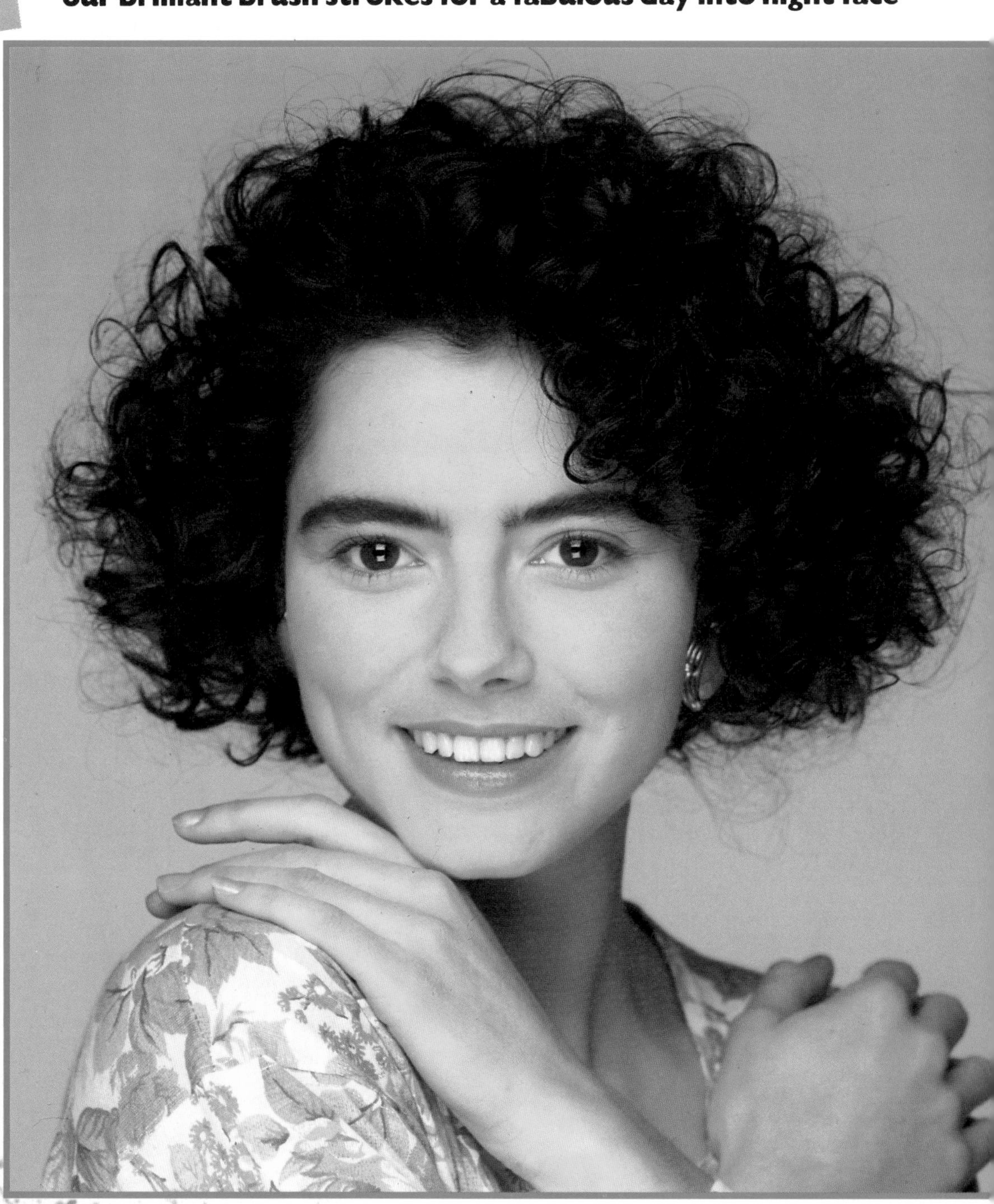

Photographs: IAN HOOTON/Hair and make-up: KIZZY HARRISON/Blouse: TOP SHOP/Earrings: MONET/Jacket: FREEMANS/Earrings: ADRIEN MANN

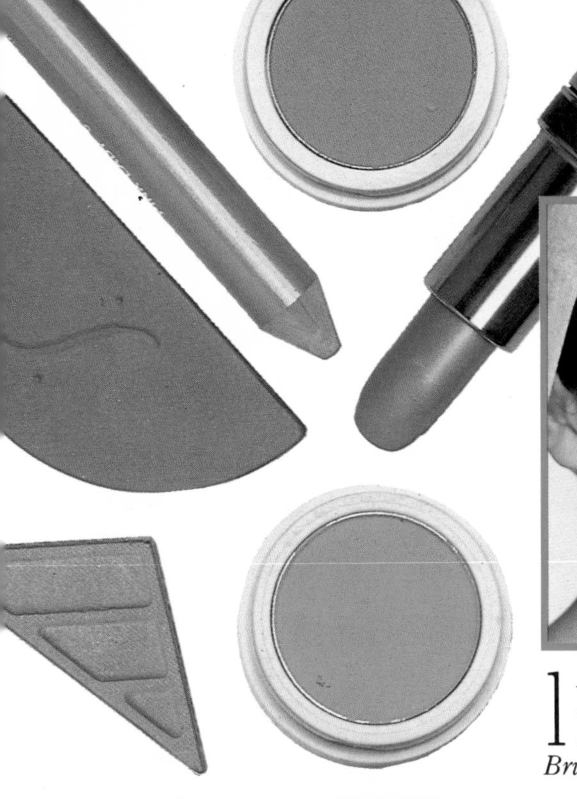

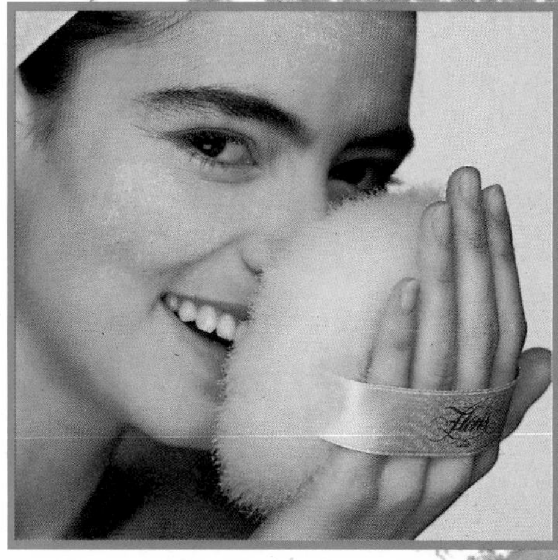

1 Dot on foundation and blend it with a damp cosmetic sponge. Use a matt formula for daytime and cover your eyelids and lips. Brush concealer over blemishes.

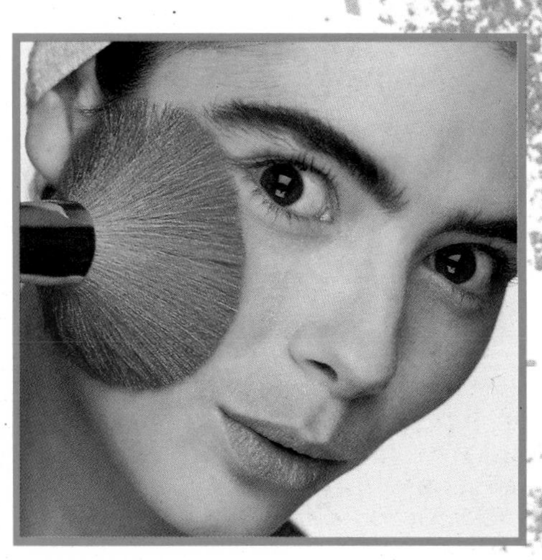

2 Dust on translucent powder with a velour or big fluffy powder puff and whisk off the excess with a soft brush.

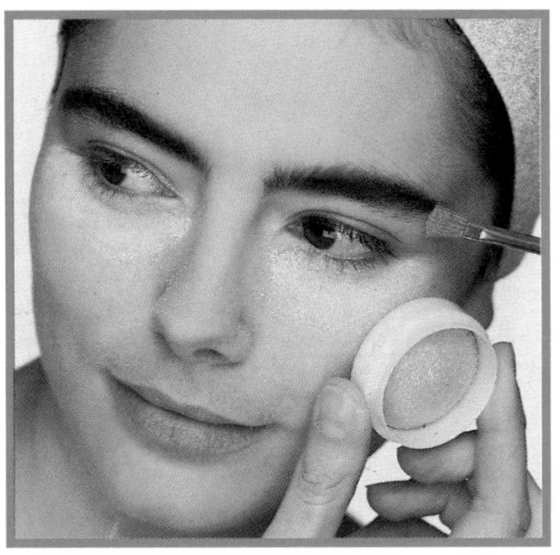

3 Pat plenty of powder under your eyes before putting on eyeshadow to collect any loose particles. Next, brush on a pale pink shadow over the whole of your eyelid.

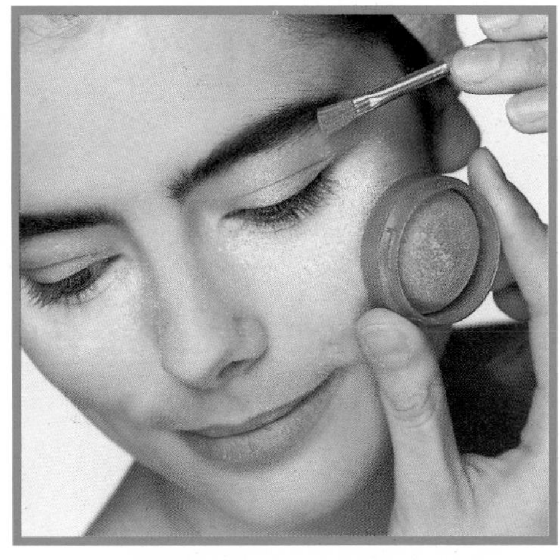

4 Stroke a dark rose pink shadow onto your browbone. Blend it well using a soft flat-edged brush. Brush a coat of colourless mascara on to lashes.

5 Flick off the powder from under your eyes with a fat soft brush using gentle strokes so you don't remove your foundation. Sweep blusher over the fullest part of your cheeks.

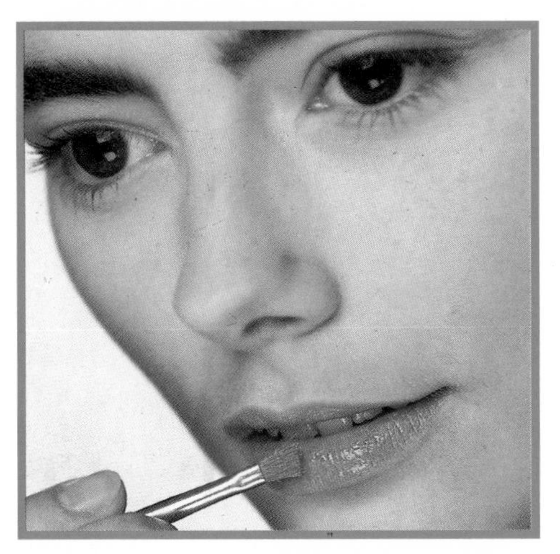

6 Brush soft pink lipstick to the edges of lips, fill in, then blot with a tissue and put on a second coat. If you have thin lips, draw an outline just outside your lips with lip liner.

PINK PEEPERS

Pale pink eyeshadow looks great with dark pink but there are plenty of really great colour combinations. Try our selection or experiment and discover your own.

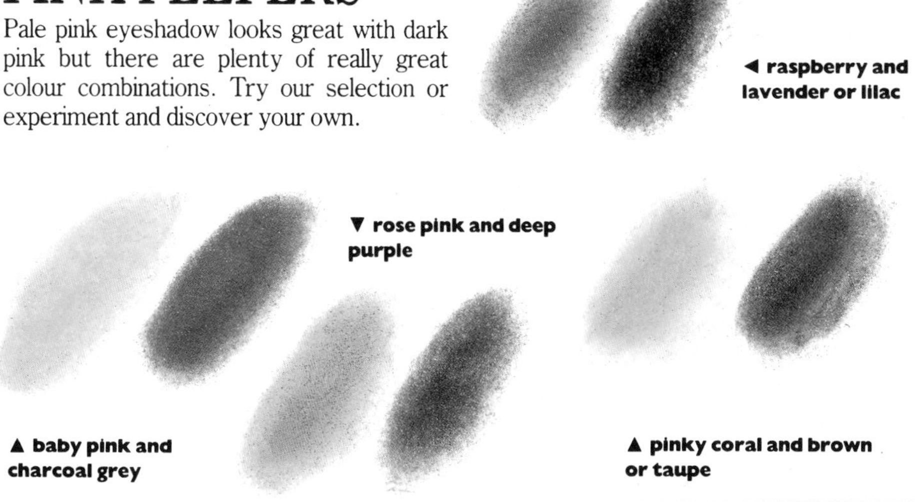

◄ **raspberry and lavender or lilac**

▼ **rose pink and deep purple**

▲ **baby pink and charcoal grey**

▲ **pinky coral and brown or taupe**

JOIN THE NIGHT CLUB

For an evening out, fix your face in a flash with this great 'going out' look.

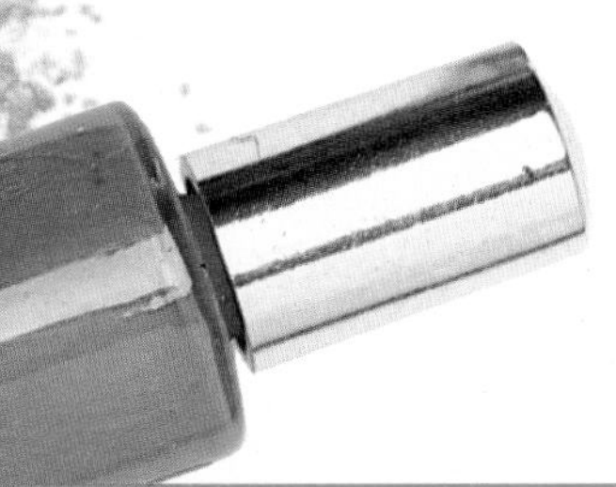

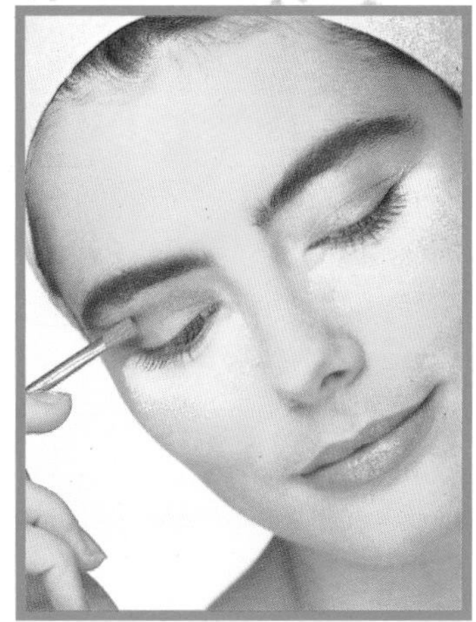

1 *Use a tissue to mop up oils, then dust translucent powder under your eyes. Brush plum pink into your socket line.*

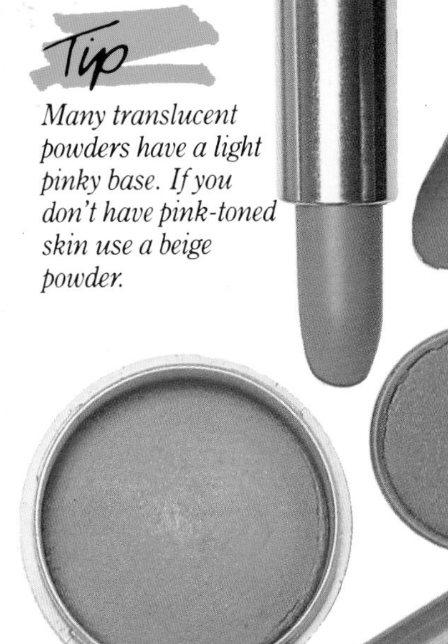

Tip

Many translucent powders have a light pinky base. If you don't have pink-toned skin use a beige powder.

Tip

Mix a pink blusher with white face powder for a natural glow. Then use a damp cotton bud to draw a smudgy plum eye line to match.

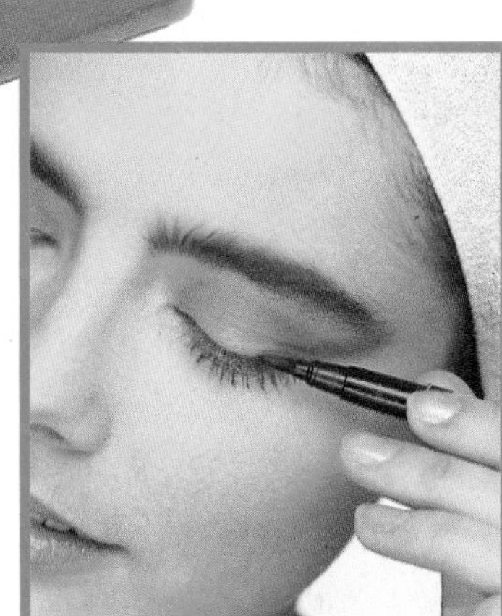

2 *Dust off the powder under eyes. Half-close your eye and draw black eyeliner from the inner corner outwards, close to the lashes.*

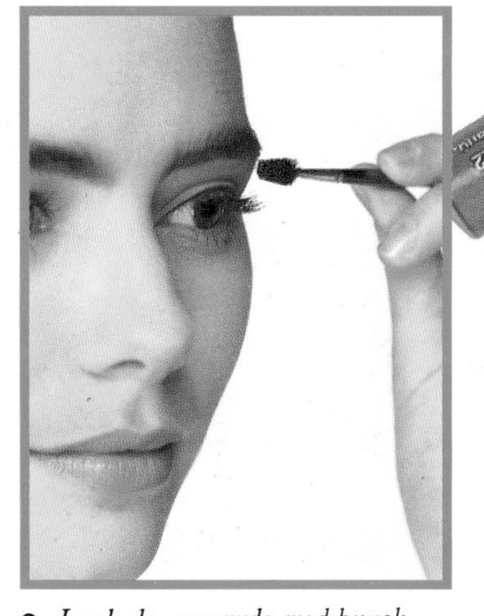

3 *Look downwards and brush black mascara on your top and bottom lashes. Use a clean mascara brush to separate the lashes.*

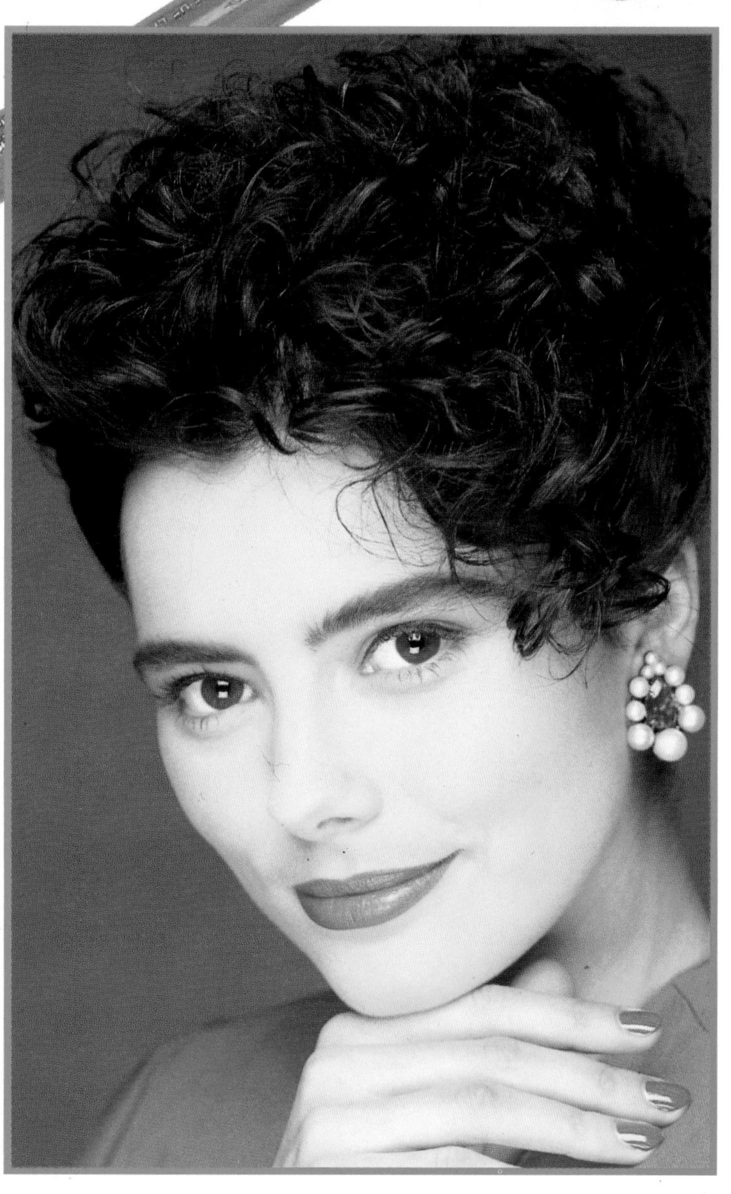

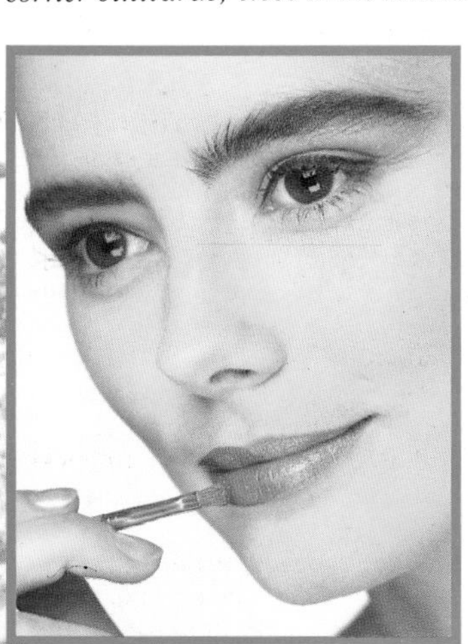

4 *Choose a bright pink lipstick (magenta or fuchsia) for the evening. Brush it on, checking the outline as you go.*

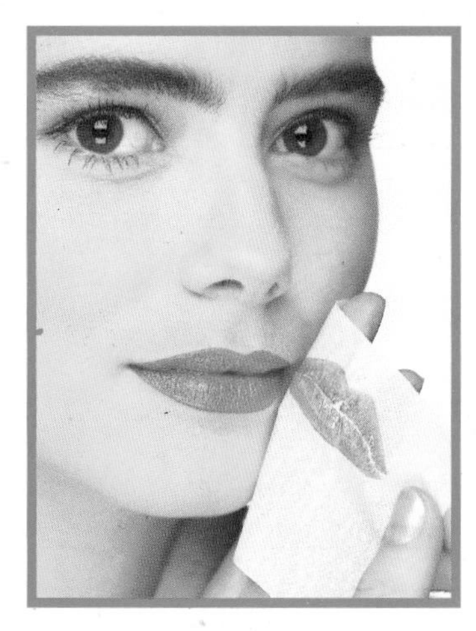

5 *Press a tissue over your mouth. Rub your finger gently across the tissue to blot excess. Re-apply for a dazzling pout.*

DARK SECRETS

Revealed, in all their glory – the tricks of the trade for making olive and black skins glow by day and positively sparkle after dark!

THE LOOK!

Create the subtle day faces (left) in soft, muted tones of brown and red.

1 Dot on foundation. We've chosen deep chocolate and warm caramel. Blend in with a sponge, easing colour around your nose and jawline.
2 Dust on matching powder and whisk off the excess.
3 Sweep a caramel blusher on the widest part of your cheeks and towards hairline.
4 Use a deep brown shadow on a blending brush to shade each eyelid, starting close to the lashes and ending at the socket line.
5 Highlight the brow area with cream shadow, taking colour up to the brow. Soften with your fingertip.
6 Use a dark kohl pencil to line the inside lower lid. Then draw a line just under the lower lashes, extending the colour at the corner, and smudge.
7 Line your lips with a pencil one shade lighter than your lipstick, then fill in with a brick red shade.

DELICIOUSLY DUSKY

SKIN SAVVY Asian skin retains moisture and feels soft and supple but tends to show dark circles around the eyes. Regular massage can help ease the problem – invest in a good eye cream and smooth on gently in the outer corner of the eyes, working in a circle towards the inner corner. Also, exfoliate your skin regularly with a facial scrub to prevent a build-up of dead skin and dull, dingy patches.

FIRST BASE: Whether it's deep olive or pale creamy beige, most Asian skin has yellow undertones which can make it look sallow.

● Choose a foundation with a hint of pink to warm up the complexion. Match it to the darkest part of your face. Light liquid formulations have better blending power. Use a damp sponge to smooth over the colour.

● Disguise dark circles with a concealer – use just a touch underneath your base, put on with a fine brush.

● Foundation shades you should go for are: taupe, sepia, caramel, mink brown. Fix base with a matt powder. Make sure you use a powder in a shade to match your skin. Too pale a powder will leave a dusty, floury look on your complexion. Even some sheer, translucent powders can have this effect.

EYES RIGHT Accentuate your almond eyes with soft and shimmering shades. Go for golden yellow, mustard, sage green, khaki and bronze.

● Shine out in soft pink, lilac and wine shades for eyes after dark, and outline them with black liquid liner or kohl pencil for a really enticing look.

● Make the most of thick lashes by curling them first then applying two coats of black mascara.

● Your eyebrows may be fairly thick and dark, but don't pluck them into a thin line – just tidy up the odd, straggly hair and comb them.

PERFECT BLUSH Soft browns and terracotta will look most natural but rose pinks and plums will give extra warmth.

LUSCIOUS LIPS Extra glossy shades look stunning. Try brown and rust shades for day and go all out for glamour with very bright colours such as fiery red and fuchsia pink tones for night.

EXOTICALLY EASTERN

SKIN SAVVY Oriental skin tends to be problem-free, usually with smooth even pigmentation. Wider cheekbones also mean that oriental-shaped faces wrinkle less quickly, too! Keep skin flawless with a regular routine. Cream away make-up and grime with a light cleanser, then use a mild toner to help close the pores. Smooth on a moisturiser under your base.

FIRST BASE Your skin will have a blue or yellow undertone – check which yours is by holding your hand up against a white card. Once you've decided, test foundations along your jawline to make the best match. Aim for matt, neutral shades rather than pink or yellow tones.

● If your skin is very good, skip the base and move straight on to colour. Use a very pale concealer to disguise any blemishes. Look out for a white colour corrective base which will fade out an uneven skin tone.

● Foundation shades to go for: olive, light beige, ivory, cream.

● A very light translucent powder or even white powder will enhance your natural skin tone. Fluff on with a soft brush.

EYES RIGHT Small eyelids need careful colouring to accentuate shape. Use a highlighter on the brow bone to open up the eyes.

● Try stunning monochrome tones of black or deep grey to emphasise your eye shape or pastel tones of pink, blue and green. Or for a super natural effect, go for 'skin tones' like gold and brown.

● Frosted shadows look great.

● Colour your top lashes only with black or charcoal-grey mascara to widen the eyes.

PERFECT BLUSH Shade those cheekbones with just a touch of blusher. Choose a shade with red or pink undertones.

LUSCIOUS LIPS Try burnt orange and chestnut or play it up in pink or red.

LITTLE GEMS

Pick the right colours to make the most of your skintone.

● Very dark and blue/black skins look fabulous in white clothes. Add sheen to your skin with a light body oil.

● Olive and yellow-based skins can look muddy in earthy tones. Try contrasting blue-based pinks and mauves.

● Accentuate ebony skin with dramatic red and black – keep your make-up simple but gloss lips a brilliant red.

● Silver sings out against a black skin – try two or more chunky, linked necklaces.

● Olive-toned skins look good in gold – choose bolder shapes that stand out.

● Dark skin sparkles at night in crystal and diamanté. Wear long drop earrings or a shimmering pendant.

● Warmer skin looks super-natural in polished wooden beads, amber gem stones and twisted coral.

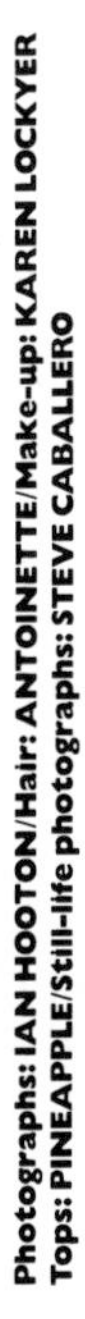

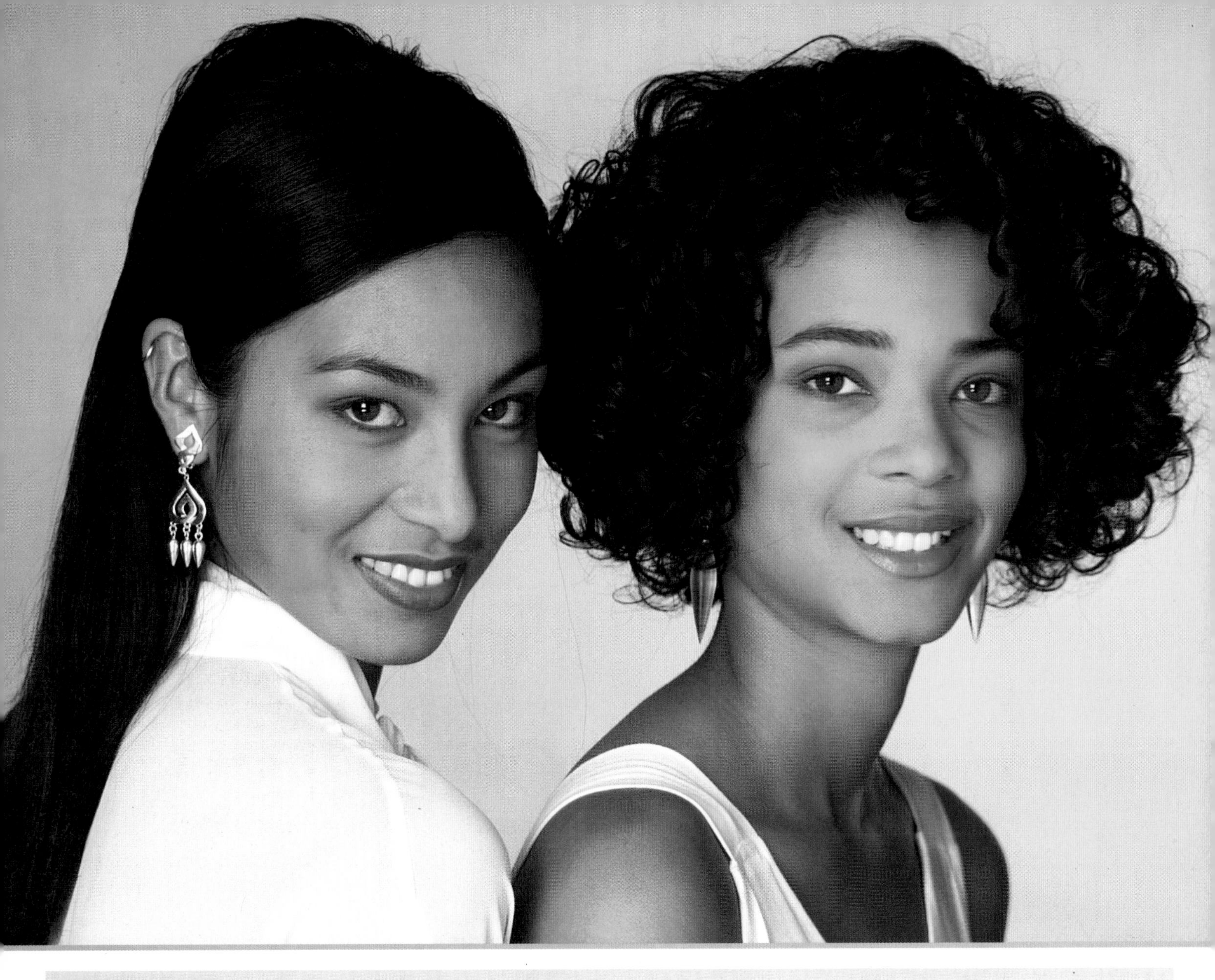

DRAMATICALLY DARK

Finding the make-up shades that work for you takes time since dark skin-tones can vary from olive to caramel, brown to black. But once you've made the perfect match the end results can be quite sensational. Read our guide and then have fun experimenting to create your own individual look.

SKIN SAVVY Black skin has more pigment than pale skin and is naturally thicker and less prone to ageing. It's this strong barrier that helps retain moisture and filter out damaging sunlight. But be careful in cold weather as it can dry out the skin and give it a dusty grey look. Swap to gentle, creamy cleansers and no-soap facial bars which help protect your skin's natural acid balance, then smooth on a light moisturiser underneath your make-up.

FIRST BASE There are at least 38 different shades of deeper-than-white skins (compared to six white shades) which are based on red, blue, grey or yellow undertones. Most conventional foundations are too red or chalky for dark skins – so pick a product that's specially designed for your skin type.

- Test the shade on the outer part of your face where colour is darker, the centre panel is naturally lighter and you can end up with a blotchy look if you colour-match to this area.
- Disguise uneven pigmentation – particularly under the eyes – with a heavy-duty concealer in the shade closest to your skin colour.
- Water-based foundations, rather than oil-based ones, work best on dark skins since the skin tends to have more open pores.
- Foundation shades to go for: deep chocolate, hazelnut brown, golden brown, tan, coffee and beige. To reduce shine, opt for tinted powder in sheer shades of bronze or rich brown.

EYES RIGHT Brown eyes can take a spectrum of colours. Try peach and deep brown, rust and bronze or plum for day.

- Emphasise your eye shape with a crayon in a contrasting colour, such as green or gold. Draw a line from the outer corner of the eye and under the lashes, then blend it in.
- Go for jewel-bright or primary colours for evening with lashings of black mascara.

PERFECT BLUSH Try burnt sugar, russet and amber shades that complement the skin's natural undertones. Avoid pinky-red, pink and orange tones unless your skin is very light.

LUSCIOUS LIPS Glossy colours can over emphasise a full mouth so stick to creamy matt shades.

- Try bright shades of coral, tangerine, nutty browns and aubergine. Steer clear of mauves – they can turn the skin blue.
- Try spicier shades for evening, like ginger and cinnamon.

THE COLOUR PURPLE

Purple suits everyone no matter what their colouring. So choose any shade from the lightest lavender to the deepest mauve – you'll be plum crazy if you don't!

PURPLE PARTNERS

Purple eyeshadow looks great when it's mixed with lighter or darker shades. Try it with a contrasting colour for something special. Choose either warm or cool tones in the other colours and you'll find they blend together more easily.

Try the following combinations: Cool purples – contrast with blue, grey, silver or taupe.

Warm purples – mix well with any shade of pink from the palest of baby pinks to fuchsia. Apricot, gold and bronze work well too.

But take care when mixing purple with yellow or green – you could look as if you've got two black eyes!

Watchpoint

Don't use purple blusher – it'll make your face look bruised.

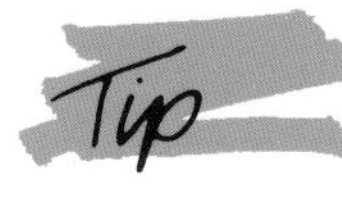

For something a bit different, try violet-coloured contact lenses. They are the ultimate accessory to purple eyeshadow!

PLUM FOR PURPLE!

Pick a purple palette to create stunning eyes, lips and nails for lasting good looks.

Stroke on heather and add matt mauve on the eye socket and under lower lashes.

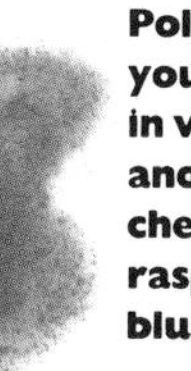

Polish up your nails in violet and get cheeky with raspberry blusher.

Intensely mauve lips can look OTT. Go for pinky-purples to complement your eye make-up.

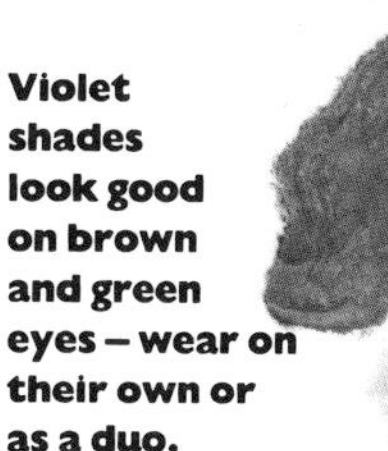

Violet shades look good on brown and green eyes – wear on their own or as a duo.

A pinky-lilac and lavender duo is great for day-time – create depth by moistening the shadows with a little water.

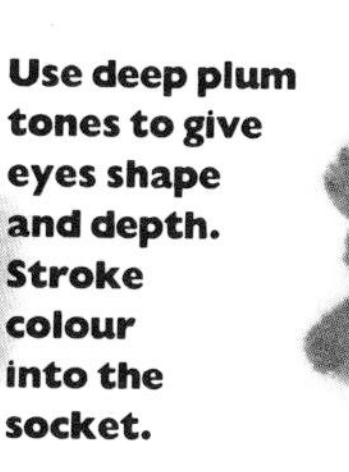

Use deep plum tones to give eyes shape and depth. Stroke colour into the socket.

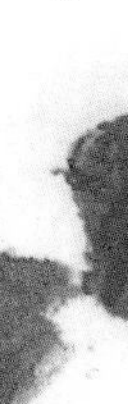

LIP SERVICE

Purple can be a difficult colour to wear on your lips – it'll make them look thinner than they really are. Wear a natural pink during the day, then jazz it up in the evening with a strong fuchsia or blood red. And if strong lipsticks aren't your style, a caramel or bronze shade will work as well.

Strong lip colours can bleed easily so condition your lips with a special lipstick fixing cream then pencil in the shape.

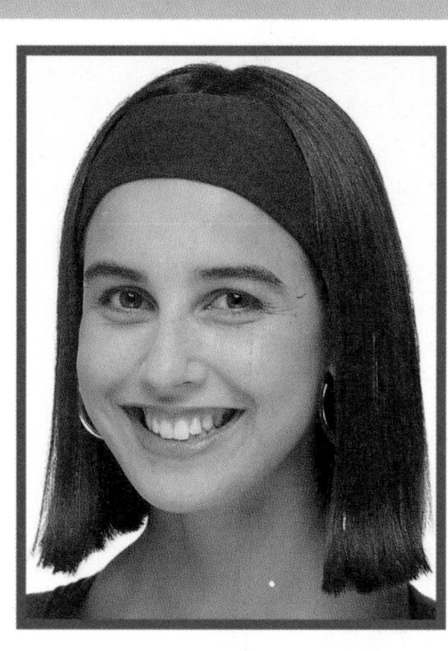

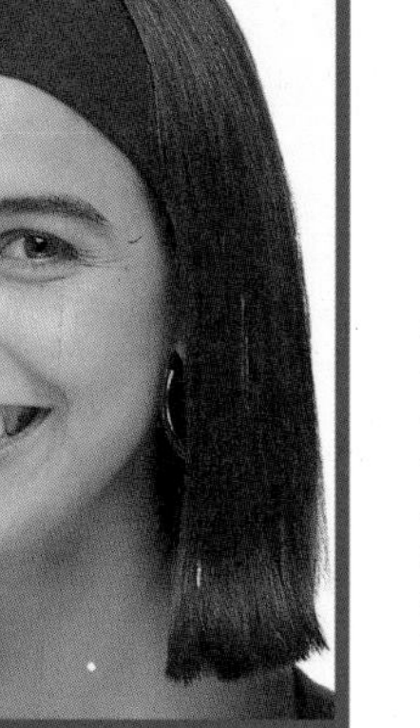

Photographs: JAMES HOBSLEY/Hair: PAULA MANN/Make-up: KIZZY HARRISON

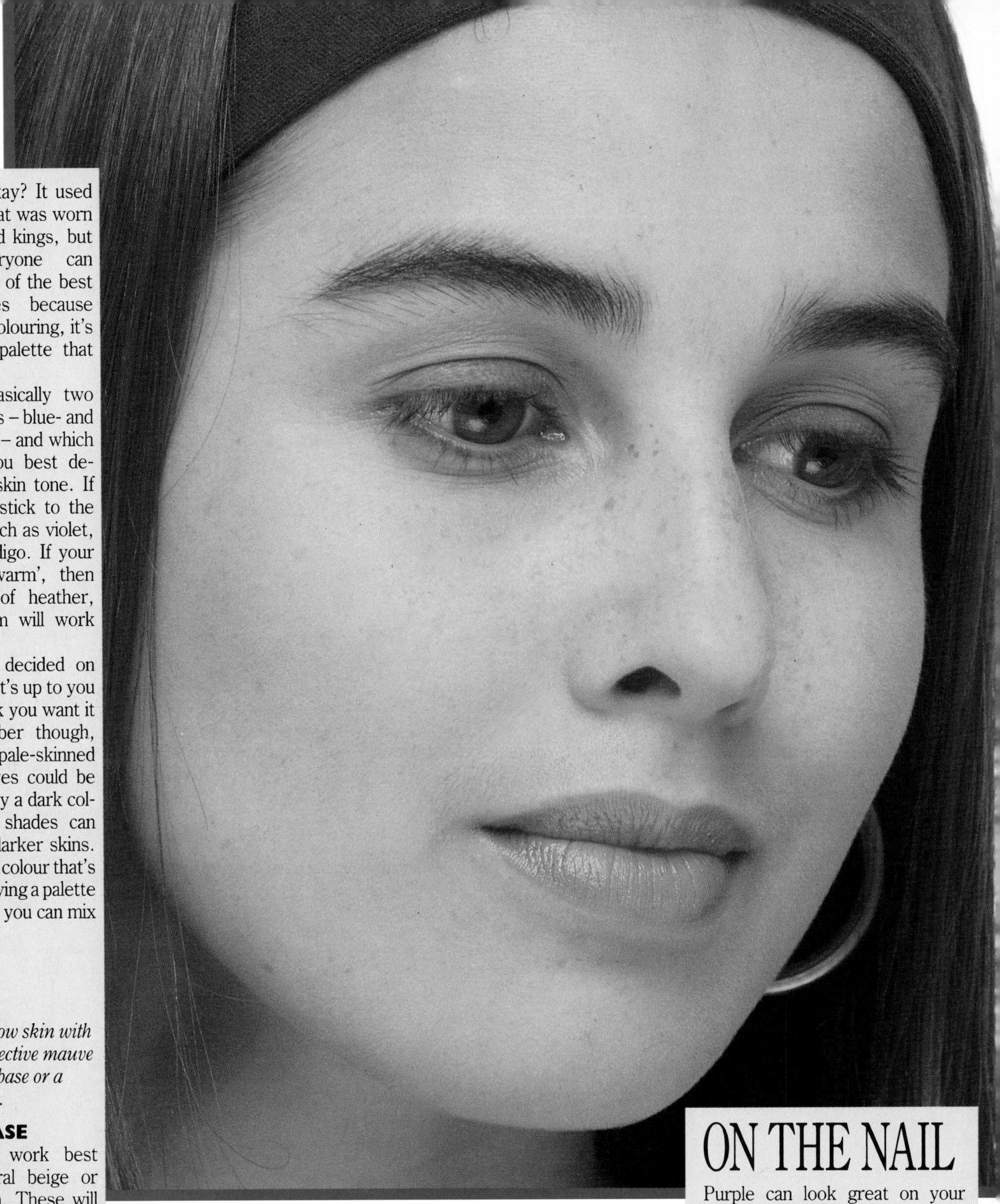

Purple reigns okay? It used to be a colour that was worn by emperors and kings, but nowadays everyone can wear it! It's one of the best make-up shades because whatever your colouring, it's easy to find a palette that suits you.

There are basically two groups of purples – blue- and pink-based ones – and which one will suit you best depends on your skin tone. If it's 'cool', then stick to the bluey purples such as violet, lavender and indigo. If your skin tone is 'warm', then pinker shades of heather, mauve and plum will work better.

Once you've decided on the shade, then it's up to you how light or dark you want it to be. Remember though, that if you're a pale-skinned blonde, your eyes could be overshadowed by a dark colour while light shades can look chalky on darker skins. If you can't find a colour that's just right, try buying a palette of purples which you can mix and match.

Tip

Brighten up sallow skin with the help of a corrective mauve cream make-up base or a lilac face powder.

BACK TO BASE

Purple shades work best against a neutral beige or ivory foundation. These will help to even out your skin tone and provide the perfect base on which to build your purple make-up. Always use a base first if your skin is very translucent or prone to broken veins since purple can emphasise these. Use concealer on under eye shadows for the same reasons. Also, opt for a colourless face powder rather than a rosy tinged one so that your skin tone doesn't clash with the rest of your purple make-up.

PURPLE PEEPERS

Practically every item of eye make-up is available in shades of purple. From eyeshadows to mascara, pencils to liner. Limit the purple to just one cosmetic if you don't want the effect to be overpowering. During the day, wear purple eyeshadow on its own and add a contrasting colour for the evening. Save sparkly shades till after dark too.

Give yourself purple peepers with a slick of a pencil across the top lids close to the lashes, then blend. Try plum-coloured mascara or violet liner for a touch of drama, or brush purple mascara on to lash tips.

ON THE NAIL

Purple can look great on your nails too. If your nails are short, choose a light shade that's not frosted. Long nails can get away with almost any shade so match it with your lipstick or go even darker. And if your nails aren't quite up to scratch, use an iridescent clear polish that'll flash purple under the light.

Tip

Paint on a base coat, then two layers of colour and top with clear varnish.

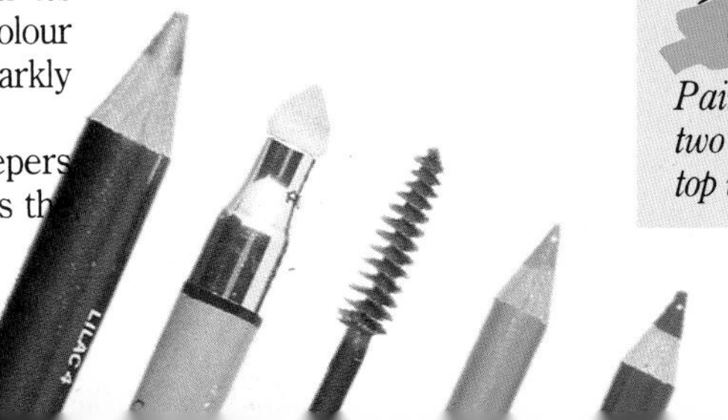

JEWEL PURPOSE

All that glitters is not gold – it could be sapphire, emerald or ruby. So dip into jewel-coloured make-up and sparkle!

It's that special night out. You've got the dress, you've got the jewellery but now you're wondering what you can do to make your face that extra bit special too.

You want something that's dramatic enough to make you stand out from the crowd but you also want to look stunningly beautiful.

This is the time to wear jewel colours. Rich, deep, strong colours like sapphire, amethyst and emerald or semi-precious stone colours like turquoise, coral and jade. All these look just as good used on your face as they do around your neck.

BE BOLD!

Many people are scared of wearing strong make-up colours because they've tried it once and thought it looked too much. You *do* need to be bold since these colours demand attention. But the secret is to keep it simple. Pick out one colour and let it dominate, keeping the rest of your make-up low key. Too many strong colours and your make-up will end up looking overdone.

PUTTING ON THE GLITZ

To find make-up that really looks like the colour of jewels you'll have to look for shades that shimmer. Matt colours, no matter how closely they match the colour of the jewel, just won't look right because they lack sparkle. Look for loose powders or cream eyeshadows since these are generally more sparkly than pressed powders.

FIRM FOUNDATIONS

With any strong make-up, and especially with the glittery colours, you need a base that's smooth and matt, and unless you have perfect skin (let's face it, few of us have), that means wearing foundation. Don't try to cover heavily with the foundation though – keep it sheer and dot concealer on any blemishes. Then powder well all over.

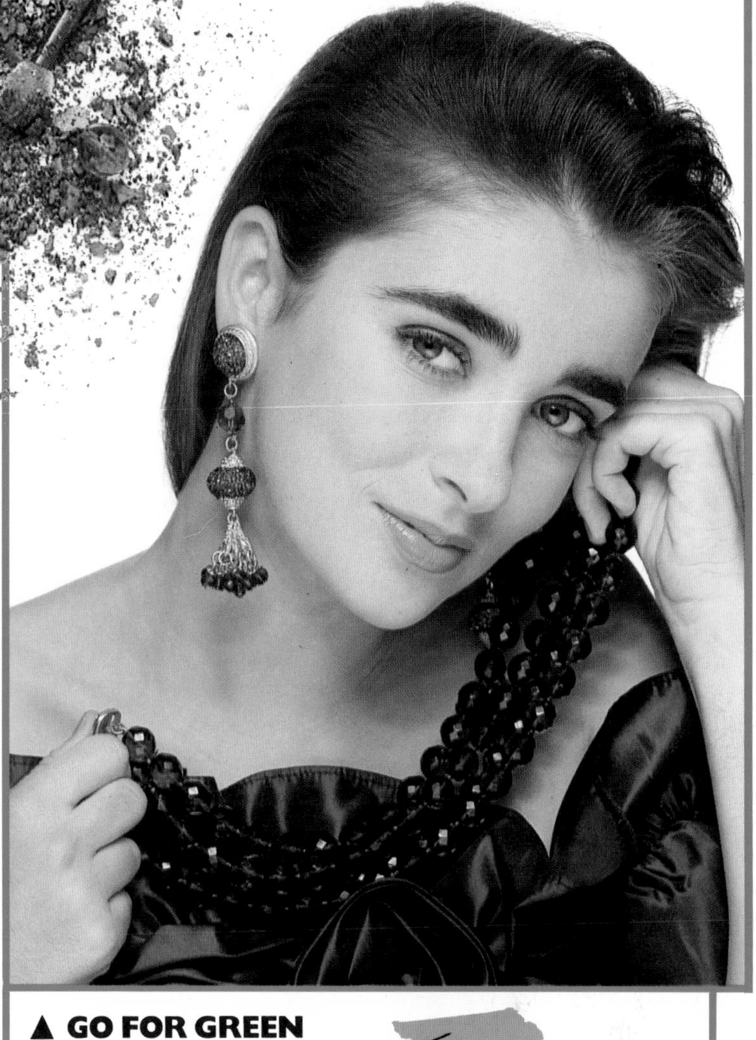

▲ GO FOR GREEN
Match your eyes to the colour of emeralds and watch your friends turn green with envy!

Choose a pale pink or caramel colour for understated lips.

SPARKLING EYES

If you've chosen a jewel colour for your eyes, keep the shape simple. A bold stroke of colour across the eyelid will have more impact than eyeshadow that's blended and shaded too much. Tap the excess powder off the brush so you don't end up with it everywhere, or try dampening your brush and then putting on your eyeshadow. Taking the colour under your eyes will be too overpowering so just line underneath with a soft pencil. Then frame the colour with dark lashes, well-shaped brows and use a muted, not bright, shade of lipstick.

LIP SHINE

Alternatively, focus on lips rather than your eyes. For lots of kiss appeal, lips should be shiny rather than matt. Choose a shade that contains glints of gold, or add your own with a touch of gold eyeshadow. Try putting your lipstick on first before making up your eyes and take time to get the shape right. Then use the softest of eyeshadows and outline your eyes with a dark liner which will balance lips.

Keep blusher to a mere hint – you don't want to look garish.

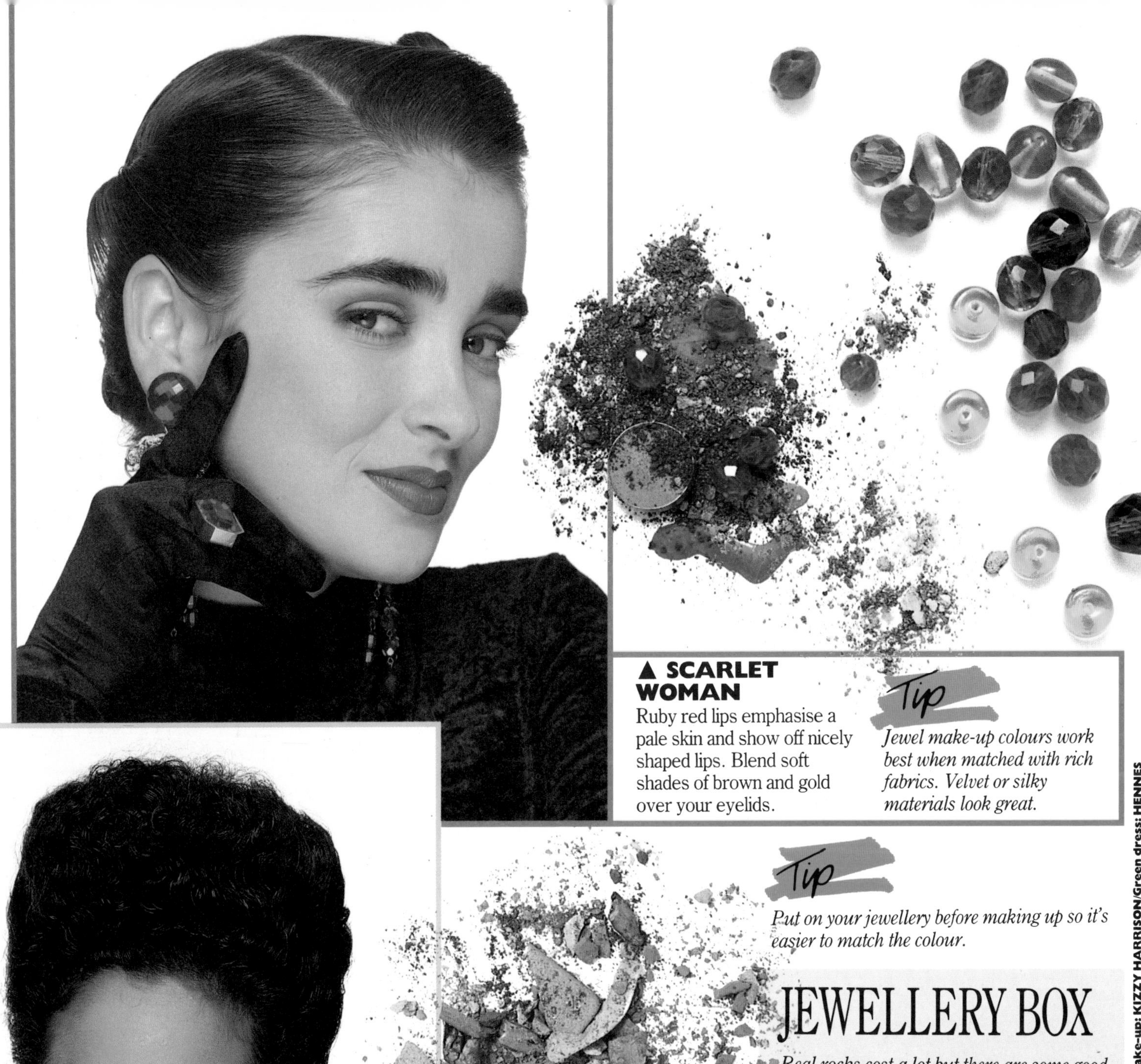

▲ SCARLET WOMAN
Ruby red lips emphasise a pale skin and show off nicely shaped lips. Blend soft shades of brown and gold over your eyelids.

Tip

Jewel make-up colours work best when matched with rich fabrics. Velvet or silky materials look great.

Tip

Put on your jewellery before making up so it's easier to match the colour.

JEWELLERY BOX

Real rocks cost a lot but there are some good fakes around so who's worrying! Match the stones to get your colour.

RUBY	**Deep red**
AMETHYST	**Purple**
EMERALD	**Green**
SAPPHIRE	**Light to deep blue**
TOPAZ	**Dark yellow**
TIGER'S EYE	**Brown**
HAEMATITE	**Metallic grey with red flashes**
PERIDOT	**Light green**
CORAL	**Pinky orange**
JADE	**Light opaque green**
LAPIS LAZULI	**Dark blue**
ONYX	**Black**
AQUAMARINE	**Blue/green**
AMBER	**Orangy yellow**
OPAL	**White with flashes of red/blue/green**
CORNELIAN	**Pink**
GARNET	**Dark red**

◄ TURQUOISE TO GO!
Brown eyes look great with a splash of turquoise across the lid. Set the look off with an amethyst shade of lip colour.

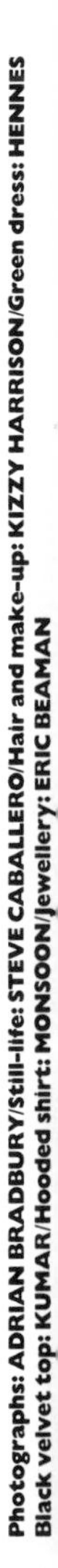

COLOUR STORY: GREEN

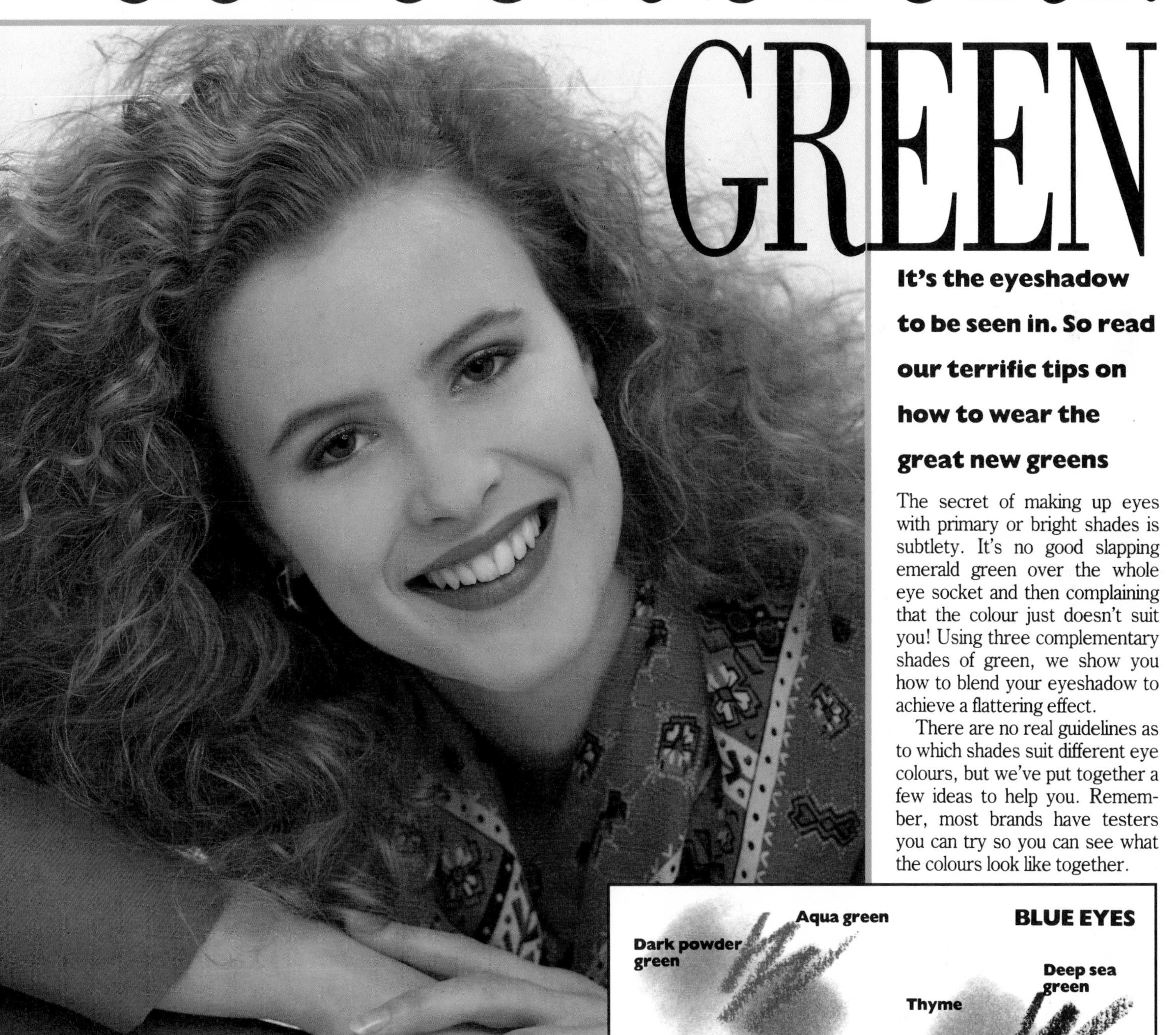

It's the eyeshadow to be seen in. So read our terrific tips on how to wear the great new greens

The secret of making up eyes with primary or bright shades is subtlety. It's no good slapping emerald green over the whole eye socket and then complaining that the colour just doesn't suit you! Using three complementary shades of green, we show you how to blend your eyeshadow to achieve a flattering effect.

There are no real guidelines as to which shades suit different eye colours, but we've put together a few ideas to help you. Remember, most brands have testers you can try so you can see what the colours look like together.

BLUE EYES

Dark powder green
Aqua green
Evening green

Thyme
Deep sea green
Smoky green

Dawn mist
Sage
Emerald

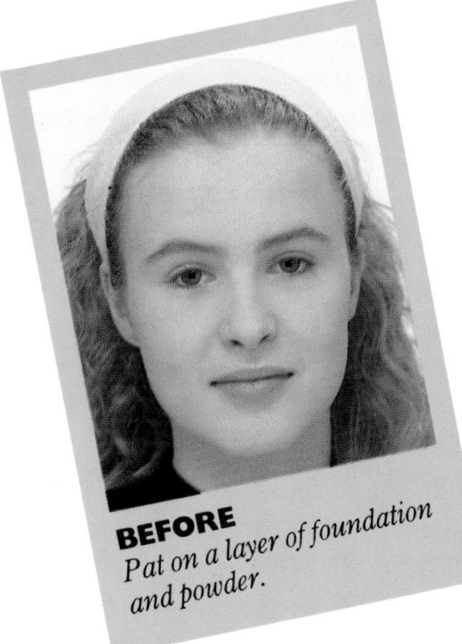
BEFORE
Pat on a layer of foundation and powder.

Make sure your hair is tied back away from your face before you start so that you have a clear view of all your features.

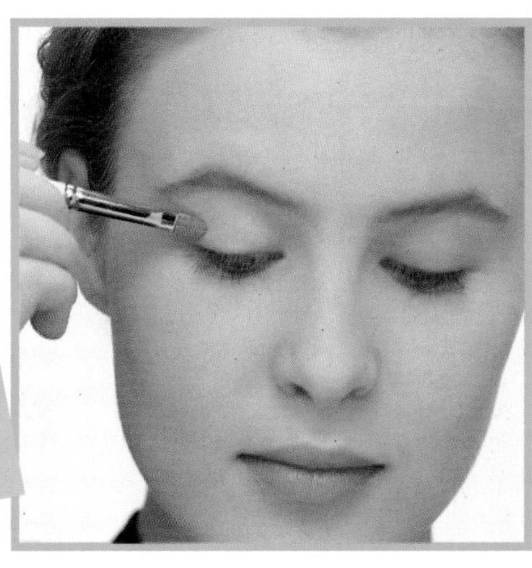

1 *Start with pale green shadow. Stroke it over your entire lid to make a base and add emphasis to darker colours.*

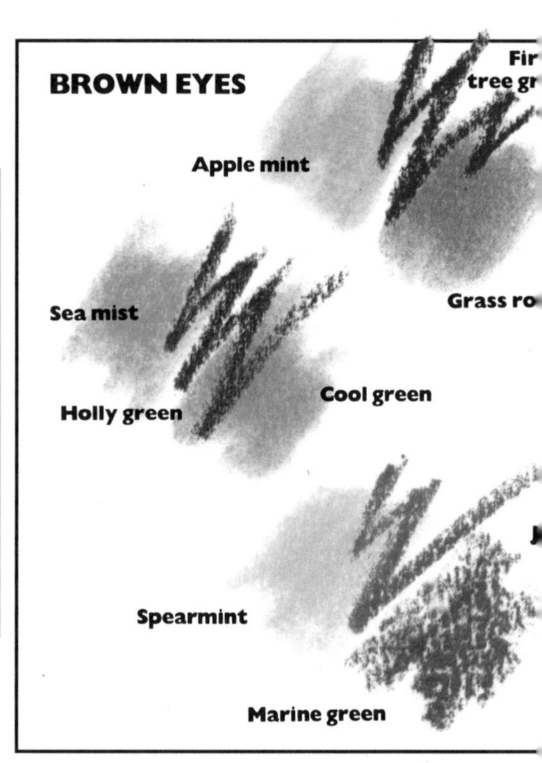

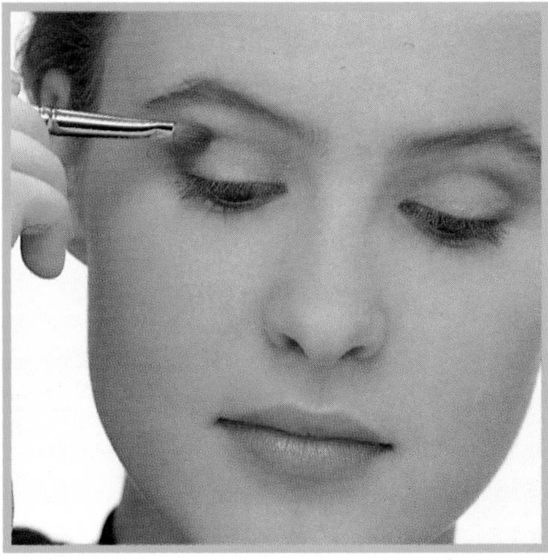

2 *Now define your eyes with a deeper shade of green. Stroke it along the socket line and into a wedge-shape at the outer corner. Then blend for a softer finish.*

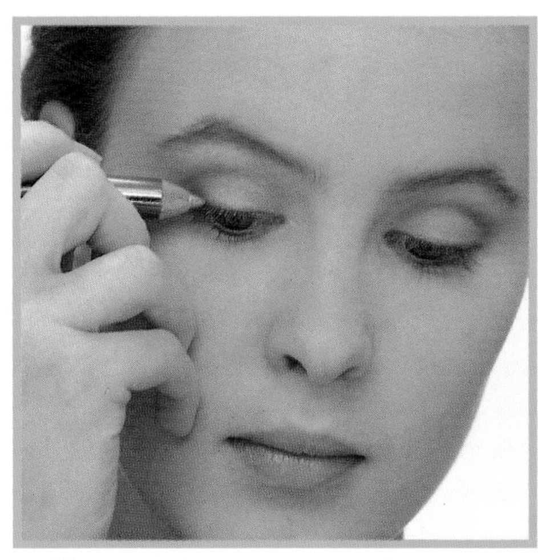

3 *Use a chunky eyeshadow pencil or crayon to draw a fine line along your upper lid close to your lashes.*

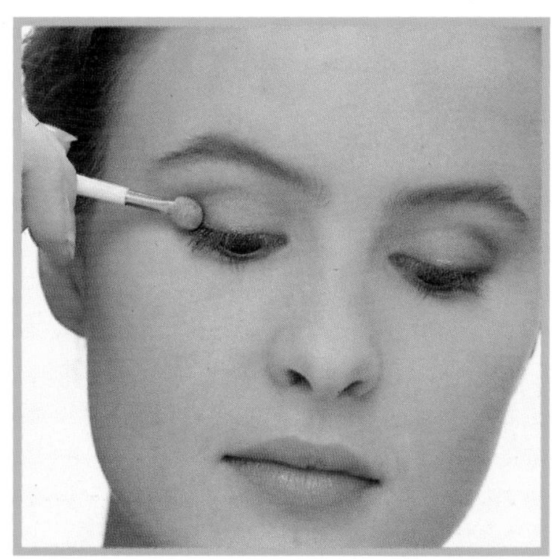

4 *To soften your eye liner and stop it from 'bleeding' off the eye, smooth a little dark green shadow over the top of the whole lid using a sponge-tipped applicator.*

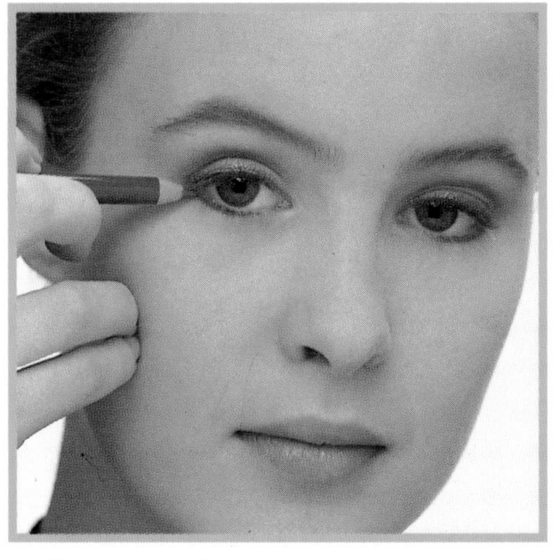

5 *Draw a pencil line underneath your lower lashes. Take the line from halfway along to the outer corner. Smudge with a cotton bud to stop it looking too harsh.*

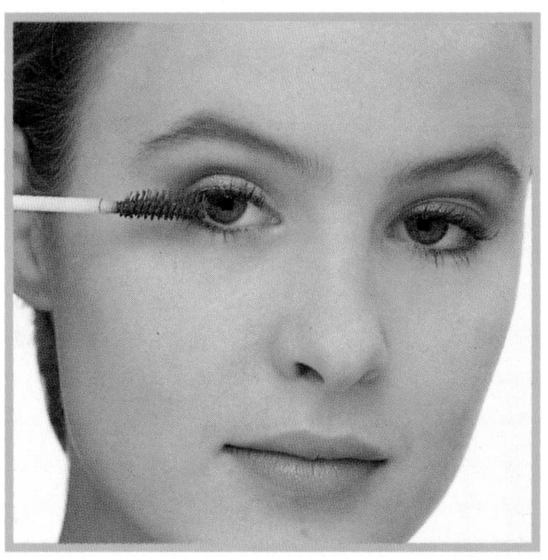

6 *Stroke mascara over and under your top and bottom lashes. Choose a shade of rich brown to complete the look.*

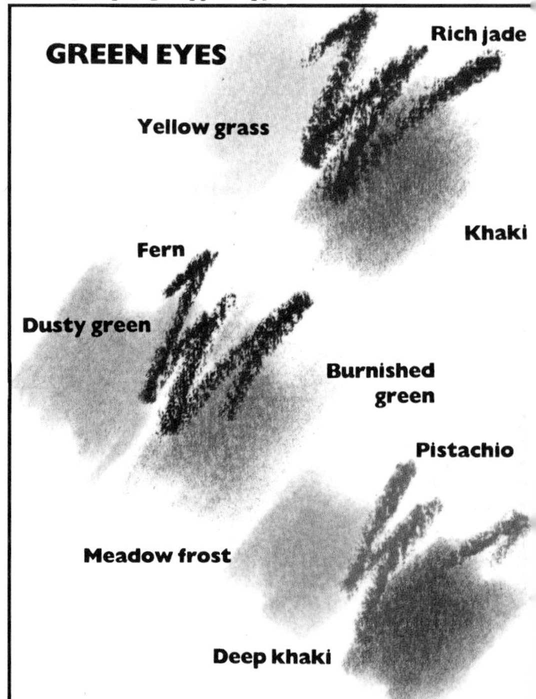

Photographs: ALISTAIR HUGHES/Hair and make-up: YA'NINA/Jacket: HOBBS/Scarf: NEXT/Earrings: MONET

TRICKS OF THE TRADE

Had a disaster with your make-up and there's only moments to go before the doorbell rings? Don't panic, we've conjured up some magic make-up tricks to fix your face in a flash!

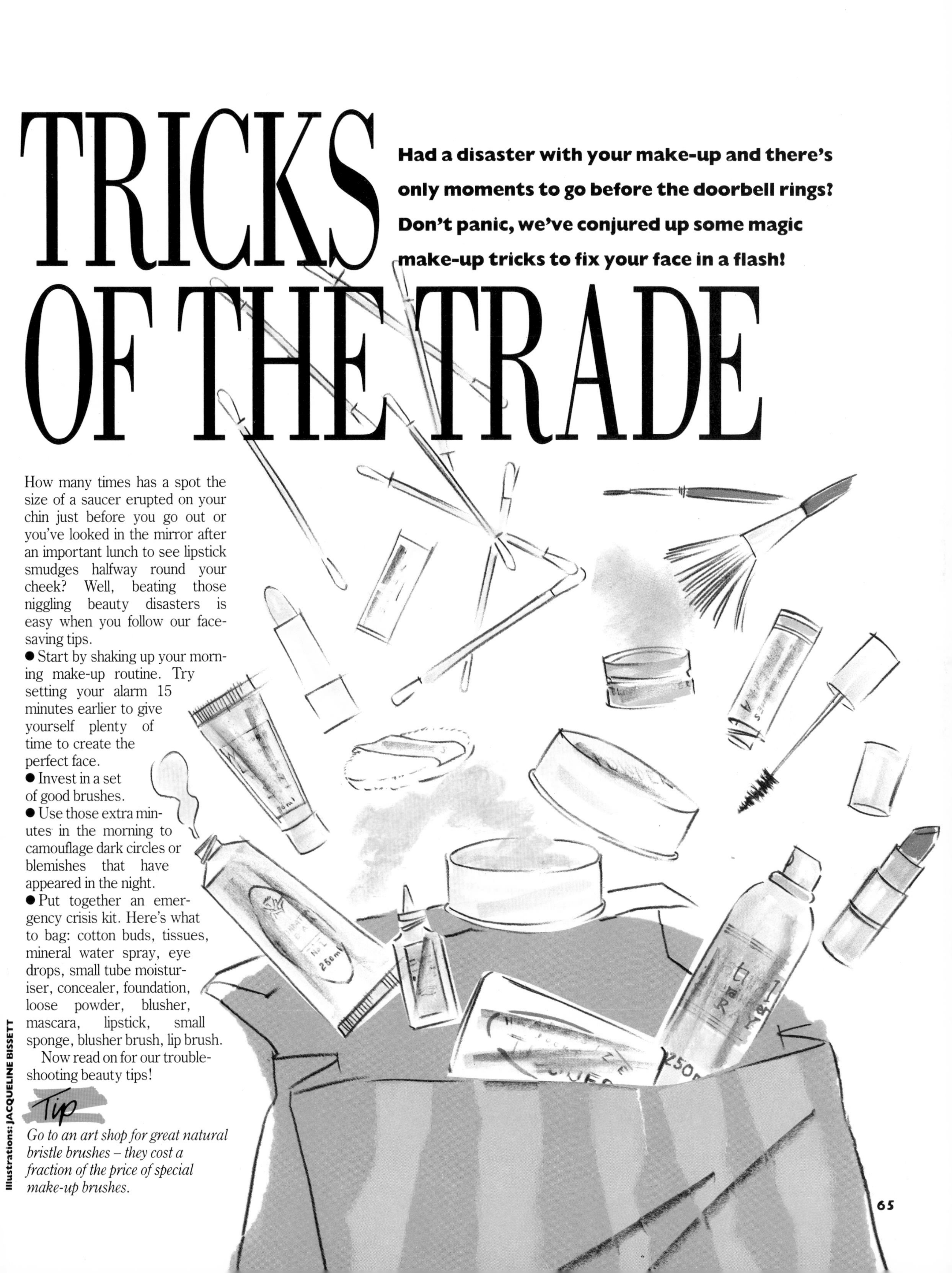

How many times has a spot the size of a saucer erupted on your chin just before you go out or you've looked in the mirror after an important lunch to see lipstick smudges halfway round your cheek? Well, beating those niggling beauty disasters is easy when you follow our face-saving tips.

- Start by shaking up your morning make-up routine. Try setting your alarm 15 minutes earlier to give yourself plenty of time to create the perfect face.
- Invest in a set of good brushes.
- Use those extra minutes in the morning to camouflage dark circles or blemishes that have appeared in the night.
- Put together an emergency crisis kit. Here's what to bag: cotton buds, tissues, mineral water spray, eye drops, small tube moisturiser, concealer, foundation, loose powder, blusher, mascara, lipstick, small sponge, blusher brush, lip brush.

Now read on for our trouble-shooting beauty tips!

Tip

Go to an art shop for great natural bristle brushes – they cost a fraction of the price of special make-up brushes.

Illustrations: JACQUELINE BISSETT

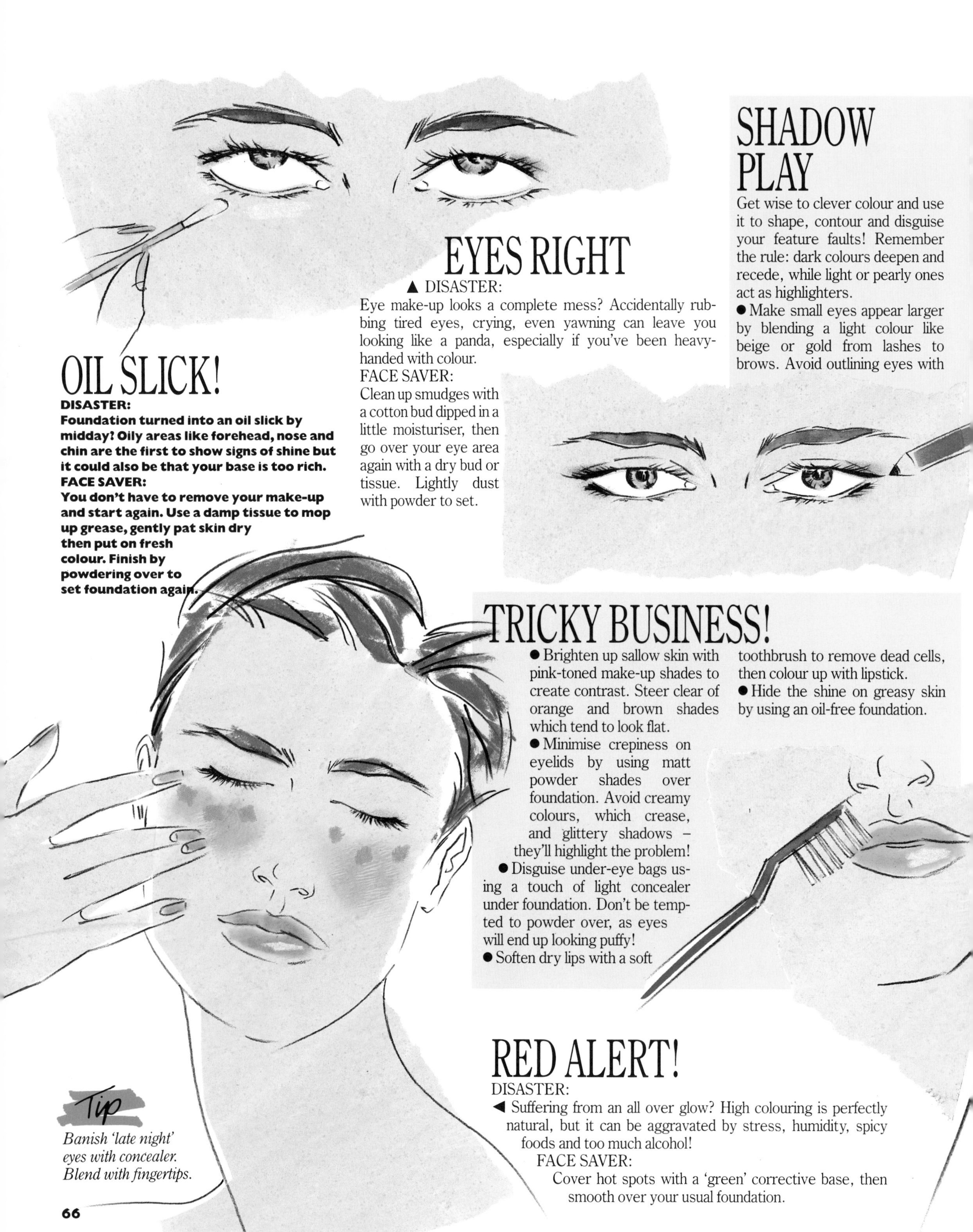

EYES RIGHT

▲ DISASTER:
Eye make-up looks a complete mess? Accidentally rubbing tired eyes, crying, even yawning can leave you looking like a panda, especially if you've been heavy-handed with colour.
FACE SAVER:
Clean up smudges with a cotton bud dipped in a little moisturiser, then go over your eye area again with a dry bud or tissue. Lightly dust with powder to set.

SHADOW PLAY

Get wise to clever colour and use it to shape, contour and disguise your feature faults! Remember the rule: dark colours deepen and recede, while light or pearly ones act as highlighters.
● Make small eyes appear larger by blending a light colour like beige or gold from lashes to brows. Avoid outlining eyes with

OIL SLICK!

DISASTER:
Foundation turned into an oil slick by midday? Oily areas like forehead, nose and chin are the first to show signs of shine but it could also be that your base is too rich.
FACE SAVER:
You don't have to remove your make-up and start again. Use a damp tissue to mop up grease, gently pat skin dry then put on fresh colour. Finish by powdering over to set foundation again.

TRICKY BUSINESS!

● Brighten up sallow skin with pink-toned make-up shades to create contrast. Steer clear of orange and brown shades which tend to look flat.
● Minimise crepiness on eyelids by using matt powder shades over foundation. Avoid creamy colours, which crease, and glittery shadows – they'll highlight the problem!
● Disguise under-eye bags using a touch of light concealer under foundation. Don't be tempted to powder over, as eyes will end up looking puffy!
● Soften dry lips with a soft toothbrush to remove dead cells, then colour up with lipstick.
● Hide the shine on greasy skin by using an oil-free foundation.

RED ALERT!

DISASTER:
◀ Suffering from an all over glow? High colouring is perfectly natural, but it can be aggravated by stress, humidity, spicy foods and too much alcohol!
FACE SAVER:
Cover hot spots with a 'green' corrective base, then smooth over your usual foundation.

Tip

Banish 'late night' eyes with concealer. Blend with fingertips.

eye pencil; you'll only end up emphasising the problem.

- Widen close-set eyes with a touch of shimmering shadow on the inner socket area. Then play up the outer corners of the eye with a dark kohl pencil to create an illusion of width.
- Slim down a round face using blusher just below the cheekbones, sweeping it out towards the centre of the ears in a soft arc. Use a warm and flattering bronze shade then define the chin with a sweep of blusher just below the jawline.
- Soften the definition of a heart-shaped face by dusting matt blusher on to cheekbones and under jaw.

BAN THE BLEMISH

DISASTER:
Hit a trouble spot? Break-outs tend to be caused by excess oil blocking pores. Stress, allergies, and topsy-turvy hormones can also be to blame.
FACE SAVER:
Use a medicated concealer under foundation to help disguise blemishes. Dab just a tiny amount on a make-up brush, then blend.

GLOW AHEAD!

DISASTER:
More flush than natural blush? Going overboard with cheek colour is a result of bad brushwork. Check the colour is a good match with your skin tone.
FACE SAVER:
Carefully blot off excess colour with a tissue, then lightly dust with powder. Sweep colour over cheekbones and up to temples using a large, soft brush.

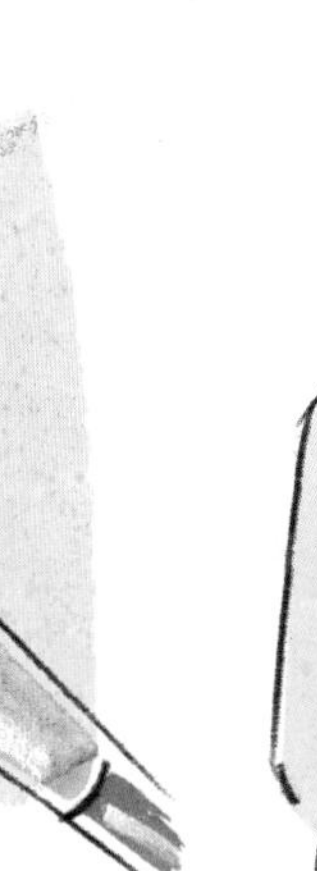

LUSCIOUS LASHES

▲ DISASTER:
Lashes sticking together? Could be that your mascara's too thick, or else you've put on too much in one go.
FACE SAVER:
Dust lashes with powder for a longer-lasting base. Sweep on two thin coats of mascara.

BROW BEATER

► DISASTER:
Brows look bushed? Over-plucking can spoil the natural line, leaving them looking straggly and uneven.
FACE SAVER:
Fill in patchy brows using a soft pencil with short, light upward strokes following the natural brow line. Or use a little matt powder on a slant-edged brush.

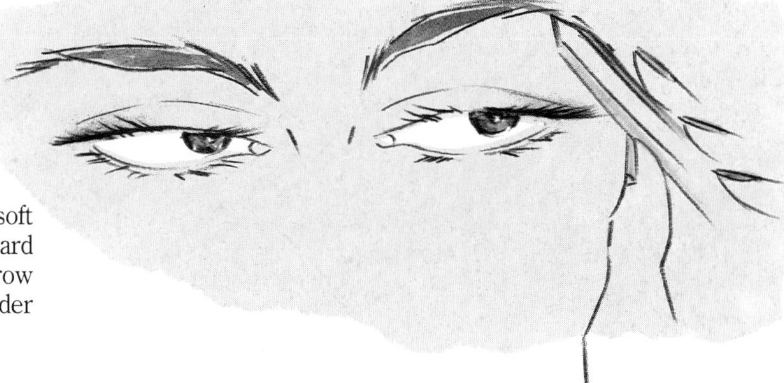

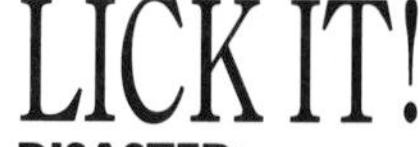

LICK IT!

DISASTER:
More lipstick on your glass than your mouth? Smudged or 'bleeding' colour can mean you haven't primed your lips first!
FACE SAVER:
Ensure staying power by taking foundation over your lips, then pat on a little loose powder. Outline mouth with a toning lip pencil to stop colour bleeding. Fill in with your favourite lipstick using a lip brush, blot and re-apply.

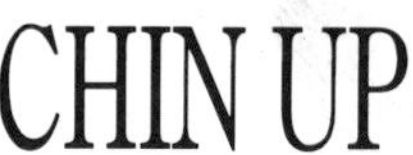

CHIN UP

▲ DISASTER:
A tell-tale 'join' around the jawline where foundation has failed to cover the skin is a common make-up mistake. Bad blending can give a hard, obvious edge, so make sure the colour isn't more than two shades darker than your natural skin tone.
FACE SAVER:
Use a wedge-shaped sponge to smooth on colour, starting from the middle of your face and working outwards. Blend carefully.

Always use a damp sponge when putting on foundation – you'll find it easier for smooth, even coverage.

Photographs: FRANCIS LONEY/Hair: PENNY ATTWOOD/Make-up: KAREN LOCKYER/Personal stereo and telephone: BOOTS/Frames: FIRST SIGHT OPTICIANS/Maroon sweater: MARKS & SPENCER/Black and white shirt: FREEMANS/Black blouse: WAREHOUSE/Earrings: ACCESSORIZE

BIG DATE

Looking your best on a big date doesn't mean hiding your face under layers of make-up – instead play up your good points with a look that is flattering, not overpowering.

- Apply a beige eyeshadow over your lids and take it up to your eyebrows.
- Blend a slightly darker, but still soft colour, over your eyelids and up to your brows.
- Draw a black eye-pencil across your lids, close to your lash roots. Take the line just longer than each lid and finish with a thick stroke that copies the upward flick of your eye lashes. Draw a fine line under your lower lashes and soften it with a cotton bud.
- Put two thin coats of mascara on your top lashes. Leave the bottom ones bare.
- Add only a touch of blusher.
- Your eyes are the focal point of this look so don't over-do your lips. Stick to pretty colours that complement your skin tone. Blondes should go for rose pinks, and brunettes for warm orange or russet tones.

Hairwise: opt for a softly swept-back style, so that he can really see your face – no hiding behind a heavy fringe! Create soft waves with a hot brush and back-comb the front hair. Pin hair on crown and spritz with hairspray.

If you never seem to have enough time to put on powder and *foundation, use a powder and foundation-in-one.*

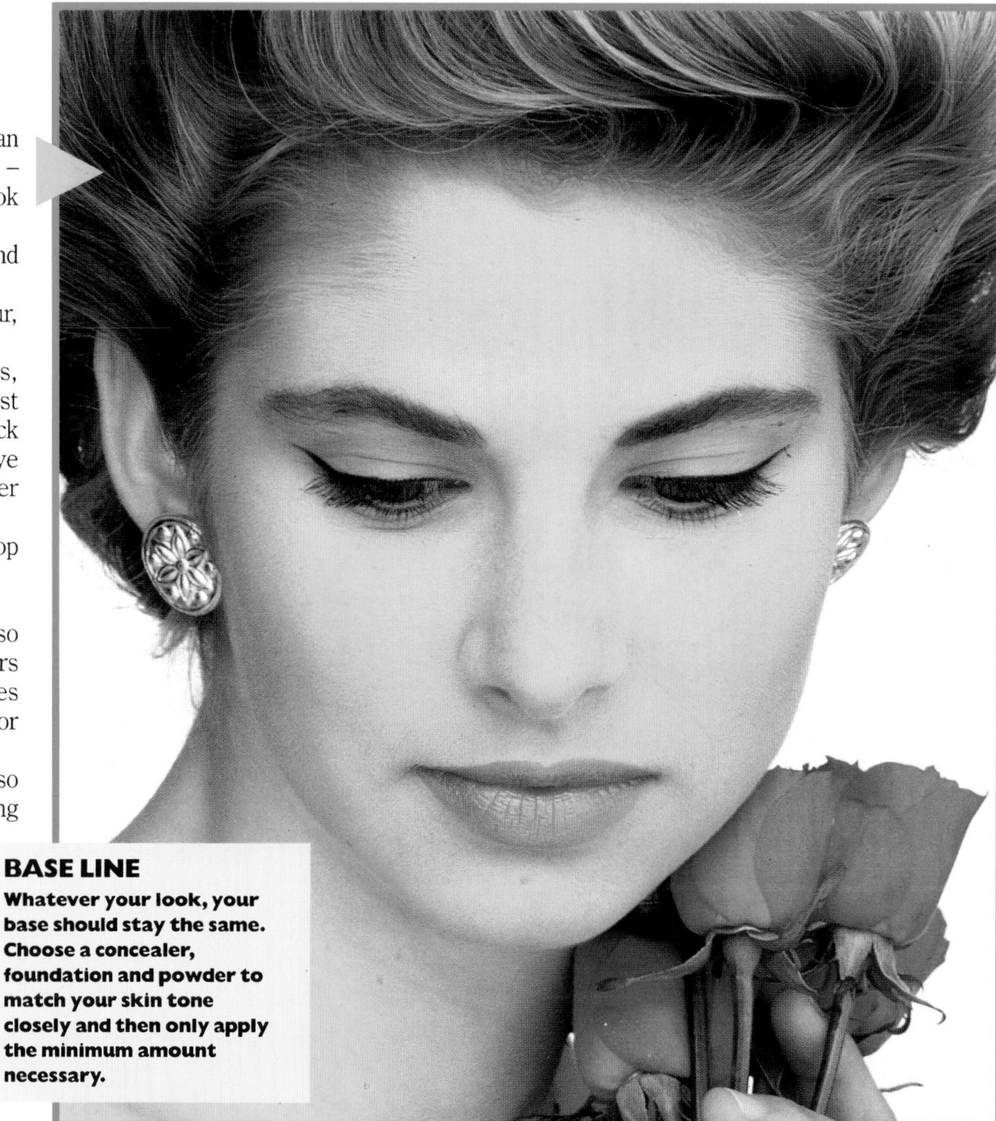

BASE LINE

Whatever your look, your base should stay the same. Choose a concealer, foundation and powder to match your skin tone closely and then only apply the minimum amount necessary.

FOUR-FACED

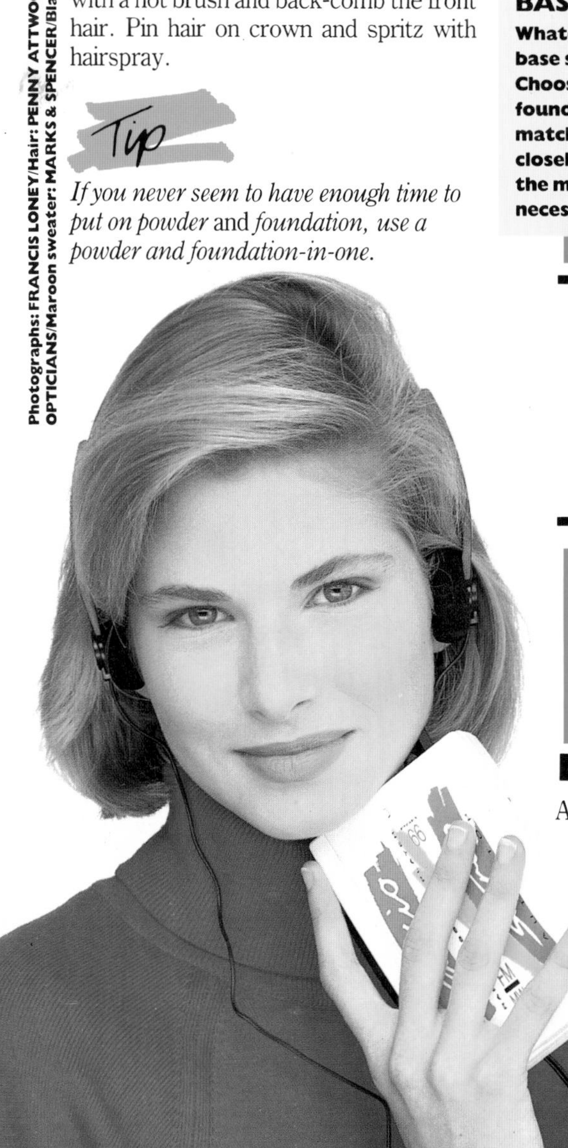

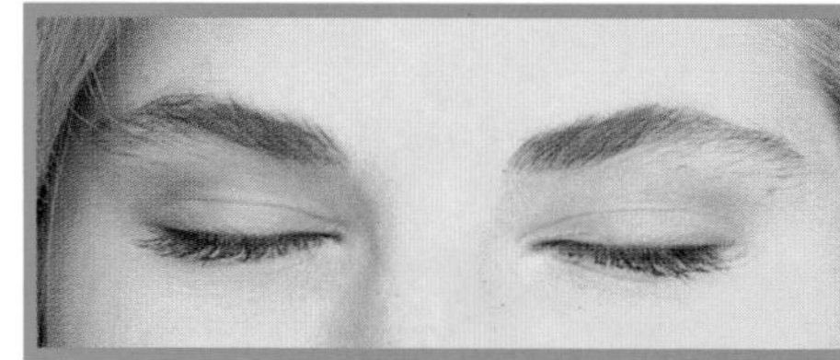

DAY OFF

A relaxed, understated look is great on your day off and gives your skin a chance to rest! If you are going out-and-about stick to a simple make-up.

- Use a pale beige eyeshadow.
- Blend a darker shade such as terracotta or gold in your socket crease and take it out to the corners of your lids.
- Stroke a touch of the darker colour under your lower lashes to widen your eyes.
- Finish with a coat of mascara.
- Keep blusher natural. Use a matt bronzing powder to give your skin a healthy glow and dust it on to the fullest part of your cheeks.
- Use a clear lip salve to protect lips or go for a lip gloss to add a touch of colour.

Hairwise: keep your hair neat and simple. Wash, condition and blow-dry it smooth using a flat-backed brush. Or, if you don't want to wash it, slick it back with gel and wear it in a ponytail or bun decorated with brightly-coloured scrunchies. Simple but very stylish!

It's not what you wear, it's the way that you wear it! Whether you're facing a dinner date or a day off, make sure you pick the make-up colours that work for you whatever you do

Have you got stuck in a rut with your make-up? Do you reach for that same old brown eyeshadow whatever you're going to do? It's much more fun to be two-faced or even four, and you don't need to spend a fortune on a drawer full of new cosmetics. Look out for versatile palettes that you can match with old favourites, or remix easily to create stunning new shades. You can then look every situation in the face – and make your make-up do the same. Just brush up on technique!

TOOL TRICKS

The key to professional-looking make-up is using the right tools to apply it:

- **Apply foundation with a damp cosmetic sponge for really smooth coverage.**
- **Use a range of sponge-tipped eyeshadow applicators and fine blending brushes – one for each different colour!**
- **Keep eye liner pencils sharp.**
- **After putting on mascara, brush your lashes through with a clean, dry mascara wand to stop them clogging up.**
- **Use a thick, soft blusher brush to make sure the colour is put on lightly and evenly. The bigger the better!**
- **Keep your lipbrush clean! Dirty brushes attract fluff that will prevent smooth application. Wipe it with a tissue.**
- **Brush your eyebrows into shape using an eyebrow brush or clean mascara wand. Follow the natural arch of your brow.**

Watchpoint

For a professional finish, always use make-up with the same textures – matt with matt and cream with cream.

PARTY PARTY!

Party make-up is fun, so why not experiment with those make-up colours you thought you'd never wear! Bring your eyes to life: use mainly matt colours, with a hint of shimmer as a finishing touch.

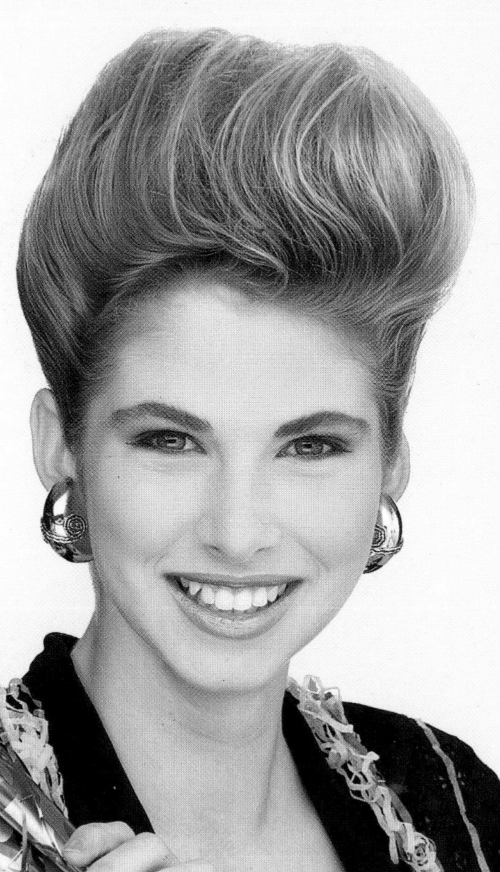

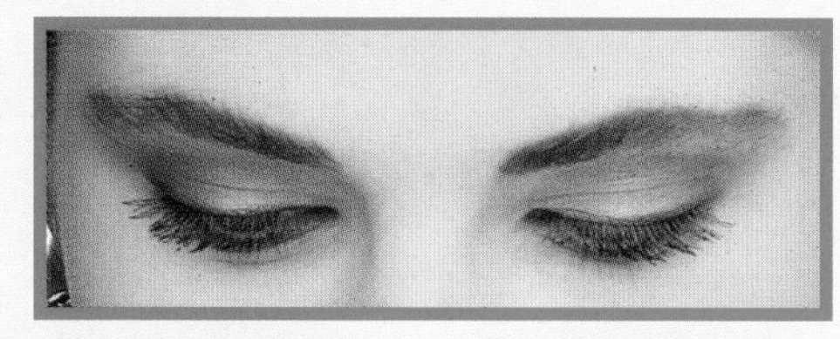

- Put a beige base eyeshadow over your lids and blend it well with a brush.
- Stroke a darker matt gold colour in the socket line to define your eyes.
- Next, stroke a shimmering colour in the fleshy area under your brows, winging it upwards for a dramatic look.
- Put on a dark eye shadow, creating a soft, smudged line above and below your lashes at the outer corner of the eyes.
- Stroke on two coats of black mascara.
- Go without blusher, or keep it very light, so your eyes and lips stand out.
- Lipsticks with a pretty shimmer are perfect for parties! Blot the colour then top it off with a touch of lip gloss in the centre of the bottom lip. Then get out and pout!

Hairwise: a mane of waves looks glamorous, as does a style with lots of height. This variation on a beehive is perfect. Just blow-dry your hair straight and back-comb it on top. Gather your hair high on top of your crown fold the back into a pleat and pin. Spray with hairspray.

Choose an eyeshadow which matches or complements your dress and use it to highlight your eyelids discreetly.

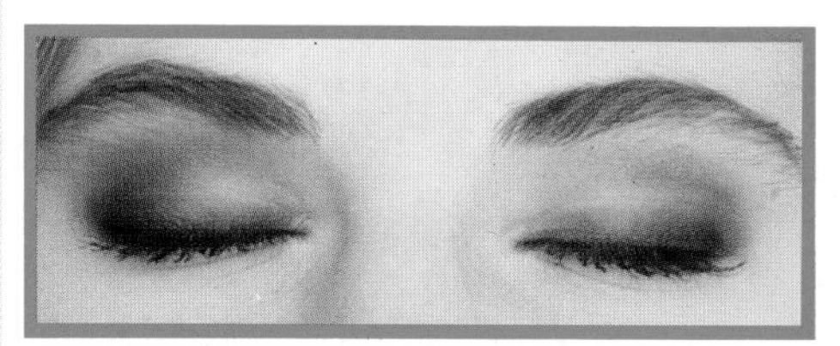

OFFICE HOURS

At work, your make-up needs to give you a look of sophistication, neatness and efficiency. Go for a flattering range of complementary colours – simple make-up is easier to keep looking good during the day.

- Start with your pale beige eyeshadow colour. Blend it all over your eyelid.
- Blend a dark smoky-grey shade of eye-shadow into your socket crease and wing it out at the edges.
- Draw a fine line across your lids close to the lash roots using a black eye-liner pencil.
- Take the pencil just underneath your bottom lashes. Blend the top and bottom lines together at the outside edge.
- Curl your lashes with eyelash curlers. Then coat with two coats of black mascara.
- Stroke rose or peach blusher over your cheeks using a big fat blusher brush.
- Choose a matt, russet or dark rose lipstick that looks understated. Blot it to avoid smudges – especially on coffee cups!

Hairwise: choose a fuss-free hairstyle, such as a bob which you can blow-dry straight before you set off for work and then revive by tipping your head forwards and spritzing the roots with hairspray. Back-comb the top hair for a bit of extra body.

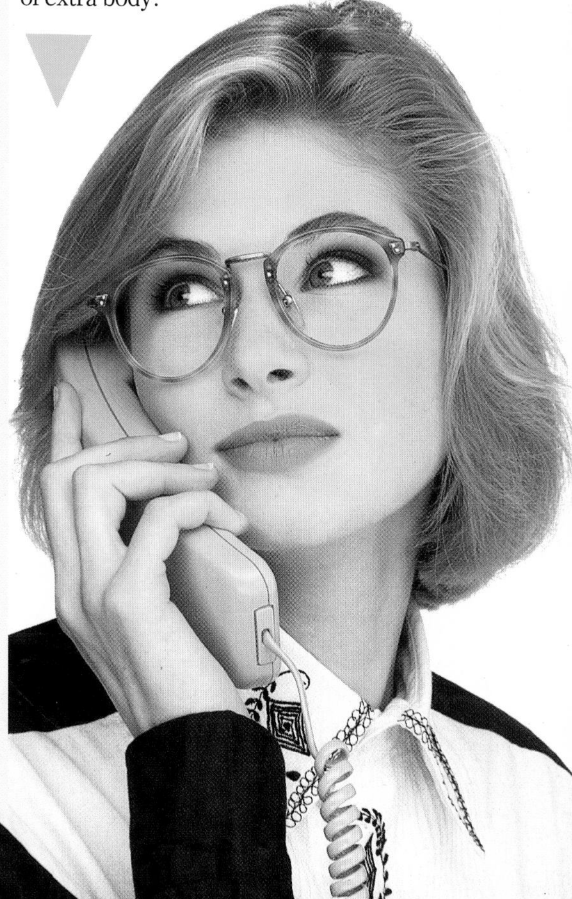

DAY INTO

Plan ahead for a night out with a nine-to-five face that'll see you through the evening with the least amount of effort

Photographs: PAUL MITCHELL/Hair and make-up: YA'NINA/Lingerie: KNICKERBOX/Polo neck and bag: PINEAPPLE/Toothbrush: BODYSHOP/Telephone: BOOTS

RISE AND SHINE

Start the day with a simple make-up routine, using carefully chosen colours for lasting good looks.

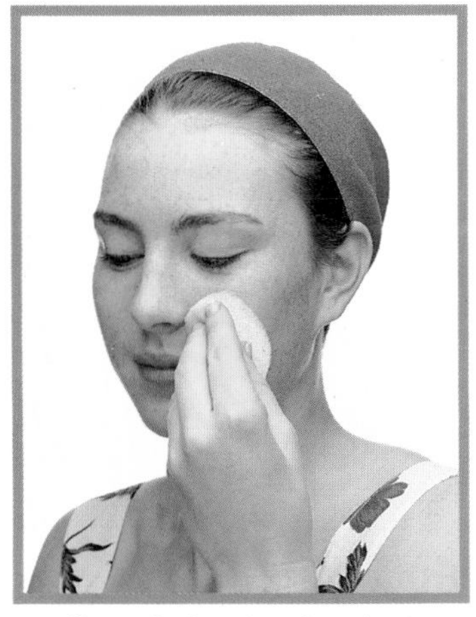

1 *Smooth tinted moisturiser over your face instead of foundation for a light, sheer finish. Put it on with a sponge to save time.*

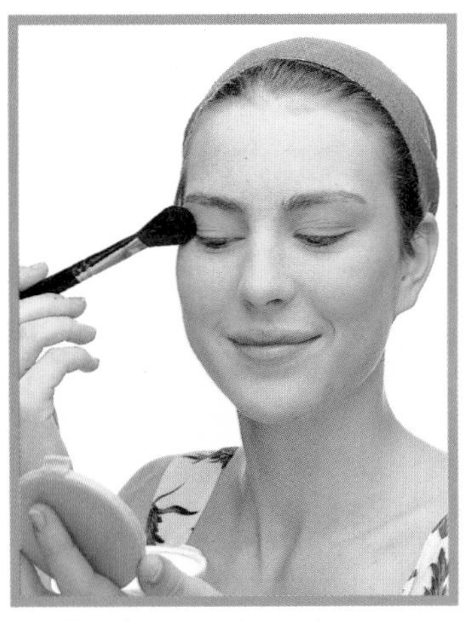

2 *Don't waste time with eyeshadow kits – use a neutral shade of blusher and brush a little over your brow bone after you've done your cheeks.*

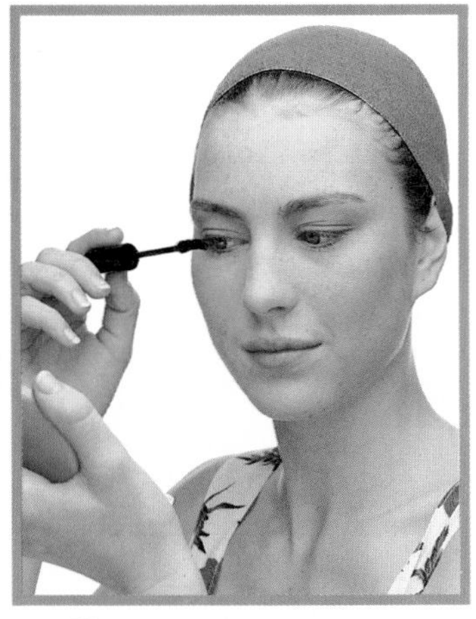

3 *Use an eyelash curler for longer looking lashes, then finish them with a single coat of brown or navy mascara.*

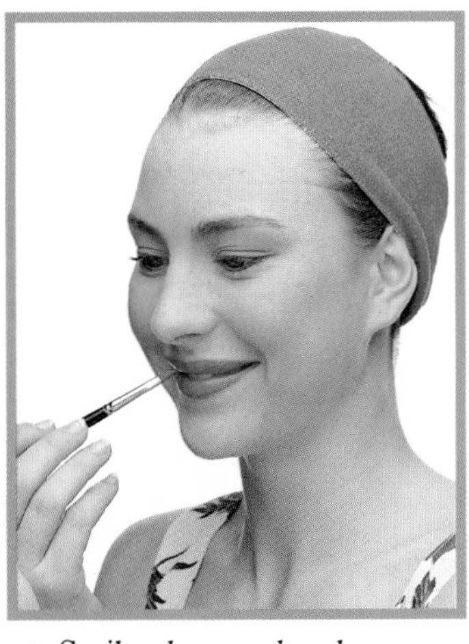

4 *Smile when you brush on your lipstick to get a perfect line! Stick to a subtle shade to complement your eyeshadow.*

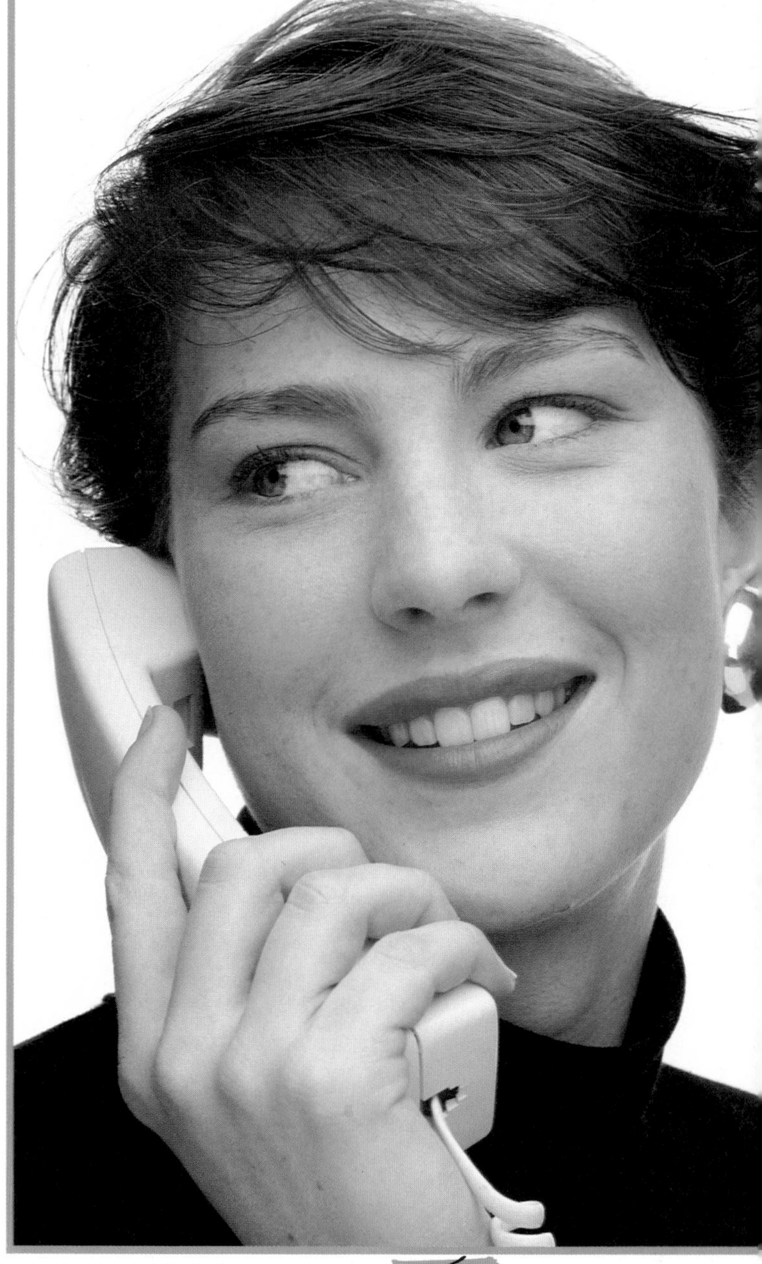

5 *Comb your hair then run your fingers through it to create lift, put on your earrings and off to work you go!*

Tip

Need a bit more cover? Just dot on concealer exactly where you need it, then dust with loose powder.

NIGHT

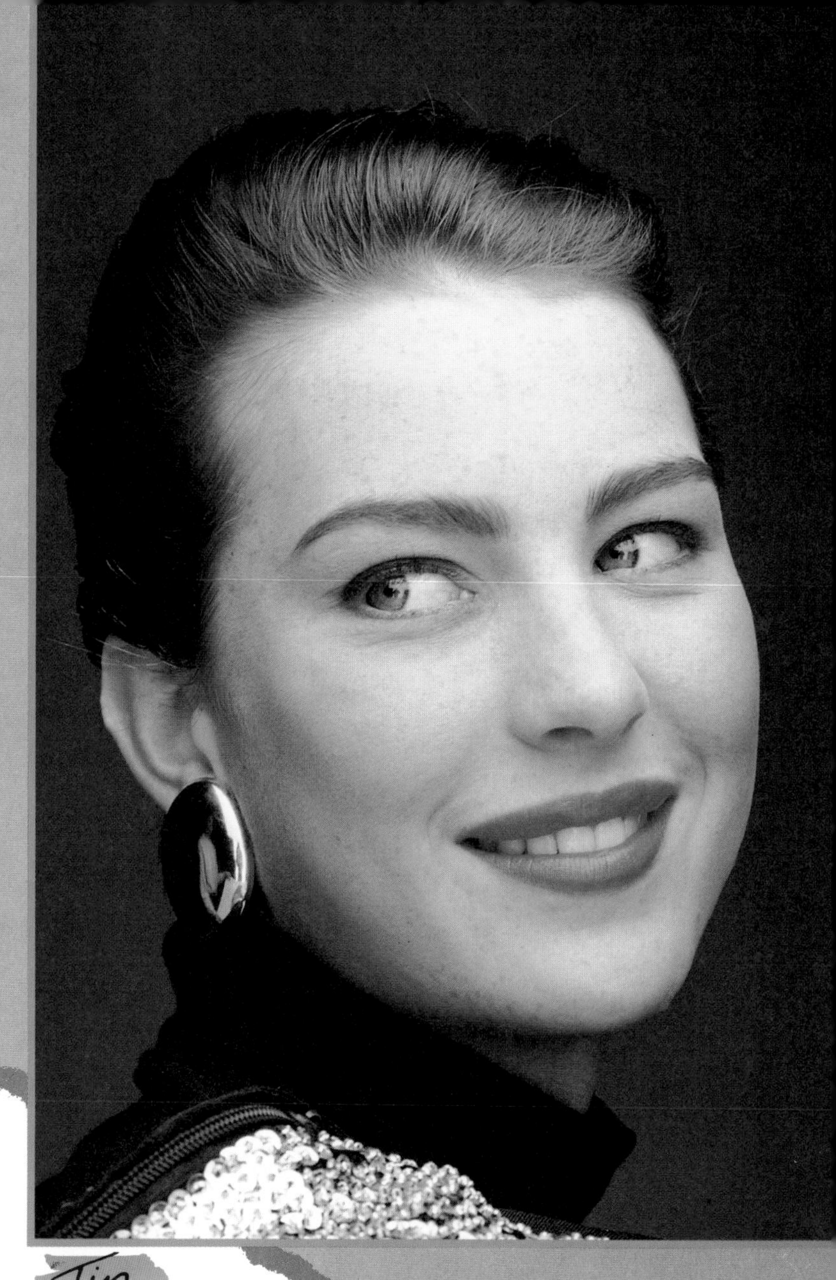

THE TWILIGHT ZONE

No time to make up all over again? Then just touch up the make-up that's lasted you through the day!

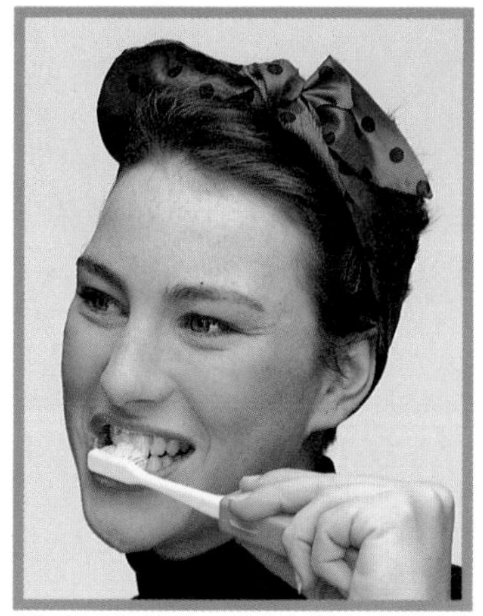

6 Romantic encounters are out if you've got stale breath, so brush up your chances with a travel toothbrush and toothpaste and make your mouth minty-fresh.

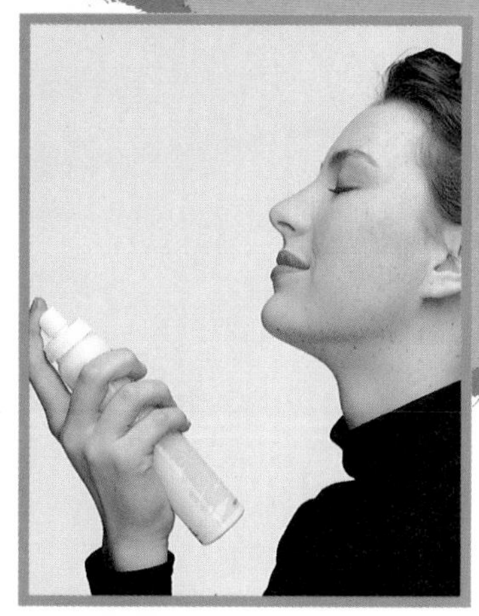

7 DRY SKINS need extra moisture. Spraying your face lightly with water will provide moisture without disturbing your existing make-up.

Tip

In a real rush? Put on your lipstick first – then you can see how much other make-up you really need.

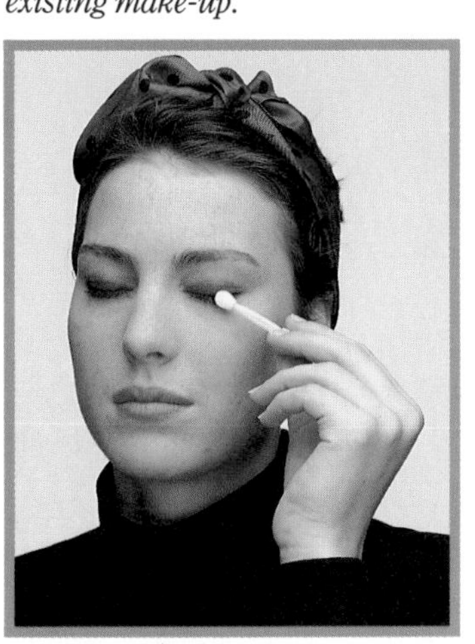

8 OILY SKINS can be blotted to take away shine. For a really matt finish use translucent powder or a powder foundation.

9 Eye make-up is best kept simple – use a little brown or grey powder shadow on a brush and blend over your lid to avoid a hard line.

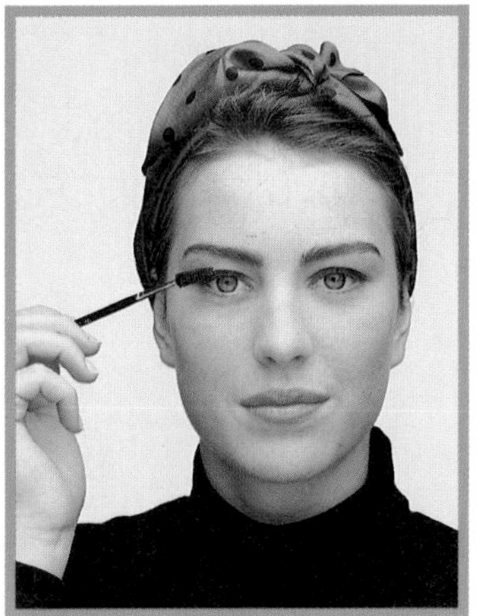

10 Brush on another coat of mascara, then use the wand on your eyebrows to comb and darken them slightly.

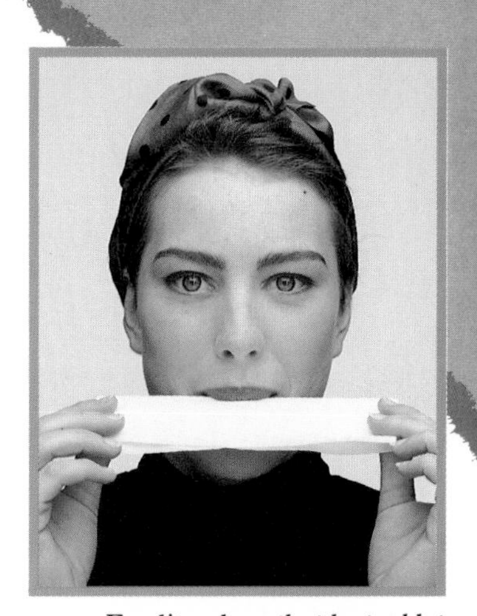

11 For lip colour that lasts, blot off all traces of your daytime lipstick and put on a new, fresh colour to brighten up your whole look.

DARE

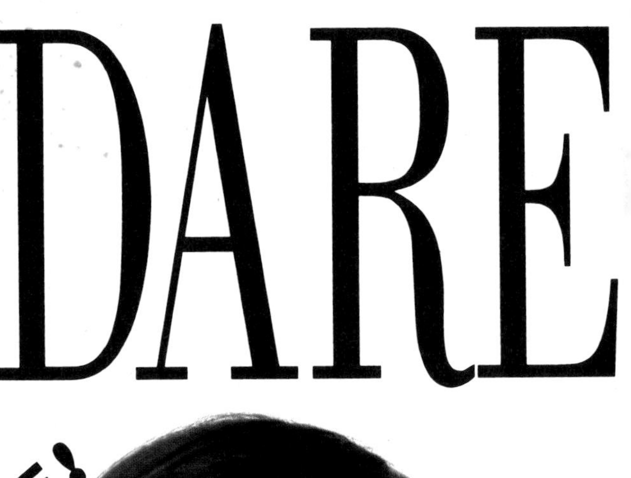

Express yourself! Clash with dash – or just be bold! Say no to neutral shades and make your make-up that bit mad, bad and dangerous to wear!

It's fun being outrageous from time to time. And that applies to your make-up too. After all, there's nothing that says you *have* to stick to neutral shades and 'barely there' make-up. Keep the colours that suit you, but branch out too. Try mixing your favourite shade of eye, lip or nail colour with a bright contrasting one or, better still, go all out – lock, stock and barrel – for a complete change!

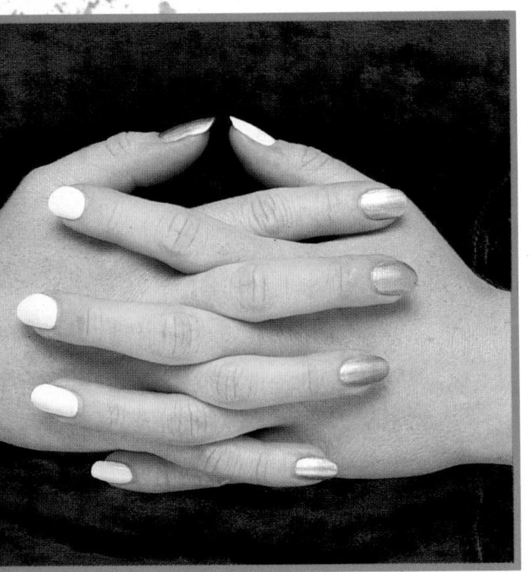

NAIL DARE!

▲ If pretty pink nail varnish or killer red talons aren't your scene, try out white nail colour or go for space-age silver and paint on a couple of coats. If you're feeling really daring, do one hand in one colour and the other in a different one. Or paint each nail a different colour.

ROCKING THE FOUNDATION

The key to using bold or unusual shades successfully is to get your base just right first. Choose a foundation that's as close to your own skin tone as possible. Experimenting with your foundation colour – going a few shades lighter or darker – will only look unnatural and won't provide the right base on which to build your new look.

And go easy on the blusher too – or alternatively don't use any at all. Your aim is to get your total make-up looking good, not garish. Use a hint of concealer to hide any blemish and dust your skin with translucent powder then get to work brightening up your eyes, lips and nails.

BRAVE NEW AGE!

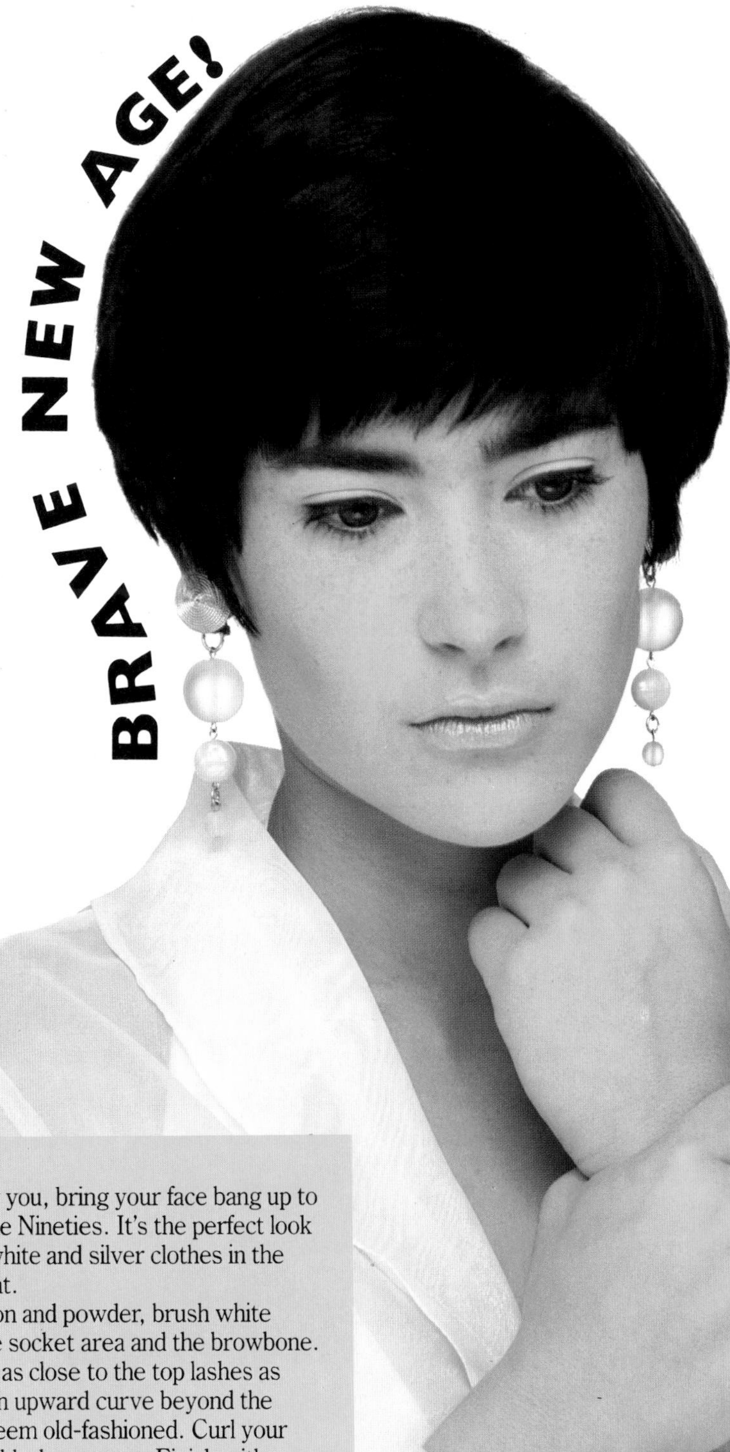

BRAVE NEW AGE!

► If browns and greys aren't for you, bring your face bang up to date with the New Age look of the Nineties. It's the perfect look to complement all the futuristic white and silver clothes in the shops and makes you look brilliant.

After putting on your foundation and powder, brush white eyeshadow over the whole of the socket area and the browbone. Draw a thin line of black eyeliner as close to the top lashes as possible. Don't draw the line in an upward curve beyond the lashes. This will make the look seem old-fashioned. Curl your lashes and brush on two coats of black mascara. Finish with a quick slick of silver lipstick.

TO BE DIFFERENT

GOBSMACKED

◀ Forget the pastel pinks and the barely-there lip glosses and splash out on a fluorescent lipstick like this orange one. Fill in your lips using a lipbrush, then press a tissue over your lips. Rub a finger gently across the tissue to blot any excess. Then put on another coat.

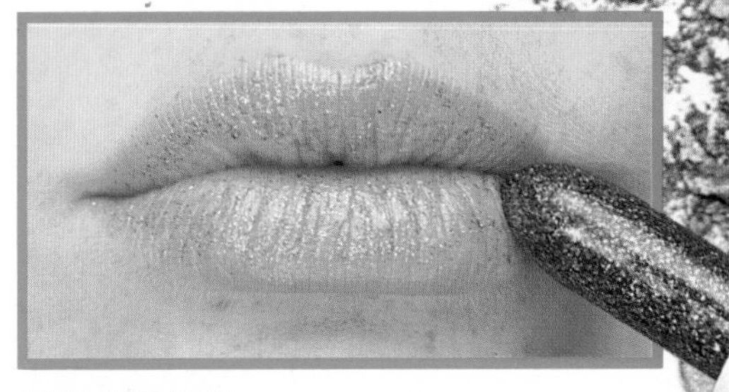

GLITTERATI!

▲ Put a bit of extra sparkle into your lips by running a glittery lipstick over a pale pink colour. A fab party look!

HOT METAL

◀ Look on the bright side! Swap your usual blue or black liner for a liquid silver eyeliner. Paint a thin line above your top lashes with an eyeliner brush.

FIZZY ORANGE

▼ Broaden your colour range and boldly go for bright, bright orange. It looks spectacular and wonderful whether you're fair or dark.

Put on your foundation and powder. Brush a tangerine colour over the whole of the socket area and then blend a line of brighter, darker orange into the socket line. Give your top lashes a couple of coats of black mascara. Sweep just a hint of orange blusher over the widest part of your cheeks using a big fat brush. Finish off by carefully putting on bright orange lipstick. Blot on a tissue and re-apply the colour.

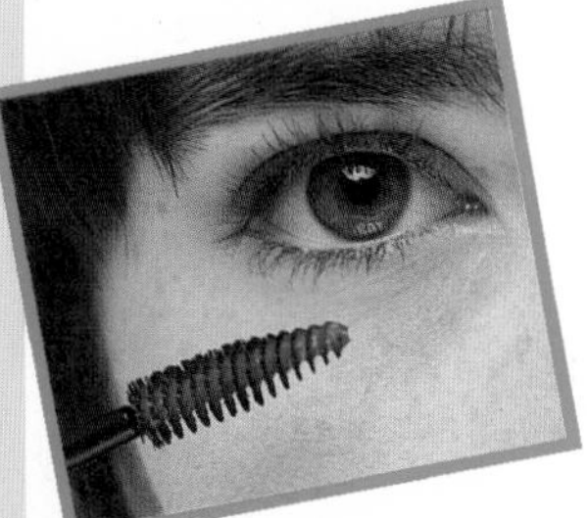

RED ALERT

▲ Hot up your usual eyelashes by tipping the ends of them with a red mascara. It'll draw attention to your eyes!

After brushing on coloured mascara to the tips of your lashes, coat them with clear mascara as a seal.

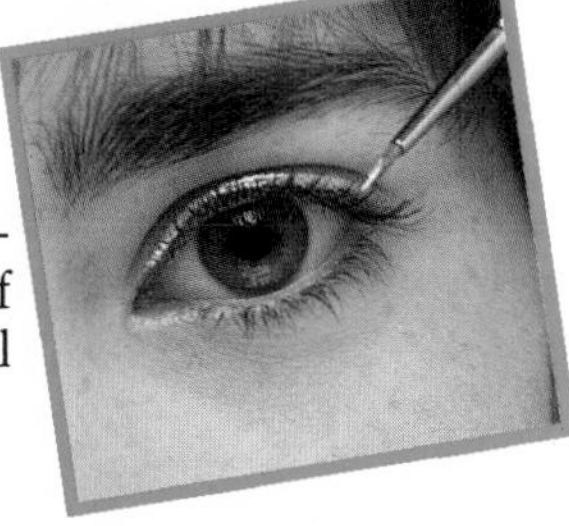

MELLOW YELLOW

▼ Don't be a coward! Give banana yellow eyeshadow a go. It's fun and looks great with pink.

Put on your foundation and powder. Brush yellow eyeshadow over your browbone. Then blend a line of bright pink into the socket line. Coat the top lashes with either clear or brown mascara and finish with a lipstick that's a similar shade of pink to the eyeshadow.

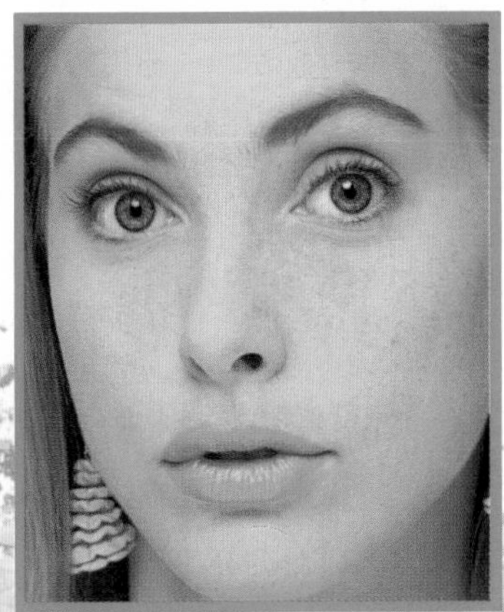

FIZZY ORANGE

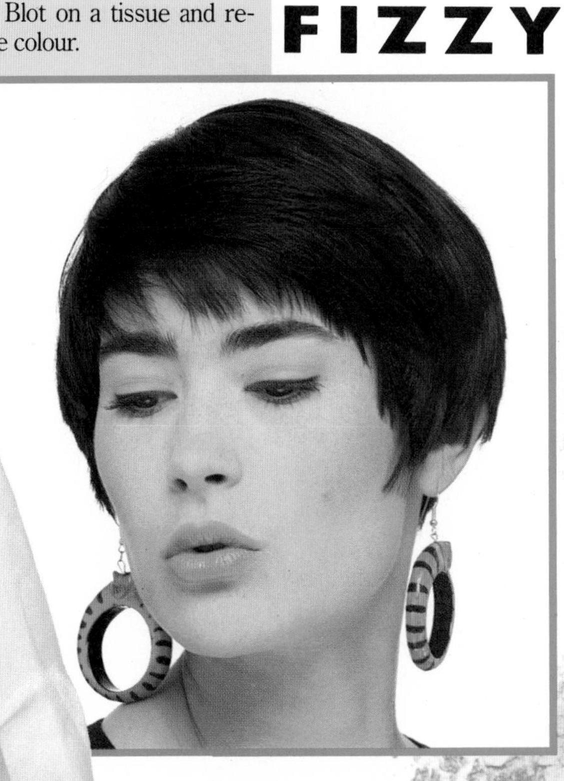

GET THE BRIGHTS RIGHT!

- **Bear in mind what light you're going to be seen in when you make up. If it's candlelight or a dimly-lit disco you can get away with brighter or glittery shades, if you're going to be out in daylight tone it down.**
- **If you've overdone it with the eyeshadow or the lipstick, dust over your eyelids or lips with translucent face powder.**
- **Experiment with new colours *before* you get ready for that big date.**
- **Put a generous amount of translucent powder underneath your eyes when you apply bright shadows. Excess shadow will collect in the powder not on your face. Dust it away when you've finished.**
- **If you really want to be different, mix and match different make-up textures. Use creme shadows with powder shadows, use glittery lipsticks with plain ones or add a bit of glitter to translucent powder and dust over your shoulders and back.**

Photographs: JAMES HOBSEY/Make-up: KIZZY HARRISON/Hair: PAULA MANN

Still life: IAN HOOTON/Halter-neck top: PINEAPPLE/Earrings: ERIC BEAMON/Hoop earrings and yellow earrings: REX INTERNATIONAL

NINE OF THE BEST!

Slim down your cosmetic kit to a nifty nine essentials! Take the weight off your handbag with a few well-chosen colours and products and get more mileage from your make-up

Is your make-up bag jam-packed with products and colours that you hardly ever use? Then it's high time for a clear out! You may find it hard to believe but all you really need to create a complete make-up is just nine basic items. Then by adjusting how you use each one, you'll be able to look your very best morning, noon and night!

BUY THE BEST

When you're buying the basics, it's worth spending as much as you can afford on each item. The more expensive brands generally have sturdy packaging so they won't fall apart in your handbag. Look out for packaging and design which is innovative too – like products that double-up to do more than one job. Take time to test colours before you buy too. Aim to get a selection of versatile colours that suit your skin and clothes. If in doubt stick to a basic palette of matt shades for eyes, lips and cheeks.

CONCEALER

Use to hide spots, blemishes, under-eye shadows and black-heads around your nostrils or in the crease of the chin. Apply on a clean fingertip or a brush and blend in gently.

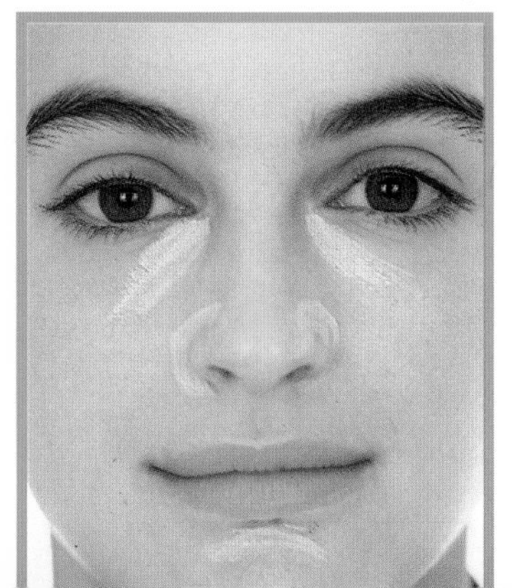

Look for:

- Texture – most come as a cream or a stick. You want one that covers well and is creamy enough to blend easily. Avoid concealers with a 'chalky' texture.
- An exact colour match to your skin. Test it on your face, not your wrist, go a bit lighter rather than darker.
- A medicated concealer, if spots are a problem.

FOUNDATION

Always worth investing in a good one. Even if you don't normally wear it during the day, foundation can give a flawless base for more dramatic evening make-up.

Look for:

- A light, liquid formula that won't look too heavy or artificial.
- The right colour to match your skintone. Don't go for darker ones thinking they'll make you look healthy. They won't!
- A fragrance-free formula, if your skin is sensitive or prone to spots and blemishes.

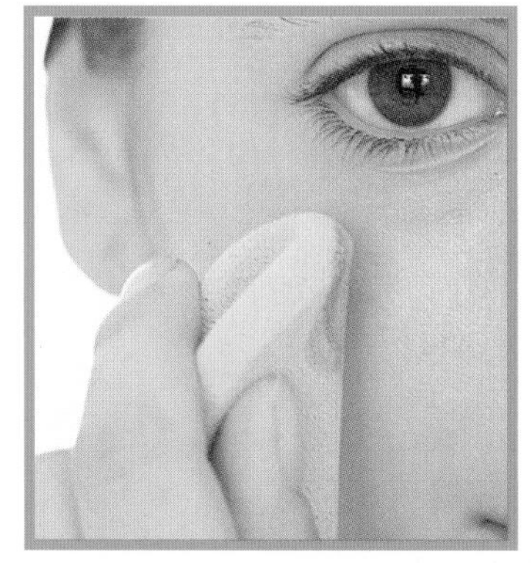

LOOSE POWDER

Even if you want to cut out everything else, a touch of powder is essential to take the shine off your skin and to 'set' your foundation and concealer.

Look for:

- Transparent powder, which is colourless. Even up your skin tone with your foundation rather than a coloured powder.
- Loose powder. Professional make-up artists always use it to set foundation and reduce shine. Pat it over your skin on a powder puff until your complexion is quite floury and then whisk off the excess using a big, soft brush. Use pressed types for retouching.
- Matt powders. They give a more natural finish.

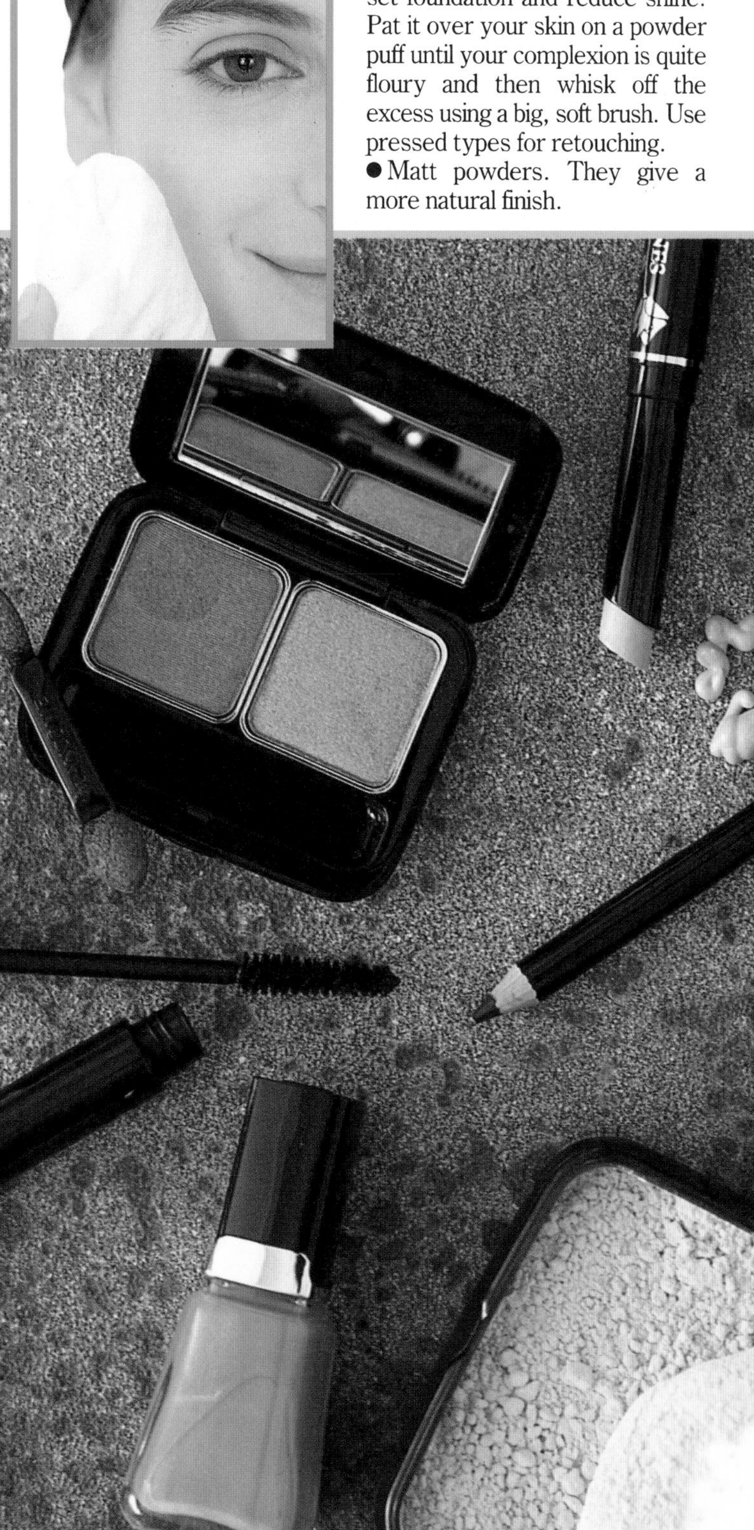

Photographs: WILL WHITE/Hair: SHIRALEE LAW/Make-up: VIRGINIA NICHOLS/Make-up from LANCÔME

EYESHADOW

Choose a range of matt neutral shades like greys or browns. Go for colours that'll blend with what you're wearing too. Choose bolder colours for evening.

Look for:

● A palette of two or three complementary shades. The darkest one should be matt for shading but the others can be slightly shimmery which look good at night.

● A large-sized sponge-tipped applicator or a small eyeshadow brush.

● A set of eyeshadows with a mirror inside the lid – so you don't need to carry a separate one.

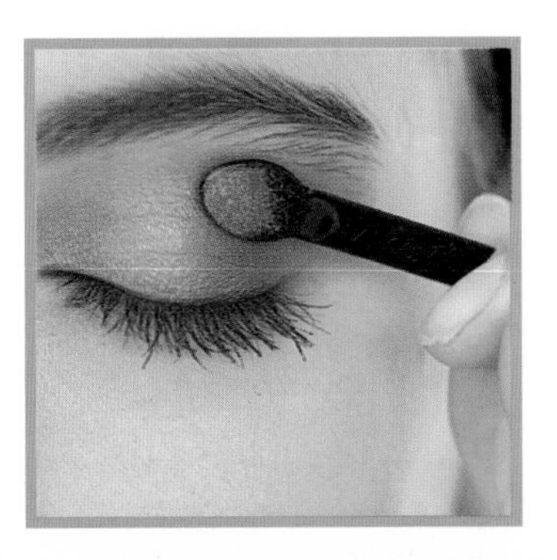

EYE PENCIL

Your eyes will look larger if lined in a dark shade and you can also use it to darken brows as well. For best results, keep the pencil sharp and rest your elbow on a table to prevent a wobbly line when putting it on. Use firm strokes.

Look for:

● Dark brown pencils. Only ever buy black pencils if your natural colouring is very dark.

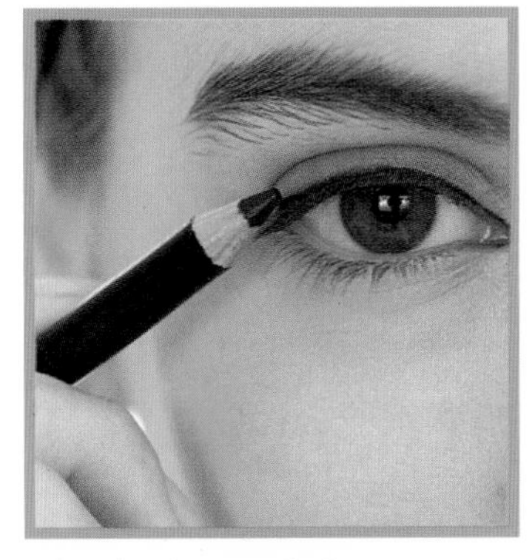

● Soft pencils that won't drag across the skin of your eyelid, or over the delicate skin underneath the eye.

● A great value double-ended pencil that has another colour and either a sharpener or a smudging sponge at the other end.

MASCARA

Everyone's favourite cosmetic! It makes your eyes look instantly made-up and bigger. Brush on both sides of your top lashes. Let each coat dry before applying the next, and brush the lashes between applications with a clean, dry mascara wand to prevent clogging. There's no need to mascara bottom lashes.

Look for:

● Waterproof types to resist tears and rain!

● Cream formula. Fibre ones can smudge and make you look panda-eyed after a day's wear.

● Mascara without fibres if you wear contact lenses.

● A long bristled brush at one end to separate the lashes.

BLUSHER

Dusted on correctly, it can add warmth to your skin and help to create the illusion of high cheekbones. As a shade guide, go for a rose-pink or a peach, depending on your underlying skin tone. Smile with your lips closed and dust colour outwards along the fullest part of your cheeks, fading it out at the temples.

Look for:

● Matt formulations – glittery ones can look clown-like!

● Powder types which look more natural and are much easier to apply than cream ones.

● A natural bristle brush – the bigger the better – to go with the blusher compact. This will help you to blend the blusher well.

NAIL POLISH

Long plum or red talons aren't really practical and show up any chips too. Keep nails neat and try a sheer shade rather than a pearly or heavily pigmented colour. You can always add an extra coat to brighten it up. Use firm, even strokes and paint the polish down the centre of the nail, then fill in on each side. Let each coat dry thoroughly before putting on the rest.

Look for:

● A smooth, quick-drying formula. Test out lots of brands on your nails before buying.

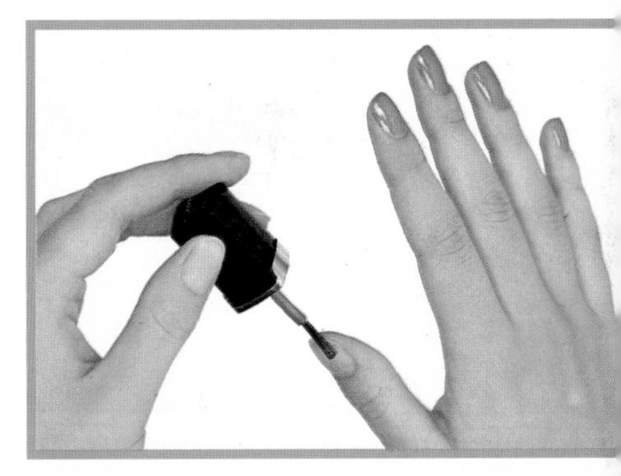

LIPSTICK

The one essential none of us would be without! There are literally hundreds of shades to choose from, but your best buy is a creamy rose pink. It'll flatter all skin tones and will make the most of your mouth, even if your lips are not a perfect shape.

Look for:

● Creamy formulas. Blot the colour down for barely-there stain. Add another coat and a touch of gloss for a night-time pout.

● Lipsticks with built-in moisturisers or sun screen.

● A matt texture.

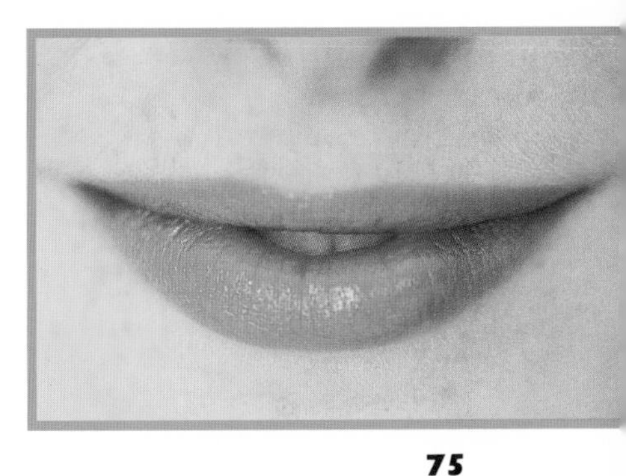

BEAUTY HELPLINE

Brow-beaten by plucking? Spots making you see red? End your problems with our professional help

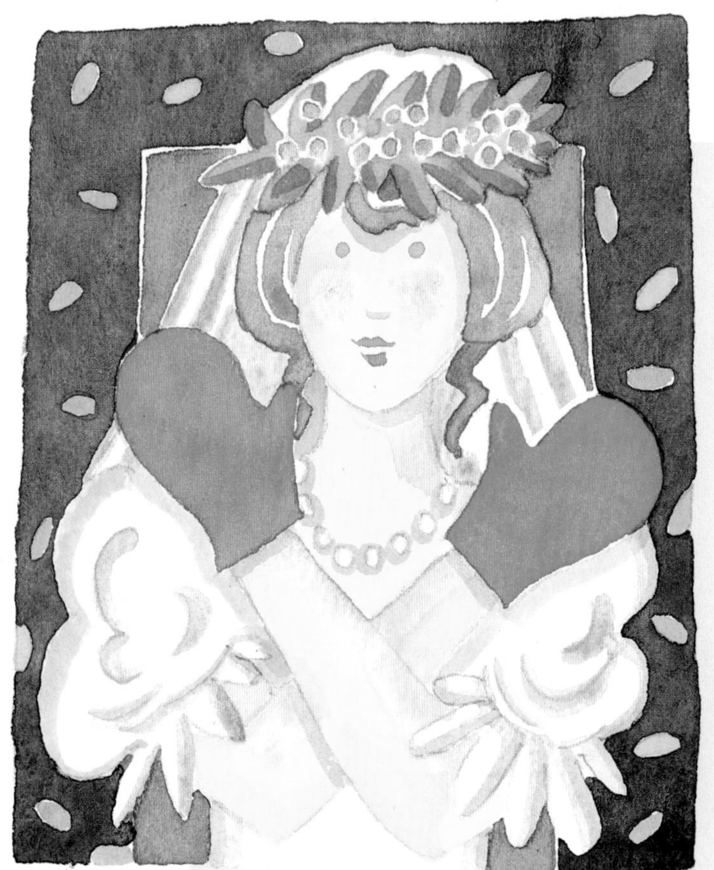

NAILING THE PROBLEM

Q I'm getting married soon, and I'm worried about my nails. I've stopped biting them, but they grow so slowly that I know they won't be very long for the wedding. How can I make them look their best?

A Try a French manicure. The finished look is perfect for a bride, and works just as well on short nails as long. Start by gently pushing back the cuticles using an orange stick or special cuticle pen. Then paint the whole nail with a pale pink matt polish. Allow it to dry, and then use a white polish to paint the white tips of your nails. When this coat is dry, go over the whole nail again with a couple of coats of clear polish.

Alternatively, you can get the effect of a French manicure by buffing your nails with a chamois buffer and buffing cream.

SORE POINT

Q I'm always getting cold sores on my lips. Is there anything I can do about them?

A Cold sores are caused by a viral infection often triggered by exposure to sunlight. You can also get them if your resistance is lowered by an illness like a cold. One precaution you can take is to wear a sunscreen on your lips whenever you go out. Similarly, buy lipsticks with a UV sunscreen – most ranges have them now.

Your pharmacist should be able to recommend a lotion to help dry up cold sores and these work best if applied as soon as you feel the tell-tale itching and before the sore actually appears. If you can't get to the chemist in time, some sufferers swear by strong, cold black coffee dabbed on to the itch at hourly intervals!

FAST FACES

Q I'm starting my first job soon and I want to look my best. But I'm really bad at getting up early in the mornings. Can you give me some quick make-up tips?

A No problem! With a bit of practice you can have perfect make-up in ten minutes. Try these few simple tips:

- Start with an all-in-one foundation that provides base and powder in one. Cover any spots or under-eye shadows with a concealer stick.
- Apply two coats of mascara to top lashes – choose brown or grey if you're fair, black if you're dark. Use a matching pencil to define brows and lower lash line.
- Dust a little powder blusher onto the fattest parts of your cheeks, blending the colour up towards temples.
- Use a lipbrush to outline your lips carefully, then fill in colour. Blot with a tissue and reapply. This does need to be done with care, so on days when you're really rushed, choose a tinted lip gloss instead since it doesn't require such precise application.

The finished result is a natural-looking make-up using neutral tones. If you want to vary your look, invest in a range of lipsticks to tone with all your different outfits. And to save time, have the make-up you need, laid out ready for the morning. In fact it helps if you can buy two identical make-up sets and keep one in your bag for repairs during the day, and the other one wherever you put on your make-up in the morning.

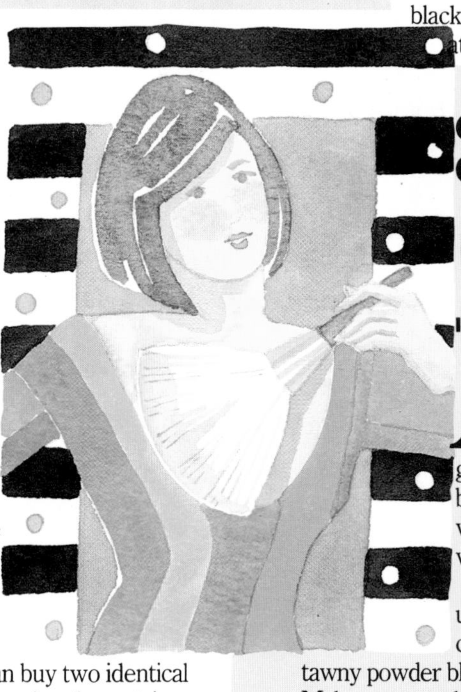

GLAMOUR OR BUST

Q My new dress has a plunging neckline but my cleavage doesn't look too good. Any tips?

A First, get your skin into tip-top condition. Use a gentle body scrub at bathtime, and then moisturise well. Also, clear up any spots with a spot cream.

On the night, wear an underwired bra and create a cleavage by dusting a matt tawny powder blusher between your breasts. Make sure you blend it well and finish off by dusting your shoulders lightly with a white or lilac loose powder.

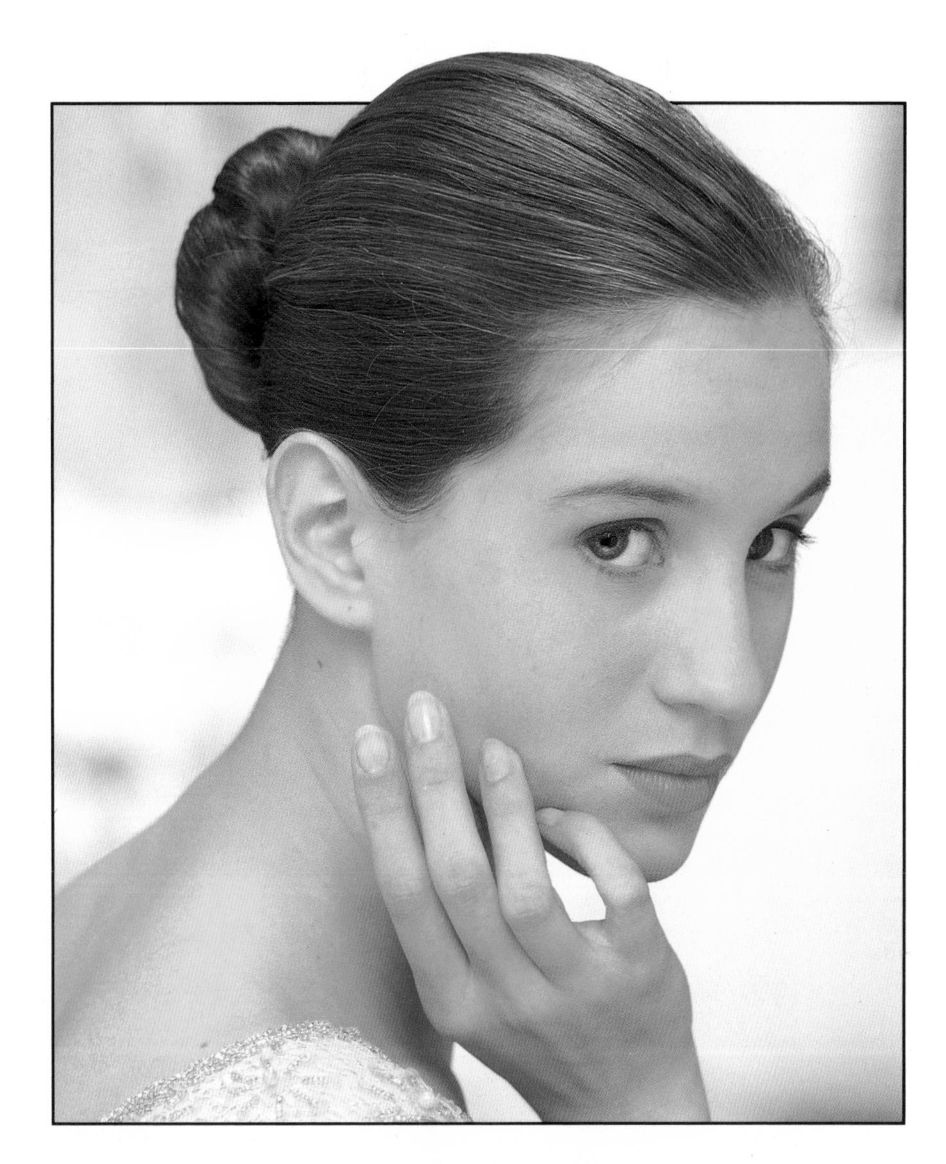

CHAPTER THREE

Skin Deep

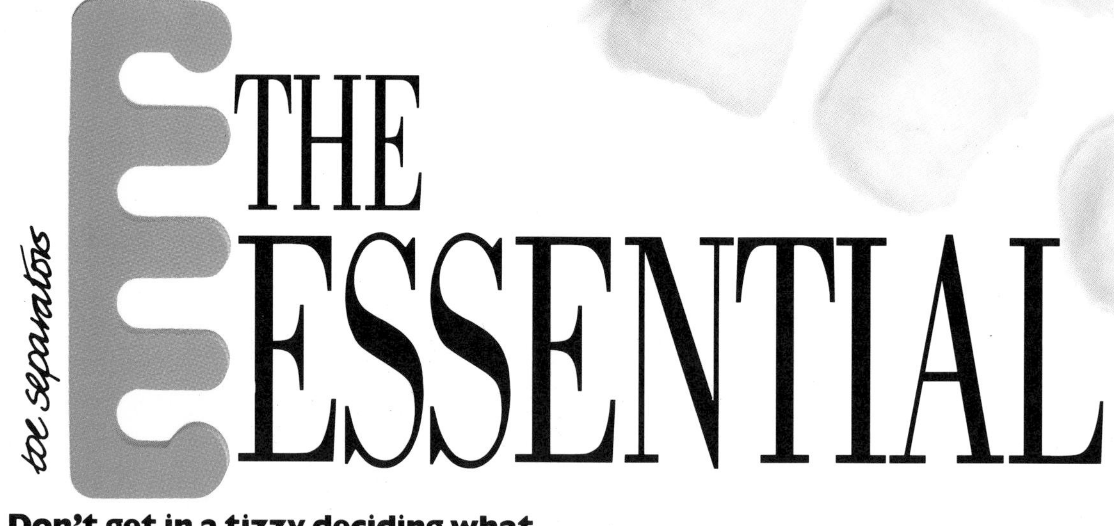

THE ESSENTIAL

Don't get in a tizzy deciding what you need for top-to-toe good looks. These basic tools of the trade will keep your body beautiful

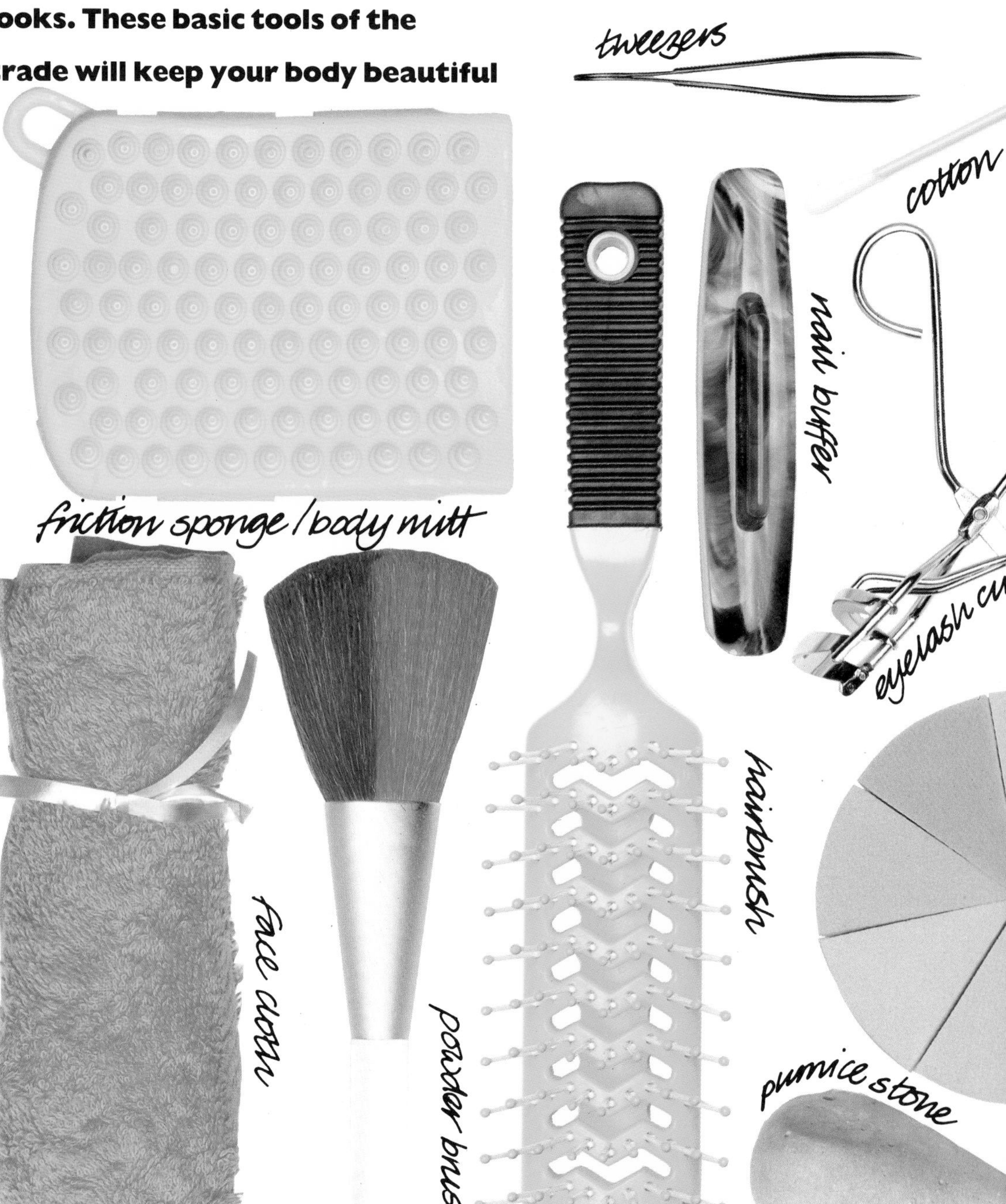

- **BACKBRUSH** – for bare-back beauty, use a brush to cleanse the parts of your back that you can't otherwise reach. Use an anti-bacterial wash on the brush if you suffer from spots.
- **COMB** – choose a wide-toothed comb for combing through wet hair, applying conditioner and styling hair.
- **COSMETIC SPONGE** – use a latex wedge-shaped one to put on foundation evenly and to get into the awkward little crevices on your face – like round your nostrils. Wash out sponges every time you use them.
- **COTTON BUDS** – really handy all-purpose tools. Use them to clean away eye make-up smudges or to soften eyeliner so that you're not left with a harsh line. And dip them in nail polish remover and use to take off nail colour mistakes.
- **COTTON WOOL** – for 101 different uses! Soak a ball in toner and wipe over face and neck to refresh after cleansing. Use a pad of it covered in baby lotion or cleanser to remove make-up or clean your face. Use a big wodge to dust translucent powder over your face.
- **EMERY BOARD** – essential for filing fingernails. Use the coarser-grained side to shorten the nail and use the finer-grained side to shape the nail. File from side to centre rather than backwards and forwards.
- **EYELASH CURLERS** – these give you lovely curly lashes. Just clamp the eyelashes carefully in the curlers for a few seconds then release them gently.
- **EYESHADOW BRUSH** – use this flat-edged brush to put on and blend eyeshadow or to dab on concealer for covering up spots and dark shadows under the eyes.
- **FACE CLOTH** – use this with cleanser for a clear complexion or to rub dead skin cells from your body with coarse sea salt or a body scrub on the cloth.
- **FRICTION SPONGE** – a body massage with a friction sponge (also called a body mitt) before or during a shower or bath increases circulation, relaxes muscles and helps stop cellulite forming.
- **HAIRBRUSH** – grooms, styles and keeps your hair in tip-top condition. If you only buy one make it an all-purpose vent brush.

Photographs: DAVE DENT

BODY KIT

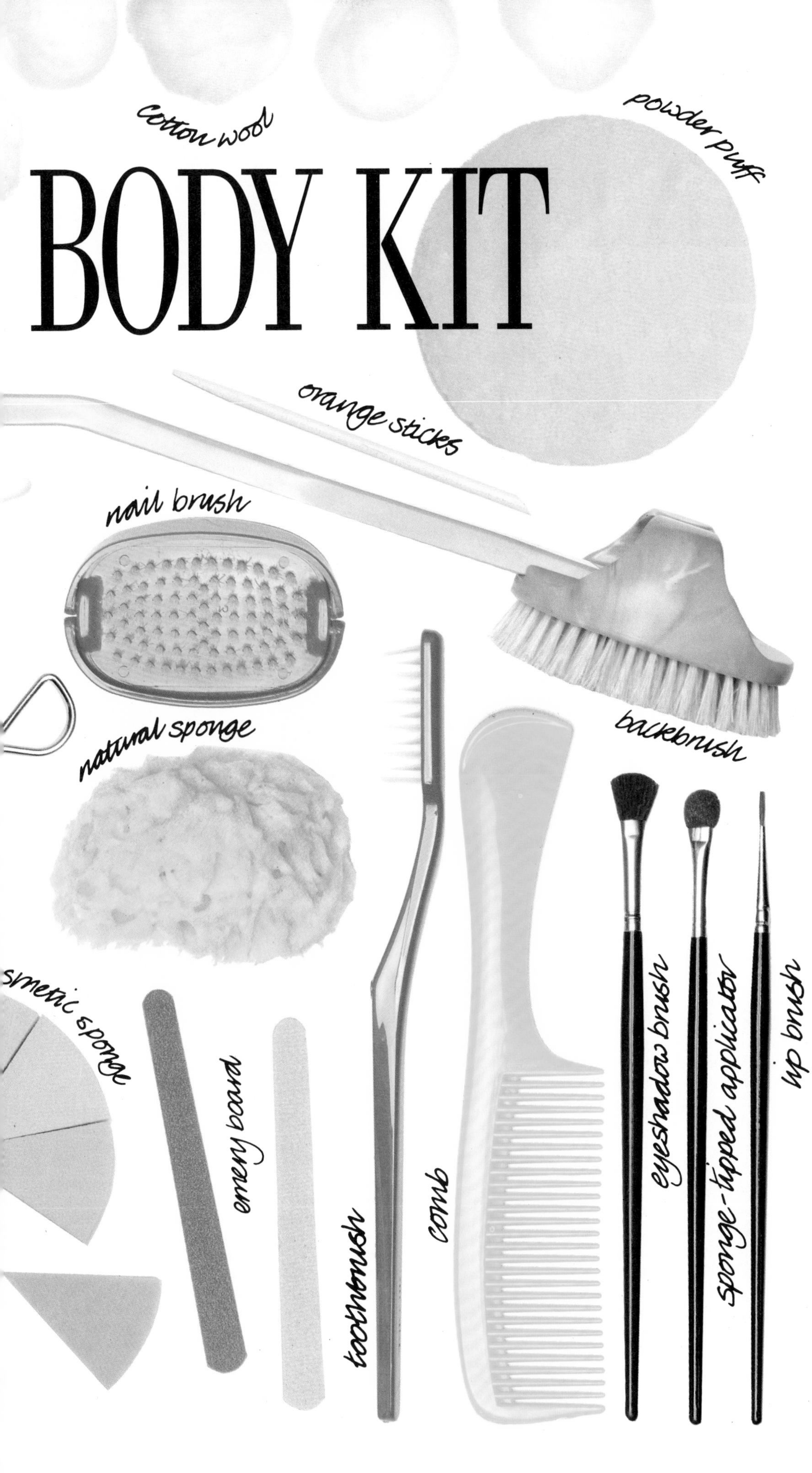

● **LIPBRUSH** – put on lipstick the professional way – it will look better and last longer. Outline lips using the edge of the brush with the shade of your choice, then fill in the colour. Blot your lips with a tissue, then re-apply colour with the brush.

● **NAIL BRUSH** – ideal for cleaning dirt from under your nails.

● **NAIL BUFFER** – rub it backwards and forwards across unvarnished nails to give a healthy gloss.

● **NATURAL SPONGE** – real sponges are the super-absorbent skeletons of a type of marine animal. Use a large one to wash yourself in the bath or shower and a smaller one to put on your foundation. Always rinse them out every time you use them.

● **ORANGE STICKS** – use for all-round nail care. The horseshoe shaped end pushes back the hard white skin at the base of the nail (cuticle) and the pointed end cleans under the nails.

● **POWDER BRUSH** – a fat powder brush can double-up as a blusher brush. Pat on translucent powder and dust off the excess with a big brush. Use powder blusher in gentle sweeping movements across your cheeks to prevent any harsh lines of colour.

● **POWDER PUFF** – this works wonders with face powder. Dust translucent powder on to your face or use it to dab bronzing powder over chest and shoulders if you are very pale.

● **PUMICE STONE** – this is actually volcanic lava which has cooled to form a soft stone – perfect for getting rid of scaly skin. Soak hard skin on your feet or elbows in warm soapy water then gently rub with pumice stone. Dry the skin and smooth on moisturiser.

● **SPONGE APPLICATOR** – useful for putting on powder eyeshadow or blending lip liner into your lipstick.

● **TOE SEPARATORS** – put the finger-shaped ends in between the toes when you're painting your toe nails. It'll stop the colour going where you don't want it.

● **TOOTHBRUSH** – regular and thorough brushing helps prevent plaque and tartar building up. Brush your teeth for about three minutes at least twice a day.

● **TWEEZERS** – use them to pluck hair from straggly eyebrows and fit fiddly false eyelashes.

SQUEAKY CLEAN

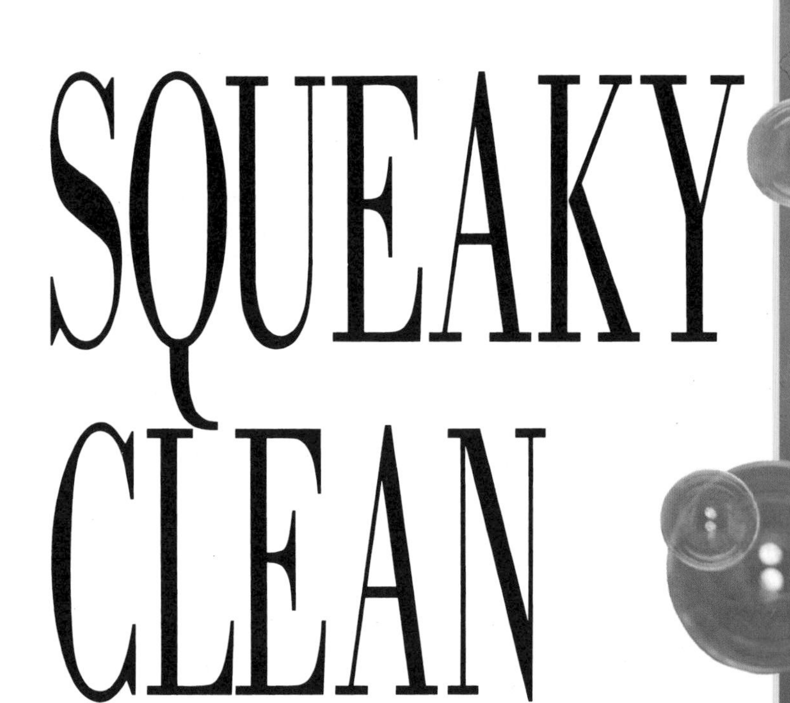

If you're all in a lather over whether to choose a cream cleanser or stick to soap for a super soft skin, read on for the bare-faced facts

There are many ways to clean up your act, and all have their good and bad points.

The basic recipe for soap is usually a mixture of animal or vegetable fat and caustic soda, plus added extras such as perfume, colour and natural extracts. Although it's one of the most efficient formulas for removing grease and grime from the skin, it also tends to dry it out. The problem is soap's alkaline, while skin tends to be slightly acidic. Therefore, for a while after washing, the skin's protective acid mantle is upset and your face may feel taut and dry. But, within a couple of hours, your skin will have rebalanced itself, so there's no lasting damage.

Cream cleansers are put on with cotton wool and don't have this reputation for being harsh or drying. This is because the cream is a liquid formula which feels more gentle and gives the manufacturers a chance to add other ingredients which help to moisturise your skin. The one disadvantage is that your skin tends not to feel as squeaky clean afterwards as when you've washed with soap and water.

Just to confuse matters further, there are other grime busters too. Cleansing bars are solid cleansers for those who like the feel of washing with water, but don't want to use real soap. They're often called soapless soaps! Facial washes can be used in exactly the same way as soap to give you the best of both worlds – a refreshing, water-rinsable product that isn't too drying. But which type is best?

The truth is that there is no single, perfect method. Some tissue-off cream cleansers contain such a high proportion of detergents and other additives that they could be a lot more irritating and dehydrating than a soap packed full of moisturising oils which counteract the drying effects of the basic ingredients in the bar. Steer clear of cleansing products that leave your skin feeling uncomfortably tight or dry and flaky. It may be a case of trial and error but go by what suits you. The final message is, if you've got a great complexion and enjoy using soap, then there is no reason at all why you shouldn't stick with it!

PICKING THE BEST BAR

If you're a soap and water fan, this simple and clear guide will

SOAP BOX *Here are a few surprising soap facts*

- **Soaps start off in the form of noodles just like pasta, or sometimes as flakes. Then the special ingredients such as perfume and moisturisers are added and all are put through a mill to mix them up. Triple milling is the secret of good quality soaps and if you ever see this term on the label, it means the milling process has been repeated three times so the soap is less likely to crumble and fall apart when it's used. After this the soap goes through a hopper and is formed into the final shape.**
- **Good soaps are left to harden for at least a couple of weeks before being sold.**
- **To make sure your soap lasts, keep it in a dry place. In a drawer of clothes is a good place, since it will help to keep them smelling sweet and fragrant.**
- **The poshest soaps are usually curved so they don't lie flat in soggy pools of water and droplets of moisture can drain off.**
- **Glycerine soaps attract moisture from the atmosphere and tend to go soft very easily, so keep them in a soap box.**
- **Although you may cringe when you receive yet another set of soap bars for a present, it's estimated that each person uses about 10lbs of soap a year – that's a lot of lather!**

WASHING UP

Follow these four simple tips for a perfect soap-and-water cleansing routine.

1 Only use tepid water – if it's too hot or too cold you could make the tiny blood vessels just below the skin's surface contract or expand, leading to broken veins.
2 Rinse, rinse and rinse your skin again, because if you leave even the tiniest scrap of soap on your skin it could very easily cause irritation.
3 If you use a flannel, buy several so you can put one in the wash every day.
4 Treat your skin gently. Just pat it dry with a towel after washing.

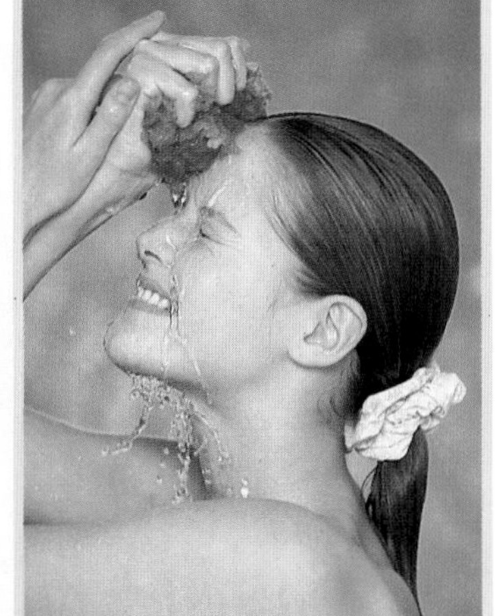

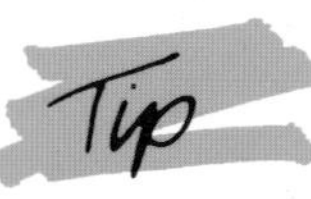

Once a week, or more if you have greasy skin, give your skin a treat by gently massaging it with a facial brush (or even a soft shaving brush) while lathering up with soap. Apart from making your skin glow by boosting your circulation, it will also remove dead cells that dull your skin, and also give it a good deep-down cleanse.

help you find the best formula to suit your skin type.

OILY
Don't make the mistake of buying a strong soap and washing too often. Opt for a mild formula to remove grime and oil but without damaging your skin. Look out too for soaps containing exfoliating granules, such as oatmeal, to help unplug blocked pores and slough off dead skin. Gel facial washes are another good choice. If your skin looks oily during the day, just blot it with a tissue.

SPOTTY
There are lots of medicated soaps around with anti-bacterial ingredients to help fight the germs that combined with excess oil lead to spots. But take care! These may be too harsh for you. There's the possibility they can remove the 'good' bacteria on your skin that keep it healthy as well as the 'bad'. Again, try out a mild formula first and don't be tempted to wash your face too often as this could do more harm than good.

DRY
You need a gentle soap packed full of moisturising ingredients such as a glycerine soap. They can be enriched with coconut or jojoba oils, or equally effective synthetic moisturisers. Of course, since you rinse the soap off, there will be no long-lasting moisturising effect. Also check out creamy facial washes and cleansing bars. If your skin is very dry, you could just wipe your face with toner or splash it with warm water in the morning, then use soap at the end of the day.

SENSITIVE
If you have sensitive skin, you'll find lots of soaps, facial washes and cleansing bars designed for this. They should contain nothing which is likely to cause irritation or allergy, so will probably be free from perfume or colourants as these are common irritants. Soaps which are pH-balanced are supposed to match the acidity of the skin, so there's less chance of upsetting the delicate balance.

NORMAL/COMBINATION
Shop around and you'll find rinse-off cleansers formulated specifically for your skin type but those formulated for dry/sensitive skins will probably be all right too.

ANY QUESTIONS?

Q I regularly wear quite a lot of make-up. Will soap remove this adequately?

A It should do but some are better at removing make-up than others. You can put it to the test by wiping your skin with cotton wool moistened in skin toner after washing. If there are any make-up stains left behind, you'll need to switch to a different soap, or try a facial wash or cleansing bar. Alternatively, you could pre-cleanse your skin using a special make-up solvent or cleanser, followed by a gentle soap.

Q Can soap be used around your eyes?

A It's best to avoid lathering up close to your eyes since the skin here is very delicate and sensitive. When you rinse off your soap, this will be enough to clean up the area. If you wear eye make-up, you should always use a special eye make-up remover before washing.

Q Are deodorant soaps necessary?

A Not really, providing you wash thoroughly each day and use an anti-perspirant deodorant afterwards, then you should stay sweet-smelling and fresh. Also deodorant soaps contain anti-bacterial ingredients to prevent the breakdown of perspiration which causes BO, and these can irritate some skins.

Q Are bath/shower gels better than soap?

A They usually claim to be kinder to your skin than soap but this isn't always the case. Bath/shower gels are probably more convenient to use, however, soaps tend to be cheaper, and good quality moisturising brands shouldn't do your skin any harm. If you're not allergic to perfume, a highly-scented soap can make bathing a luxurious pleasure, but it is best used on your body rather than your face.

Photographs: SARAH HUTCHINGS/Hair and make-up: KIZZY HARRISON

THE GREASE FACTOR

If you've got greasy skin you probably think it's the bane of your life, but in fact you should think yourself lucky!

There's no denying that greasy skin can cause problems – blackheads, spots, and make-up that goes shiny. But as long as you look after it properly it's a great skin type to have since the oil protects it from drying out. This means you'll get fewer wrinkles as you get older and so stay looking younger.

OIL CHECK

You probably think you know what type of skin you've got, but if you use creams and lotions these can create a false impression. To discover your true skin type, cleanse your face thoroughly last thing at night but don't use any toner or moisturiser. In the morning halve a tissue and press one piece against your forehead. Use the other half for the centre of your face and your cheeks. Hold the tissue halves up to the light and see if there are any traces of oil. If both tissues have oil on them – then you have an overall greasy skin. If the centre tissue is oily but not the cheeks – you have a combination skin. If neither tissue shows signs of oil then your skin is normal or dry and you won't need to read this article!

WHAT CAUSES GREASY SKIN?

Unfortunately greasy skin is usually caused by factors that are beyond your control. The main causes are:

Hereditary factors – if either of your parents has greasy skin, then it's highly likely that your skin will be greasy too.

Hormonal factors – if you have an imbalance of hormones due to puberty, periods or pregnancy.

Whatever the cause, it results in the sebaceous glands producing increased amounts of the skin oil called sebum. If this oil is allowed to build up on your skin it will attract dirt and block pores, leading to the formation of blackheads and spots. This is why it is essential to keep greasy or combination skin scrupulously clean at all times.

GREASY SKIN HAS ONE OR ALL OF THE FOLLOWING:

- An overall shininess.
- A sallow colour.
- A coarse texture.
- Blackheads and spots.
- Less reaction to beauty products.

CLEANSING GREASY SKIN

Since greasy skin tends to attract dirt which can lead to spots it's essential that you keep your skin as clean as possible. However, this doesn't mean using the strongest medicated lotions or the most abrasive face scrubs you can find. Putting these on your skin will only aggravate the situation by degreasing the skin so much that it steps up oil production to compensate. This just leads to a vicious circle.

The most important thing to remember when cleansing greasy skin is that it's done gently, regularly and thoroughly. Try to cleanse your face in the morning and evening and also at lunchtime if your skin is very greasy – it'll make your skin look and feel very much better.

Facial soaps and washes are best for greasy skin and an antibacterial cleanser will help prevent spots. Give your face a two-minute gentle massage while foaming up your cleanser and rinse it off with plenty of lukewarm water. Follow this with splashes of cold water to tone up your skin. If you use a shop-bought toner, choose one that doesn't contain alcohol since this will dehydrate your skin rather than cure the greasiness.

Even greasy skins benefit from a moisturiser. Choose a light lotion or oil-free cream and use it on your skin before you go to bed.

BEAT THE GREASE

- Dilute your toner by using it on cotton wool dampened with a little water.
- Exfoliating scrubs are good for greasy skins so long as you don't get carried away. Choose a scrub with dissolving grains since they are much gentler.
- If you've got greasy skin on your face it's likely that you'll also have oiliness on your back, chest and shoulders. Treat these areas the same way you treat the skin on your face, cleansing regularly with a facial soap or wash.

OIL-FREE COVER

Greasy skins need a bit of extra care when you use make-up.

- For oily/combination skin use an oil-free or water-based foundation to minimise shine (the high powder content in water-based foundations gives a matt finish).
- If your skin is spotty or blemished use a concealer. Dot it onto the areas you want to cover and blend using a brush. Dust with translucent powder to minimise shine.
- Use powder make-up that's less likely to smudge.

GREASY HAIR

Anyone with greasy skin will probably have greasy hair too. As with your skin, wash it as often and as gently as possible. Choose a mild frequent-use shampoo and put conditioner on the ends only.

Illustration: BILL PIGGINS

HOME FACIAL

When your skin's looking sallow and spots are on the verge of breaking out treat yourself to a home facial to get you glowing again!

Sometimes your normal cleansing routine just isn't enough and your skin cries out for some extra loving care. Maybe you've been ill and have more spots than usual, or maybe you want to look your best for a special occasion. Whatever the reason, when you want to pep up your skin, nothing works better than a deep-down cleanse and a little pampering. There's no need to pay for an expensive facial in a salon – doing it yourself at home is quick, cheap and often as effective. The facial won't take you much longer than half an hour but the benefits to your skin last much longer! Your complexion will look instantly clearer and brighter. And with regular facials, you'll help prevent future spots and blemishes by getting rid of the grime before it causes problems. Try to fit a facial into your beauty routine at least once a fortnight if you've normal to dry skin, or once a week if it's oily or prone to spots. Just follow our five-step facial for a fresher looking face!

Step 1

Start the facial by getting your skin scrupulously clean. Tie all your hair back, keep it out of the way with a wide hair band and remove any make-up with your normal cleanser. Then use a facial scrub with tiny abrasive grains to remove dead skin and boost blood circulation. Alternatively, a facial wash with a soft brush, or a gently abrasive sponge will have the same effect. Don't forget to include your neck in this too, especially the often neglected areas behind the ears and around the jaw which are prone to spots.

Helps unclog pores and remove dead, dull, dingy skin. Also peps up the circulation and revitalises your skin making it look clearer and more radiant.

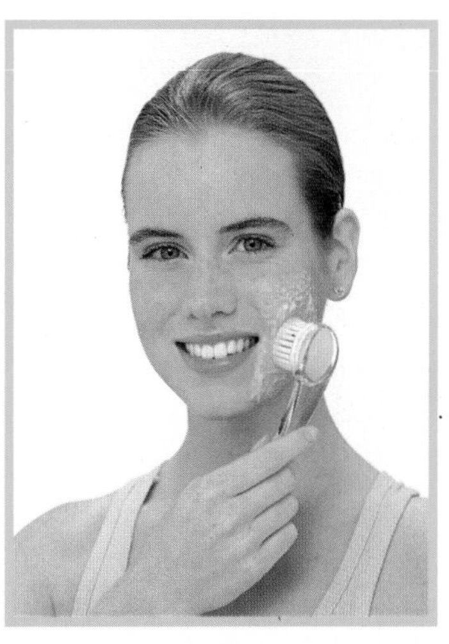

Step 2

Next boil a couple of pints of water and pour this into the sink or large bowl. Add a pinch of dried herbs to make the water fragrant. Some, such as sage and parsley, have antiseptic properties which when released via the steam can help spotty skin. Lean over the bowl and cover this plus your head and the water with a towel – forming a type of 'tent' to trap the steam. Remain like this for 5-10 minutes until the water starts to cool and your pores are open.

Helps the skin to sweat out impurities. Opens the pores and softens blackheads making them easier to remove.

Step 3

Once you've finished steaming, pat your face dry with a towel and stand in front of a mirror with a strong light on your face. With clean hands very gently squeeze any blackheads, working quickly before your skin cools and the pores close. You'll find that the blackheads come out easily after steaming but if they don't, leave them until your next facial. Don't try to force them out as you risk damaging the skin and also you may force the blackhead into becoming an extra unsightly spot.

Helps: Prevent spots that are caused by blocked pores and blackheads. Leaves skin smoother and clearer.

Step 4

Wipe your skin with a freshener or toner, then smooth on

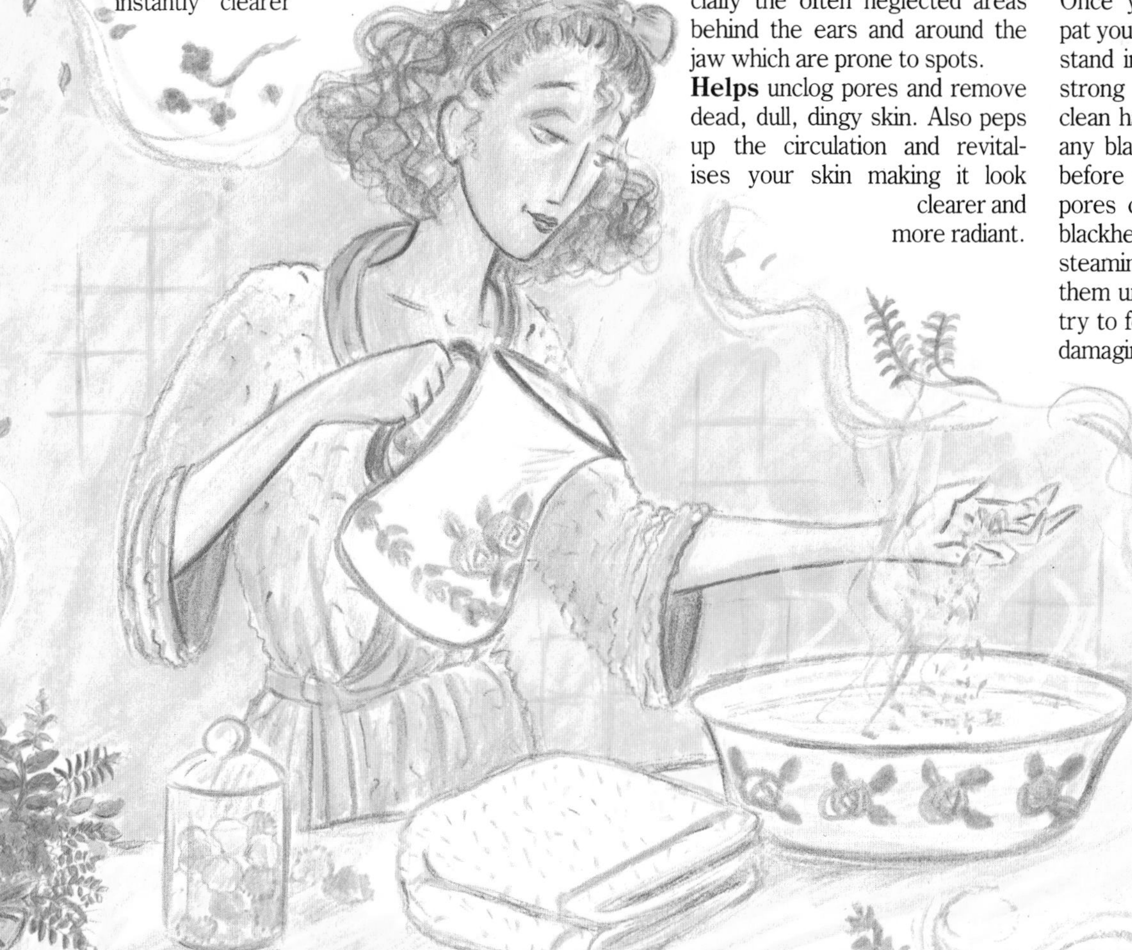

a mask using your fingers or a brush, making sure you get right around the corners of the nose but avoid the delicate eye area. A clay mask is the best for deep cleansing as it draws out impurities from the skin as it dries. On problem areas, leave the mask to dry for five minutes, then apply another layer on top for an ultra-effective treatment. If your skin is sensitive, go for a non-drying plant-based mask. Smooth it on, leave for five minutes, then rinse off with lots of tepid water. Lie down and relax your face muscles while the mask is on. Refresh your eyes too by covering them with cotton wool pads soaked in

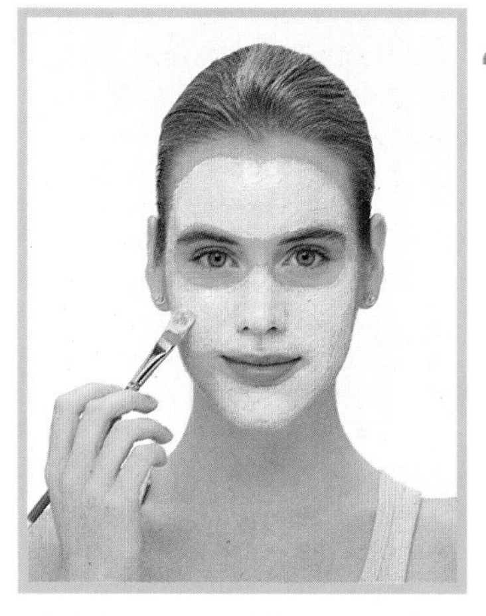

witch-hazel, or cold water with a couple of eyedrops on each one. When the time is up, rinse off the mask with plenty of clean, tepid water, then pat skin dry using a soft towel.

Helps draw out impurities, tightens and tones the skin, and stimulates circulation.

Step 5

Re-hydrate your skin after the facial using a generous amount of moisturiser. Follow the steps for a light face massage to help the moisturiser soak in.

Helps: tone up the muscles of the face; makes the skin more supple and elastic.

Finally . . .

A complete home facial can draw out nasties such as spots, so don't worry if your skin looks a bit worse for a few days before it gets better.

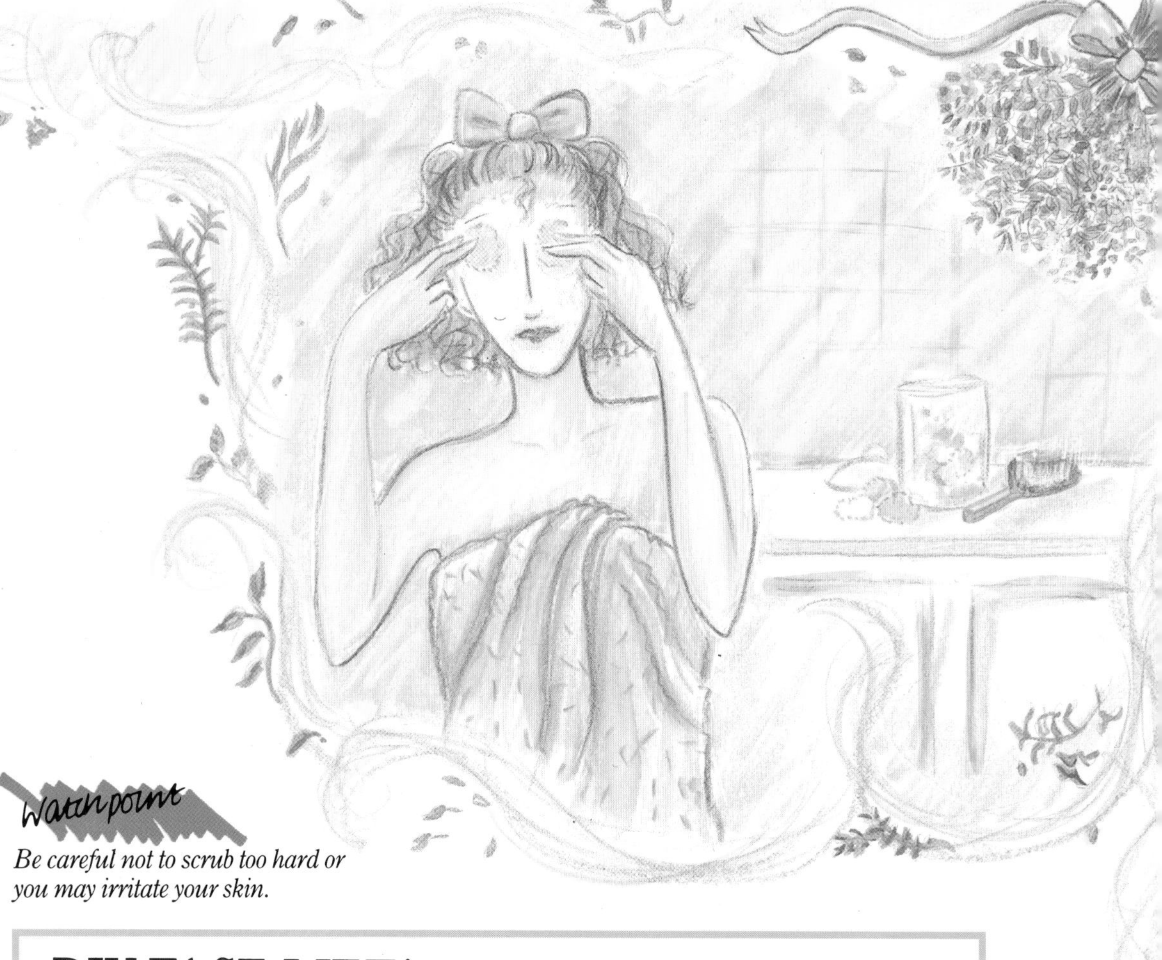

Watchpoint

Be careful not to scrub too hard or you may irritate your skin.

DIY FACE LIFT! *For a firmer face.*

Here's a mini face-lift that's totally painless which you can do yourself at home! Learn the simple moves and you'll have a massage routine that's perfect as part of a facial but it can also be done every day. If you can, do this massage in the evening. Before bed is the best time, as it will also help you wind down. Use a moisturiser as you massage to avoid dragging your skin.

1 Start by smoothing the moisturiser all over your face and neck. Then add a generous blob of moisturiser to the backs of both hands and rub them together. Now place the back of one hand at the base of your neck and stroke firmly up to the jaw, following with the other hand. Repeat all around the neck 25 times. Then starting at the jawline, repeat the move, first up and over one cheek to just under the eyes, then on the other cheek. Repeat 15 times on each side of your face.

Watchpoint

Make sure your fingernails are short so that you don't scratch your skin, and that your hands are scrupulously clean to avoid spreading germs onto your face.

2 Pinch the skin all along the jawline and under the chin very gently using the thumbs and bent forefingers of both hands. This exercise should help to tone up and smooth the skin.

3 Place your fingers flat, together, on either side of your nose. Stroke out firmly along the cheekbones, finishing up in front of the ears. Repeat this about 15 times.

4 Now rest your fingers lightly on the skin just under each eye. Lift gently as you slide the fingers up over the eyes until you reach the eyebrows. Then press several times along the brows and very lightly sweep fingers underneath the eyes. Repeat 10-15 times.

5 Complete the massage with gentle upward and outward stroking movements over the forehead, starting between the eyebrows and finishing at the temples. Repeat this 25 times and your skin should look and feel lovely and smooth.

Tip

When massaging around the delicate eye area, it's a good idea to use your ring finger to ensure the lightest touch.

Photographs: ALISTAIR HUGHES/Hair: ANTOINETTE/Make-up: KAREN LOCKYER
Top: KNICKERBOX/Earrings: H SAMUEL/Illustration: CHERYL TARBUCK

SPOT CHECK

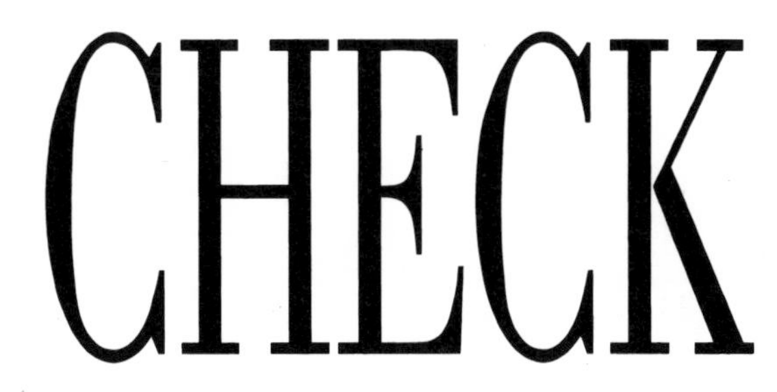

Are you plagued by pimples or having a spot of bother with acne? Help is at hand, so take that paper bag off your head, and find out how you can blitz those zits!

Over 85 percent of people aged between 12 and 25 suffer from spots to some extent – which is great if you're one of the lucky 15 percent, but not so wonderful for the rest! But the good news is that we're learning more and more every day about what causes spots – and how to prevent and cure them.

WHERE SPOTS COME FROM

Sebaceous glands, which make the skin's natural oil, are found under the surface of the skin, particularly on the face, back, shoulders and upper chest. Spots occur when these glands go into overdrive and produce too much oil. Normally, the oil flows out of the narrow openings in the skin called pores. But when there's an excess the pores can become blocked, resulting in blackheads or pimples.

Blackheads are caused by dead skin cells and oils plugging the pores. Pimples occur when oil trapped under the blocked pores seeps into surrounding skin tissue. You can see this activity on the surface of your skin as redness and inflammation when the normally harmless bacteria in your skin get to work and an infection sets in. The white part of a spot is actually made up of sebum, waste and the white blood cells which fight off the infection.

ZAP THOSE ZITS!

If you thought the only effective treatment for spots was a paper bag over your head, think again. Today's spot treatments really do work. Ask your pharmacist to recommend a cream containing benzoyl peroxide. It works by drying up the oil and dissolving the plugs blocking your pores. Benzoyl peroxide can work quickly – you might see an improvement in a matter of days – but it's strong stuff and can leave some skins red, sore and irritated. Follow the label instructions carefully, and don't apply it to large areas of skin.

Other over-the-counter spot treatments work by controlling the bacteria which, when combined with oil, can cause spots. You might also like to try taking zinc supplements – though it hasn't been completely proven, some experts believe this mineral helps reduce skin inflammation and it could work for you.

DESTROYING THE EVIDENCE

The scars left behind after severe acne can be almost as distressing as the spots themselves, but there are several medical treatments which can reduce or even get rid of them, although these are drastic measures used only in serious cases. Collagen injections can be used to plump up pitted scars, while dermabrasion involves removing the top layers of skin to reveal smooth new skin beneath. For deeply pitted scars, there are techniques such as punch excision, where the scar is removed with a small punch-type instrument, and the wound closed with fine stitches. All these techniques must be performed by qualified practitioners, and not all are suitable for every type of scarring. In addition, some skin treatments can have serious side-effects, so it's essential to see your GP who can refer you to a skin specialist at your local hospital.

SPOT THE MYTH

There are probably more myths about spots than about any other beauty problem. Here are the four most common fables:

Spots are caused by dirty skin You can have the cleanest skin in the world, and still develop acne. Kids, no matter how grubby, don't get spots because the hormonal activity that increases sebum production hasn't begun for them.

Chocolate, chips and other greasy foods cause spots There is no evidence to suggest that any food causes spots – but that doesn't mean you can binge on egg and chips or gooey chocs too often! A healthy skin relies on a healthy diet. And it *has* been proven that eating a sensible well-balanced diet with plenty of fresh vegetables and fruit does improve the condition of the skin. As does drinking about 10 glasses of water every day.

Oily skin needs cleansing with strong medicated products Over-enthusiastic, harsh cleansing can make things worse. When the skin is stripped of oil, it may over-compensate and produce even more. Or else you'll make your skin dry, sore and chapped, and even more vulnerable to infection.

Sex causes spots Having or not having sex has no effect on spots – it just seems to for some people because they discover sex just when spots are discovering them!

DO'S AND DON'TS

Very few people go through their teens and early twenties spotlessly, but there are steps you can take to avoid the worst.

DO

- **Use a gentle wash-off cleanser or mild soap on your face morning and night. Try a medicated soap on spotty areas of your body.**
- **Try a very gentle facial scrub once a week to get rid of dead cells – but don't scrub spotty areas or you might spread infection, and stop if your skin becomes irritated or too dry.**
- **Treat yourself to a professional facial to help get rid of blackheads and spots.**
- **Eat a balanced diet and get sufficient amounts of essential vitamins and minerals – vitamins A, B and C are particularly good for the skin.**

DON'T

- **Squeeze, pick or touch your spots – you could cause infection and turn a single blemish into a nasty crop of pustules.**
- **Use heavy moisturisers and foundations – light powder/cream or medicated brands are the best make-up choice.**
- **Wear tight-fitting clothing or let bra straps dig into your skin. Stick to natural fibres so that your skin can breathe.**

Illustration: BILL PIGGINS

THE SPOT-FREE ACTION PLAN

Spots make life a misery. Whether it's hormones or stress that's causing them, we can help

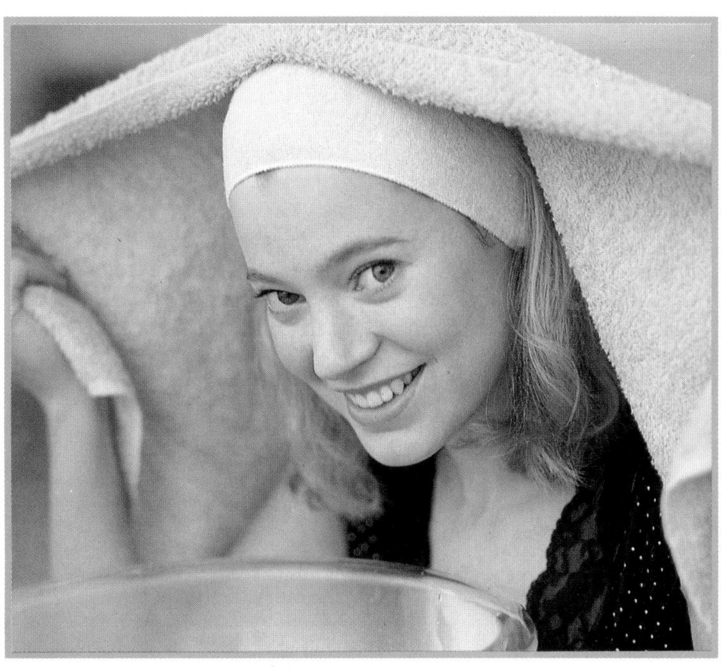

Everyone knows what a spot looks like but not quite so many people know what causes one. In fact a spot is formed when the natural oils (sebum) produced by your skin become trapped inside a pore. This causes swelling and you get a spot. If the spot then becomes infected, the surrounding skin will also turn red and pus may develop. Spots are also largely due to hormone activity within the body. This explains why the problem gets worse around the time of your period, during puberty and pregnancy. These are all times when hormones are in turmoil and it's quite natural that the effects show on the skin.

Stress is another factor that plays an important role in spot development. Have you ever wondered why, on an important day, you wake to find a brand new spot – just when you really didn't want it? This is because your stress levels are higher at such times and these seem to affect the hormones controlling oil production in the skin.

SPOT CHECK

•**Spots** – these pop up in the form of swellings and reddening of the skin caused by infection. Only one pore is involved for each spot. Spots most frequently appear on your forehead, nose and chin where your skin is oiliest.

•**Blackheads** – these are not dirt under the skin, but caused by a blockage of sebum at the surface of the pore. Once the sebum comes into contact with the air it turns darker in colour. If a blackhead becomes infected it will turn into a spot.

•**Whiteheads** – these are not spots that contain pus but tiny rounded lumps under the skin's surface. They are usually found across the upper cheeks and under the eyes. They are caused by cysts in the glands that produce the sebum. Do not be tempted to squeeze whiteheads as you would spots. It's best to seek professional advice and have them removed by a beautician.

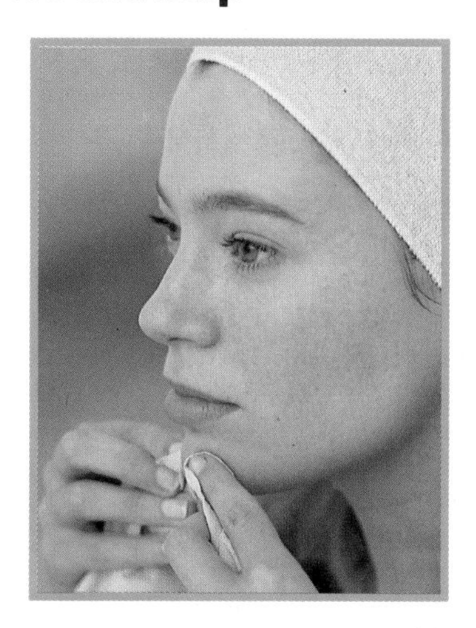

STEAM TREATMENT

Steaming is the best way to prepare your skin for squeezing out a spot or blackhead. Pour some boiling water into a large bowl, tie your hair back, and put a large towel over your head to catch the steam. Keep your face in the steam for the recommended time for your skin type. If you

ANY QUESTIONS?

Q Are spots and acne the same thing?

A Acne, as opposed to the odd eruption, is when you've got lots of spots. It is a very distressing problem and the spots can appear not only on your face and neck, but across your shoulders and over your back and chest as well. It's well worth a visit to your doctor as there are quite a few recommended treatments which are now available, like tetracycline, a form of antibiotic. Many forms of the contraceptive Pill can also help. If your doctor can't advise you, he may decide to refer you to a skin specialist.

Q I've just started wearing make-up. Will I be more prone to spots?

A Wearing make-up doesn't give you spots or make them any worse, providing you clear it off thoroughly at the end of the day. In fact, wearing make-up to help hide spots will probably make you feel a lot better and less self-conscious. If your skin is greasy, choose an oil-free foundation and use powder eye-shadows and blushers rather than cream. If you suffer from spots use a concealer and use loose face powder to help stop skin looking greasy and shiny.

Photographs: LIZ McAULAY/Hair & Make-up: YA'NINA/Top: NEXT

have any broken veins but want to steam your face – do remember to cover the veins with pads of moistened cotton wool to protect them during steaming. Add a pinch of dried herbs to the water for a refreshing smell. The heat opens your pores and increases blood circulation. This method will make the blackheads a lot easier to remove.

To make a spot easier to squeeze, apply a pad of cotton wool soaked in hot water to the spot and hold it there until it cools. This will act as a poultice and help to bring the infection to the surface.

Make sure your fingers and face are clean before you start to squeeze. Wrap your fingers in tissue paper to reduce the risk of spreading the germs to other parts of your face.

When you do squeeze, the most essential thing to remember is to be gentle. Squeezing hard will damage the deeper layers and may result in scarring. If the spot doesn't come out easily, it is obviously not ready and the best thing is to leave it alone for a day or two.

Finally, always tone your face after steaming to close the pores, and no matter how oily your skin is, make sure you use a light moisturiser.

Tip

Spotty skins usually improve during the summer. An occasional short session with a sun-ray lamp may help you in the winter.

COMING CLEAN

Keep your skin clean by cleansing twice a day. Be careful not to overclean or you may strip away the skin's natural bacteria and make it even more prone to outbreaks. To remove the dead cells that can block pores and lead to spots, use an exfoliator.

For best results use the method that's best for your skin type. Follow our guide below:

Tip

Avoid too vigorous scrubbing with facial scrubs – it'll actually stimulate oil production.

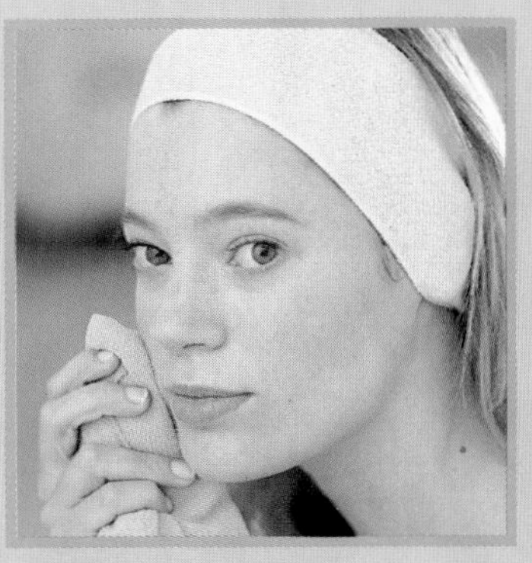

•Sensitive skin: use a clean, damp flannel.

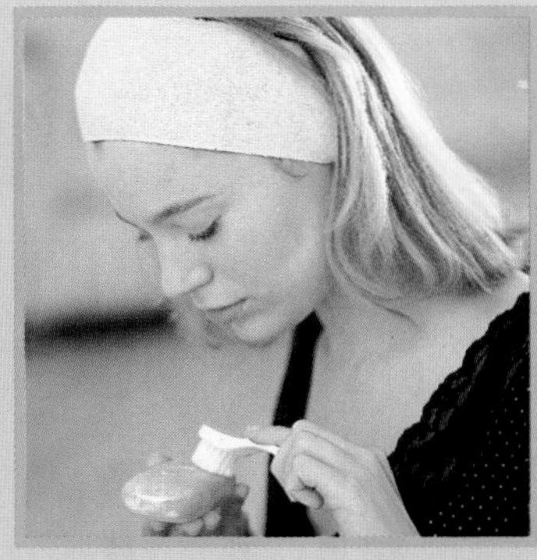

•Dry skin: use a facial brush with soap or cream cleanser.

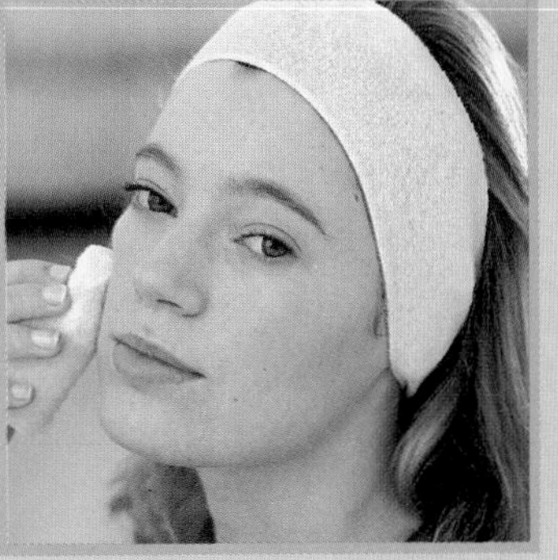

•Combination skin: use a friction sponge for oily parts and a brush for dry.

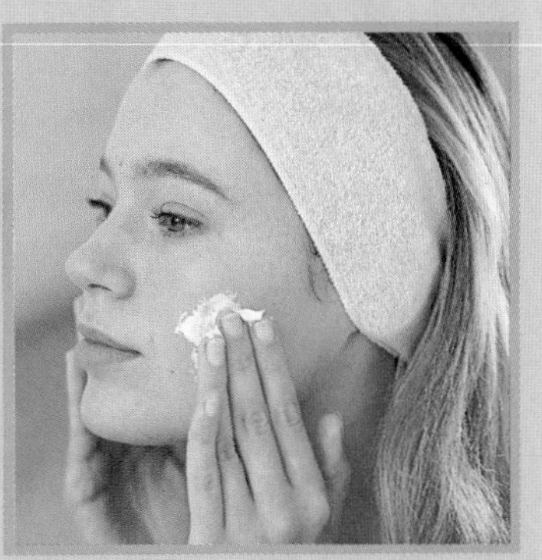

•Oily skin: use a facial scrub or an abrasive sponge.

SKIN TYPE	EXFOLIATION	STEAMING	TONING	MOISTURISING
Oily with frequent spots	Any type of facial scrub with non-dissolving grains	Five to ten minutes	Toner containing alcohol	Non-greasy lotion
Dry	Cream cleanser and a facial brush	Three to five minutes	Toner without alcohol	Rich cream
Sensitive	Cream cleanser or facial soap using a flannel	Not recommended	Mild toner such as rosewater lotions	Hypo-allergenic formulation
Combination with oily centre panel and normal/dry cheeks	Any type of facial scrub with dissolving grains	Five minutes – use moisturiser to protect drier areas	Toner containing alcohol for centre panel – diluted with water for cheeks	Non-greasy lotion with cream on dry patches

HIDE THAT SPOT

If you have a spot and don't want the rest of the world to know, use a concealer to cover it up. It's essential that the concealer matches your skin colour exactly, so try it out on the inside of your arm before you buy. If it's too light or too dark, your spot will be more noticeable than if you hadn't used it in the first place.

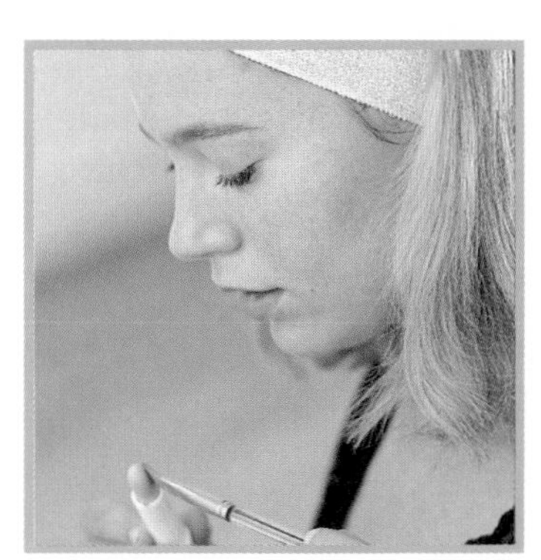

1 *Use a brush to apply your concealer, it's more hygienic than putting it straight onto your skin. Remember to wash your brush after use too.*

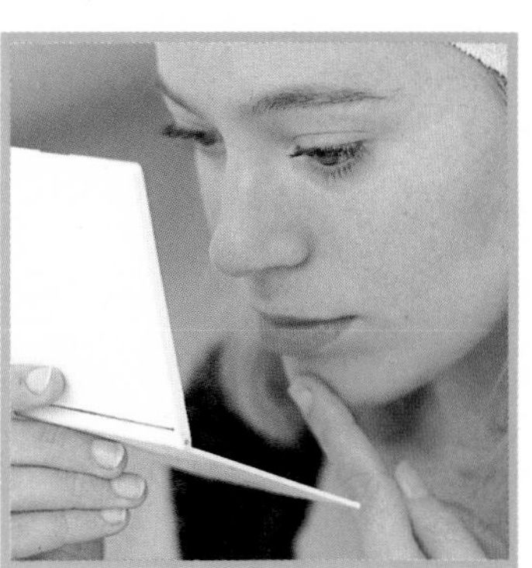

2 *Use a clean finger to blend in the edges. As you blend, only touch the area around the spot, not the spot itself.*

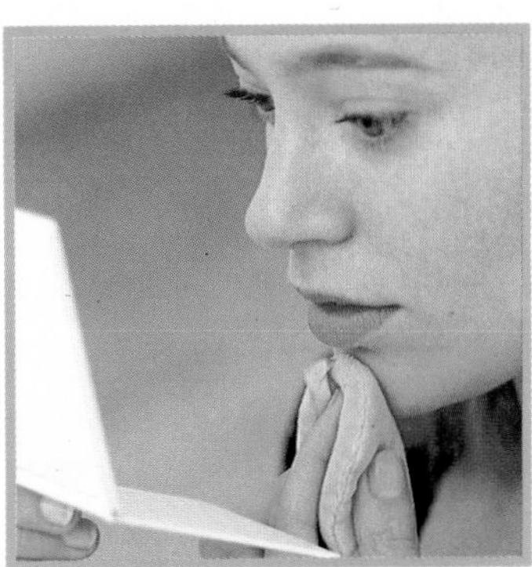

3 *When you have blended the edges until you can't see them, set with a little dab of loose powder. This will also help prevent breakthrough shine.*

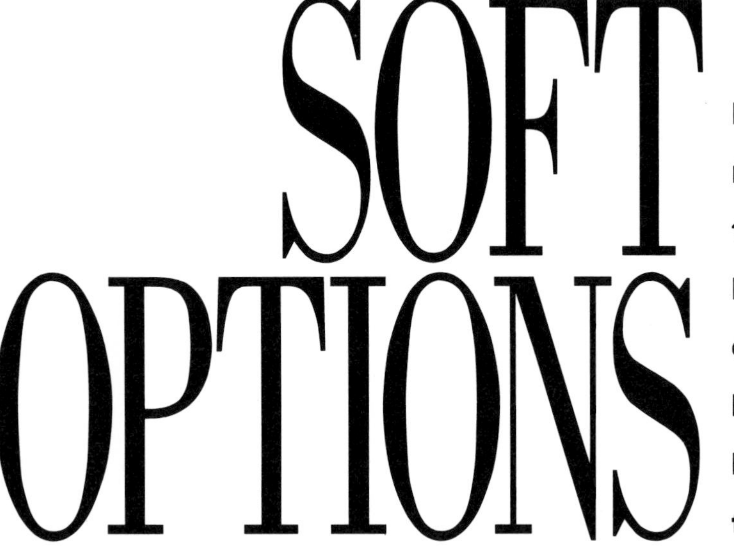

SOFT OPTIONS

Moisturiser is a must if you want your skin to be a soft touch. Make it part of your daily routine and keep your skin looking younger – for longer!

Come rain or shine, your face is under attack from the elements. And the only real protection you can give it is moisturiser, make-up or a sunscreen. Moisturiser is your first line of defence. It is by far the most popular skincare product – and the easiest to use.

Moisture plays an important role in keeping your skin looking young. As a child your skin has almost double the amount of moisture as when you're an adult, which is why moisturiser is a must as you get older.

But don't expect a moisturiser to work miracles – it won't be able to turn back the clock. To understand its limitations it will help to know a little about how your skin actually works.

Tip

If your moisturiser still hasn't been absorbed after a few minutes, dab off any excess with a tissue.

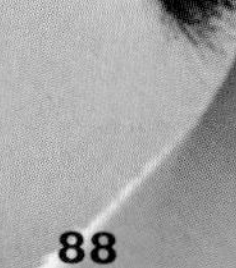

SKIN DEEP

Your skin helps to regulate your temperature and protects your body from harmful bacteria and the environment.

Like the rest of your body, your face is covered with an outer layer of skin which is actually dead. This outer layer is almost impossible to penetrate except by cuts or injury so forget those claims on some of the more expensive creams!

Your skin is made up of about 15 per cent water and is constantly losing moisture. Sebaceous glands continually secrete oil, or sebum, which mixes with sweat to form a protective film.

Harsh soaps, detergents, the weather and central heating can affect this protective film, as well as illness or poor diet. And once you hit your twenties your skin's oil production starts to slow down which is great if you suffer from acne, but not if your skin is normal or already dry!

HOW IT WORKS

Moisturiser helps keep your skin supple by forming a protective

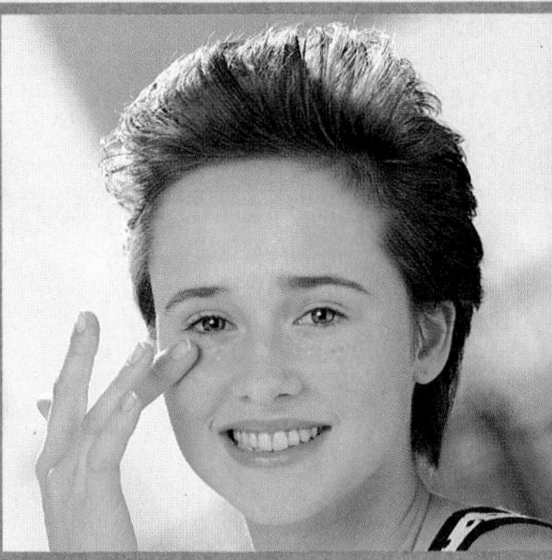

EYE OPENERS

The skin around your eyes is very thin and tends to wrinkle easily into fine lines, often called crow's feet.

Eye moisturisers are very light creams or gels which contain very fine oils. This area can go puffy if a cream is too heavy or oily. Start with a gel to refresh your eyes in the morning and graduate to a cream last thing at night to help nourish them.

Go gently! Use your ring finger and dot tiny amounts of moisturiser under your film on the surface to keep moisture in. It also adds moisture, which helps plump up the top layer of skin cells, making fine lines less apparent. As an extra bonus the smoothing action of putting on moisturiser stimulates circulation which can help speed up skin cell renewal and keep your skin looking younger.

SPOILT FOR CHOICE?

All skins, except very oily and acne-troubled, need a light daily moisturiser. To find out which one is right for you, it's important to know your skin type.

● **Normal skin:** If this is your skin type, then lucky you! It's not too dry or oily and needs minimum care to keep it looking good. Try an oil-in-water moisturiser with a light texture.

● **Dry skin:** If your skin feels tight and uncomfortable after cleansing then it's dry. You'll need a heavier, water-in-oil moisturiser. These are generally creamier and contain more oil.

● **Oily skin:** You know when your skin's oily – make-up just seems to slide off! And within half an hour of cleansing, you notice that familiar sheen of oil. Unless your skin is exceptionally oily, you'll still need extra moisture. Look out for oil-free or non-comedogenic moisturisers which don't contain ingredients that block the pores so are less likely to cause spots or blackheads.

● **Combination skin:** This is the most common skin type. It means an oily 'T-zone', the centre panel of your face, combined with dry cheeks. You may need to use two moisturisers – an oil-free one for the T-zone and a water-in-oil formula for your cheeks.

● **Sensitive skin:** Over 40 per cent of us think we've got sensitive skin. Search out hypo-allergenic moisturisers which match your skin type. These contain the minimum of ingredients and avoid allergens.

WHAT'S IT MADE OF?

Most ingredients aren't stated on the label. More expensive products do contain more sophisticated ingredients, but this doesn't necessarily mean they will perform any better.

● Lanolin used to be the most common ingredient in moisturiser and comes from the oil in sheep's wool. It is still often used but it can irritate sensitive skin.

● Petroleum jelly is included in some heavier creams.

● Cocoa butter is made from cocoa seeds and is particularly good as a skin softener.

● Aloe vera comes from a cactus-like plant. It heals, soothes and can stimulate circulation.

● Jojoba comes from the beans of a plant and is especially good for sensitive skins.

● Evening primrose oil soothes and revitalises the skin. It's also good for eczema and dry skin.

● Vitamins are often used. Vitamin A can relieve dry skin. Vitamin E is good for burns and is known as the 'anti-ageing' vitamin because it helps neutralise the effects of pollution. Vitamin F helps smooth the outer skin cells.

PUTTING IT ON

Always apply moisturiser first thing in the morning and last thing at night, after cleansing. Dot small blobs on your forehead, cheeks, nose and chin and smooth upwards in light movements.

Give it a few minutes to sink in before you put on foundation – or it may just slip off!

NIGHT, NIGHT

Night creams are just another type of moisturiser. They're usually heavier than day formulations and are designed to help skin regenerate, rather than just protect it. Unless you think your skin needs an extra boost, you can use an ordinary moisturiser all the time and leave night creams until your late twenties.

BODY BASICS

The rest of your body needs moisture too! And don't neglect your skin during winter just because it's covered up.

Body moisturisers contain the same ingredients as those for your face, but are usually in a slightly heavier formulation because your body doesn't have as many oil glands as your face. They are often strongly perfumed so it's best not to use them on your face as they may irritate your skin.

Put on body lotion after a bath when your skin is warm and slightly damp. Smooth it on with strong upward movements to get your circulation moving.

Your skin takes 21 to 28 days to renew itself, so you can't truly see whether a moisturiser is effective for about a month.

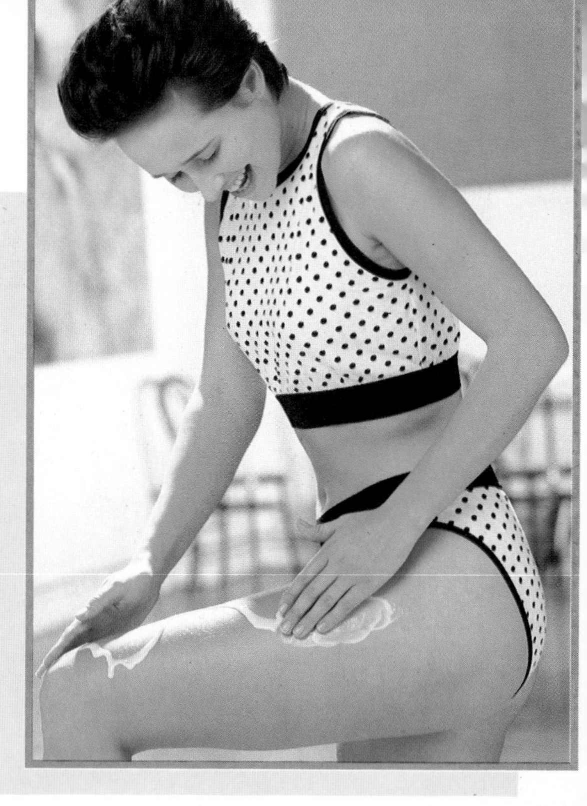

eyes and above your eye crease. Don't pull the skin, tap it gently until the product sinks in.

NECK NEXT

It's easy to forget your neck, but the skin here is quite dry and can go very wrinkly when you get older. You can buy specially enriched throat creams, but your usual moisturiser is good enough – as long as you remember to include your neck!

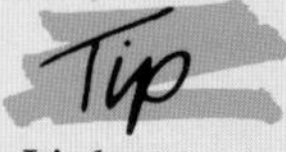

It's best to start moisturising when you're in your late teens and even younger if your skin is dry.

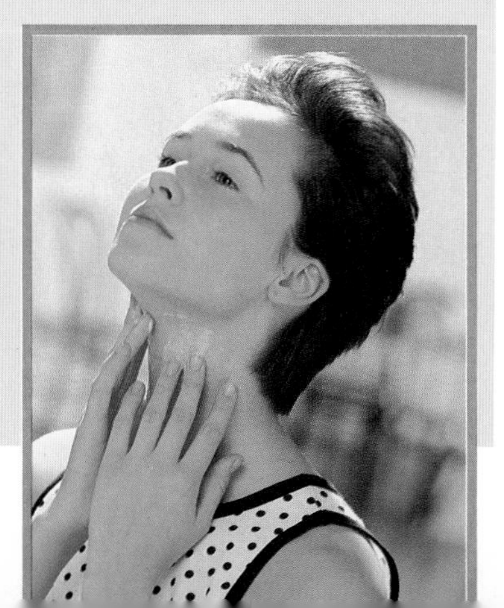

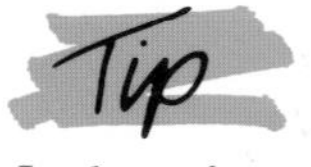

Look out for a moisturiser that contains UV filters to protect your skin from the damaging effects of the sun. But don't use it instead of a sunscreen.

HOLDING BACK THE YEARS

Moisturisers will definitely make your skin look and feel good and can help prevent premature ageing. What they can't do is actually get rid of wrinkles, despite the claims of many manufacturers!

Your other most important weapon in the wrinkle-war is being really sensible about sunbathing.

Too much sun on unprotected skin will give you wrinkles and make you look old before your time. So when you're out in the sun always use a sunscreen.

A high protection sunscreen is one product you can't start to use too early – 70 per cent of sun damage is caused during childhood.

Most suncare ranges now include a product specially developed for the face. These are lighter, perfume-free and less likely to cause irritation and spots than sun creams for the rest of your body.

Photographs: ALISTAIR HUGHES/Hair and make-up: YA'NINA/Lingerie: MARY QUANT

SUPER NATURALS

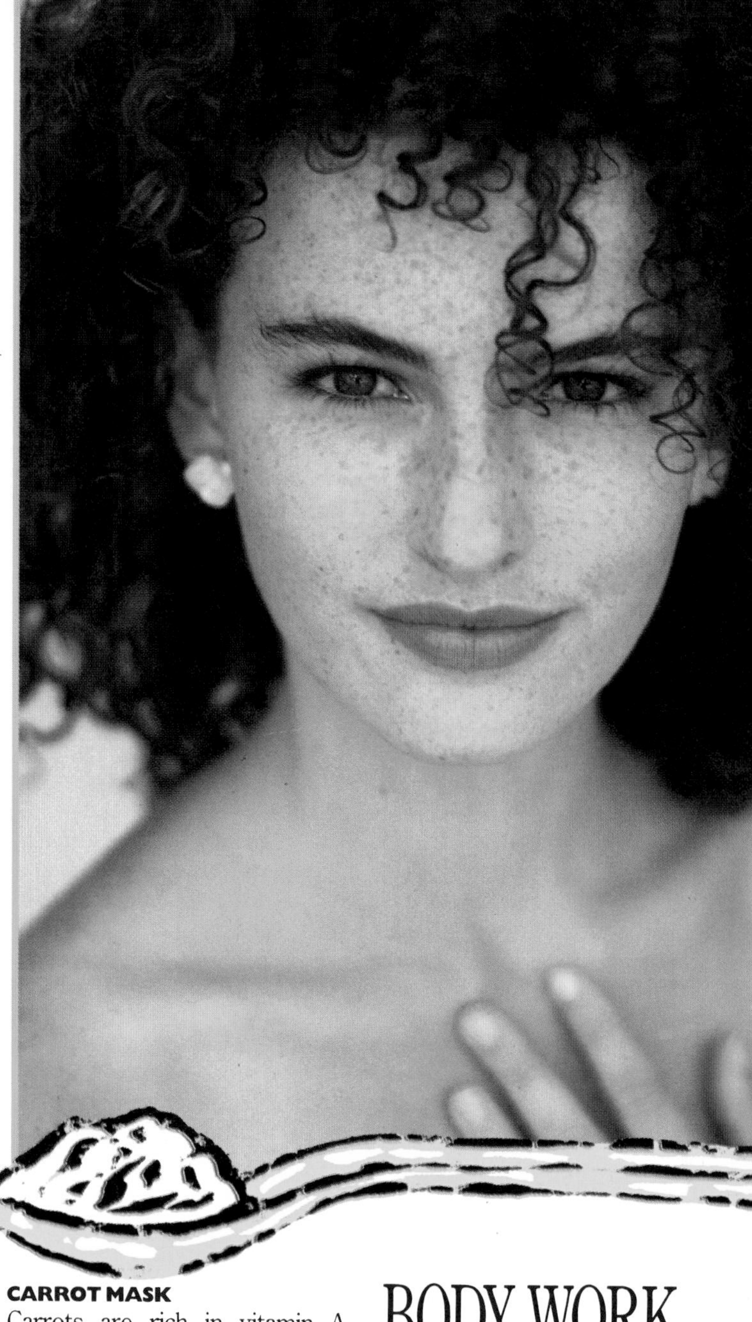

Try our down to earth, top-to-toe beauty treats for out of this world good looks from the fridge and larder

Nature's goodies have been used for centuries to put a shine on hair and a glow in your cheeks. At a fraction of the cost of expensive beauty products you can raid the larder to solve many of your beauty problems.

Milk, for instance, will help to soothe dry skin; egg whites tighten open pores and a puréed carrot mask will work wonders for even the most troubled complexion.

But remember, unlike manufactured products, they won't have any preservatives so you'll be better off only making up small quantities and storing perishable items in glass jars with screw-top lids in the fridge till you've used them all up.

FEED YOUR FACE

ZIPPY LEMON CLEANSER

Lemon juice used either on its own or mixed with other ingredients makes a powerful antiseptic cleanser for oily skins.

Ingredients:
1 lemon
1 egg white

Squeeze the juice out of the lemon and strain to get rid of pips and pith. Whip up the egg white until frothy and heat with the juice in a saucepan until the mixture thickens. Allow to cool then smooth over face. Leave for a few minutes and remove with damp cotton wool.

CARROT MASK

Carrots are rich in vitamin A which is useful for treating all kinds of skin problems and allergies. Mix up and use this soothing face mask.

Ingredients:
2 large carrots
1 tsp honey

Purée raw carrots in a food processor or cook them and mash through a sieve. Warm the honey until runny then mix with the carrots. Smooth over damp skin for five to 10 minutes then wash off with cool water.

BODY WORK

SUGARY SCRUB

Buff up body skin with a nifty scrub which helps slough off dead cells and leaves skin gleaming!

Ingredients:
1 cup granulated sugar
2 tsp vegetable oil

Mix sugar with oil to make a light paste. Massage it over your body paying attention to dry areas like elbows, knees and thighs. Rinse off with cool water and moisturise with body lotion.

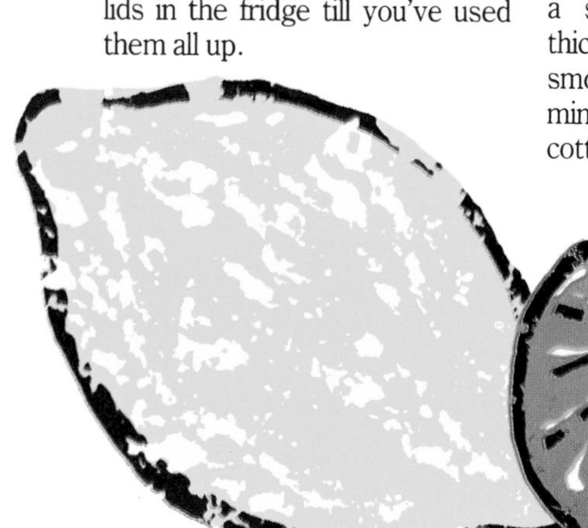

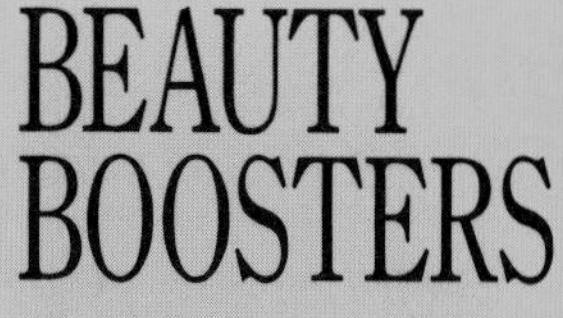

HONEY BATH SOAK

Honey makes a great skin soother and milk acts as a perfect moisturiser. Try this bath when you're in need of a boost!

Ingredients:

600 ml/1 pt boiling water
100 g/4 oz honey
600 ml/1 pt milk
4 tbls salt

Pour half the boiling water into a pan with the honey, stirring well to dissolve. Add the milk and whisk well, dissolve the salt in the rest of the water and pour into a saucepan. Stand up in a bath of warm water and rub some of the liquid over your body. Leave it on for a few minutes then pour the rest of the liquid into the bath and relax for 15 minutes.

ROSE LOTION

This is a great dry skin treat.

Ingredients:

6 tbls rosewater
2 tbls glycerine

Mix and massage into skin.

HAIR TONICS

FRUITY HAIR RINSE

This tingling hair rinse helps put a shine on lack-lustre locks. It also controls any oily build-up.

Ingredients:

1 orange
1 apple
1 small slice of melon
1.2 l/2 pt water
600 ml/1 pt cider vinegar

Peel and slice the orange, apple and melon. Put both the fruit and peel in a pan with the water. Bring to the boil, cover and simmer for 10 minutes. Take off the heat and let it stand for one hour. Strain well and add the cider vinegar. Bottle and leave for 24 hours before using as a rinse.

YOGHURT AND EGG SHINE

Flyaway hair needs the right kind of conditioner to help reduce static and give it sheen. Use this recipe once a week.

Ingredients:

6 tbls natural yoghurt
1 egg

Whisk yoghurt and egg together in a bowl until well blended. Massage evenly into the scalp and hair for four minutes. Wrap the hair in a warm towel and leave for 10-15 minutes before rinsing the hair thoroughly.

COCONUT COCKTAIL

A nourishing, penetrating treat for dry or damaged hair.

Ingredients:

1 tsp honey
2 tsp coconut oil

Mix ingredients together and massage into your scalp. Leave on for 10 minutes, then rinse out and shampoo your hair.

HANDS UP

OATY HAND CLEANSER

Whiten and soften rough hands with this simple cleanser.

Ingredients:

2 tbls oatmeal
2 tbls milk

Pour a few of the oats into the palm of one hand. Add just enough milk to moisten and rub over hands. Then rinse off and repeat. Leftover porridge can also be used as a hand cream.

FIVE-HERB FOOT MIX

Treat tired, aching feet to this soothing foot bath.

Ingredients:

5 tbls dried marjoram
7 tbls dried mint
3 tbls dried thyme
1 tsp dried mustard
4 tbls dried rosemary
1.2 l/2 pt boiling water

Put the herbs in a saucepan then pour in boiling water. Cover and simmer over a low heat for five minutes. Remove from heat and leave to stand for 20 minutes. Strain and soak feet for 15 minutes.

BEAUTY BOOSTERS

Zap those trouble spots with these natural remedies.

- **Tired, dry elbows? Slice a lemon in half and place one elbow in each for five minutes to help whiten and soften skin.**
- **Swap your usual shaving cream or soap for sesame, sunflower or peanut oil – your legs will be silky smooth after shaving.**
- **Brew a cup of extra-strong black coffee and use as a shine-boosting finishing rinse for dark hair.**
- **Pour a cup of dried skimmed milk into warm bath water for silky soft skin.**
- **Strain cold tea and use as an instant leg stain or to liven up a fading tan.**
- **Rub the inside of pineapple skin over face as a skin-tingling tonic.**
- **Take a handful of chopped mixed nuts and gently massage them all over face to get rid of dead skin cells. Then rinse off and pat face dry.**
- **Soothe an itchy gnat bite by rubbing it with a clove of fresh garlic – a great antiseptic healer.**
- **Blend an egg yolk with a blob of ordinary conditioner to make a nourishing treatment for dry or damaged hair.**

Illustrations: DAVID CARTER

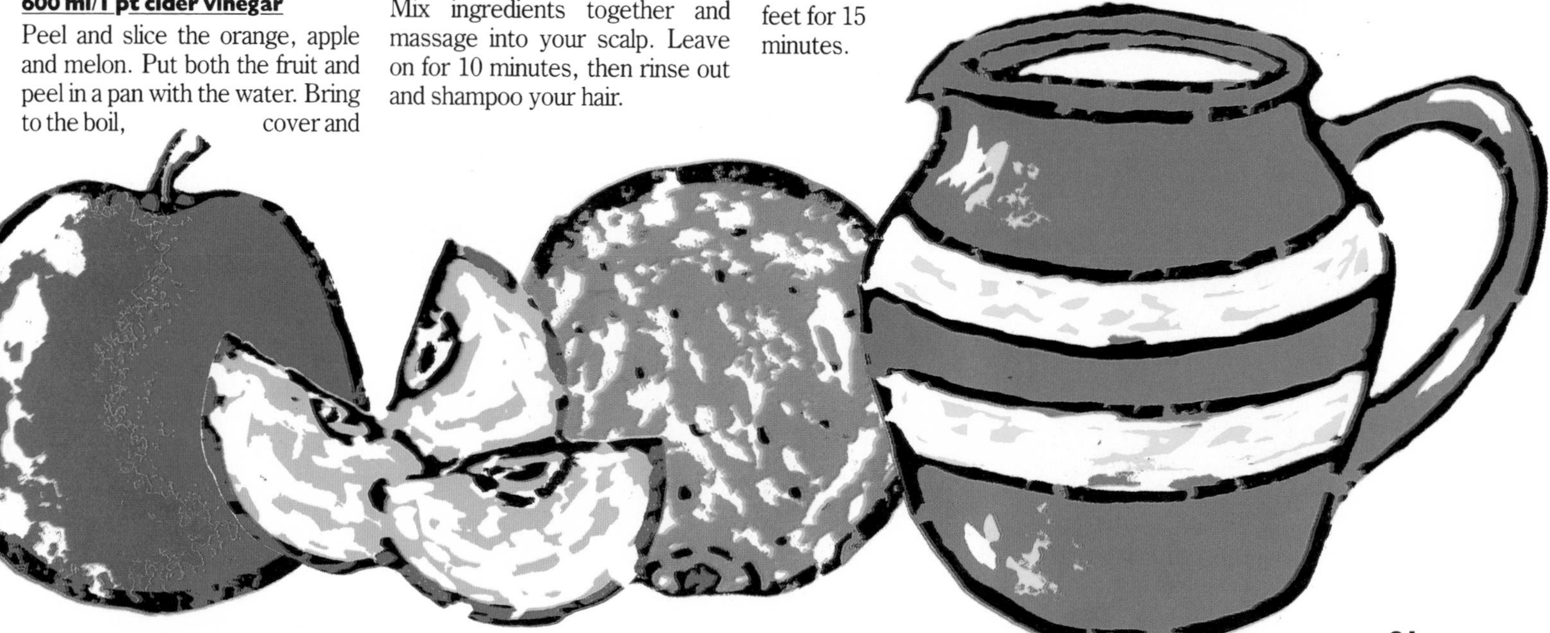

NECKS

Even if you're up to your neck in skincare creams, does your beauty routine ever venture below chin level? If your neck is dull, dingy, lined or neglected, follow our neck-care know-how

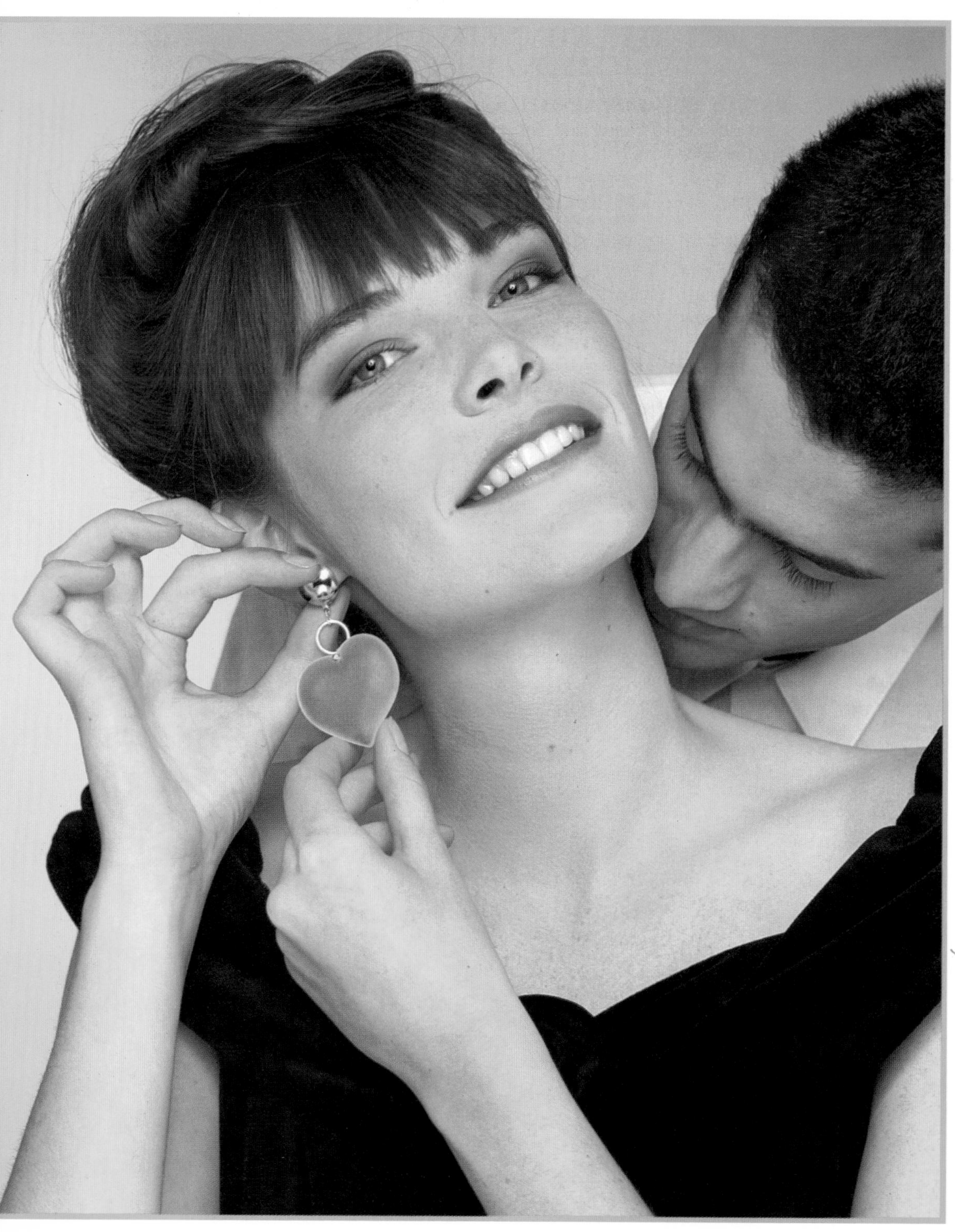

The neck can certainly show signs of ageing sooner than any other feature – and this isn't surprising when you think of how many times your neck moves, how exposed it is to the elements which contribute to ageing, and how little care and attention you probably give it.

To look good, your neck needs to be pampered as much as your face. Every cleansing session should include the neck and it must be moisturised regularly, too. In cold weather, extra applications of an emollient cream – both before *and* after outdoor exposure – will help to protect your skin and to recover from the drying effects it has faced. In hot weather, your neck needs a different kind of protection.

Exposure to strong sunlight is known to trigger the formation of early lines and wrinkles, so a sunscreen must be applied, to shield your skin. Be sure to extend this protection down on to your chest, too – that triangle of skin which few clothes cover, even in winter, gets more than its share of sun. And the effects soon show – you'll see a grainy texture, criss-crossed with fine lines. Be sure to apply a good aftersun lotion to rehydrate the skin and soothe any soreness.

Necks don't always come as clean as they could and this means marks on collars and necklines. As well as cleansing regularly, a deep cleansing treatment will help remove dirt and dead skin cells; try a gentle exfoliating scrub, applied to already-damp skin to prevent reddening and soreness. Or use a face mask, which will both cleanse and exfoliate, leaving skin softer and smoother. Remember to reach around to the back of your neck and ears, too!

PLEASE

NECKLINES

● If jewellery tends to leave ugly black marks on your neck, go without it on particularly humid days. Enamel, pearls and beads tend not to mark the skin as much as silver, gold or nickel.
● Long hair can make the back of your neck sweat, and that may mark clothes. Use a roll-on anti-perspirant if this is your particular problem.
● Make-up should stop where your neck starts. Take foundation just over the jawline. If the contrast in colour between neck and face is too obvious, you're wearing the wrong colour foundation and need a shade closer to your skin's own tone.
● Dabbing neat perfume straight onto your neck can cause sun damage or irritation to your skin if the fragrance contains light-sensitive ingredients – and many do. Wear it on pulse points – wrists, inside elbows, behind knees – or shake a few drops on to a cotton wool pad and tuck it into your bra instead to help save your skin!

SMOOTH IT!

The texture of the skin on your neck may not be as smooth as you'd like. Moisturising will help to keep it supple, which in turn will soften and minimise the appearance of ageing lines. But a more intensive treatment can help, too – try this simple routine once each week and see the difference it makes:
● First wash your neck well with warm soapy water, and rinse thoroughly.
● Next, wipe over with a cotton wool pad soaked in your favourite skin toner.
● Wet a small towel in warm water, wring out, then wrap it around your neck for 2-3 minutes and relax.
● Remove the towel and quickly rub in a rich moisturising cream.
● After you've left this to soak in for 20 minutes, wipe away any excess.

Prone to a spotty neck? Try using a medicated skin wash, regularly once a week, to help dry them up.

UP OR DOWN?

Not all the beauty experts agree on the right way to apply creams or lotions to the neck.

Some say *upward* strokes will fight the natural tendency of ageing skin to sag downwards; others are positive that, as the skin is going to pull down anyway, due to gravity, creams and lotions should be applied with firm downward strokes, too.

It's probably best to avoid strong, firm strokes in either direction, since they will simply subject your skin to *more* movement.

Apply moisturising creams and lotions with a light patting action instead. This will get them onto the skin, where they're needed – and don't kid yourself that as strong a force as gravity can be deflected with fingertip movements!

Always use cotton wool or soft tissues to apply and remove your cleanser.

When you're concentrating on your posture don't forget your neck and chin. Your chin should be parallel to the floor and tucked back – not jutting forward. Now you're well ahead!

These three easy exercises will help your neck muscles to keep their tone and elasticity:

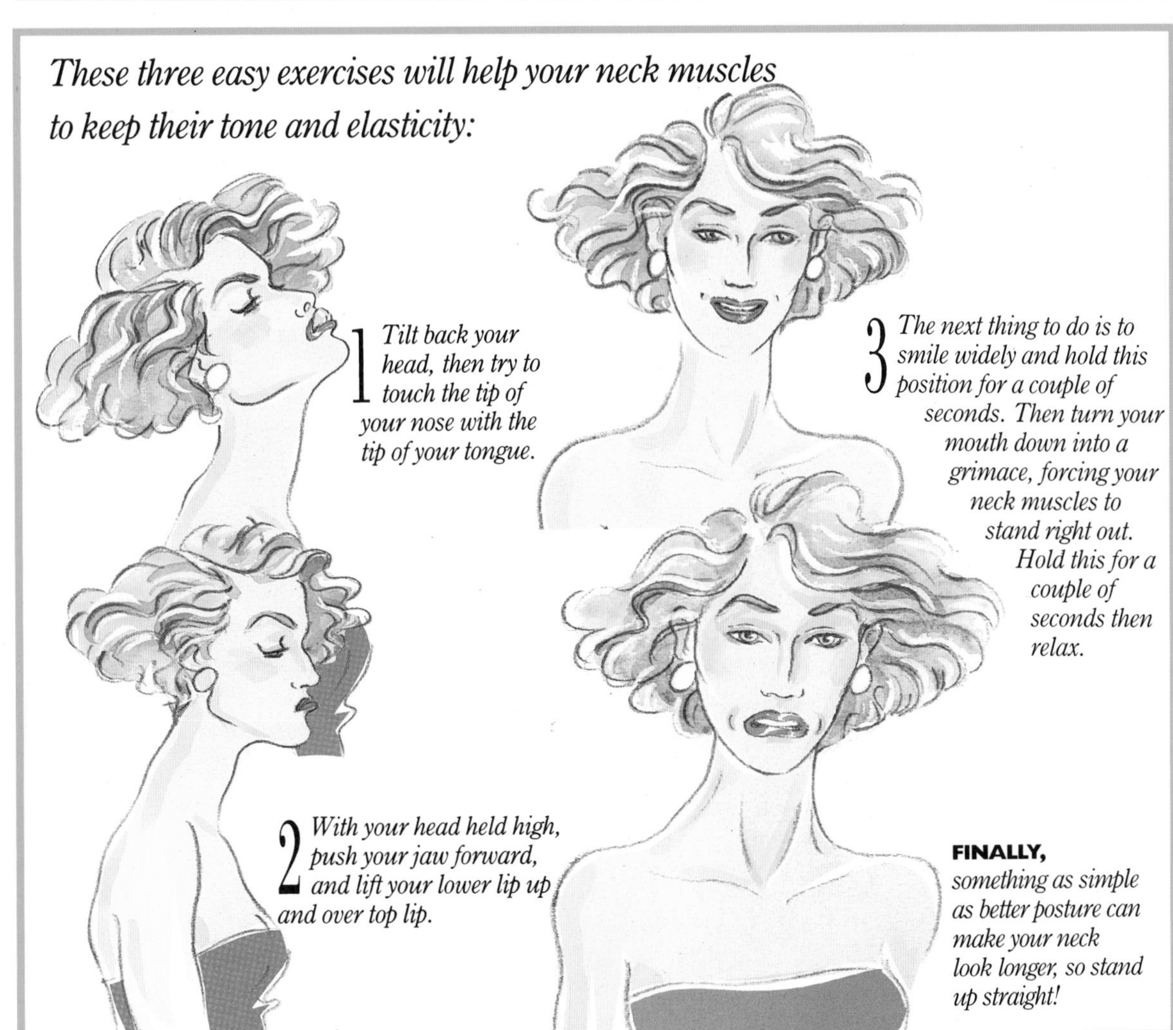

1 *Tilt back your head, then try to touch the tip of your nose with the tip of your tongue.*

2 *With your head held high, push your jaw forward, and lift your lower lip up and over top lip.*

3 *The next thing to do is to smile widely and hold this position for a couple of seconds. Then turn your mouth down into a grimace, forcing your neck muscles to stand right out. Hold this for a couple of seconds then relax.*

FINALLY, *something as simple as better posture can make your neck look longer, so stand up straight!*

Photograph: ADRIAN BRADBURY/Hair: PAULA MANN Make-up: KAREN LOCKYER/Dress: FREEMANS/Earrings: $AM UBHI/Illustrations: TERRY EVANS

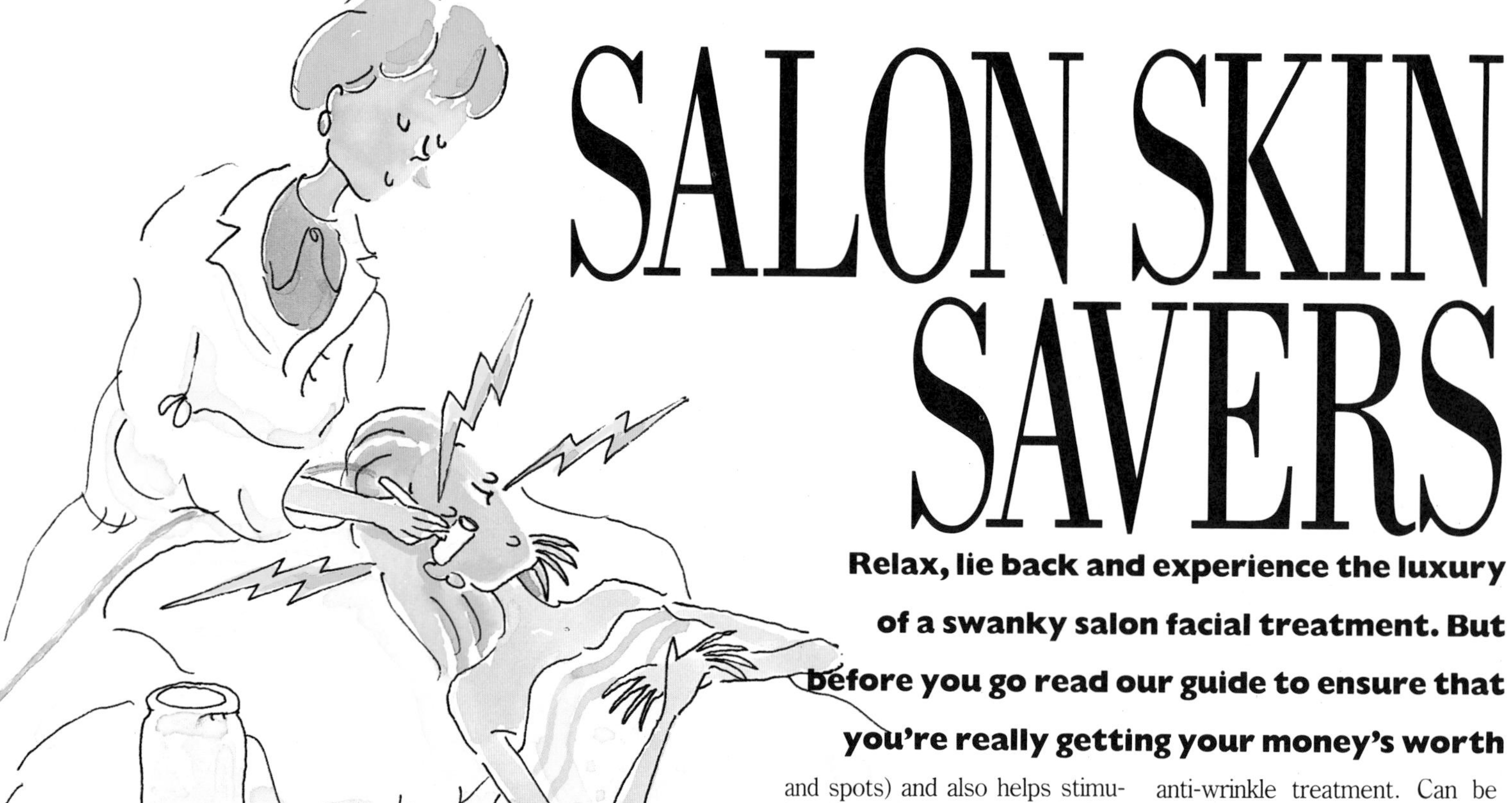

SALON SKIN SAVERS

Relax, lie back and experience the luxury of a swanky salon facial treatment. But before you go read our guide to ensure that you're really getting your money's worth

Having a facial in a beauty salon isn't just a luxury and a pleasure. It has a practical purpose too, supplementing your usual daily skin care routine with the type of deep cleansing, intensive moisturising and massage only a professional can offer.

Using high-tech gadgets and a multitude of special salon-only products, a facial could be just the boost your skin needs. And the more troublesome your skin is – whether you suffer from spots, excessive dryness or oiliness – the more it will benefit from the additional attention.

WHO NEEDS THEM?

Everyone can benefit from a professional facial no matter what your age or skin type. A deep cleansing facial is especially beneficial for younger skins as it is an effective means of helping to control a troublesome complexion. (However, if you have acne it is advisable to consult your doctor who may recommend you see a dermatologist first for specialist treatment). For older skins, (age 30-plus) moisturising facials smooth and soften the skin.

Professional treatments can be expensive, so it's worth remembering that you can save yourself considerable expense if you treat yourself to a facial at home.

PARIS MASSAGE FACIAL

The basis of this treatment is the dual-action massage used in the application of all products. It helps what is known as lymphatic drainage (or cleansing the skin of the toxins which can cause puffiness and spots) and also helps stimulate blood circulation (which gives you a rosy glow and boosts all natural skin functions).
Recommended: Monthly for all skin-types and ages. Weekly for problem skins.

CATHIODERMIE

A treatment which uses two kinds of electric currents which have a combined deep cleansing, rehydrating and stimulating effect. First a gel is applied to your skin to help the electric current work more efficiently, then a treatment gel is applied to suit your skin type. This may include camphor to check sebum or oil production, for instance, or soothing orange blossom for dry skin. The current is then applied through special rollers which glide smoothly over the gels activating the special ingredients in them.

The gel is removed, blackheads are carefully extracted and then a cream and a second high-frequency current is used which has an antibacterial effect, warms the skin and helps stimulate cell renewal. A massage and moisturiser complete the treatment – which takes around 75-90 minutes. Because of the electric current used, you shouldn't have Cathiodermie treatment if you suffer from epilepsy.
Recommended: As a monthly treatment for problem skins, such as acne, or for ageing skins as an anti-wrinkle treatment. Can be adapted for use as a treatment for spotty backs, or as a neck or bust treatment to tighten and firm-up the skin.

COLLAGEN FACIAL

Most of the products in this facial contain collagen, a protein found in the skin which helps maintain its suppleness. A pure collagen mask is said to stimulate the production of natural collagen in your own skin. Critics say that collagen molecules are too large to penetrate and reach your natural collagen levels but there's no denying its softening effect. The immediate result is that of a plumper, less-lined complexion.
Recommended: Regular six-weekly treatments have a cumulative effect. Best for the over 30s. Not suitable for very sensitive or oily skins.

MUD FACIALS

There are many types of mud used: Dead Sea mud from Israel, Le Moor, derived from rotting vegetation from the banks of the River Danube and Parafango, volcanic mud from the lakes of Padua in Italy. Mud is rich in minerals and treatments have been found very beneficial for eczema and psoriasis sufferers, as well as for acne.
Recommended: Once a week for particular skin problems or as an occasional pep-up treatment.

FACE FACTS

DO

- **Have a salon facial regularly to reap the full benefits.**
- **Book a course of treatments to save money.**
- **Be inquisitive! Find out why the therapist is using each product. The price of a treatment includes as much skin care advice as you want. So ask exactly what's going on and then you might be able to use some of the same steps in a home facial.**

DON'T

- **Go back to using products that are too astringent or oily for your skin type. Your therapist can advise you.**
- **Apply a thick layer of make-up immediately afterwards – let your skin rest overnight.**

Illustration: BILL PIGGINS

SOAK OPERA

Linger a little longer in your bath tub at least once a week and just soak up our top-to-toe beauty treatments

There's nothing like a lovely luxurious bath to soak away the stresses and strains of the day. It relaxes the muscles, eases tension and is a good excuse to lock yourself away for 30 minutes of pure indulgence. The bath is also the best place to catch up on all those little beauty chores that can often get neglected in a busy schedule. From smoothing away rough skin to tidying up your nails, get busy in the bath and you'll emerge feeling and looking great.

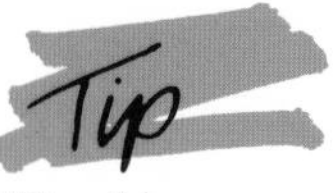

The skin on your face and neck is very delicate, so use a soft, wet complexion brush to clean away dirt and dead skin. Coat the bristles with unperfumed soap or a special cleansing bar, then work up a lather over your face with gentle circular movements.

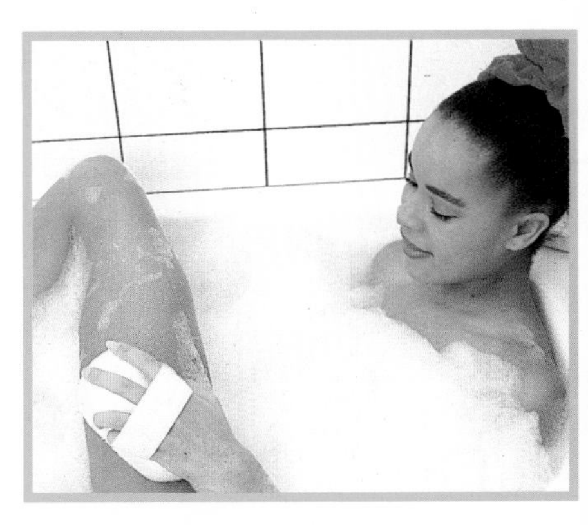

▲ **MASSAGE MAGIC** *Start off with a gentle massage. Treat yourself to a special massage mitt or glove with rounded nodules and work over fatty areas prone to cellulite – especially thighs, buttocks and upper arms – to improve circulation and help to disperse the fat deposits.*

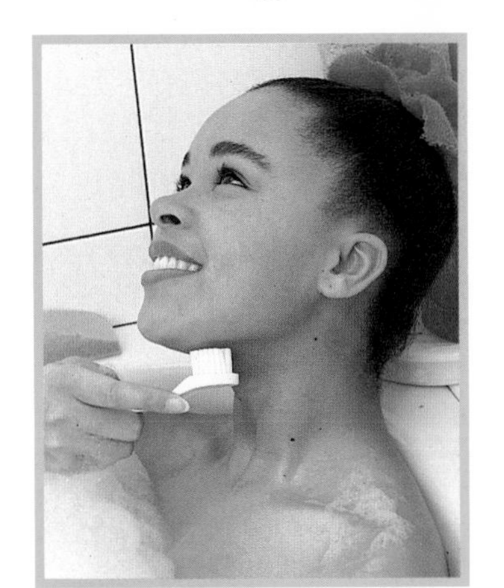

◄ **RUB A DUB SCRUB** *Exfoliating is essential for deep-cleansing and softening the skin. It removes stale make-up and grime that can leave your skin looking dry and dull. As your skin varies in thickness, your sloughing tools need to suit each part of the body!*

WASHED UP

- After a bath, wait 15 minutes to allow your skin to cool before using deodorant – it'll be more effective.
- Unless you're going to make use of the hot atmosphere to give your hair a hot oil treatment, it's best to wash your hair after bathing as the steam can make it go flat and lank.

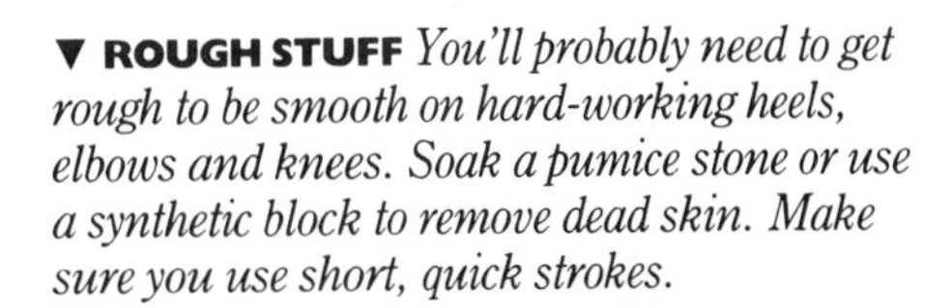

Keep the pumice wet so that you don't make the skin sore.

▼ **ROUGH STUFF** *You'll probably need to get rough to be smooth on hard-working heels, elbows and knees. Soak a pumice stone or use a synthetic block to remove dead skin. Make sure you use short, quick strokes.*

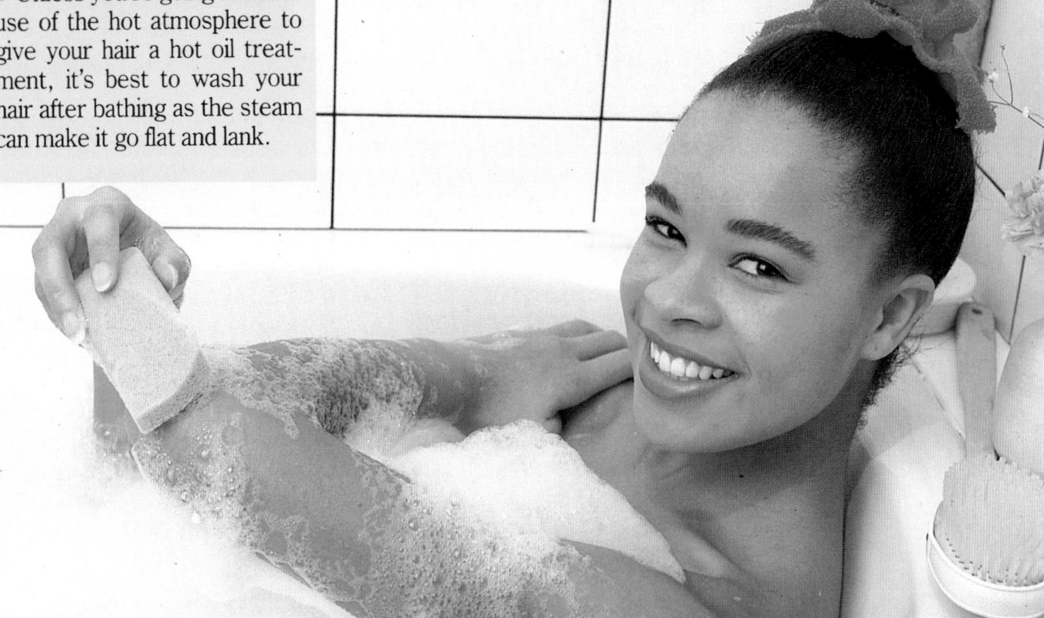

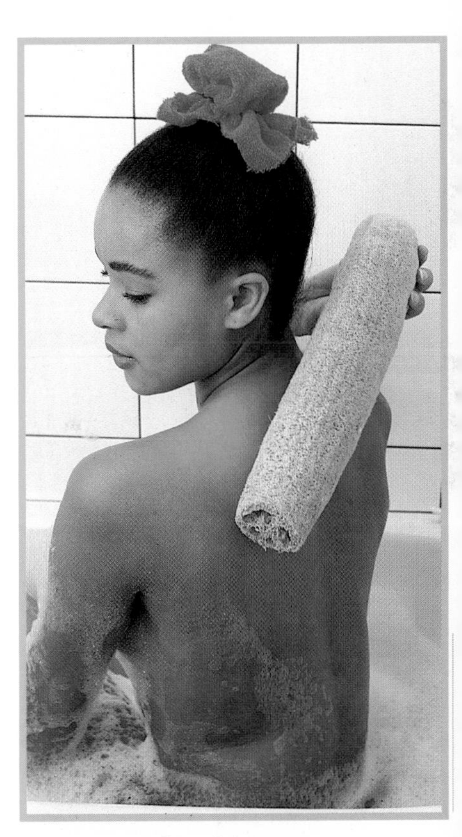

▲ **BACK UP** *Out of sight and hidden under thick clothing, your back can often be neglected in your beauty routine. Stop those spotty outbreaks and get to the tricky bits with a wet loofah or long-handled body brush.*

Treat your back to a face pack. Get Mum or your sister to smooth it on, leave for the recommended time, then rinse off.

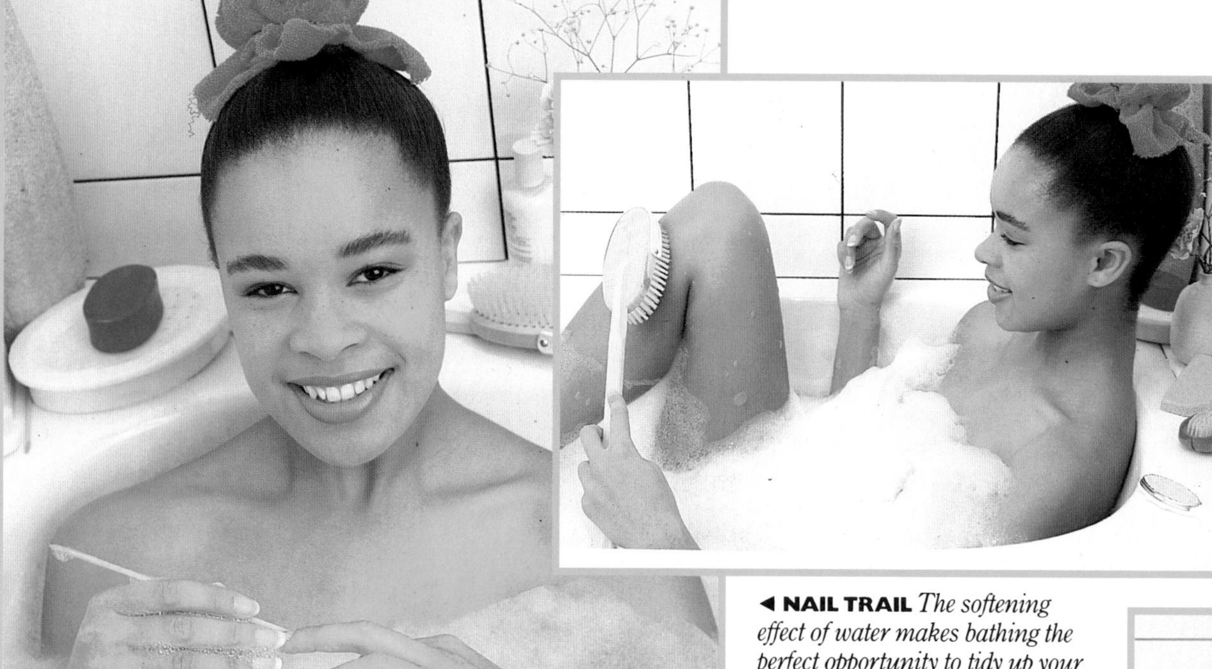

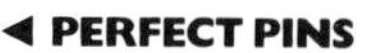

◄ PERFECT PINS *Next, move on to your legs. Use a body brush to remove dead, flaky skin and help soften the hairs if you're going to shave them afterwards. Use long, firm strokes and don't forget to do the backs of the legs.*

Watchpoint

Shaving? Don't lather with a scented soap – you could get a rash on sensitive skin.

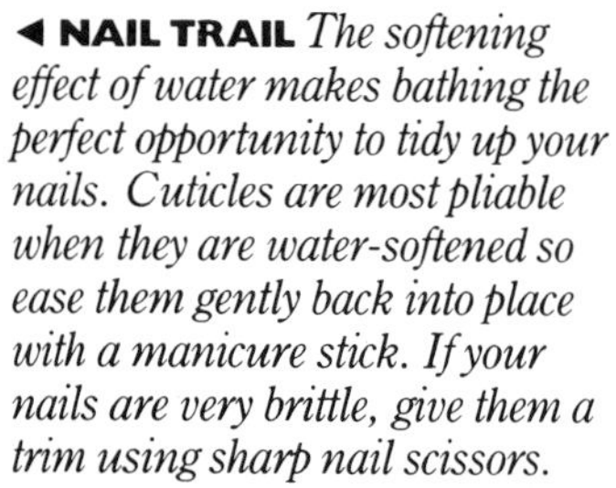

◄ NAIL TRAIL *The softening effect of water makes bathing the perfect opportunity to tidy up your nails. Cuticles are most pliable when they are water-softened so ease them gently back into place with a manicure stick. If your nails are very brittle, give them a trim using sharp nail scissors.*

◄ BRUSH WORK *Now come clean with a nail brush – the easiest and gentlest tool to unclog the dirt and grime that can become trapped behind your finger – and toe – nails.*

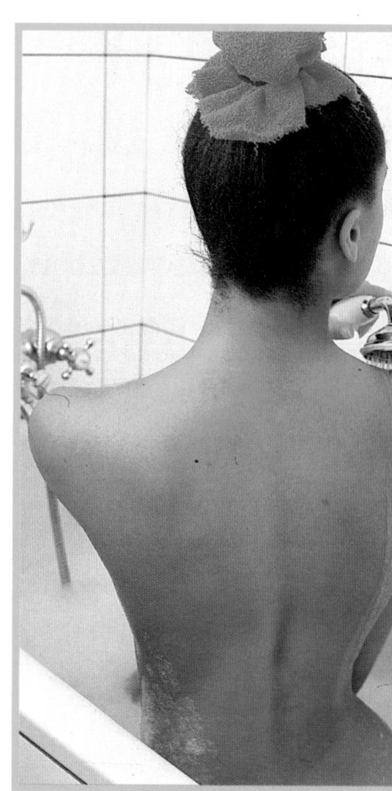

► SHOWER POWER *Lying in bath water leaves a soapy scum which can dry out or irritate sensitive skin. To keep your skin clear, drain the bath before you get out, then thoroughly shower yourself down in lukewarm water for a couple of minutes.*

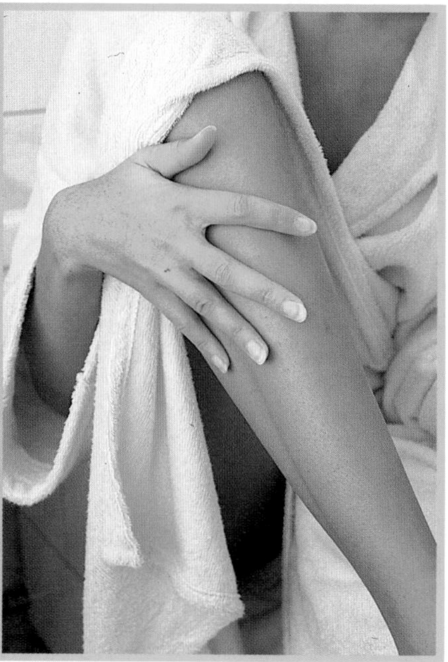

◄ SMOOTH MOVES *Next, dry yourself off with a big fluffy towel. Give yourself a vigorous rub over fleshy areas such as thighs, buttocks and upper arms. You should now be feeling totally refreshed and ready to finish off your routine with a luxurious moisturiser – all over. Dot small blobs on each part of your body, then gently massage in with fingertips, until it's all absorbed. Use light, upward strokes.*

Dry between your toes thoroughly, then condition nails with a few drops of almond oil.

SPLASH OUT

- Put a DO NOT DISTURB notice on the door.
- The water should be comfortably warm – too much heat can dehydrate the skin and cause thread veins. Also, avoid letting the water get tepid so you don't get a chill!
- Baby yourself and test the water by dipping your elbow in first.
- Don't fill the bath too full as immersing yourself in too much hot water can make you feel faint. When you lie back in the tub the water should reach slightly above your waist.
- Add a capful of moisturising bubble bath or bath oil to the water to keep your skin soft and supple. Alternatively, tie a muslin bag filled with herbs or pot-pourri under the tap and let the water run over it for an aromatic bath.
- Make sure everything you need is within arm's reach!
- Take off old nail polish in preparation for some pampering!
- Put a large fluffy towel to warm ready to dry you off afterwards.
- If your face is in need of a deep down cleanse, now's the time to put on a face pack.

Photographs: PAUL MITCHELL/Hair and make-up: LIZZIE COURT

SENSUAL HEALING

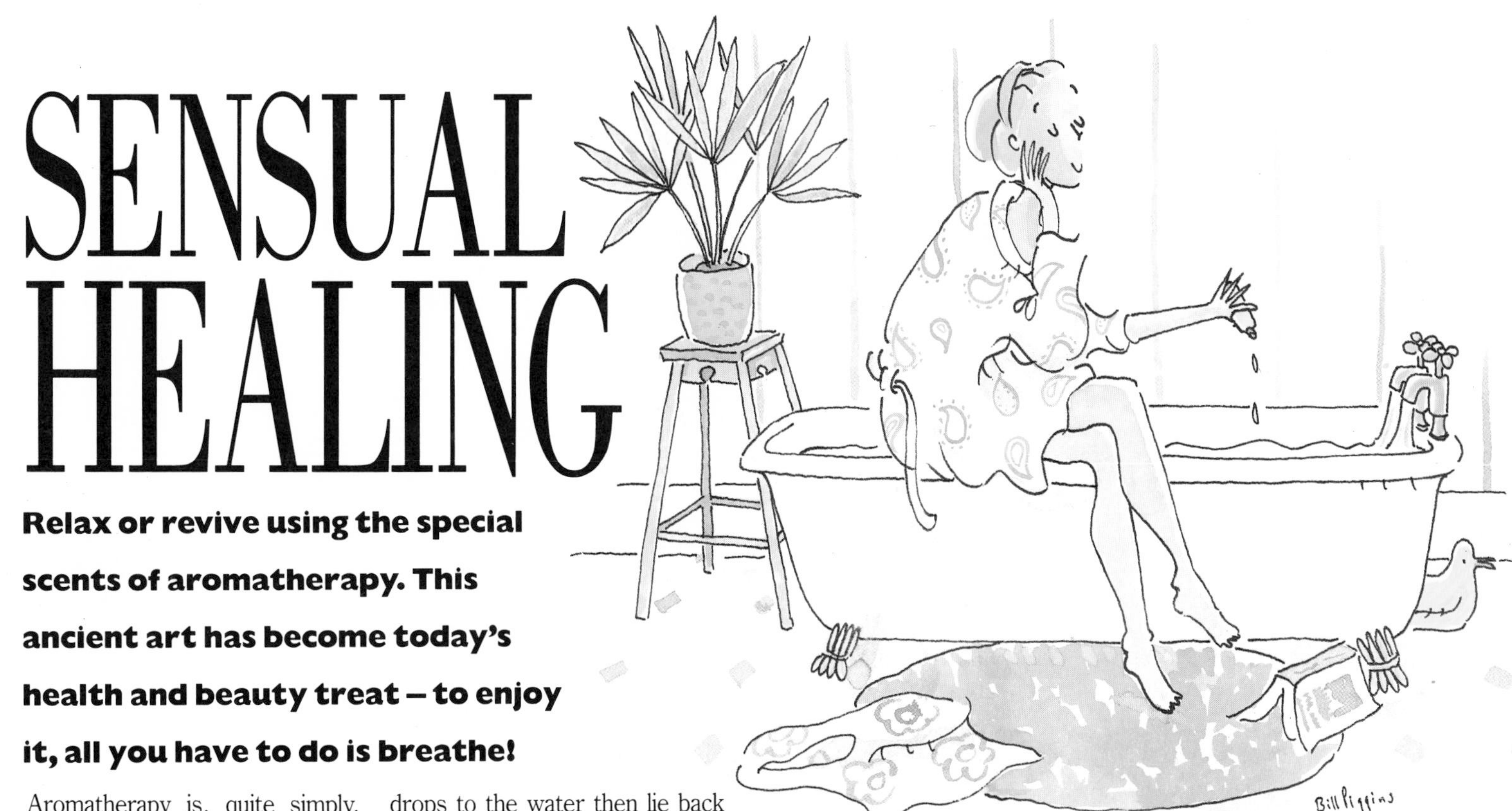

Relax or revive using the special scents of aromatherapy. This ancient art has become today's health and beauty treat – to enjoy it, all you have to do is breathe!

Aromatherapy is, quite simply, the use of scented oils extracted from plants to improve health and well-being.

The fragrant, pure essential oils from the plants are extracted by various processes and these oils form the basis of the treatment. Essential oils work mainly through smell but they can also be applied directly to the skin and absorbed into the bloodstream. Either way, their potent aromas will have a soothing and relaxing effect on you, easing both emotional and physical problems.

Aromatherapy dates back to 3,000 BC but has been revived recently, and essential oils are now widely available. They are highly concentrated and very potent so shouldn't be applied directly to the skin. If you want to use them as part of a massage they should be diluted in a carrier oil, such as almond oil, or with water in a bath.

A little really does go a long way so measure the oils by the drop. Most oils come in bottles with a 'dropper' so it's easy to be very specific about the amount you use.

TREAT YOURSELF

You can enjoy aromatherapy at home in a number of ways.

Aromatic baths: add about five drops to the water then lie back and relax, breathing slowly and deeply for 10-15 minutes. Keep all doors and windows closed and don't have the water too hot or the oil will evaporate. Choose an invigorating oil in the morning and a relaxing oil at night.

Massage: making essential oils part of a soothing massage will certainly help you to relax. You can either buy ready-diluted aromatherapy massage oil or mix up your own. To make your own massage oil you need to mix an essential oil with a pure carrier oil (not a refined oil like baby oil) such as sweet almond, wheatgerm, soya-bean or grapeseed oil. Add 15 drops of essential oil to every 30 ml of carrier oil.

Inhalations: turn a facial into an aromatic treat by adding 10 drops of oil to a bowl of very hot water. Inhale the steam deeply for about five minutes. If you've got a cold or a sore throat try 'steaming' by adding drops of eucalyptus oil to relieve the symptoms.

Air freshener: freshen the air in a stuffy room by adding a few drops of oil to water in a plant spray and spraying it into the air. Alternatively, add a few drops to a bowl of water and place this on a shelf above a hot radiator.

You can also make aromatherapy part of your skincare routine by choosing ready-made products which contain essential oils.

THE PROFESSIONAL TOUCH

To appreciate the full potential of aromatherapy you may like to visit an aromatherapist for a massage. Having been given some idea of your general health and lifestyle he or she will choose the essential oils to help you most.

Skin conditions like eczema, psoriasis or acne may be eased and an aromatherapist can mix up a lotion for use at home. But do consult a doctor first.

If you have any doubts about the power of an inhaled substance, just think about the effect that gas at the dentist's has on you. But aromatherapy's far more pleasant, we promise!

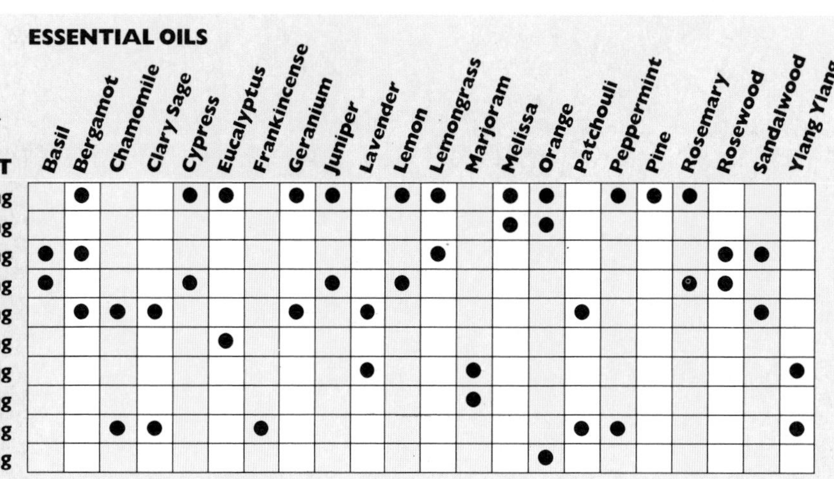

SCENTSATIONAL

There are a huge number of essential oils to choose from, here's what a few of them offer.

ESSENTIAL OILS

EFFECT	Basil	Bergamot	Chamomile	Clary Sage	Cypress	Eucalyptus	Frankincense	Geranium	Juniper	Lavender	Lemon	Lemongrass	Marjoram	Melissa	Orange	Patchouli	Peppermint	Pine	Rosemary	Rosewood	Sandalwood	Ylang Ylang
Refreshing		●			●	●		●	●		●	●		●	●		●	●	●			
Reviving														●	●							
Uplifting	●	●										●								●	●	
Stimulating/Invigorating	●				●				●		●								●	●		
Relaxing		●	●	●				●		●						●					●	
Head-clearing						●																
Calming										●			●									●
Fortifying													●									
Comforting/Satisfying			●	●			●									●	●					●
Restoring															●							

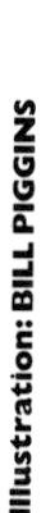
Illustration: BILL PIGGINS

BACK CHAT

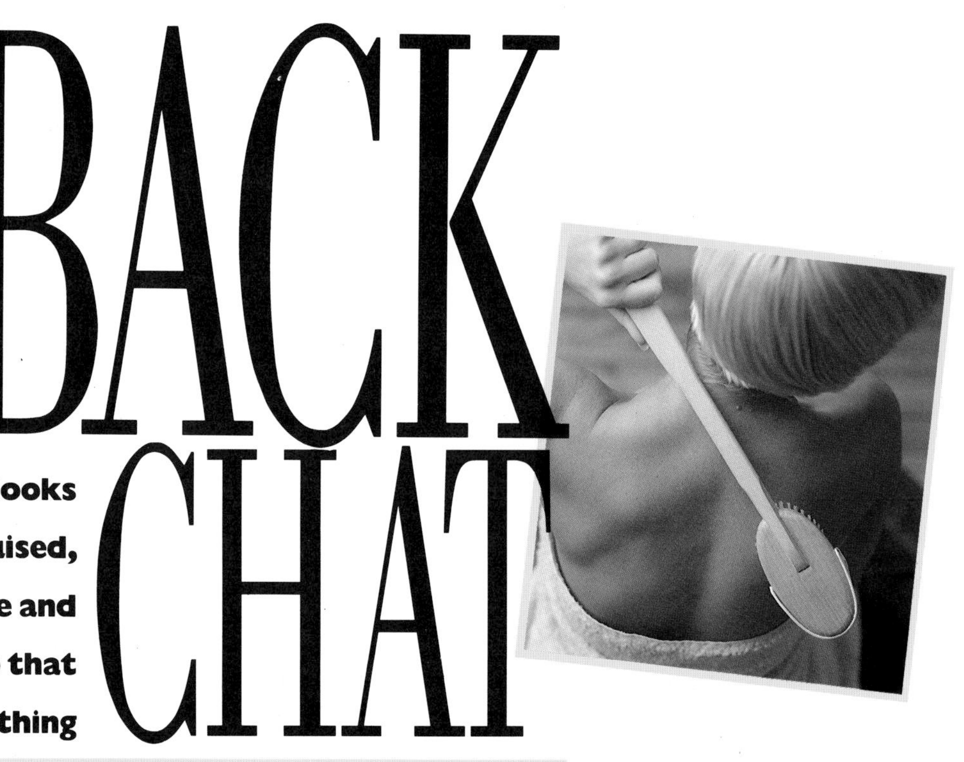

A beautiful back is a must if you want your exit to be as good as your entrance! All it takes is a little time and effort and you can dramatically improve the way your back looks and feels. Blemishes can be disguised, dull skin given a new lease of life and you can even fake a tattoo that looks as good as the real thing

A beautiful back is a great all year-round asset that can be flaunted in bikinis, backless party dresses or glamorous silk lingerie. So if your attitude to back care has always been 'out of sight, out of mind', then now's the time to get to work and start spending as much time on your back as you do on your facial skincare routine.

Start by adding just a couple of extra steps to your general cleansing routine. When you take your bath or shower use a loofah, an abrasive sponge or a long bath brush to cleanse your back. If your skin is greasy and prone to spots and blemishes, then use an antibacterial face wash on your back too. If the spots don't respond to cleansing alone, then use a spot cream on them. If you have dry skin on your back then use a moisturiser (you may need a friend to help you put it on).

You'll also improve the condition of the skin on your back if you stick to wearing natural fibres like cotton and wool. These allow the skin to breathe, whereas synthetic fibres cause the skin to sweat and will only make a greasy or spotty skin worse.

Avoid the dehydrating effects of water by adding a few drops of baby oil to your bath.

SPECIAL EFFECTS

If you really want to draw attention to a beautiful back, then decorate it for the evening. Add some stars or fake a tattoo if you really want to cause a sensation.

The easiest ones to use are the ones that can be pressed onto the skin. They work rather like a transfer giving you the outline of the design you have chosen and you just have to paint it in. (The paint is supplied with the transfers.) Get a friend to help you as it's impossible to apply one yourself! To remove the tattoo afterwards you simply rub it off using an alcohol-based toner on a cotton pad.

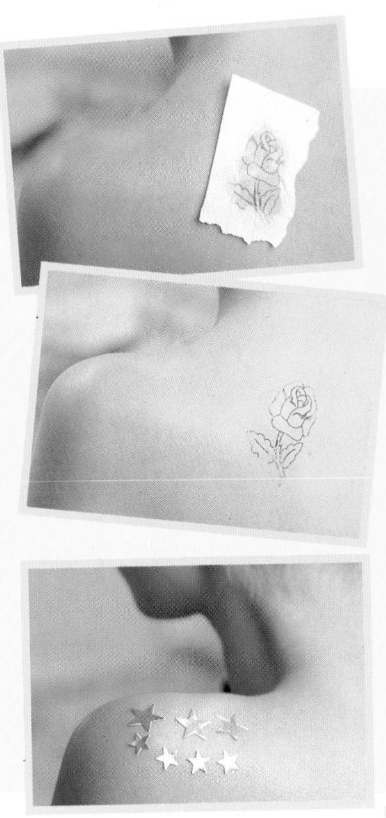

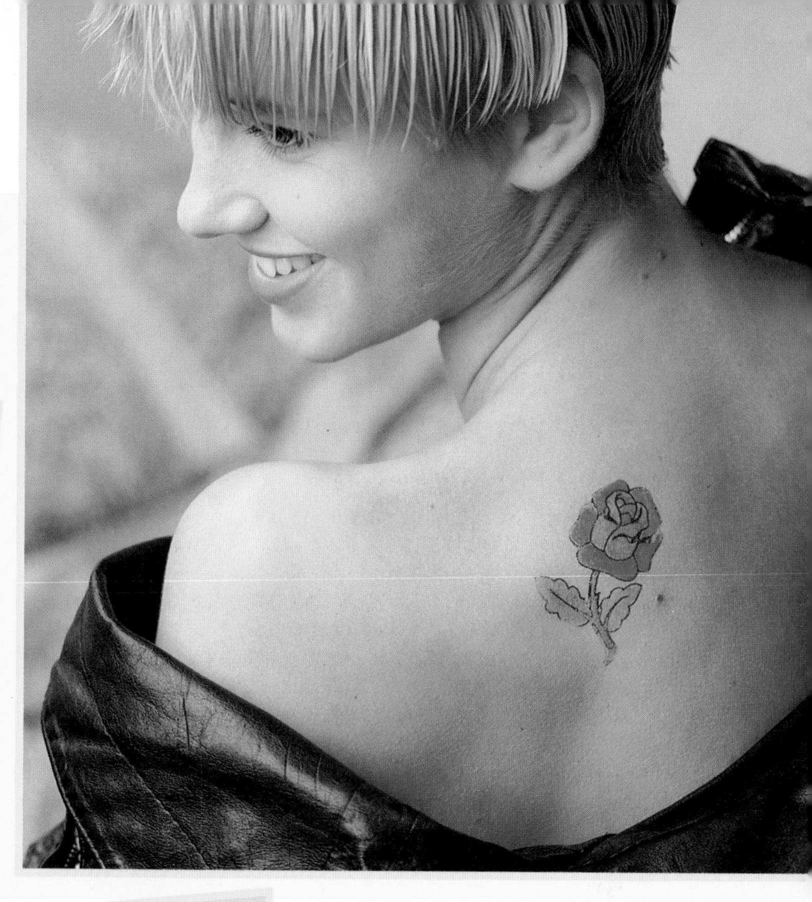

SPOT COVER

If you break out in a blemish just before that important occasion, don't panic, cover it up. Use a liquid rather than a stick concealer (some of them have quite long wand attachments which make it easier to reach awkward areas). Choose a medicated variety to hide and heal at the same time. Dab the offending blemish with a small amount of concealer, then blend it in well so that there are no harsh edges.

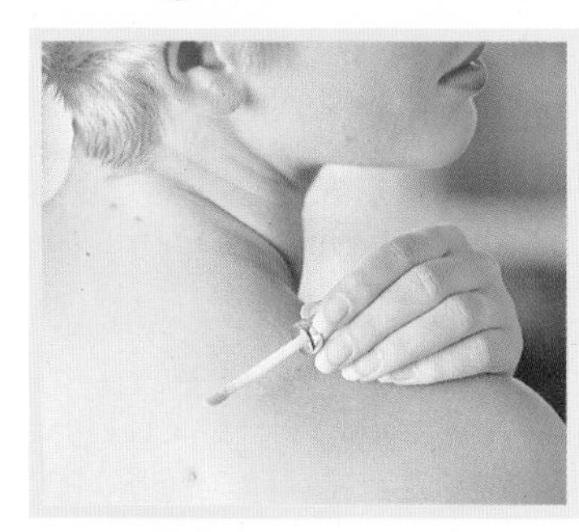

Watchpoint

Check that any foundation or body tint used for cover-ups will wash off your clothes.

Tip

If you have very bad spots on your back a course of sunbed treatments may improve the condition or your doctor may prescribe a course of antibiotics to ease the problem.

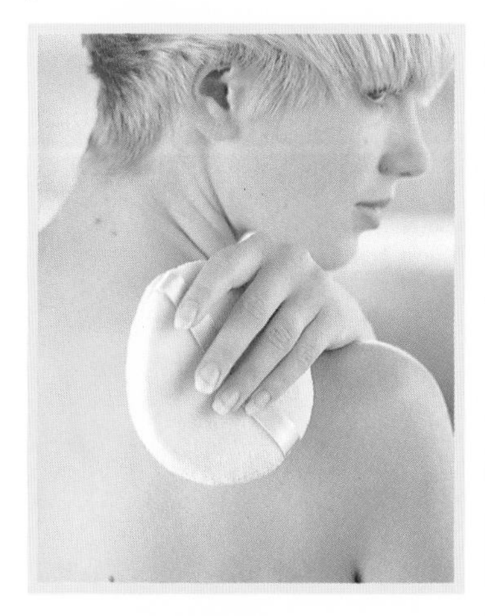

A PERFECT FINISH

After tackling any problem areas with concealer, dust all the skin that's going to show with loose translucent powder. To get the best finish use a large flat powder puff to lightly press the powder into your skin. This will create a velvety-soft appearance as well as evening out skin tone. Loose powder is messy so make sure it doesn't mark your outfit.

NO MORE LINES

Strap marks, caused by the sun having tanned around the outline of your bikini, can ruin the effect of an otherwise lovely tan. Cover them up by blending fake tanning lotion, foundation or body tint over the visible lines using a damp sponge or a piece of cotton wool and then cover with translucent powder.

ANY QUESTIONS?

Q I really love wearing halter necks and backless tops, but my back is so white and never goes brown. Is there anything I can do about it?

A Yes, fake a tan! Use a tanning lotion – you'll need someone to help you put it on. It develops after a few hours without natural sunlight. You can add another coat if you want a darker colour. Alternatively, you can use a bronzing powder which can be brushed over a clean, smooth back using a large powder brush. Again, get a friend to help.

Q I sit at a desk all day and find by the time I go home, my back is really aching, what can I do about it?

A Try to avoid bending over a typewriter or slouching in front of a computer screen all day. Bad posture puts unnecessary strain on your back and causes backache. Aim to sit up as straight as you can, or try relaxation exercises to improve your posture. And remember, if you do suffer from persistent and unexplained backaches, see a doctor.

Q The skin on my back looks a bit grey. What can I do about it?

A The grey appearance is probably caused by dead skin cells which, if they're not removed, can give a dull look. To get rid of the dead cells and to revitalise your skin, use a loofah or a grainy exfoliator to gently massage your back. If you have dry skin rub a back brush in circular movements over your skin. This will exfoliate the skin, increase the circulation and make your back look clear and smooth.

Photographs: PAUL MITCHELL/Hair & Make-up: LIZZIE COURT

A CLOSE SHAVE

Although some methods may seem more feminine and others may last longer – for rapid, regular removal of excess body hair – a blade beats all. There's no truth to the rumour that shaving makes more hairs grow, or that it makes hair grow faster. However, as shaving does slice hair off at the skin's surface, regrowth does appear rapidly. And, because shaving leaves blunt ends rather than tapered tips, regrowth may look coarse and heavy.

WET VS DRY

Wet razors are cheaper and easier to use, but don't do as close a job as electric shavers. You're also more likely to nick yourself with a razor.

WET, WET, WET

Wet shaving's easy – all you need is a few extra moments after a bath or shower – and a razor! Choose either a disposable one or a razor with a fixed head and changeable blade. Each blade should last for about ten shaves on underarms, but fewer if used on legs. Take care of your razor: after use, rinse the blade in warm water, then store upright. If there's any sign of rust on the razor blade, replace it. And for reasons of hygiene *never* share your razor with anyone else.

Use soap, shaving cream, foam or gel – rather than just water – to wet hair and keep it wet. Always shave with hot water – cold water won't soften the hairs enough.

Watchpoint

Avoid using any deodorant for at least four hours after shaving – your skin is extra sensitive and it'll sting! Dust with talc instead.

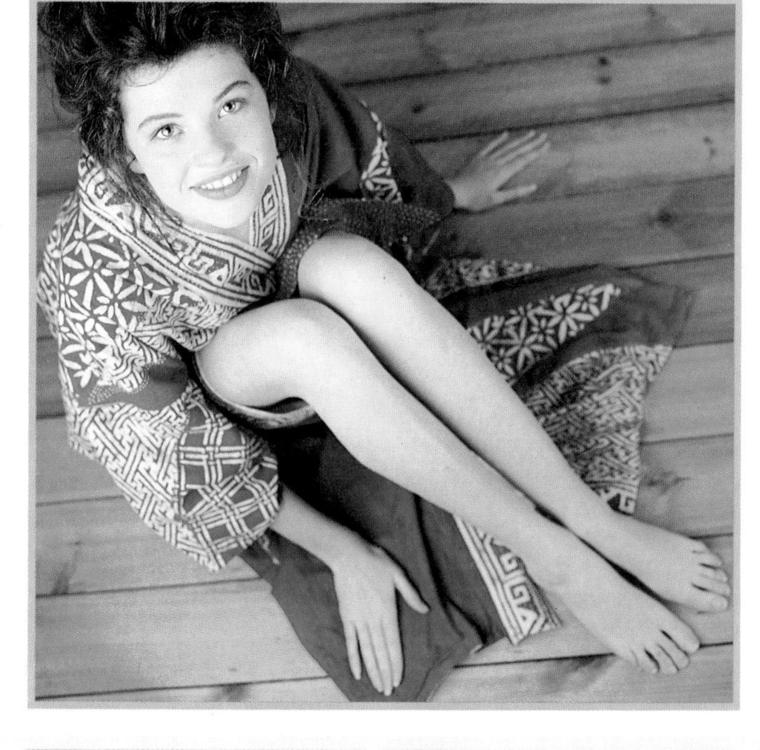

LEGWORK

Silky smooth legs don't just happen – so leave yourself plenty of time when you wet shave. Perch on the edge of the bath and do one leg at a time. Shave slowly and you'll avoid nasty nicks!

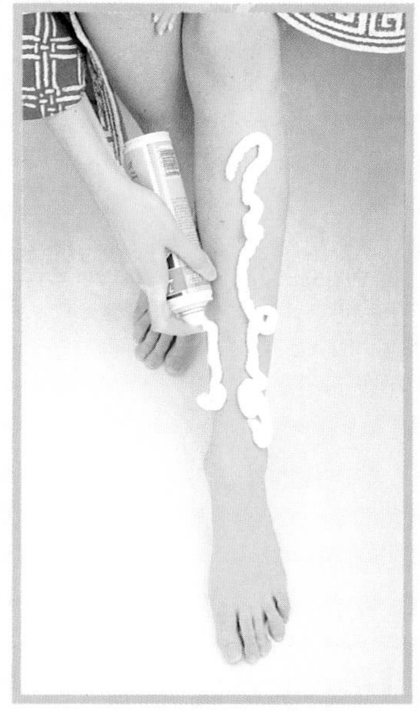

1 *First, exfoliate with a body scrub to get rid of dead skin cells. Then lather your leg with a shaving preparation or soap.*

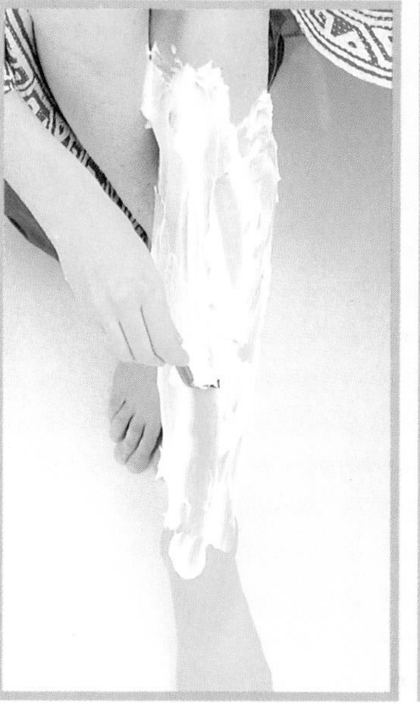

2 *Shave up to and including your knee, going against the direction of hair growth. Keep the razor at an angle of 45°.*

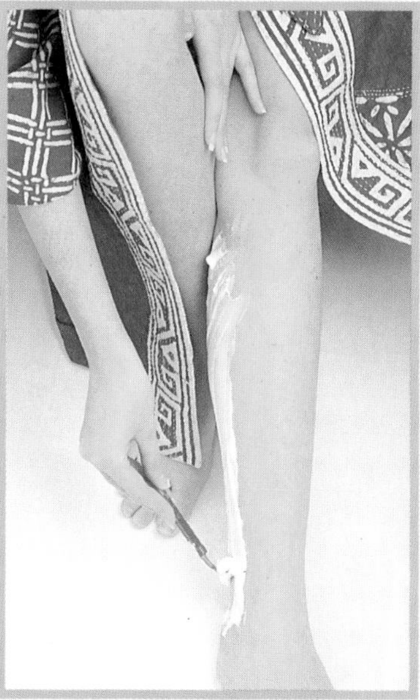

3 *To shave the back of your leg, flex your foot upwards to tighten the calf muscle. Rinse the razor to stop it getting clogged.*

Photographs: PAUL MITCHELL/Hair and make-up: LIZZIE COURT

Ignore all those old wives' tales about heavy regrowth – the fastest, easiest way to get rid of unwanted hair is with a wet razor or a dry shaver. Follow our sharp instructions on shaving and you'll be well on your way to smooth success

BIKINI LINE TIME

You may need to remove hair from the tops of your thighs to look good in high-cut swimsuits or bikinis. You can wet or dry shave, but do treat skin here gently, as any irritation will be aggravated by friction from clothes. It's a good idea to shave your bikini line just before going to bed.

Bikini line hair grows in different directions, so make sure you shave against the growth.

WET SHAVE: lather well with shaving preparation or soap and shave with a new, sharp blade.

DRY SHAVE: take a bath or shower and dry thoroughly, then apply talc. Pull skin to be shaved taut with your free hand.

AFTERCARE: when you've finished shaving rinse with warm water, dry and dust with talc.

UNDERARM TACTICS

Be a smooth operator! Shave just before bedtime so you don't need to wear deodorant.

WET SHAVE

- Wash your armpit first to remove all traces of dirt and deodorant, then lather well with soap or a shaving product.
- Lift arm up and back to pull skin taut, then shave against direction of hair growth.
- Rinse and pat dry, then dust with talc.

DRY SHAVE

Use a slim-headed battery shaver for underarms. It can cope more easily with awkward contours, and its comb-and-clip action is kinder than a hard blade.

- Wash and dry thoroughly. Dust armpit with talc to help razor glide over skin.
- Lift arm up and back to pull skin taut, then shave against direction of hair growth.

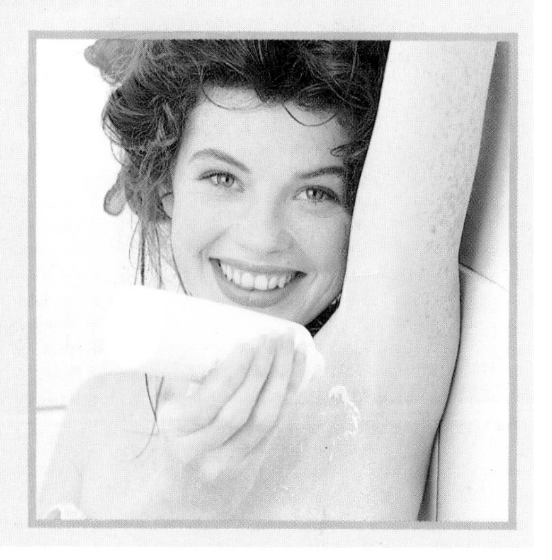

DRY RUN

For best results skin must be completely dry, so wait a few minutes after a bath or shower before using a shaver.

1 Holding the shaver at an angle of 45° work up from your ankle to your knee, against the direction of hair growth. This allows the trimmer head to remove the longest hairs.

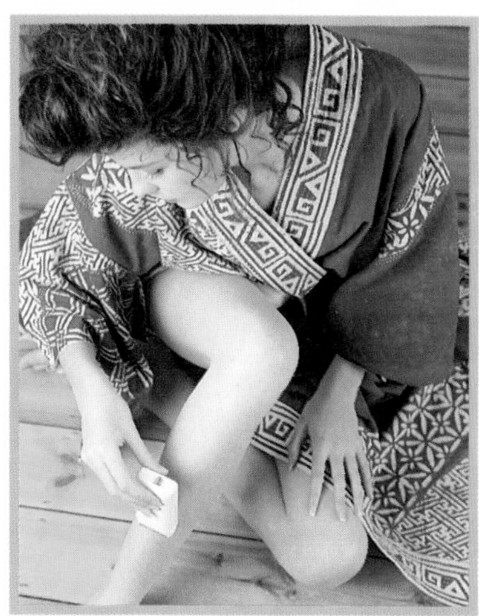

2 Flex your foot forward to tighten the calf muscle while you shave the back of your leg. Keep it flexed while you shave the back of your ankle.

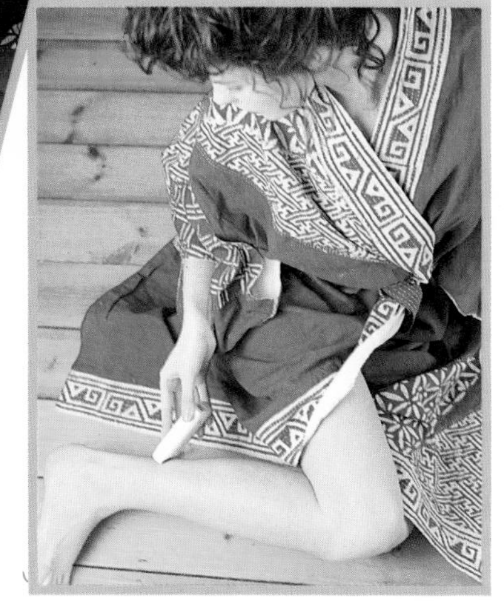

Tip

Shaving the leg a second time will give a final closer shave and get rid of hairs you may have missed. This time hold the shaver at a right angle to your leg and shave with a light but firm pressure.

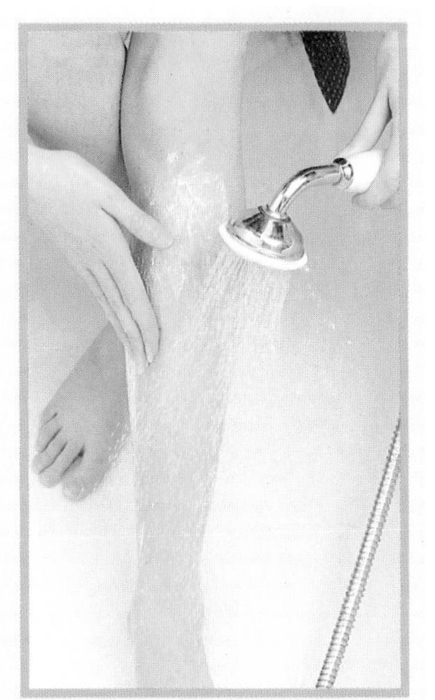

4 Rinse your leg with warm water. Check for remaining hairs. If you find any, lather them and then shave.

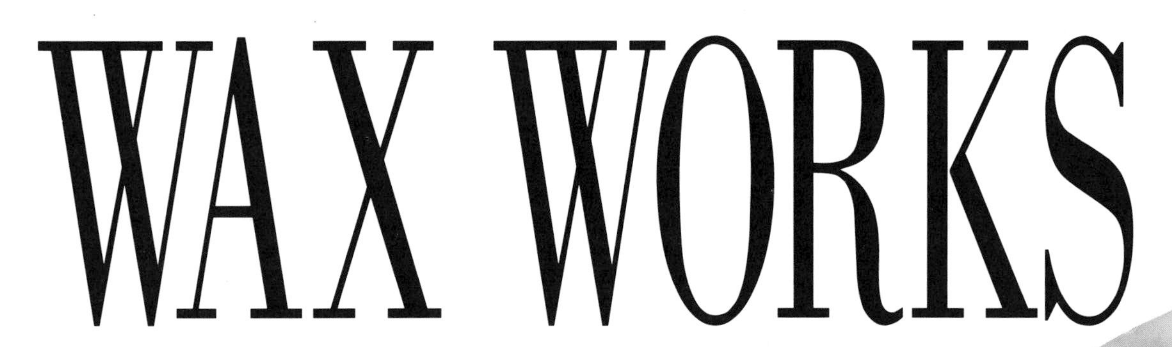

WAX WORKS

If you fancy being happily hair-free but the thought of leg waxing makes you wince, try it out in the comfort of your own home. You could find wax works for you

Waxing is one of the most effective ways to remove unwanted hair. The principle is simple: wax-coated strips are used to pull hair out from the roots, so re-growth is much slower than with any other method. Depending on the speed your hair grows, you should be hair-free for about four to six weeks.

Home waxing kits are convenient and easy to use, and if you follow the instructions, are as effective as professional salon treatments.

There are two basic methods: cold strip wax and hot wax. The choice is very much up to you. A strip wax pack contains a number of disposable ready-waxed plastic strips which you just smooth over your legs and peel off, along with all the unwanted hair. A hot wax kit is more expensive but is reusable and should last for years. It contains a thermostatically controlled heater, cloth strips and a roller applicator which holds the liquid wax. This takes around 40 minutes to heat up.

Waxing can be painful, especially the first few times, but gets easier the more you do it. The way you wax will also make it less painful – it's important to hold the skin taut so that the hairs, not the skin, are pulled by the strips. With practice, you should feel only slight discomfort, and the results are definitely worth it!

BE PREPARED

Before using either waxing technique, remember:

- Read the instructions through before you start.
- Carry out a patch test on your ankle to make sure that your skin is not too sensitive.
- The hair to be removed must be over 4 mm/1/6 in long.
- You shouldn't take a hot bath or shower for at least four hours before or after waxing, because high temperatures leave the skin extra sensitive.
- Waxing can make your skin blotchy for a few hours afterwards so don't attempt to wax just before a special occasion.

FIRST STEPS *Getting ready to wax.*

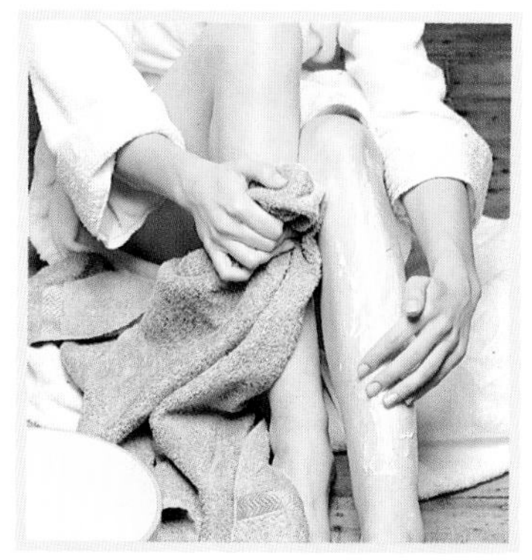

1 *Before using wax, wash your legs with warm, not hot, soapy water to remove any oil or creams. Then dry with a towel.*

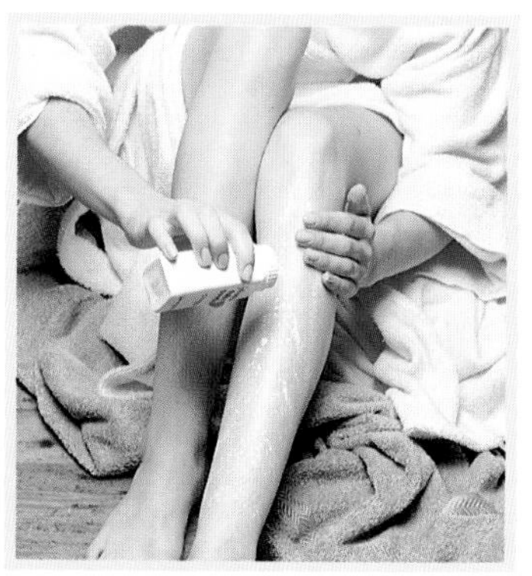

2 *Dust talc generously over the bottom half of your leg where you're going to wax and smooth with your hands.*

HOT WAX TREATMENT

A do-it-yourself wax treatment that gives salon results. Just plug in the heater, switch on and in no time at all you'll have fuzz-free skin.

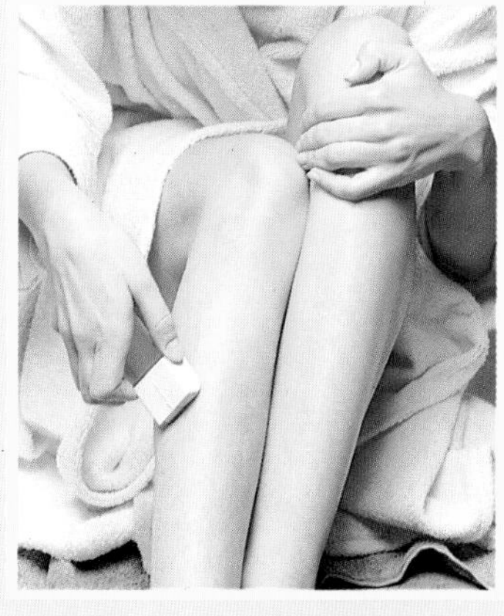

1 *Roll the applicator down your leg in the direction of the hair growth. Put on enough wax to be covered by one strip.*

Main photograph courtesy of CLAIROL, step-by-step photographs: PAUL MITCHELL

COLD STRIP WAX

Quick, cheap and easy to use strip wax is the instant answer to unwanted hair. Start stripping just below the knee and work down the whole of the lower leg.

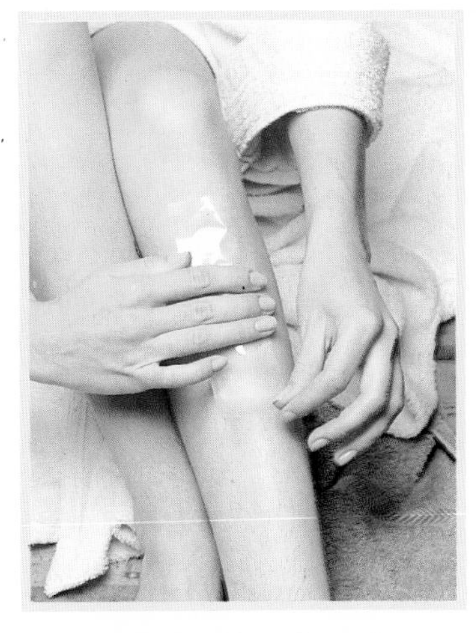

1 Peel the backing sheet away from each strip and gently stroke the wax-coated plastic onto your skin, wax side down.

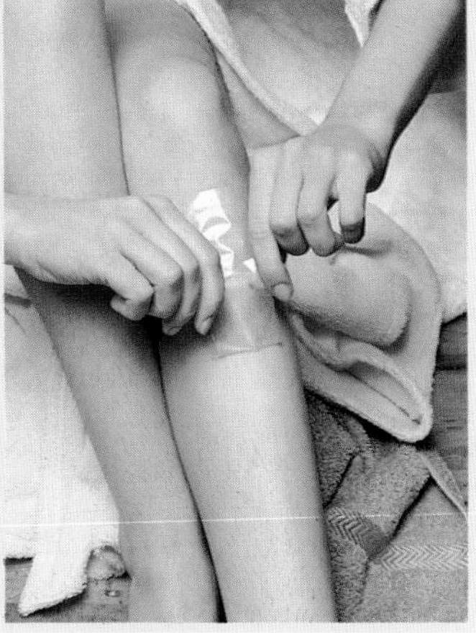
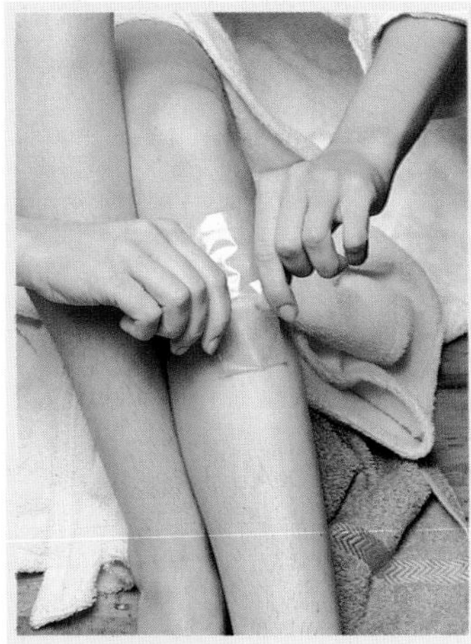

2 Immediately and in one swift movement, pull the strip back in the opposite direction to the hair growth.

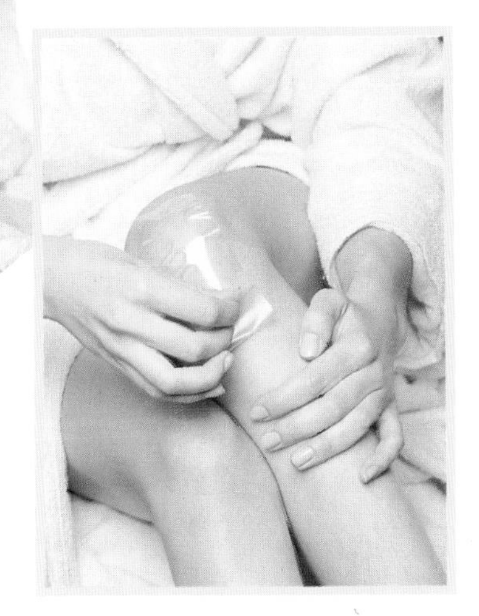

3 Wax your knees by bending your leg slightly so that the skin is taut. Hold this position as you use the strip.

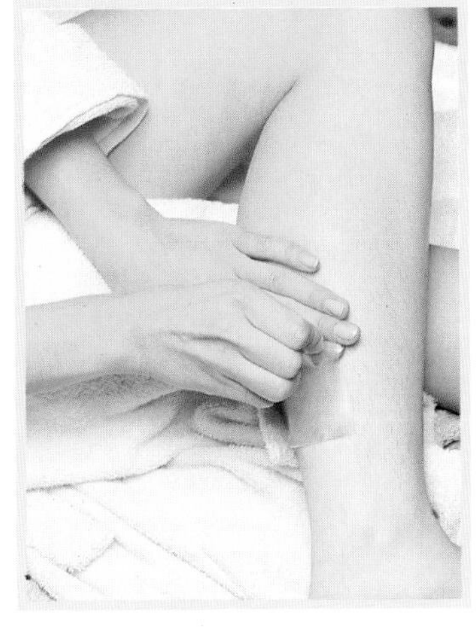

4 Wax the back of your leg by flexing your foot so that your skin is pulled taut when you remove the strip.

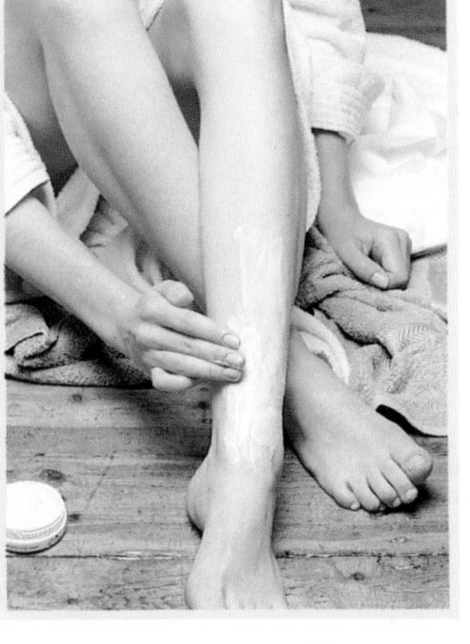

5 Let your skin settle down after waxing, then generously smooth unscented moisturiser all over your legs.

Watchpoint

After waxing, your legs may still have a few blobs of wax on them. Get rid of these by using baby oil on a piece of cotton wool.

Tip

In warm weather or centrally heated rooms, cold wax strips may go tacky, so pop them in the fridge for half an hour before use.

BIKINI LINE WAX

The bikini line is the name for the pubic hair that grows on the inside of your legs and stomach which sometimes shows around the line of your bikini. You can use either hot or strip wax to remove this hair, but if the length is over 12 mm/½ in long, you may find it easier to trim it first.

Wash the whole area with soapy water, dry thoroughly and put on plenty of talc. Sit down on the floor, bend your leg outwards and apply the strip in the direction of the hair growth. Hold the skin taut and pull the strip off quickly in the opposite direction.

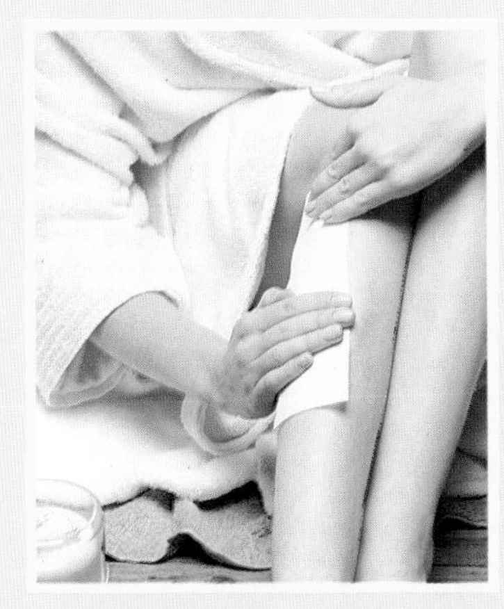

2 Return the applicator to the heating container then smooth one of the strips down over the wax. Rub the strip for even coverage.

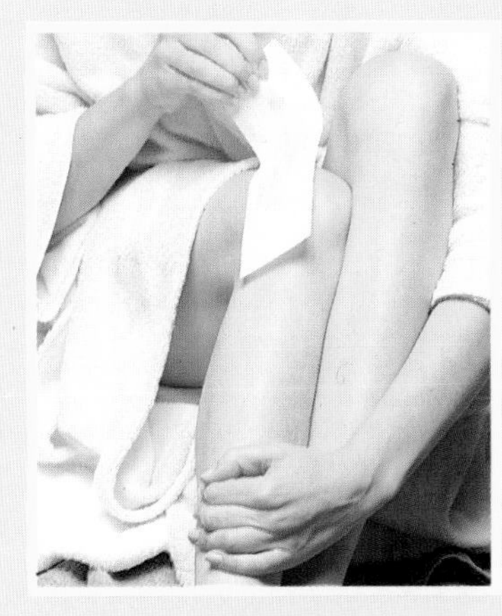

3 Hold your skin taut with one hand, and pull the strip back on itself as quickly as possible with the other one.

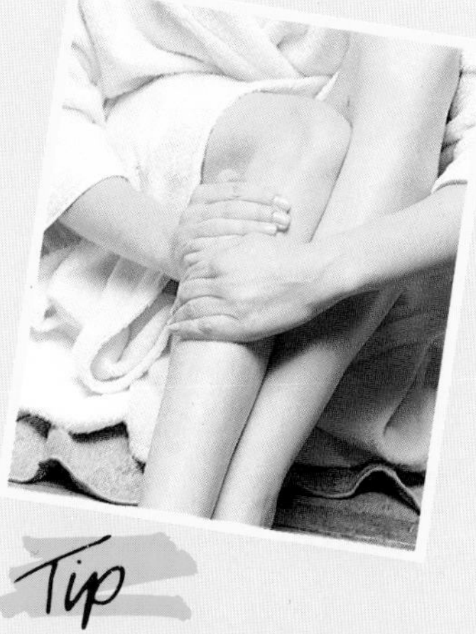

Tip

Press your palms over the newly waxed area for a few seconds to help reduce stinging.

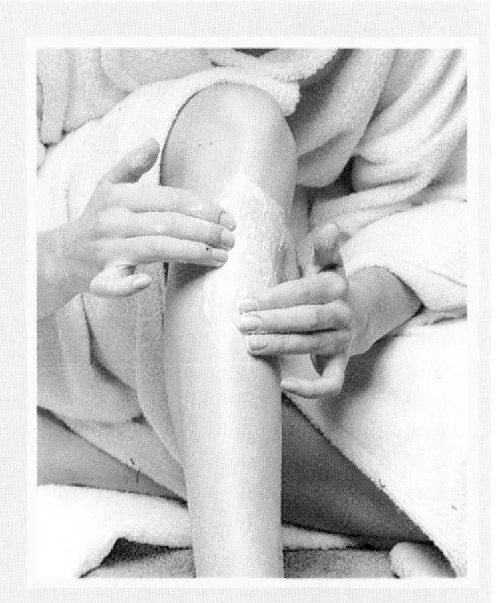

4 Continue waxing down each leg. Your legs may now feel sensitive, so let them settle down before moisturising.

WHAT IS CELLULITE?

Cellulite is a special type of fat: it has very little to do with actually being overweight and can be a problem even if you're pencil slim. Cellulite trouble-spots are usually the hips, bottom, thighs and knees. As you get older. It can also affect the upper arms and between the shoulders. The skin looks dimpled like orange peel and is sometimes wrinkly – not the prettiest sight! It doesn't feel good either. In the early stages, your skin will be flabby and spongy. As the cellulite develops, hard nodules and bumps can form.

If you could see under your skin, you'd find that cellulite is actually made up of pockets of fluid and toxins as well as fat trapped in a network of thickened skin fibres.

THE CULPRITS

- Hormones dictate your fat distribution and whenever there's an upheaval such as during puberty or pregnancy that's when cellulite tends to appear.
- Sitting around and living a lazy lifestyle slows your circulation down, so it can't do the job of nourishing skin cells and carrying away waste as efficiently. And don't forget that smoking, and even wearing tight jeans or underwear can restrict your circulation.
- Bingeing on junk food means your body fills up with all sorts of unnecessary rubbish. Some of this waste will be eliminated but sometimes your poor body just can't cope and the toxins are stored away.

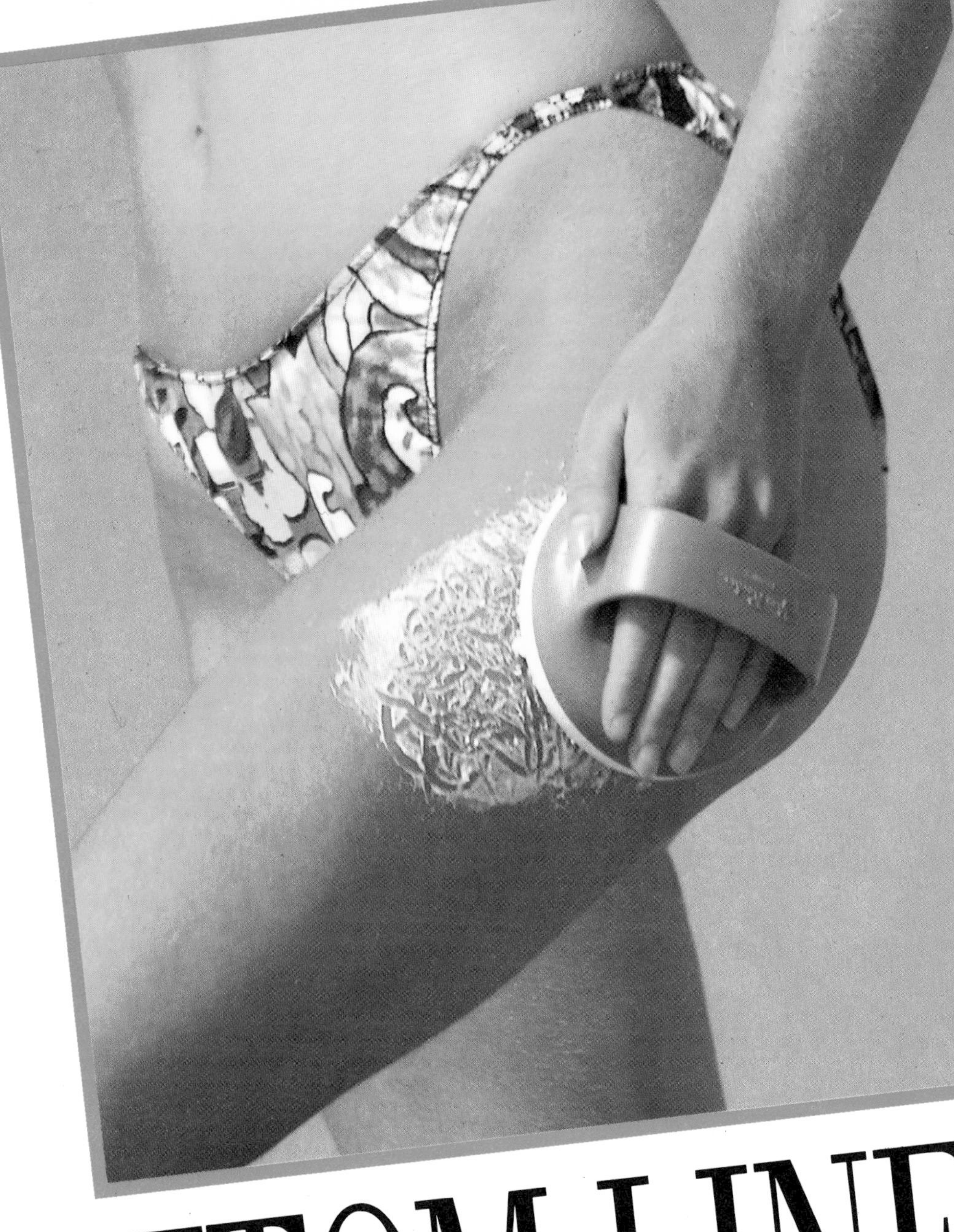

THE BOTTOM LINE

Are your BLTs – bottom, legs and thighs – in great shape or do you run for cover under a towel rather than bare them on the beach? Give that dimpled, dingy-looking skin the rub with our anti-cellulite work out and dare to show a toned new you!

SIMPLE SOLUTIONS

Basically, if you want to rid your body of cellulite, you need to boost your circulation and encourage your body to flush away excess fluid and toxins. By doing this the pockets of fat can then break down, leaving you with smooth, toned skin.

PLAN OF ACTION

Start by following our straightforward, four point action plan. Just set aside a few minutes each day and – that is all it takes – in no time you'll have a body beautiful!

DID YOU KNOW?

As cellulite can be painful, it was once thought to be a type of inflammation. Hence its name: 'cellule' (of the cell) and 'ite' (inflammation).

1 BRUSH YOUR BODY

Begin by stroking your skin with a soft bristle body brush to get the lymphatic system moving. Sweep the brush upwards over your skin, starting at the ankles, then move over your legs, knees and thighs. You can rub more vigorously with circular movements over your bottom. The brush should be used *dry* but don't worry, it's not as painful as it sounds. Don't be over enthusiastic, however, and avoid sensitive, broken or irritated skin.

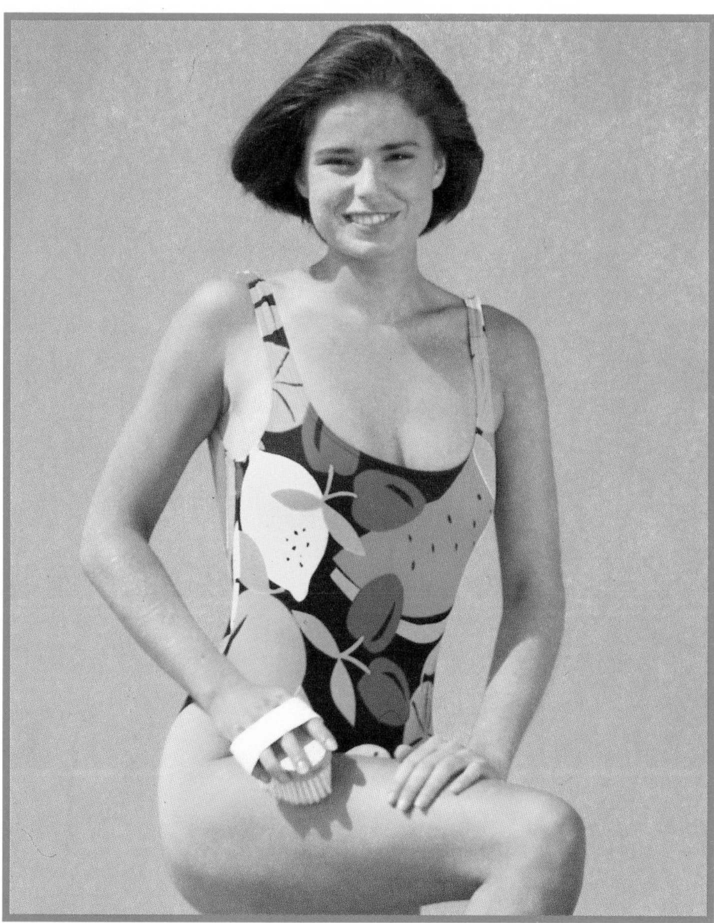

2 DEEP CLEANSE AND DE-TOXIFY

The next step is a bath sprinkled with anti-cellulite ingredients.

- **Seaweed-based bubble baths**, for instance, are renowned for their invigorating and deep cleansing properties. Horsetail, horse chestnut and ivy are other herbal ingredients with skin toning and fluid-flushing properties that are found in many 'contouring' bath products.
- **Aromatherapy oils** are another alternative. These are very concentrated so you only need use a few drops. Try juniper, which encourages your body to get rid of water although it shouldn't be used by pregnant women or those with kidney problems. Rose geranium is uplifting and again helps relieve fluid retention, or try rosemary, which boosts circulation.
- Don't get out of the bath without blasting your cellulite with a stimulating spray of cold water – it's one of the best ways to wake up a sluggish circulation and it really does seem to have a skin tightening and toning effect.

DIET DO'S AND DON'TS

Now you've pampered your body from the outside, think about what goes on on the inside.

DO

- Eat plenty of raw fresh fruit and vegetables. Apart from being a pure and rich form of vitamins there's no need to worry about artificial additives. It also means your diet will be high in fibre, essential for helping your body get rid of waste products. Another bonus is their high vitamin C content, which helps to build up the collagen fibres which lie deep down in your skin – if these deteriorate, skin becomes slack and loses its tone.
- Cut down on fatty foods. Sometimes it's clear which foods are fatty – red meats and fry-ups for instance, but fat is also hidden in processed foods like cakes and biscuits. It's worth buying a fat unit guide, available from most newsagents, so you know you're on the right track.
- Drink plenty of water – at least eight glasses a day. Far from contributing to fluid retention, it actually helps flush excess water from your body and helps the toxic elimination process work. Watery foods like celery and cucumber have a similar effect so serve large helpings in your salad.

DON'T

- Eat too many salty foods as they encourage water retention. This includes the obvious savoury nibbles such as crisps and peanuts, but many other processed foods are also high in salt, even some cakes if you look closely at the label. Yet another reason to opt for fresh and unrefined foods when possible.
- Drink too much tea or coffee. Try and get a taste for herbal tea instead – it's much better for you. Fennel, which has a delicious aniseed flavour, is excellent because it has inner cleansing and water flushing properties.

3 MASSAGE MOVES

The next step is to massage your skin to get the blood pumping. This will be even more effective if you use a massage mitt or glove with a special preparation that stimulates circulation.

- **Massage gadgets** are specially designed, often with a knobbly surface, to get your circulation going and pummel away at the pockets of fat and thickened skin fibres. All you have to do is rub them over your wobbly bits with firm, circular movements in conjunction with a soap, cream or scrub. Or, for an inexpensive, natural body scrub, try a handful of sea salt. Massage gadgets can be used every day.
- **Loofahs and exfoliating mitts** are harsher, however, and should only be used about once a week. They're meant for removing roughness rather than attacking cellulite but they can help to stimulate the circulation.

SITTING PRETTY

Your bottom is usually the first place where cellulite strikes and besides massage, exercise is a great way of beating the flab in this area. Exercise doesn't just burn up fat. It tones up your muscles too, so making your bottom firm and pert instead of droopy! Exercise also gets the blood pumping round your circulation. If you exercise fairly briskly, 18 times more blood than usual reaches your muscles and every time you contract them you literally pump away water and toxins which helps to dislodge that fat. So stop lounging around and spring into action.

Swimming and brisk walking are ideal activities – jogging tends to jolt your joints too much. Clenching and relaxing your bottom muscles is another easy exercise that can be done at almost any time in any place, whether sitting or standing.

4 SMOOTH AND SOFTEN

Finally, once you've pummelled your skin, use a circulation-boosting gel or cream – it'll help to soften you up too!

● **Anti-cellulite creams** have had a bad press in the past but it's mainly because too much has been expected of them. You can't possibly remove fat simply by rubbing a cream into your skin. What these products can do, however, is gently tighten and tone the skin, rev up your circulation, encourage your body to get rid of toxins and, of course, moisturise so your skin feels softer. To do all this, active ingredients from plants such as ivy, seaweed, butcher's broom and even caffeine, are included.

Anti-cellulite gels are also available, which do the same job as creams but have a lighter, more refreshing feel.

Both gels and creams are used in the same way. Place a little on the fingertips, then massage into your skin using a kneading action, or roll or pinch the flesh until all the product is absorbed.

● **Aromatherapy oils** can also be used to soften and smooth the skin. Different essential plant oils have different effects ranging from astringent cypress to soothing lavender and a skilled aromatherapist can put together the perfect cocktail for you. Or try a ready-made mixture, available from health food shops.

● You can massage the oils directly into your skin once they have been diluted in a carrier oil, such as almond oil, or for a lovely bathtime treat, add a few drops to the running water. Finish your action plan by applying a blob of moisturiser using light circular strokes. There are few oil glands on the body so it's important to keep the skin super soft.

SALON SCIENCE

These treatments are fairly expensive but you may decide they're worth it to boost the effects of your home anti-cellulite regime. Check them out at your local beauty salon, sports centre or health club.

G5 – this is a massage machine which kneads your flabby bits more vigorously than you can possibly do yourself at home.

SLENDERTONE – a lazy way to work out. Electrical currents make your muscles contract to tone them up.

BODY WRAPPING – your body is smothered with stimulating ingredients such as seaweed extracts, then wrapped in hot blankets or bandages, so you sweat out toxins.

IONITHERMIE – it is claimed that this treatment can whittle away flab on thighs and knees. Special creams formulated to break down fatty tissue, boost circulation and firm skin are applied. Next, clay is smoothed on and electrodes inserted to increase absorption of the creams and exercise the muscles.

STEAM CABINETS – you sit in these with the steam circulating around you, a bit like a mini Turkish bath. It makes your body perspire, drawing out toxins. A sauna at your local sports centre might be cheaper, but the heat is dry so it doesn't leave your skin feeling so soft.

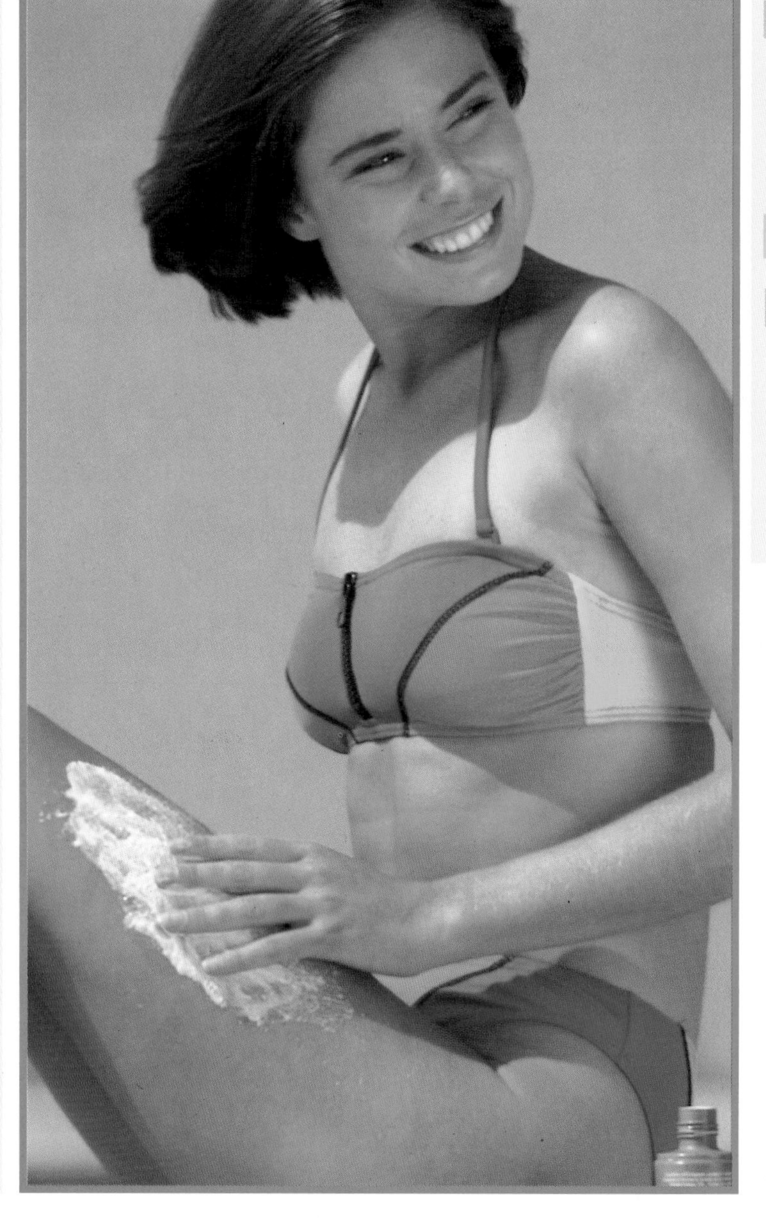

ANY QUESTIONS?

Q My mother suffers with cellulite. Is it hereditary?

A You are likely to inherit a tendency towards cellulite. Some races are more prone than others, too. Swedish women, for instance, don't seem to suffer as much as Mediterranean races.

Q Does the contraceptive pill cause cellulite?

A As it affects your hormone levels, it can encourage cellulite but not in every case.

Q Will my doctor be able to give me anything to get rid of cellulite?

A It's not a life-threatening medical condition so it's not something you should need to see your doctor about. Many doctors are sceptical that such a thing as cellulite even exists. To them it's merely fat.

Q Is it true vitamin E can help fight cellulite?

A Possibly – sunlight and stress can form toxins in our body which lead to wrinkles. One of the many jobs vitamin E does is to protect you against the effects of these toxins, which is why it's added to so many suncreams and even a few anti-cellulite products.

BEACH BUMS

A holiday by the sea can work wonders on cellulite. For instance, swimming in sea water is not only good exercise but because it's rich in minerals, it's invigorating and detoxifying too. If you can't swim, wading through the water and letting the waves break over you is an equally effective toning and invigorating exercise. And don't just sit there sunbathing with your legs stretched out in front of you, 'walk' backwards and forwards across the sand on your bottom, shuffling your hips from side to side. The sand rubbing against your skin will stimulate your circulation and help soften the skin by rubbing off dead skin cells.

Photographs: IAN HOOTON/Hair and make-up: JO GILLINGWATER/Main photo, bikini: NEXT/Small photos, swimwear: FREEMANS

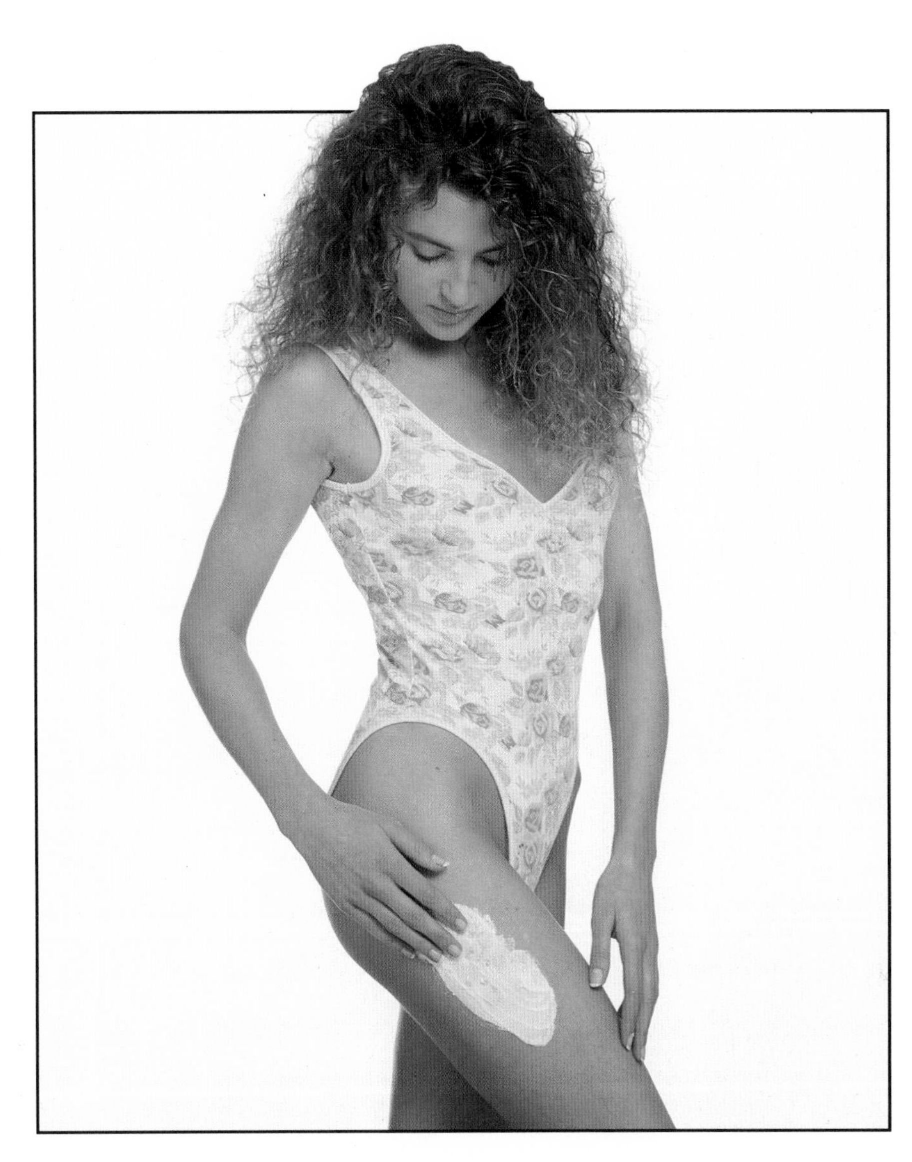

CHAPTER FOUR

The Full Body Treatment

TALON TRICKS

Hands up if your nails are broken or bitten down to the quick. Whether you want to make them stronger or longer, follow our steps for nicer nails

Nails, like hair, are made up of layers of protein (keratin), plus trace elements such as phosphorous and calcium, all bonded together by moisture. And just like hair, nails reflect the general state of your health, so if you've been seriously ill, or just feeling under par they can grow brittle and split.

Besides poor health, plunging your nails into hot water, letting them come into contact with household detergents, and everyday wear and tear can all take their toll. Luckily, there are ways you can make them look lovelier without worrying about growing pains, so take a look at our tricks and treats for lovely fingertips.

IT'S A WRAP

A silk-wrap treatment will repair a broken nail quickly or it can be used to strengthen weak or brittle nails. First, thoroughly clean each nail that you want to wrap with an oil-free polish remover. This will take away any traces of oil and dirt which could stop the silk from sticking.

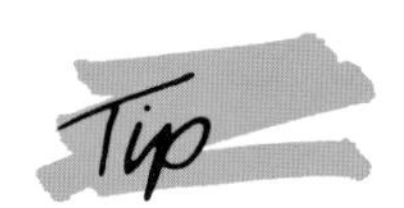

Always file gently towards the centre of your nails, not down the sides since this can cause splitting.

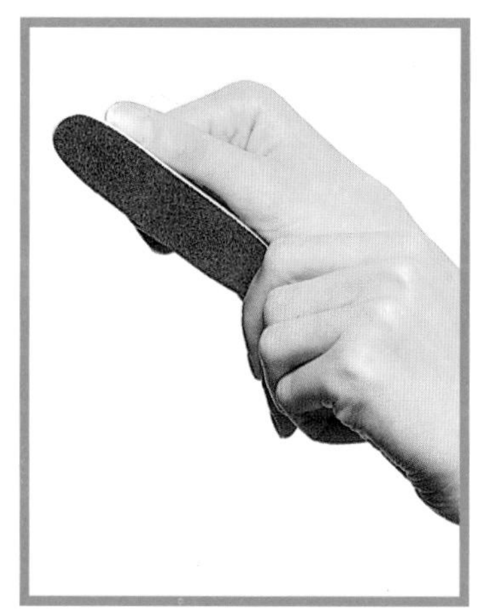

1 If a broken edge is the problem, smooth it first by filing across the top of your nail with an emery board.

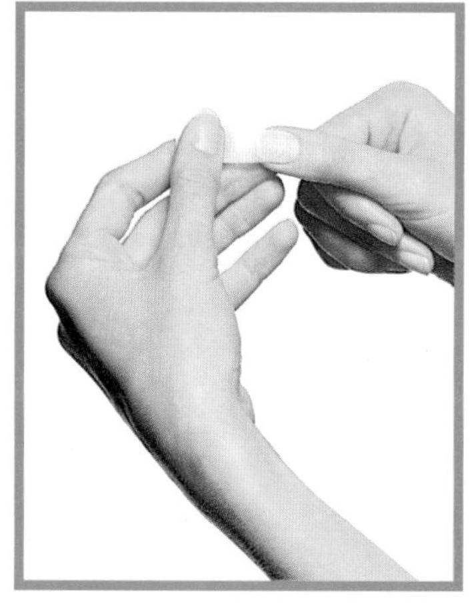

2 Select a silk wrap that fits your nail width, then peel off the backing and smooth the wrap on to the nail from base to tip.

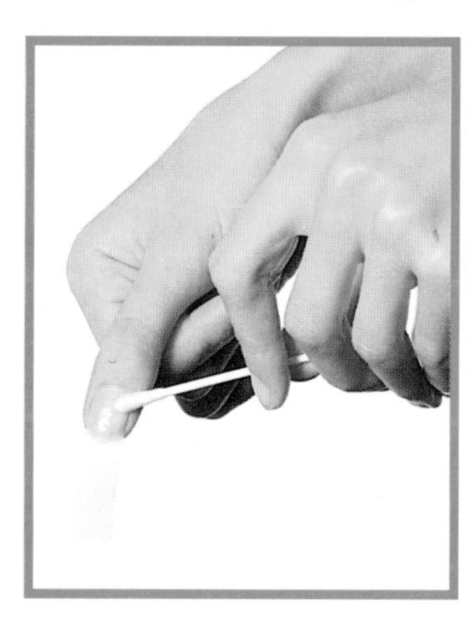

3 Spread the glue evenly over the surface of your nail with a cotton bud, avoiding the silk overhang.

STICK 'EM UP!

Ready painted stick-on falsies are the simplest and quickest way to make your nails beautiful in a flash. They're a great standby when you're going somewhere special and your hands will be on show.

Stick-on nails are available in lots of colours, or you can buy a natural finish and paint them yourself. The good news is that the nails are reusable and you'll just need to buy some more sticky tabs. With nails you've painted, always use an acetone-free nail polish remover, otherwise the false nail will wrinkle and melt.

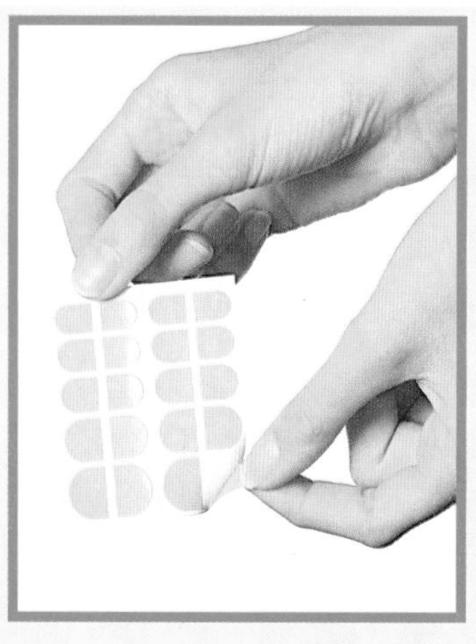

1 Choose matching-sized double-side sticky tabs for each nail then peel off the backing paper of each one.

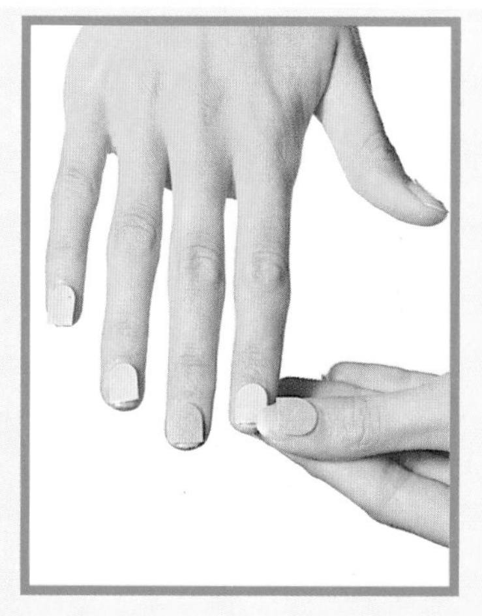

2 Position each tab sticky side down so that the rounded side is next to your cuticle at the nail's base.

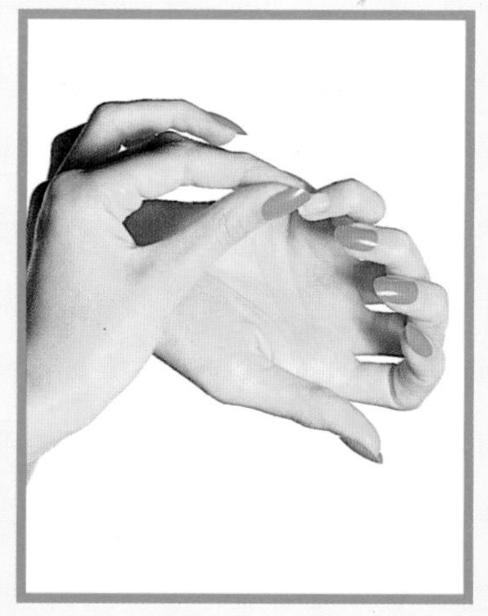

3 Peel the backing paper off the top of each tab. Press each matching false nail gently down on top.

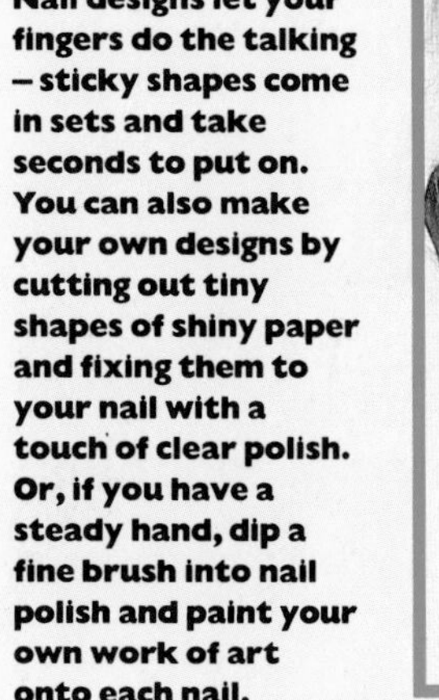

STUCK ON YOU ▶
Nail designs let your fingers do the talking – sticky shapes come in sets and take seconds to put on. You can also make your own designs by cutting out tiny shapes of shiny paper and fixing them to your nail with a touch of clear polish. Or, if you have a steady hand, dip a fine brush into nail polish and paint your own work of art onto each nail.

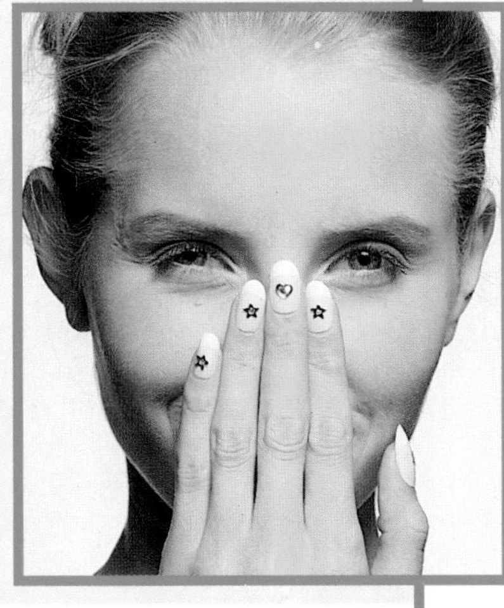

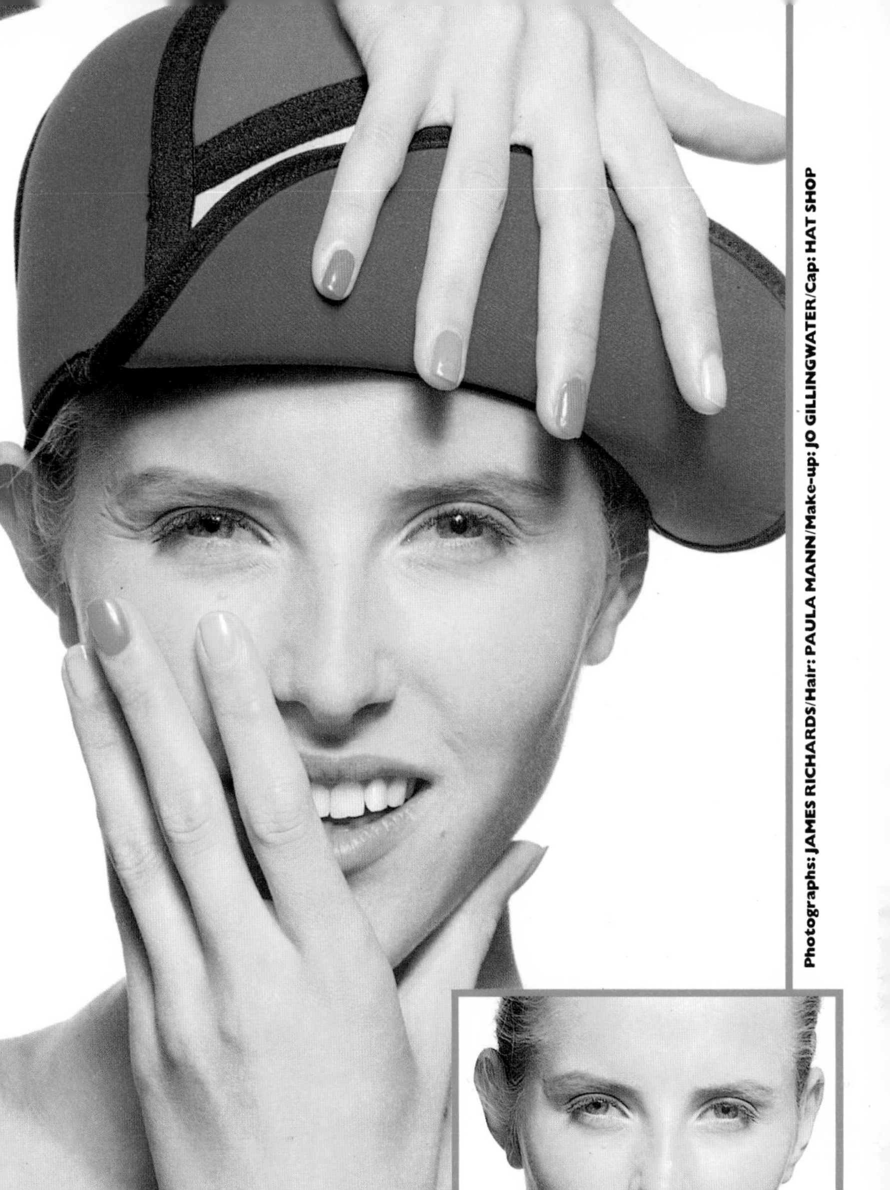

Photographs: JAMES RICHARDS/Hair: PAULA MANN/Make-up: JO GILLINGWATER/Cap: HAT SHOP

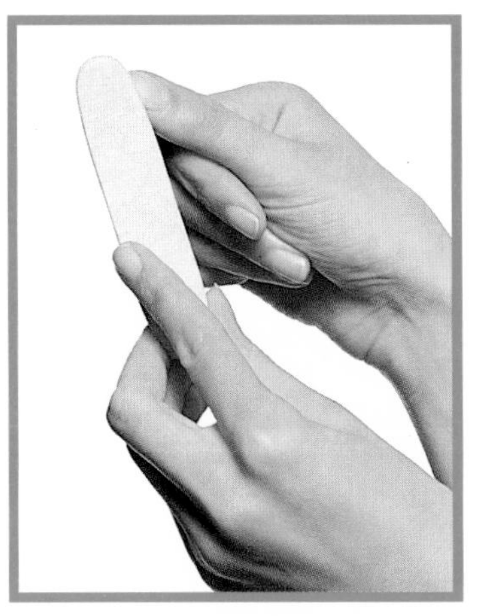

4 *Allow five minutes for the glue to dry. Trim the overhang then file it to the right length with an emery board. Now paint it.*

Buff the top of your nail for a smooth, shiny finish using a soft, suede pad.

SMOOTH REMOVAL
To take off the silk wraps, use a glue solvent from the same range as your nail kit. Afterwards, rub in a little nail cream to smooth the nail.

OOH LA LA! ▶
Cheat – a French manicure with stick-on ready-painted nails!

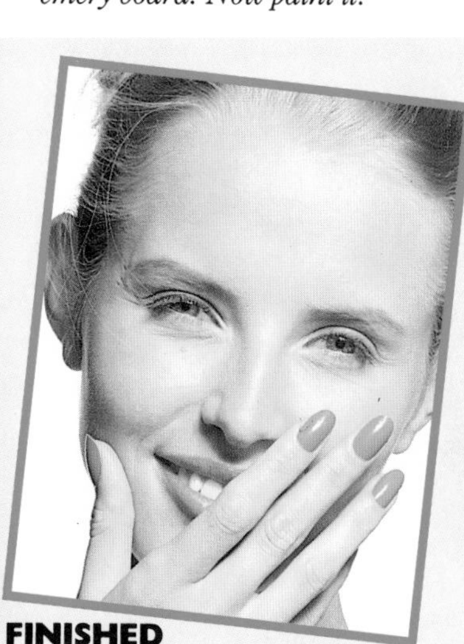

FINISHED
Perfect falsies and nobody need ever know that they're not home grown!

STAYING POWER
Keep your new-look nails in place.
- don't wear them for sport.
- don't immerse them in water.
- put your nails on only after applying your make-up and styling your hair.

SMOOTH REMOVAL
Soak the false nails in water to make removal easier. Use a manicure stick to pry them up, then peel them back.

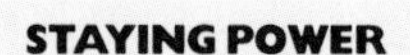

For the sake of your real nails' health, don't wear stick-ons for more than 48 hours without a 12 hour break.

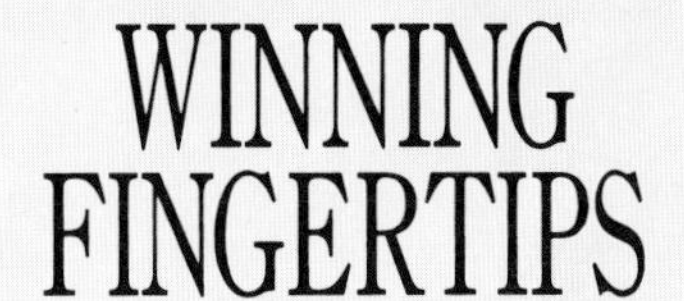

WINNING FINGERTIPS

- Avoid using silk wraps or falsies if your fingers or cuticles are sore or damaged.
- For lovelier nails, buy the basic essentials for the job – a proper pair of nail scissors or clippers and emery boards.
- Don't dig the skin around your cuticles with a sharp implement. Always use an orange-stick to help push back the cuticles.
- Nail biting a problem? Buy bitter-tasting lotion and paint on to your nails.

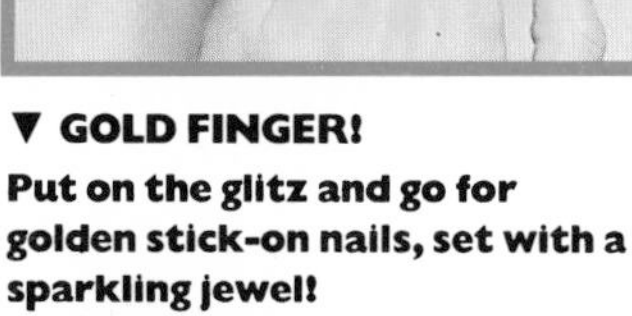

▼ GOLD FINGER!
Put on the glitz and go for golden stick-on nails, set with a sparkling jewel!

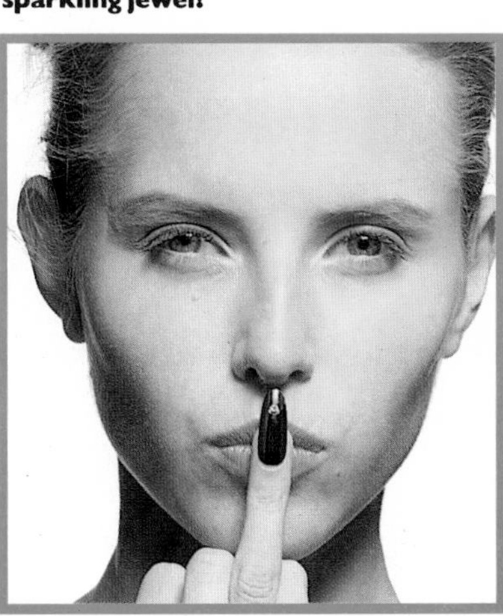

HANDIWORK

Whether you prefer your talons long and pointed or neat and natural, a manicure is the best mitt maintenance you can have. Treat yourself once a week at home!

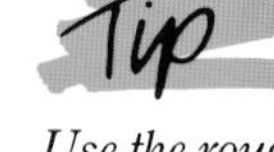

Use the rough side of the emery board if your nails need a lot of shaping. Otherwise stick to the gentler, smooth side.

IT'S A MYTH!
Eating jelly cubes won't make brittle nails any stronger. Instead, try supplementing your diet with extra vitamin A, zinc or iodine.

Tip

Add a few drops of castor oil to nail polish remover to stop your nails drying out.

DID YOU KNOW?
Nails grow about 6 mm/¼ in a month. They grow faster in the summer and on your right hand (if you're right-handed) and vice versa if you're left-handed.

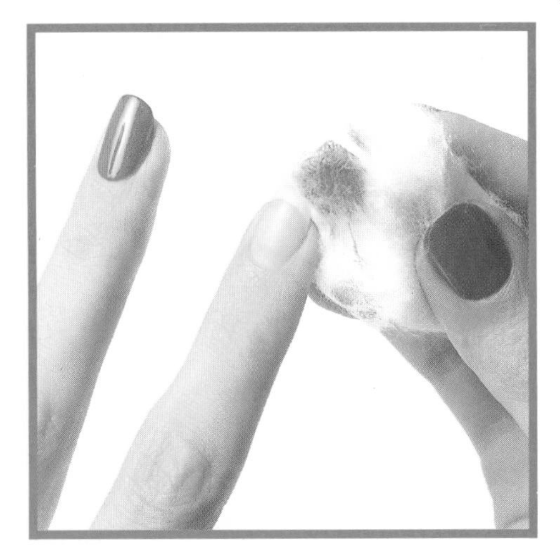

1 Remove old polish with nail polish remover. Soak a cotton wool pad, press it on to your nail, wait a few seconds then wipe off.

2 Using an emery board, file your nails in one direction from each side to the middle. Aim for rounded edges. If your nails are very long, use nail clippers first.

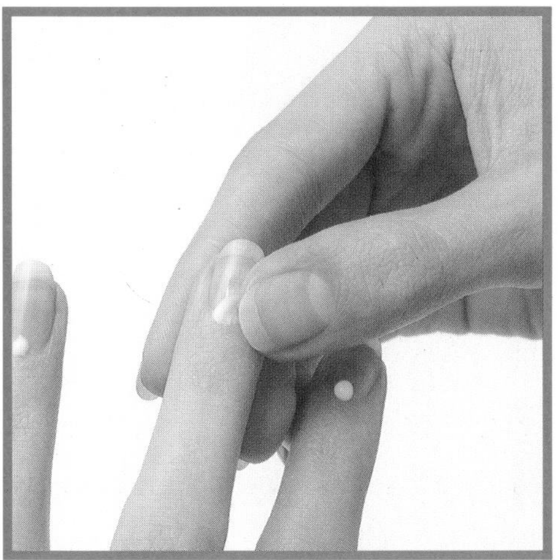

3 To soften the cuticles (the dead skin around the edge of the nails), massage a little cuticle cream or hand cream into the base of each nail and surrounding skin.

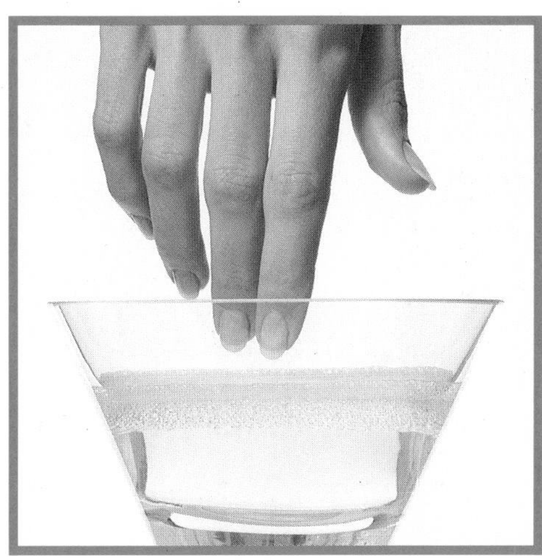

4 Dip your fingertips into warm, soapy water made with a mild shampoo as it's less drying than most soaps or washing up liquids.

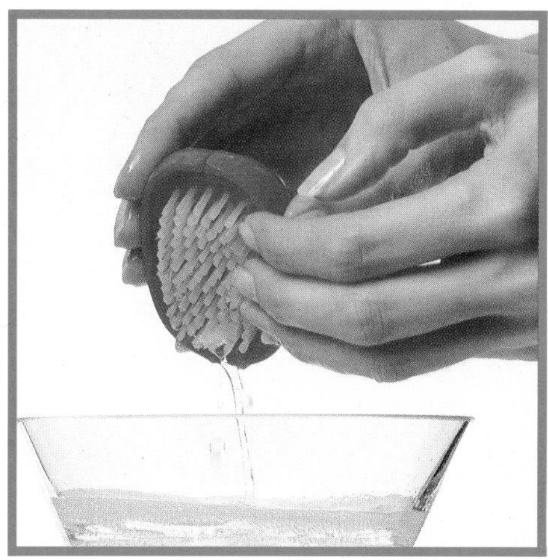

5 Using a soft brush, lightly scrub away any stubborn hard skin and clean under your nails. Afterwards, dry thoroughly with a towel.

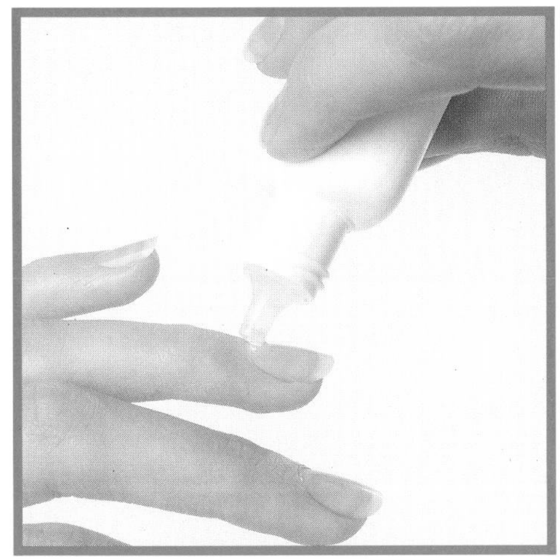

6 Next, squeeze a small drop of cuticle remover onto the base of each nail and massage in gently.

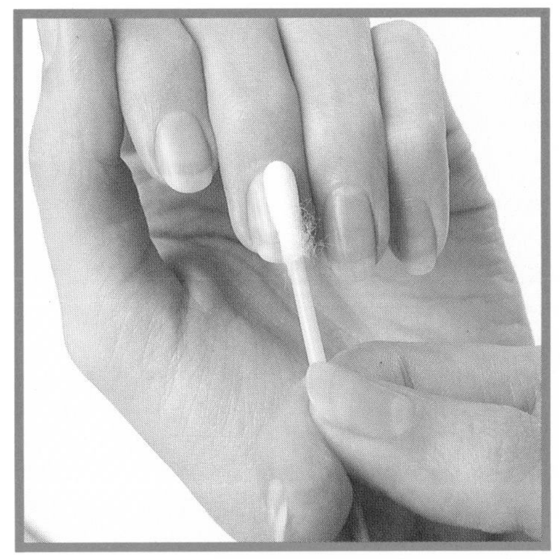

7 The cuticles should now be soft enough for you to push them gently back with a cotton wool bud or an orange stick with cotton wool wrapped round the end.

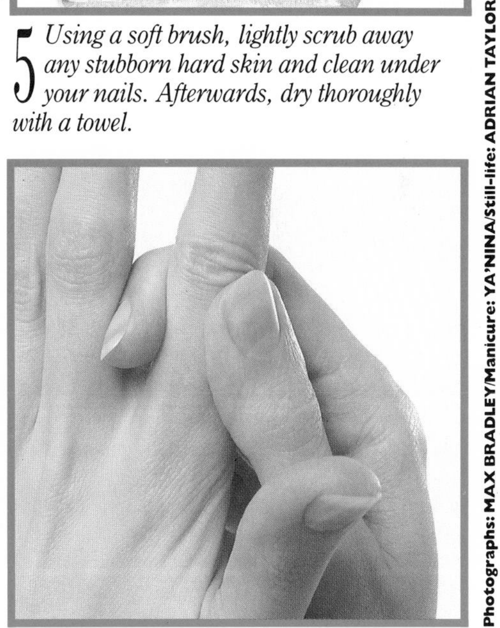

8 Massage a generous helping of rich, moisturising cream into your hands. Start by pushing towards your wrist, then work the cream down each finger.

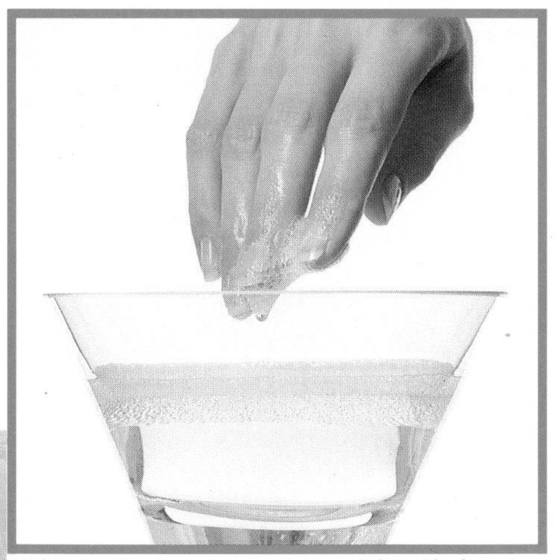

9 Give your fingers another quick dip in soapy water, washing away any excess hand cream from your nails. Dry your hands thoroughly.

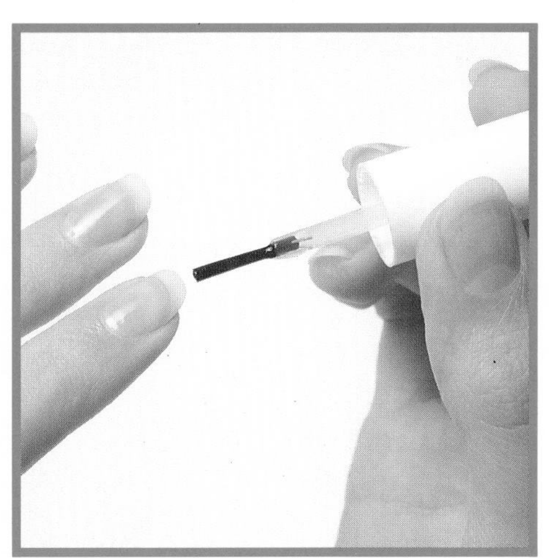

10 Protect your nails from staining by putting on a base coat. When it's completely dry, apply varnish in three strokes – middle first and then each side.

Tip

Make your own cuticle softener by mixing together two tablespoons of egg yolk and half a teaspoon of cider vinegar. Massage into the base of each nail, then rinse.

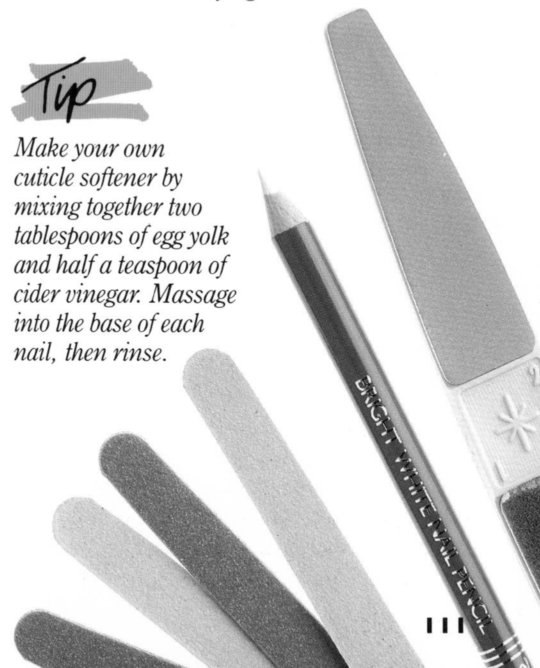

Photographs: MAX BRADLEY/Manicure: YA'NINA/Still-life: ADRIAN TAYLOR

THE NAIL FILE

What do you know about your nails? Take a tip from our nail care file and get yours up to scratch!

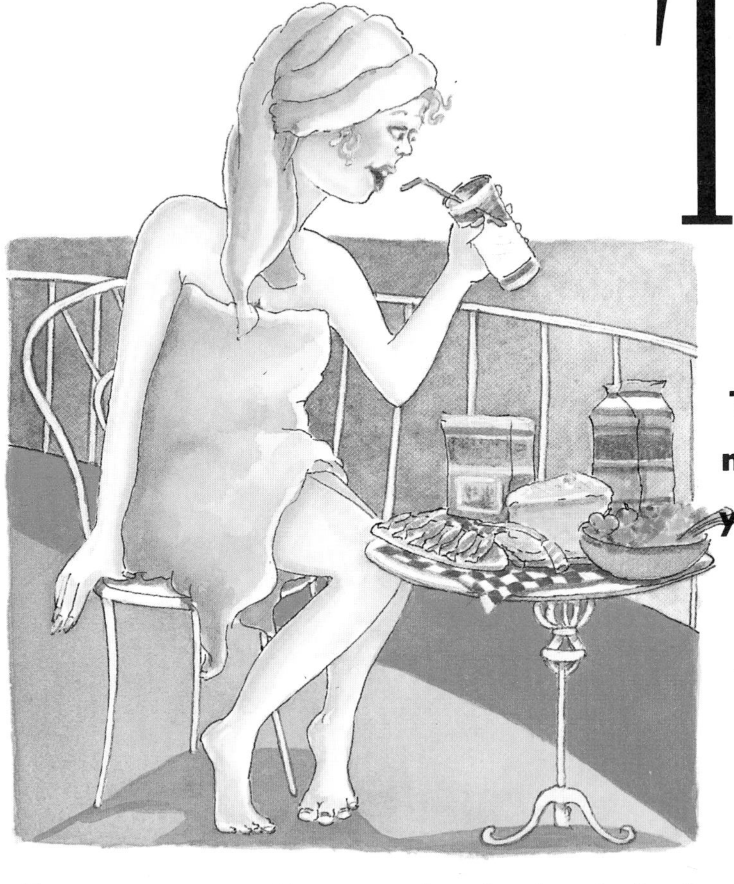

1 Your nails need a healthy diet to ensure strong growth. Step up your intake of vital nail foods rich in vitamins A, B, C and D, including cheese, milk, fruit and fish. As well as calcium, zinc is important – find both in spinach, cheese and nuts.

Like your hair, the visible nail is dead but the matrix at the base – like the hair follicle – is supplied with blood capillaries and nerve endings that need a regular and healthy diet.

2 Hangnails and tiny, painful threads of skin around the nail bed are caused by not pushing your cuticles back properly, excessive dryness, or from biting the bits of skin.

Pushing and prodding with sharp metal files will damage the nail bed. Smooth on a little cuticle cream instead to help prevent hangnails, then gently ease your cuticles back with a special rubber-tipped hoof stick or tissue-covered orange stick. Always moisturise the skin daily and snack on a carrot or some celery, instead of your skin.

3 Nails that splinter and break at the sides are caused by a heavy-handed manicure. Filing too far down at the sides weakens the edge and nails split under the slightest pressure.

Use the fine side of the emery board to file nails and never file deep into the corners – nails will appear longer and wear better when the sides of the nails are allowed to grow.

Filing to a sharp point also weakens nails and looks old-fashioned. Aim for a gentle curve to match the shape of the cuticle-end and file in one direction towards the top of the nail only.

4 Brittle nails that tend to break and split easily could be the victims of harsh soap and detergents which rob the nails of their natural moisture. Treat yourself to a moisturising soap and always wear rubber gloves when keeping your hands in water for any length of time. Keep a tub of moisturising cream by the rich sink and lavish it on after drying your hands. Don't forget to wear gloves for DIY chores.

5 White specks that appear on nails are caused by knocks and bumps or, it is thought, a zinc deficiency.

Try and keep your nails out of harm's way and protect them with gloves whenever you can.

Invest in a good manicure set to keep your nails in great shape and never poke at the nail base as this can cause the new nail to grow through damaged.

6 Your nails take between four and six months to grow from bed to tip and growth averages between 3 mm/⅛ in and 4 mm/⅙ in a month.

This means any splitting could relate to stress or illness six months ago and any further growth should be split-free. Try taking brewers' yeast or cod liver oil to strengthen nails.

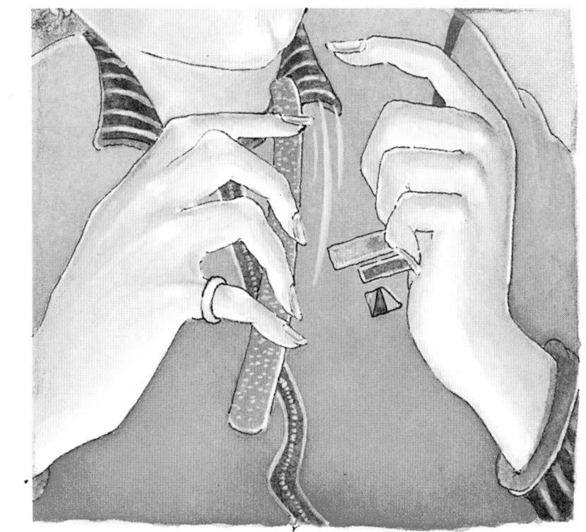

7 Acetone-based nail polish remover can dry out your nails and make them look dull as well as cause splitting, because the nail's surface is made up of layers of keratin (protein) which are banded together by natural oils and moisture.

Whisk away colour with an oil-based or conditioning remover and never peel off polish as the top layer of nail can come off too!

8 Onychophagists – that's the official name for nail biters – can't do any long-term damage to their nails but half-chewed fingertips do look ugly.

Beat biting them by trying one of the specially-formulated nail-biting solutions which are made to taste horrid to stop you nibbling! Or apply two thin coats of a good nail hardener which toughens up soft nails and makes them much harder to bite and nibble.

9 Yellowing nails are caused by wearing heavily-pigmented dark colours without a base coat. It depends on how porous your nails are as to how much they absorb.

Whiten them up a bit by soaking them in lemon juice for a few minutes or remember that there are some beauty salons which offer a special electric buffing treatment to remove any stains. Prime your nails for colour first with a clear or pale pink protective base coat. Smoking will also discolour your nails since they can become coated with nicotine – so give it up!

10 Allergic reactions to the formaldehyde which is added to some brands of nail polish is common and can lead to skin irritations.

Look out for brands that are formaldehyde-free or buff your nails to a natural high shine using a chamois-leather buffer. Rashes and redness around the cheeks and mouth can be caused by touching your face with painted nails.

11 The pill, which depletes the body's iron supplies, can affect the way nails grow. Check out health shops for supplements specially for nails and hair that help put back missing vitamins and minerals. It's a myth that chewing gelatine can make your nails grow stronger!

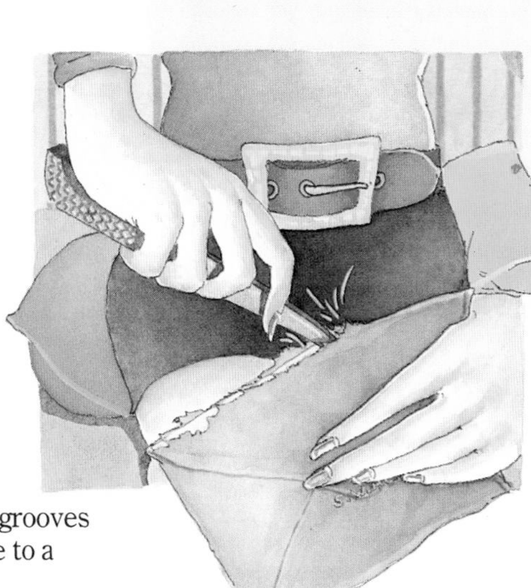

12 The development of horizontal ridges and grooves can be hereditary or due to a severe illness.

Once the ridge has formed there's nothing you can do until the nail has grown out. Buffing will help smooth the surface of the nail, but

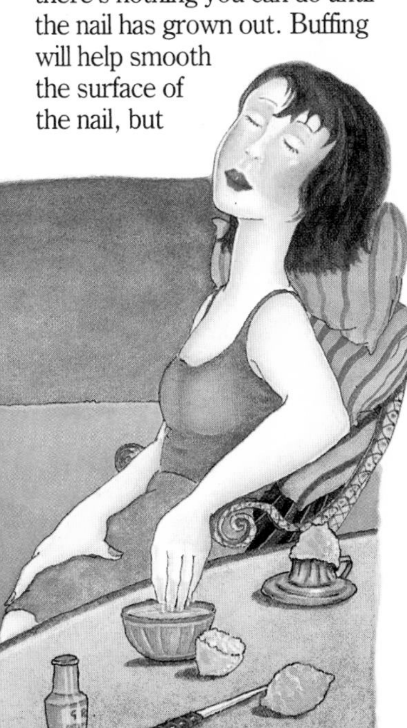

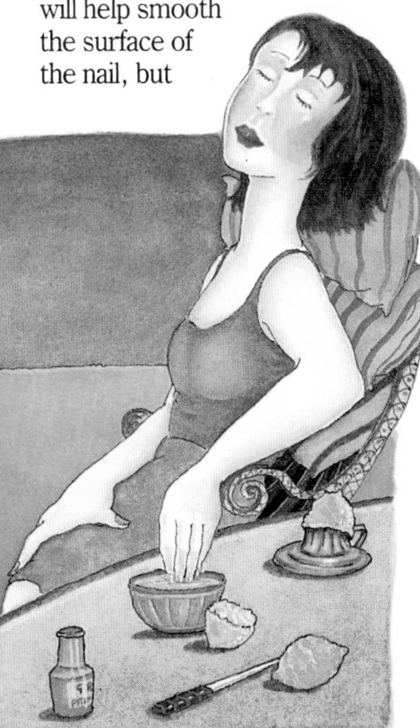

only do it twice a week. Look out for special ridge-filling creams that are worn under your nail polish and give an even base for painting on colour.

13 Very long nails shouldn't be filed and need careful cutting or clipping.

Use special nail scissors or manicure clippers and take small snips working carefully from one side to the other. Cutting off the tip straight across can severely weaken your nails.

14 Short nails look best painted in pale colours which can make them look longer and slimmer.

Choose pastel pinks, corals and gold and leave a thin strip unpainted at the sides of each nail to give the illusion of a slimmer, longer shape.

15 Regular exercise helps get the circulation going and speeds up nail growth – that's why typists, surprisingly, are often able to grow long, super-strong nails.

Try some simple hand exercises once a day; hold the tip of each finger with your other hand and work it up and down quickly five times for each finger. Now move your fingers as if you were playing the piano. Finally, clench your fingers into a fist and shoot out your fingers quickly, stretching them as far as you can. Repeat these exercises 10 times.

16 A broken nail before an important date doesn't have to be a complete disaster. Nail glue will bond a split nail in a matter of seconds or, if your nail has snapped off entirely, replace it with a substitute, plastic press-on tip and no one will ever know the difference – honest!

17 Nails need to be able to breathe to stay long and strong. When putting on your nail polish leave a tiny gap at the base of the nail to allow oxygen to get to the nail bed. Painting around the 'half moon' shape on the nail looks attractive too.

18 Nail polish lasts longer if you take time to apply it. Start with a base coat, then apply two thin coats of colour allowing each one to dry thoroughly. Twenty-four hours after your manicure, apply a top coat to fix your polish. Plunging your fingers into icy cold water when they're touch-dry will help to harden the varnish.

19 False nails are great if you're a lady of leisure, but don't expect them to be any more durable than natural nails if you insist on doing any heavy-duty housework.

Permanent acrylic tips have to be applied professionally and it's important to get a good fit to prevent any bacteria being trapped, which could lead to infection. Your own nails will continue to grow underneath, so fake tips won't last for more than four to five weeks at the most.

20 Nails on the hand you write with will always grow faster because of increased stimulation to the nail root.

Improve circulation on both hands by gentle buffing and a hand massage. Professional manicure buffers work best; or rub handcream into nails and hands.

NAIL-SAVING TIPS

- **Avoid ring-pull cans.**
- **Type letters or dial telephone numbers with the pads of your fingers.**
- **Open mail with a proper letter opener.**
- **Take care when undoing door locks or bolts.**
- **Keep your fingers as close together as possible when lifting objects.**
- **Don't attempt any chores straight after a bath – your nails will be soft and more likely to break.**
- **Keep nails well-shaped and fairly short.**
- **Paint the very tips with clear nail hardener.**
- **Never cut your nails with large or blunt scissors.**

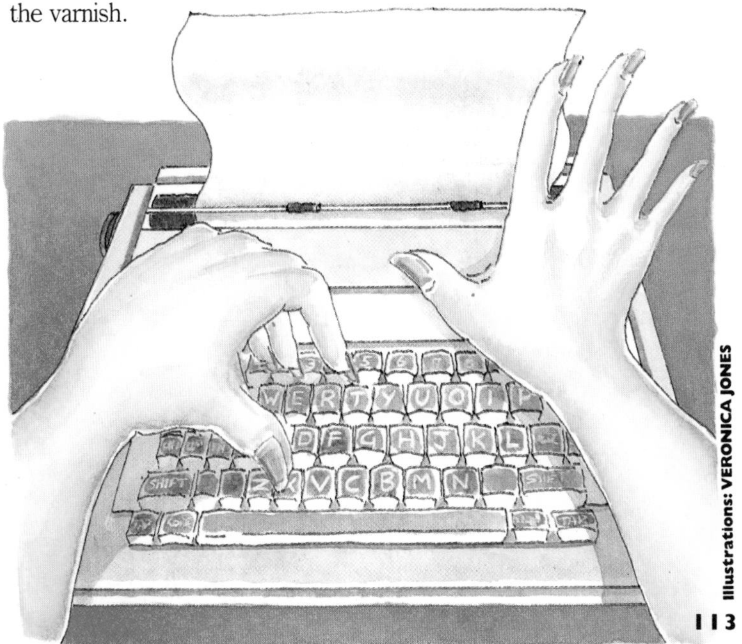

Illustrations: VERONICA JONES

ON THE MEND

Just when you manage to get your nails to a length you can be proud of, chances are one of them will split, crack or break. Here's how to master a spot of invisible mending so clever that no-one else will ever know!

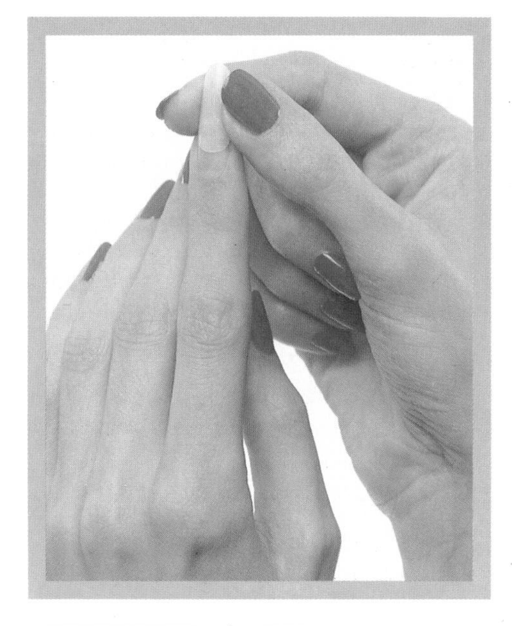

1 Buy a set of natural colour false nails and choose one that exactly covers the width of your broken nail. Keep the rest of the set for emergencies. Put a blob of glue on your clean nail and position just below the nail tip. Press firmly until stuck.

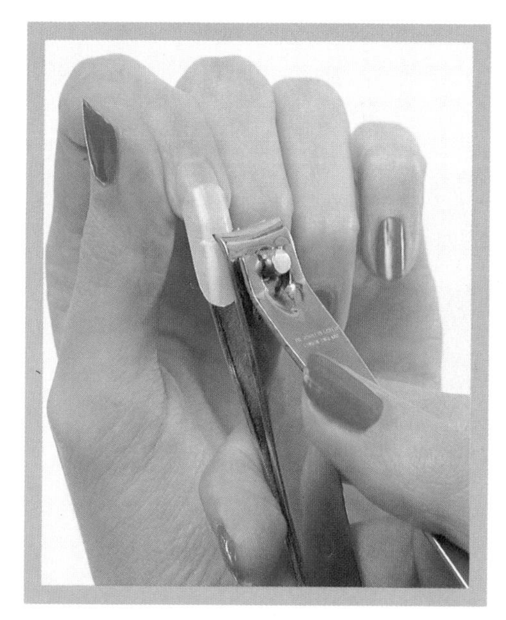

2 Use a pair of fingernail clippers, rather than scissors, to cut to length. Don't worry about cutting a perfect shape at this stage, the important thing is that the length matches the length of your other nails.

ALL STUCK UP

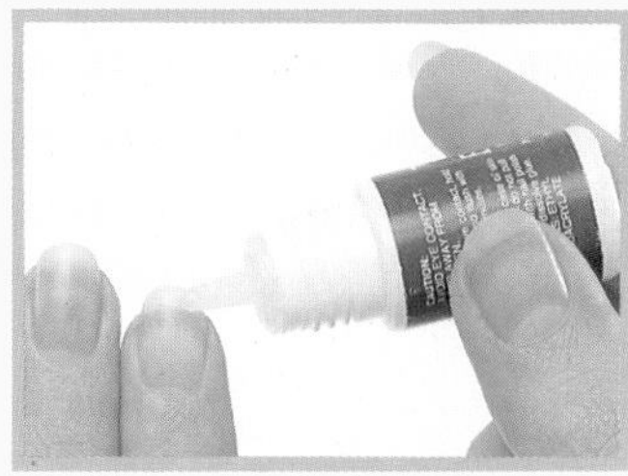

1 *If you crack the side of a nail, it's not necessary to cut off the whole thing because nail glue forms a long-lasting seal. Put a tiny blob of glue, enough to cover just the crack, onto the clean, dry nail.*

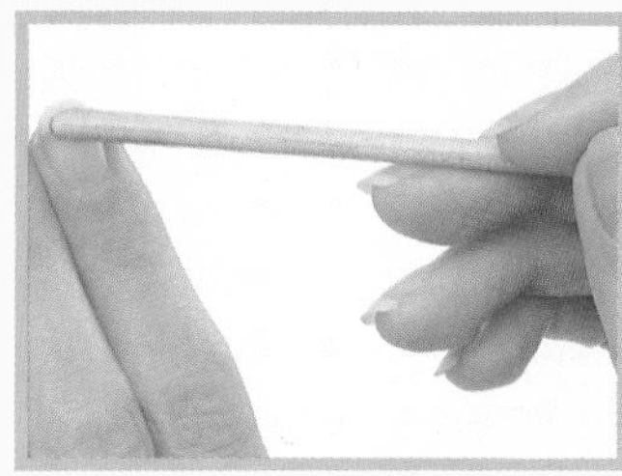

2 *To spread the glue into a thin even layer, use the end of a cuticle stick. Work quickly before the glue starts to set! Leave to dry completely then cover carefully in a layer of basecoat or polish.*

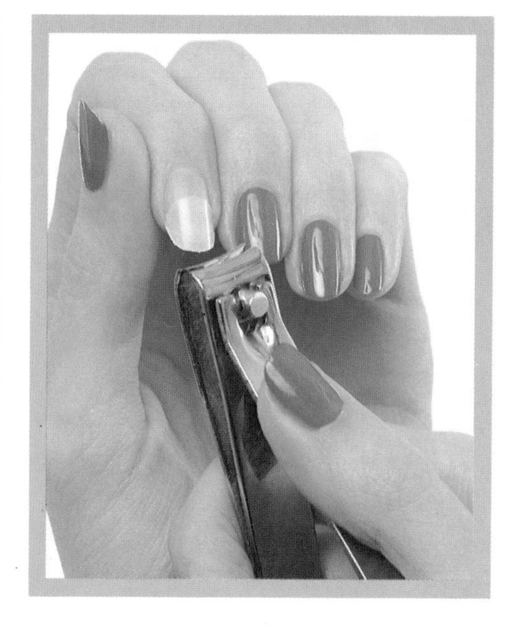

3 Start the cut from one side. Trim straight across the top of the false tip, then down the other side so that it forms a rough oval shape. Be careful that you don't pull or press too hard or the glue will come unstuck.

Photographs: MAX BRADLEY/Make-up: KARIN DARNELL

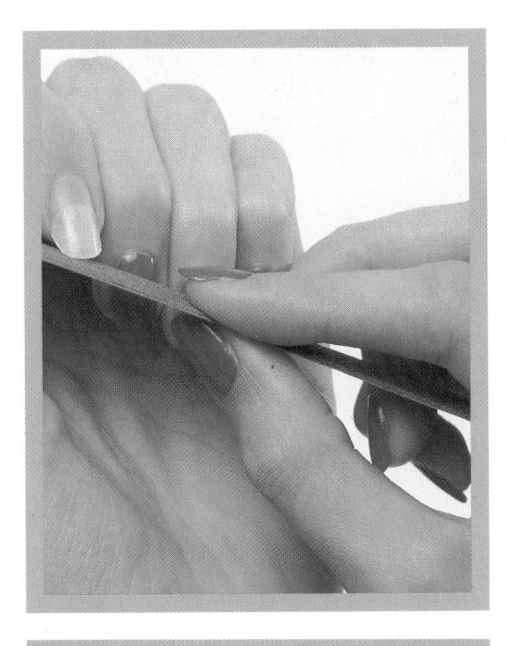

4 **Use the rough side of an emery board to file a neatly rounded shape. File in one direction only, not side to side, to avoid making any rough edges. Plastic is a bit tougher than nail, but you should still manage to get a really smooth rounded edge.**

Once you've filed your falsie into the right shape, use the fine side of the emery board to smooth it.

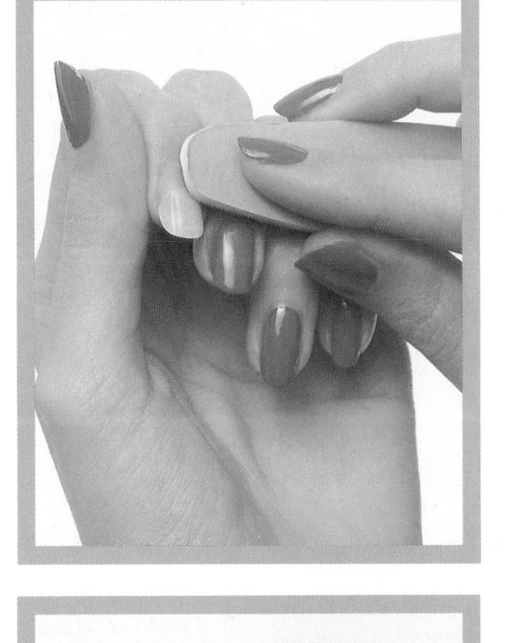

5 **To minimise the ridge where the edge of the tip and your nail meet, use the rough side of a buffer. Do this very gently to prevent damaging the nail. The ridge won't disappear completely, but you should be able to make it much smoother.**

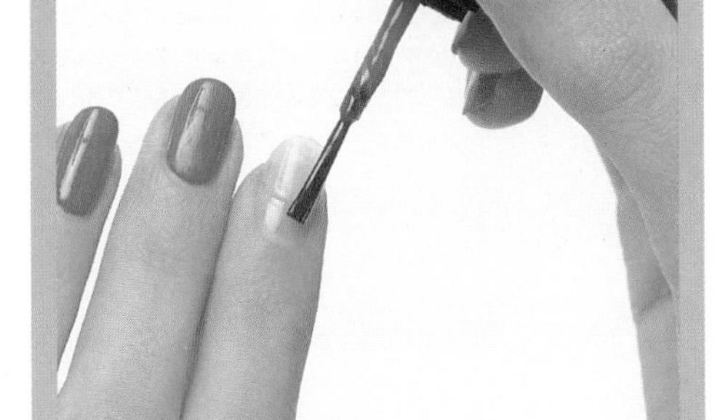

6 **To disguise the tip, choose a strongly-coloured nail polish. Begin by putting a basecoat over your nail. Then paint on the colour in a thin, even coat over your nail and the false nail tip.**

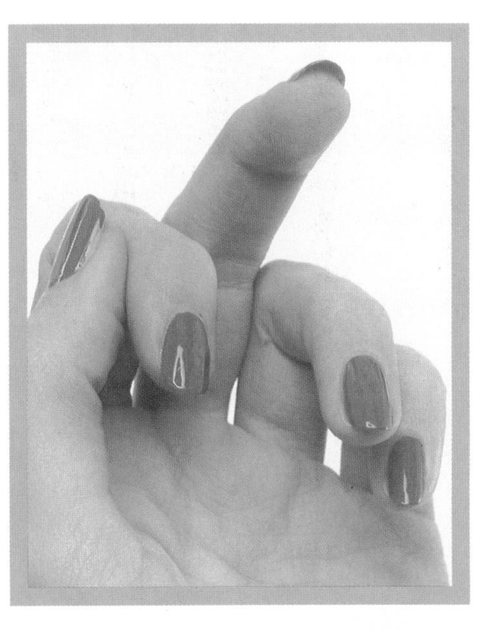

7 **Let the first coat of colour dry completely, then put on a second coat for extra cover. Once the second coat is dry it really will be very difficult for anyone to tell which nail is fake.**

THE TISSUE TRICK

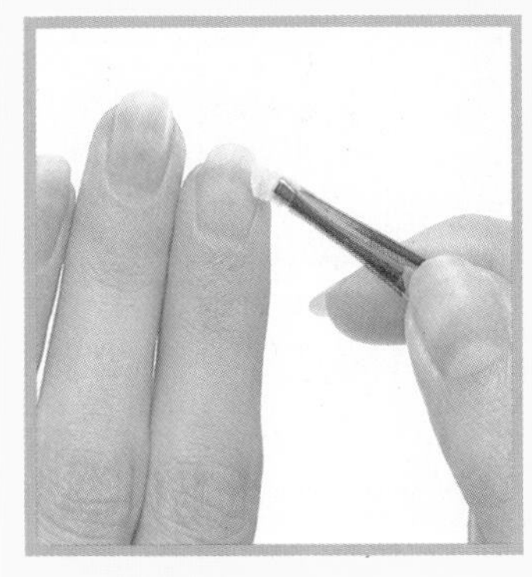

1 *If you crack a nail and have no glue, use a piece of tissue instead. Use a single sheet of either white or pale pink tissue. Paint a thin coat of clear polish over your nail and carefully position a tiny piece of tissue over the crack. Use a pair of tweezers for greater accuracy.*

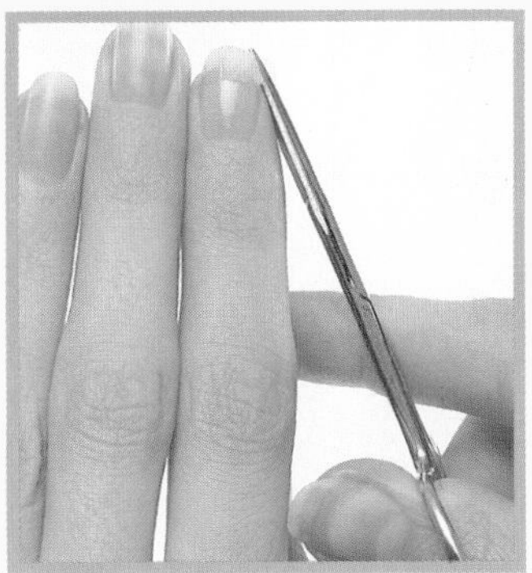

2 *Don't worry about the end of the tissue sticking over the edge of your finger, just make sure it's positioned correctly. The tissue will start to sink into the polish and then stay firmly in place. Neaten the edge of the tissue with a pair of nail scissors.*

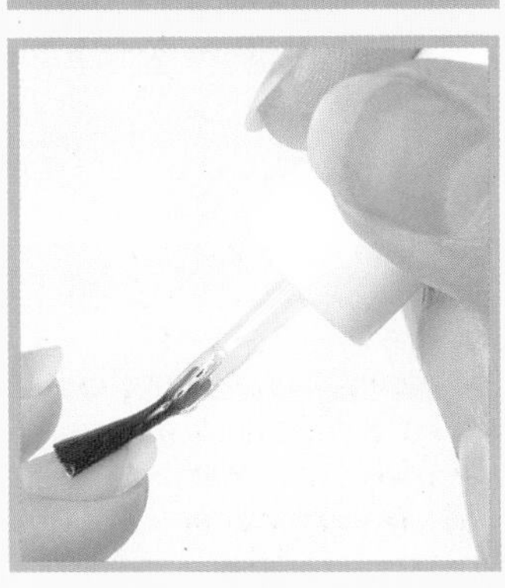

3 *To completely cover the tissue and form a long-lasting seal, carefully put on a second layer of clear polish. Paint all your other nails to match. You should find that the tissue stays firmly in place until your next manicure when you'll have to repeat the process.*

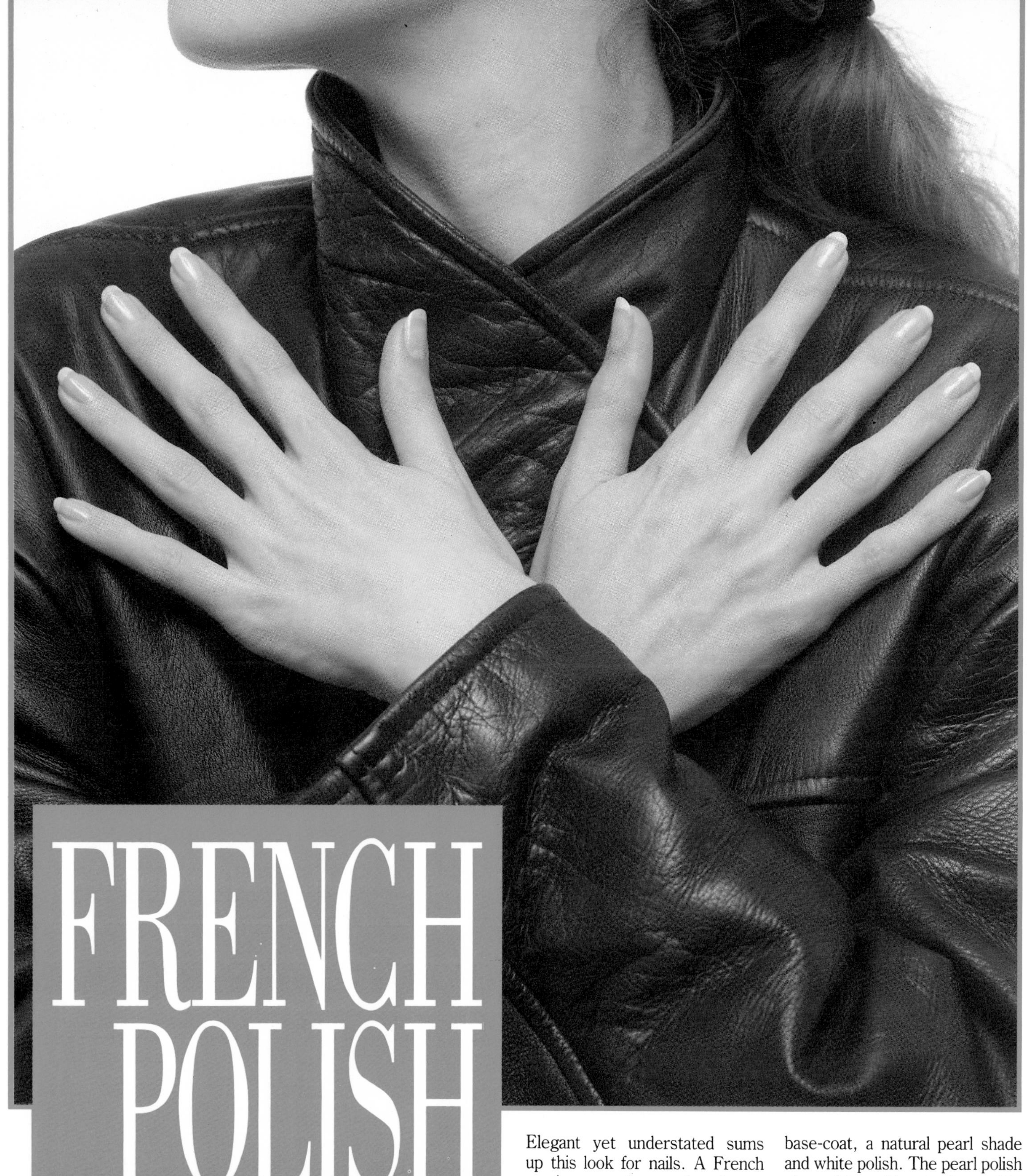

FRENCH POLISH

If scarlet talons aren't your style – why not try a French manicure? It'll flatter your fingertips with a natural finish that won't wage war on your wardrobe

Elegant yet understated sums up this look for nails. A French manicure makes nails of any length look good and goes well with whatever you're wearing – so there's no need to repaint your nails every time you decide to change your outfit!

Either buy a made-up kit from the chemist or make your own. You'll need basic nail-care items like a soft nailbrush, emery board, cuticle cream and hand-cream. You'll also need a bottle of clear base-coat, a natural pearl shade and white polish. The pearl polish gives shine without colour while the white heightens the colour of your nail tips.

For an individual touch that's still subtle, switch from neutral to nude-beige or soft pink polish, plus white tips.

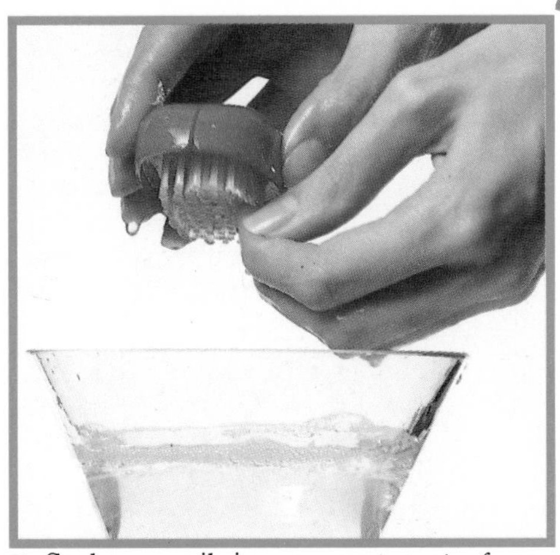

1 *Soak your nails in warm soapy water for a few moments to loosen dirt and soften cuticles. Gently scrub nail tips clean with a soft nailbrush, then rinse and dry well.*

Watchpoint

Polish won't adhere if nails are wet, or if any residue remains. Wash and dry nails thoroughly before applying polish.

You need very little white polish to paint the tips in a French manicure, so make sure you wipe off any excess on the brush against the bottle top, before you begin.

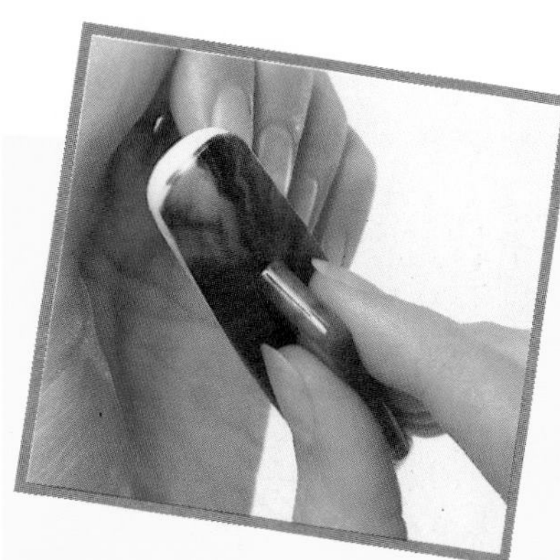

IN THE BUFF

If you've got healthy-looking nails, you can get the effect of a French manicure by buffing with a chamois buffer and buffing cream. Buff in the cream in one direction only, allowing half a minute per nail.

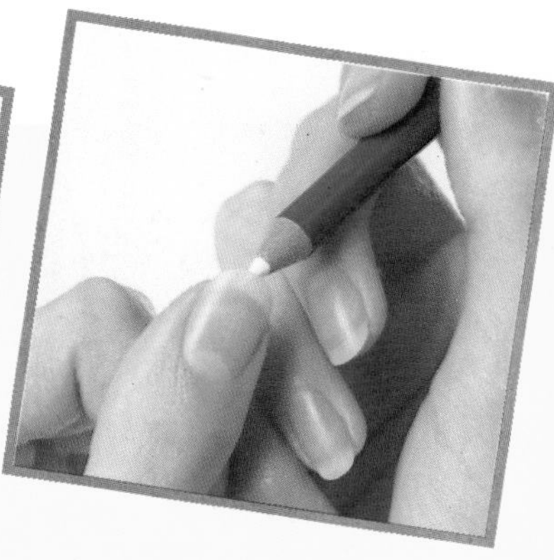

WHITER THAN WHITE

If you haven't time for a French manicure run a sharp white nail or eye-liner pencil under the white part of your nails to highlight the tips. Finish with a coat of pearly natural polish.

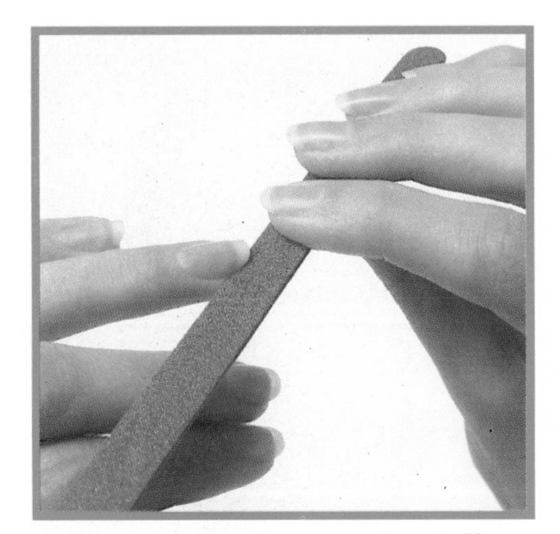

2 *File your nails with an emery board. Use the rough side to shape and the other to smooth any roughness. File in one direction, from each side to the middle.*

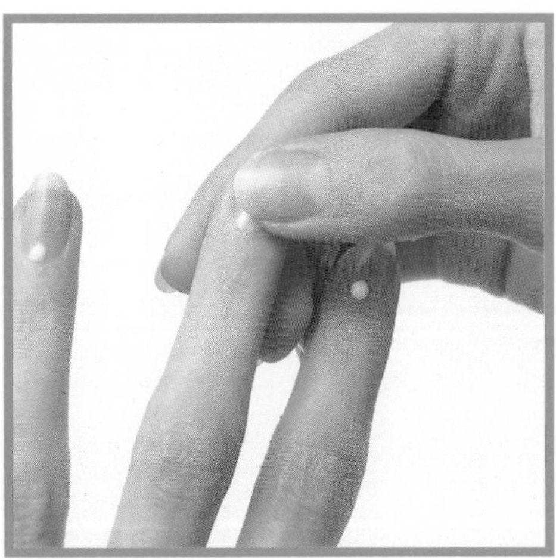

3 *Dab a dot of cuticle cream on the base of each nail and massage gently into the base and both sides of the nail with the pad of your thumb.*

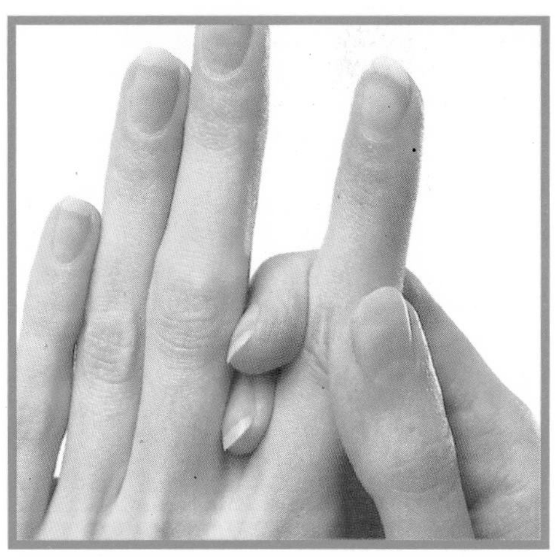

4 *Massage hand-cream into your hands, paying particular attention to finger joints and knuckles, where the skin is thinnest and most likely to wrinkle.*

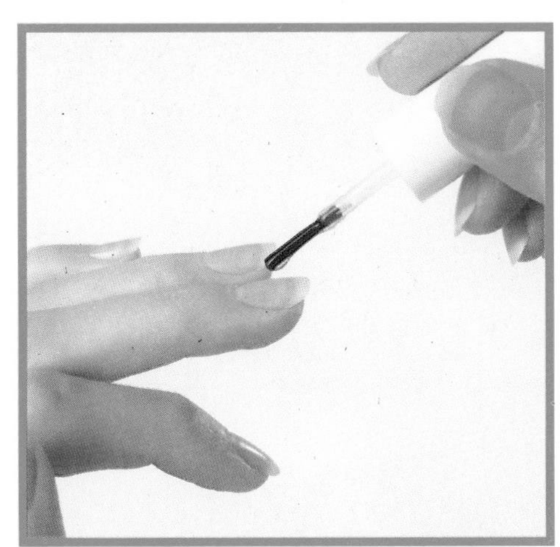

5 *Paint on a base-coat to protect your nails and provide an even surface. Then paint each nail carefully with a single coat of natural pearly polish.*

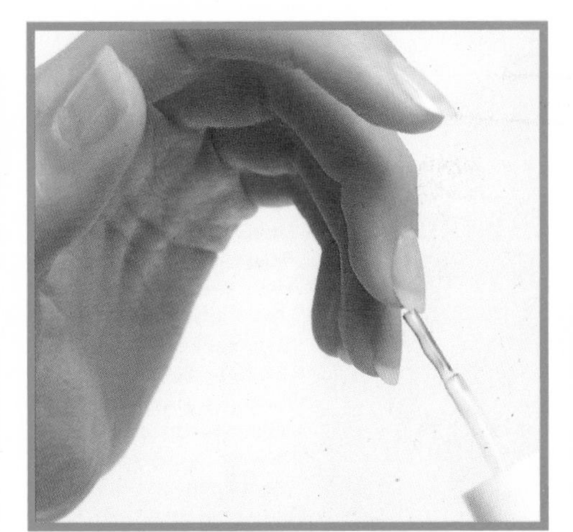

6 *Steady yourself for the tricky bit! Paint the white part at the tip of your nails only with white polish, carefully following the curved contour.*

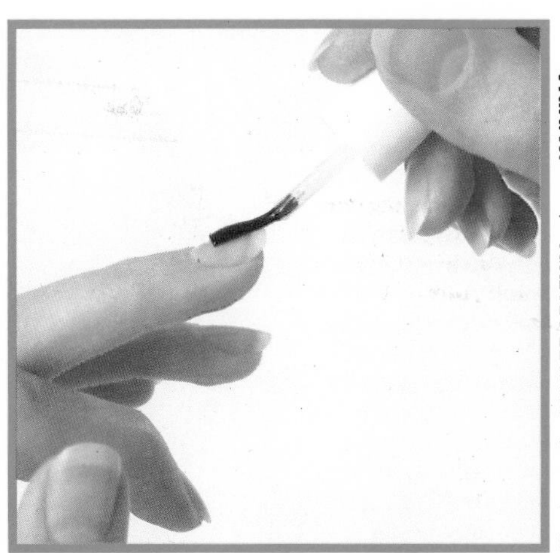

7 *Apply a final coat of pearly polish over the entire nail to protect and add shine, covering previous coats completely.*

Photographs: MAX BRADLEY/Manicure: YA'NINA

PLAQUE ATTACK

Give yourself plenty to smile about by following our step-by-step guide to teeth that look and feel squeaky clean

Everyone wants clean, healthy teeth but unfortunately most of us have to work at getting them that way. And the sad fact is that most of us will have damaged our teeth during the first 15 years of life by eating too many sugary foods that cause tooth and gum disease.

Plaque, the main culprit, is a film that forms over the teeth when remains of sticky foods and bacteria are allowed to accumulate. If this isn't removed properly it'll gradually attack the gums.

The most important part of your dental programme should therefore be to discourage plaque. Cutting down on sugary foods and drinks helps.

You should also see your dentist frequently and brush your teeth regularly and thoroughly.

The latest research suggests that cleaning your teeth before you eat may be the best weapon in the fight against decay. The moment you start to eat, bacteria already present on the surface of the teeth starts to break down the food to produce the sugary substances which form the perfect breeding-ground for plaque.

So clean thoroughly before meals and again at bedtime using an ordinary fluoride toothpaste to slow down the plaque producing process. If plaque really does become a problem, visit your hygienist for a proper scale and polish.

1 Use a disclosing tablet to show you where the plaque is. The tablet is made of a harmless dye which you swoosh around your mouth with some water for a few minutes before spitting out. Any plaque-covered areas of your mouth will be stained a pinky colour and will need a really good clean. Try using a disclosing tablet after brushing too. You'll see just how well you've cleaned your teeth.

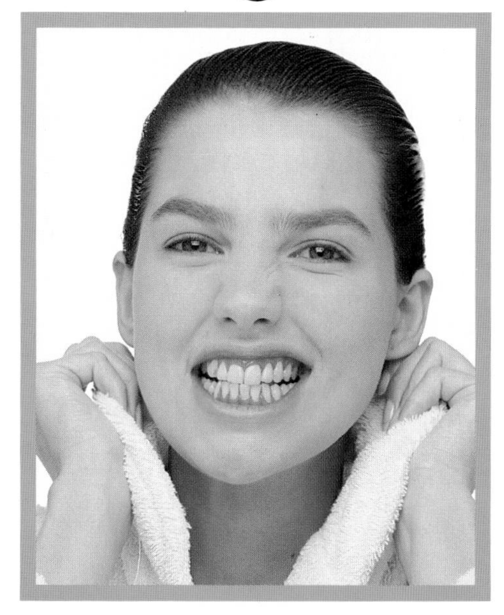

2 Squeeze a small blob of toothpaste – about the size of a pea – onto your brush. The danger with using too much toothpaste is that you may feel as though your mouth is clean before it really is. You can clean your teeth in any order, but make sure you do it properly. Regular brushing prevents plaque building up which eventually loosens teeth.

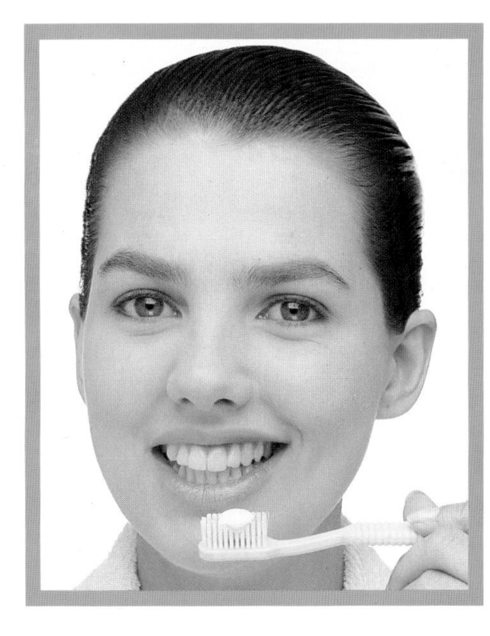

3 Put the bristles flat on the tooth's surface at the point where it joins the gum. Push the bristles down into the gum and then flick firmly outwards: this gets rid of any food which may be trapped in the gap between the tooth and the gum. And do remember to brush the backs of your teeth where plaque can also build up.

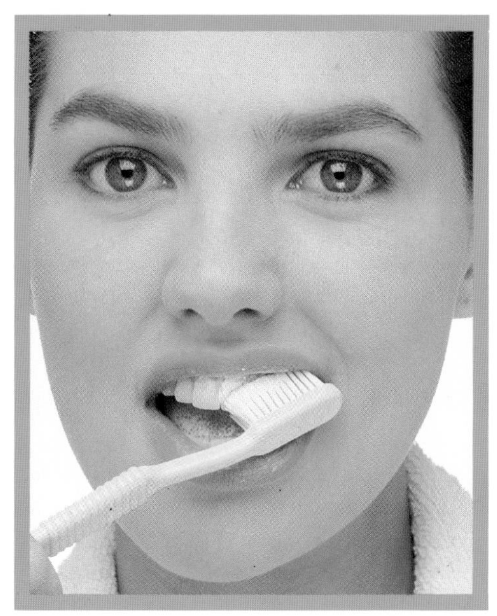

4 **Now use a brisk up and down movement to clean the front surface of each tooth.**

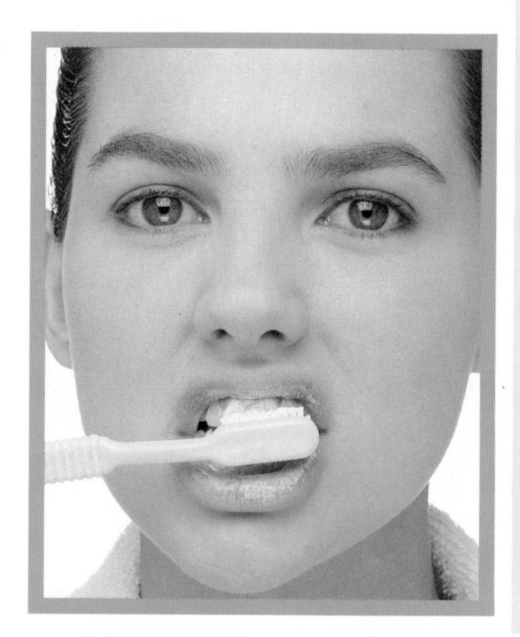

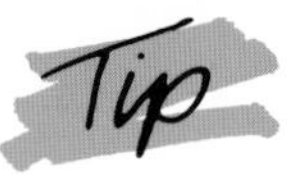

Don't just rub toothpaste round your mouth or use a mouthwash as an alternative to brushing your teeth. Brush at least twice a day for about the same time it would take to listen to a song on the radio.

BRUSHING UP

Choose a toothbrush with a medium-sized head and medium-textured nylon bristles. A large toothbrush feels clumsy in the mouth, while soft bristles can't get to grips with stubborn plaque.

Hard bristles are not a good idea either: they scratch the tooth's surface, leaving it open to decay. To reach the tricky back teeth you might need an angle-headed brush, which is designed to help you reach out-of-the-way surfaces.

An inter-space brush has only a small clump of bristles and is used to clean the teeth on either side of a gap and the line where the tooth joins the mouth. This is where most gum disease begins, and gum disease is the biggest cause of tooth loss in adults. Use a tiny dab of toothpaste, and work around the gum line using a gentle circular movement.

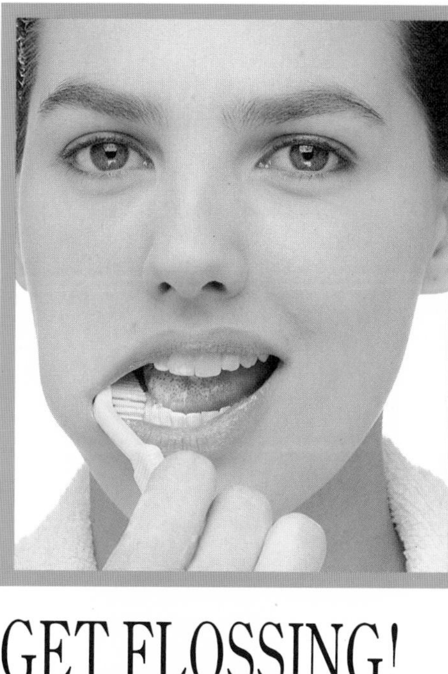

5 **When it comes to cleaning the back and edges of each tooth, you may find it easier to use an angle-headed brush.**

Pay as much attention to the gums as the teeth themselves. A staggering 90 per cent of us suffer from gum disease without realising it. If your gums bleed after brushing see your dentist.

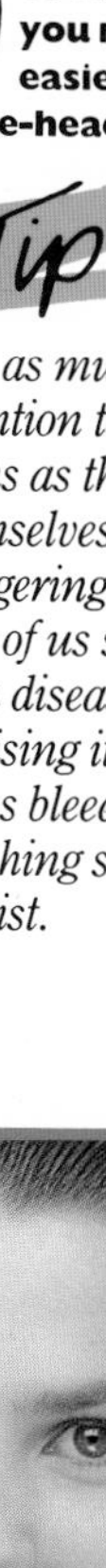

GET FLOSSING!

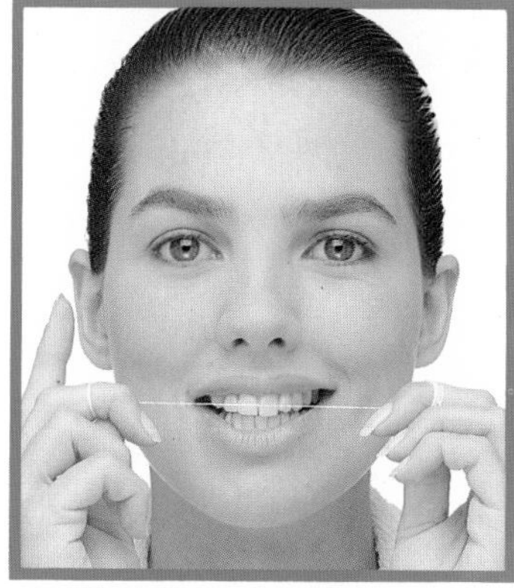

1 *Wrap the ends of floss around your two index fingers and hold them apart so that the floss is taut.*

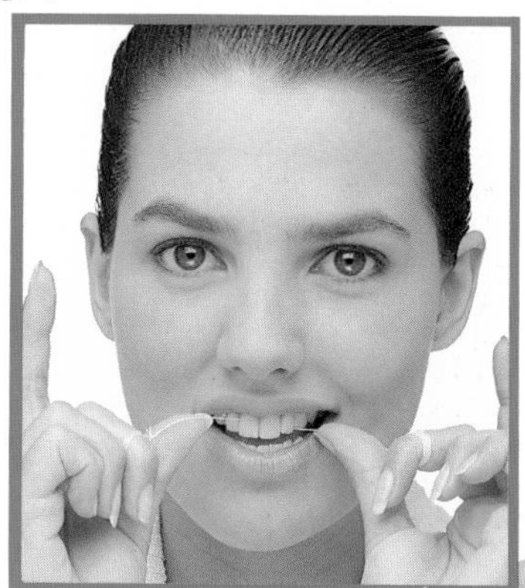

2 *Wrap the floss in a C-shape around each tooth and very gently scrape up and down over the surface.*

Photographs: PAUL MITCHELL/Still-life photographs: ADRIAN TAYLOR/Hair & make-up: CHASE ASTON

Squashed, pinched and neglected – how would you like to be in their shoes? Put your feet first and pep up those tired tootsies

SOLE SURVIVORS

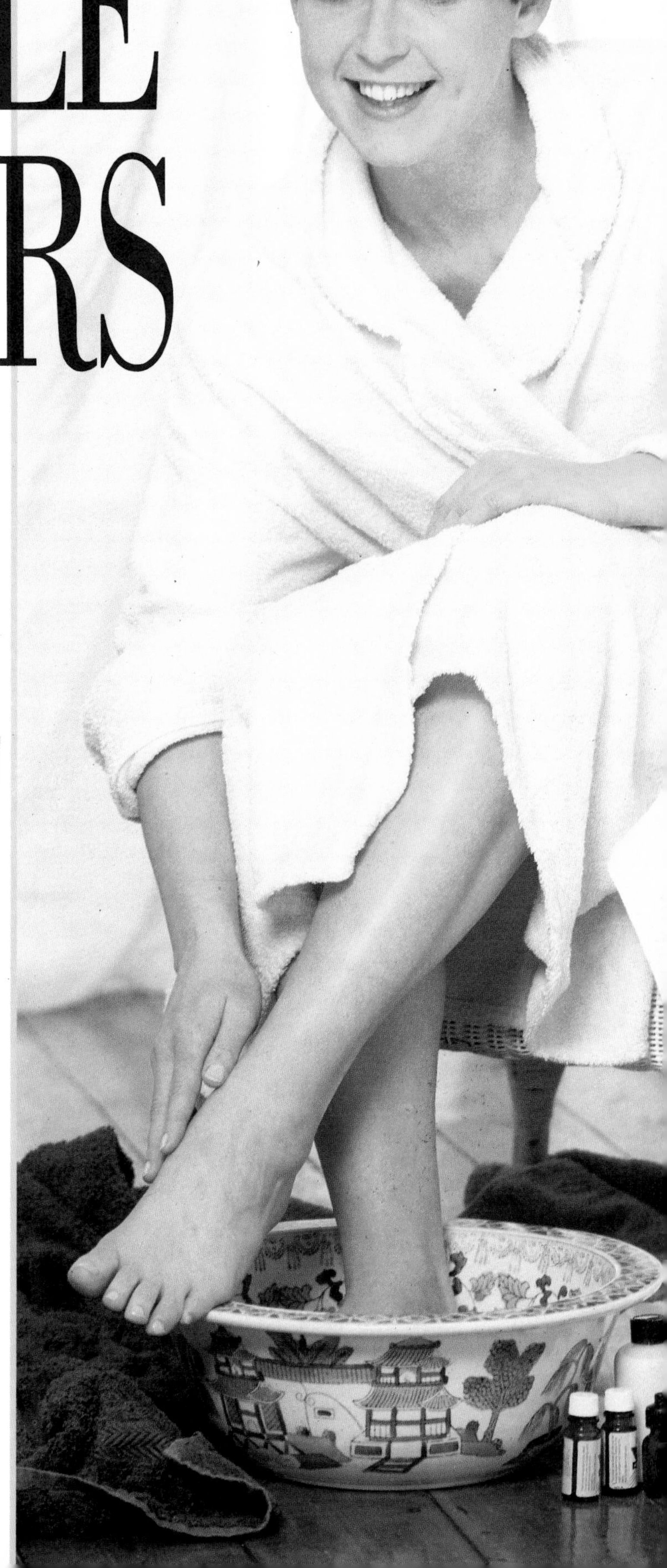

Your feet not only support your weight but will walk the equivalent of twice around the world during your lifetime. It's no wonder, then, that they need pampering occasionally! Put aside a few moments each week to try some of our soothing solutions and you'll soon feel the benefits right down to the tips of your toes. For starters, take the following steps for happier feet:

- **Avoid shoes that pinch your toes or strappy styles that cut off the circulation, otherwise your feet will be sore and puffy.**
- **On hot days, dust feet with talc if you're going without tights – it'll help to keep them cool and prevent stickiness.**
- **Walk barefoot whenever you can to firm muscles and to relax your feet after a hard foot-slogging day in shoes.**
- **Try walking barefoot on tip-toes for a minute every day to strengthen and stretch muscles.**
- **Relieve tired feet with a footsie roller massage. Place the roller on top of a thick towel so that you don't make grooves in the carpet, then sit down and roll your foot to and fro over the roller. Exert enough pressure to move it from your toes right back to your heel.**
- **Fill cotton socks with dried lentils and walk around in them for five minutes to massage the soles of your feet – it really does work! Or if you've got some spare cash, invest in a pair of exercise sandals especially designed for the job.**

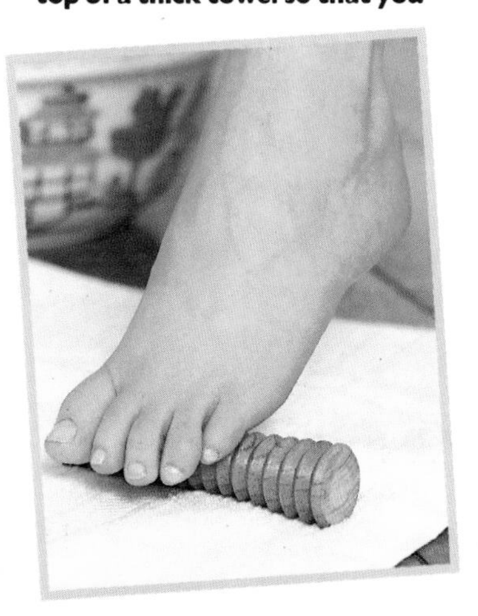

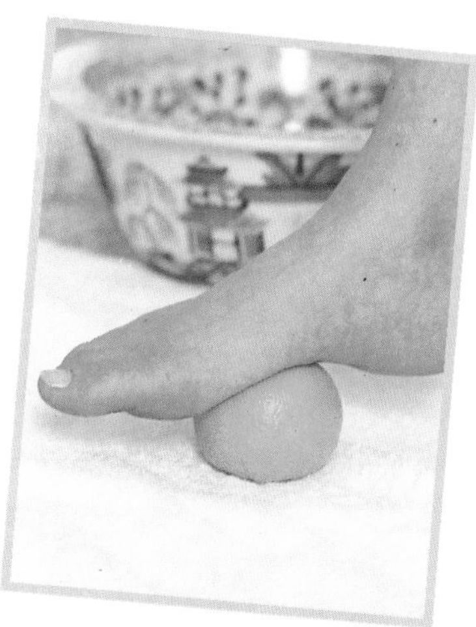

- **Roll a soft ball or an orange under each foot to keep them supple and to relieve aching arches.**
- **If you can't wait till the end of the day for some foot relief, try exercising at your desk. Remove your shoes and rotate your feet 20 times to the right, then 20 times to the left.**

DID YOU KNOW?

The heel tip of stilettos worn by a woman of average weight will exert the same amount of pressure on the ground as an elephant!

SOAK OPERA

► After a hard day on the run, soaking tired feet in a big bowl of water has to be one of the best ways to relax and revitalise them. In fact, it'll make you feel better all over.

Before you start, brush each foot with a big soft body brush to remove dead skin cells and to pep up your circulation. Concentrate on the soles of your feet and brush with firm circular strokes. Next, wash your feet in warm water with mild soap and rinse them well. Then change the water and get ready for a long luxurious soak!

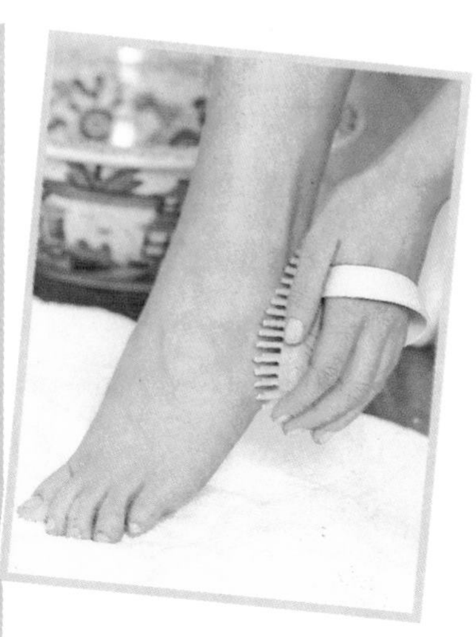

● Have a towel and moisturiser to hand, then take your phone off the hook to make sure you won't be disturbed.

● Fill a large bowl or bucket with comfortably warm water. Elbow test the temperature before you take the plunge. For a bracing foot bath, plunge feet into warm water first then into icy cold!

● To get maximum benefit, leave your feet to soak for at least 15 minutes. You may need to reheat your foot bath so have a friend at hand to top it up with some warm water for you.

KITCHEN TREATS

Step up your foot bath the natural way with a little help from some home-made standbys.

● Add a tablespoon of dried herbs like mint, yarrow, or marigold leaves, which are renowned for their soothing properties, to your foot bath.

● Try a mix of good old-fashioned ingredients to soften and smooth your skin. Fill your bowl or bucket with warm salted water, then stir in one tablespoon of borax and one tablespoon of Epsom salts.

● Add a teaspoon of mustard powder to your foot bath to pep up tired feet.

● Make an infusion – like making tea – from one tablespoon of nettles and one tablespoon of cider vinegar. Put them in a bowl then pour boiling water over and leave to 'brew' for five minutes. Sieve, then add the liquid to your bath.

AROMATHERAPY

Aromatherapy uses the pure fragrant oils extracted from flowers and plants which are renowned for their therapeutic properties. You must use genuine extracts as opposed to synthetic scents which smell the same but don't have any of the beauty benefits. Add these to your bath water.

Watchpoint

Don't put undiluted essential oils straight onto your skin – they're too concentrated and may cause an allergic reaction. Dilute the oils in the quantities given.

● To help relax tired or puffy feet, add six drops each of lavender and geranium oil, or seven drops of camomile and three drops of basil oil. Other oils known for their relaxing properties include ylang-ylang, neroli and marjoram.

● To soothe aching feet use four drops of rosemary oil, three drops of camomile oil and two drops of thyme oil.

● Soften your skin and strengthen your toe-nails with a cup of camomile tea and six drops each of lavender and geranium oil.

● Sweaty feet? Freshen them by bathing in a mixture of one tablespoon of witch-hazel and six drops of pine oil.

MOISTURISING

▼ After bathing your feet, dry them in a warm, fluffy towel – don't forget to dry between your toes – then treat them to a gentle massage using moisturiser. Rub a generous amount all over your feet in circular movements until the lotion is absorbed.

If your feet tend to get hot and sticky, look out for special foot lotions containing peppermint oil to refresh and overcome foot odour.

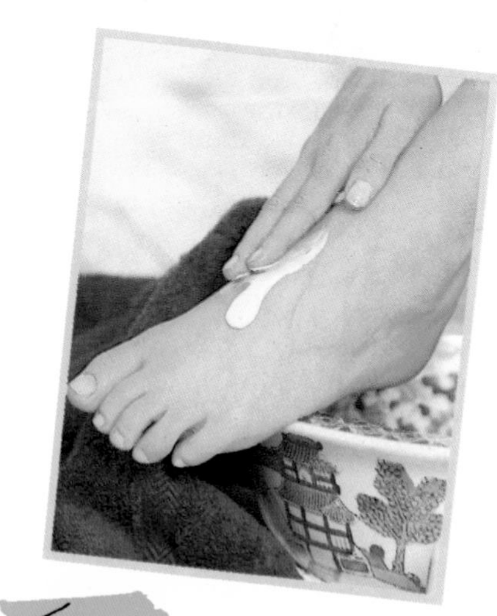

Tip

If your feet look dry and leathery from too much sun and sea, split open a vitamin E capsule and gently massage the oil into the tops of your feet.

Watchpoint

Make sure you wipe off any excess moisturiser before you walk on your carpet or slip on a favourite pair of shoes!

IF THE SHOE FITS . . .

Twenty-six bones and a network of muscles and tendons keep your feet on their feet! They'll soon start to complain – painfully – if you squash them into badly fitting shoes and over a period of time may develop bunions and corns. Follow our guide to the perfect fit.

● Going shopping for a new pair of shoes? Buy them in the afternoon – your feet swell during the day.

● Opt for leather shoes rather than man-made ones because they stretch to fit your feet and also let your feet breathe.

● Make sure you can wiggle your toes around with 12 mm/½ in between your big toe and the end of the shoe.

● If you have to claw your toes to keep your shoes on, they're too big for you.

● Don't wear high heels all the time. They shift your body weight forwards causing pressure on your soles. Save them for special occasions only.

● Vary your heel height, alternating medium-height heels and flatties to help prevent foot fatigue.

● Nylon socks and tights make your feet heat up and swell. Try to wear natural fabrics whenever possible as they allow cooling air to circulate.

Photographs: MIKE DAVIES/Hair and make-up: LIZZIE COURT/Towelling robe: MARKS & SPENCER/Foot bowl: CRABTREE & EVELYN/Moisturiser, body brush and footsie: THE BODY SHOP

BEST FOOT FORWARD

Your feet may often be well hidden, but that doesn't mean they should be forgotten. Set aside an hour or so every fortnight to pamper them and you'll never want to hide them away again

Foot-refresher sprays are the perfect pick-me-up for tired tootsies.

Old-fashioned remedies can't be beaten as far as feet go. There's nothing quite like a traditional mustard bath to pep them up. Blend three teaspoons mustard powder to a paste with a little water and add to a bowl of warm water.

Ouch! Corns really hurt. They're caused by ill-fitting shoes. Don't attempt to cut or treat them yourself – seek professional advice.

Take time out to pamper your feet. Give them a pedicure at least once every two weeks.

Never apply sudden warmth to cold feet.

Opt for aromatherapy oils to ease away tension and fatigue. A few drops of lavender oil in warm water is a perfect pick-me-up.

Try a footsie roller to relieve sore, tired feet. Just roll the massager back and forwards over the entire sole, exerting a steady pressure.

Easy does it! Be kind to your feet. Don't torture them by wearing high heels all the time.

Synthetic materials aren't good for the feet. Natural fibres like cotton are a far better choice.

DID YOU KNOW?
It's estimated that your feet travel over 70,000 miles in an average lifetime.

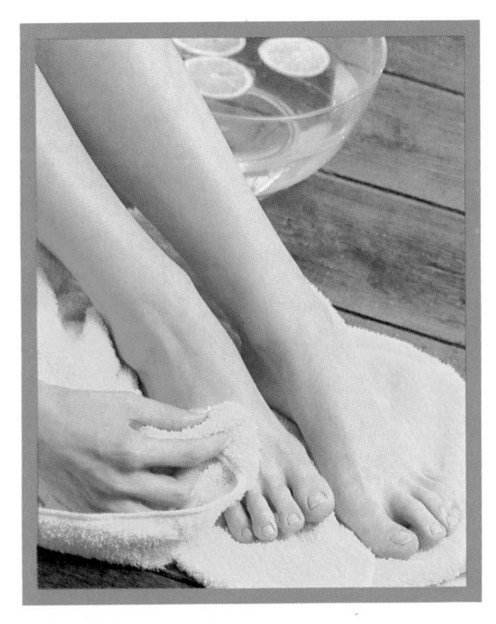

1 ◀ **Remove old nail polish. Soak your feet in a soothing foot bath of lemon slices and warm water. Make sure you dry between your toes carefully after bathing – bacteria thrive in moist, dark conditions.**

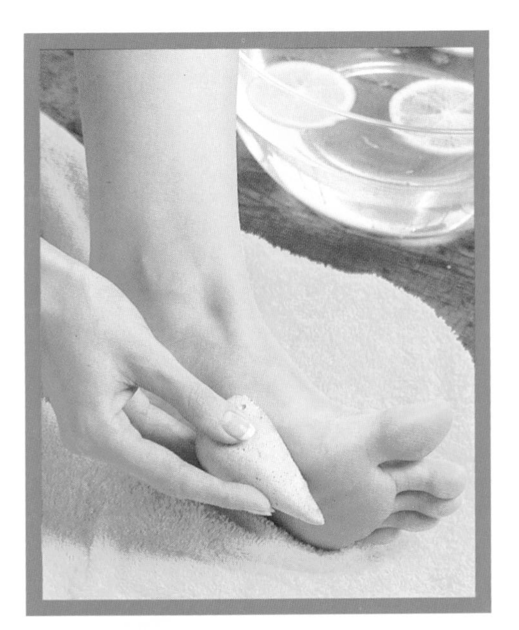

2 ▶ **Use the flat side of a pumice stone to get rid of hard skin on the soles of your feet. Don't rub too vigorously – a gentle rubbing is fine.**

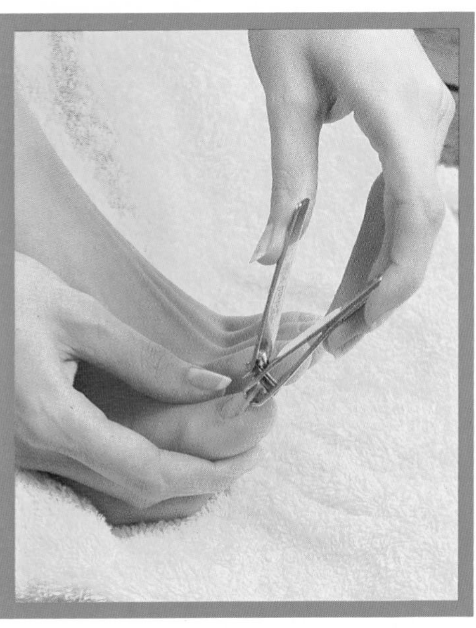

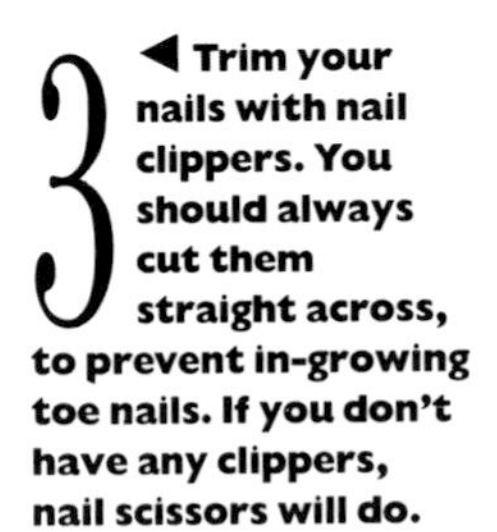

3 ◀ **Trim your nails with nail clippers. You should always cut them straight across, to prevent in-growing toe nails. If you don't have any clippers, nail scissors will do.**

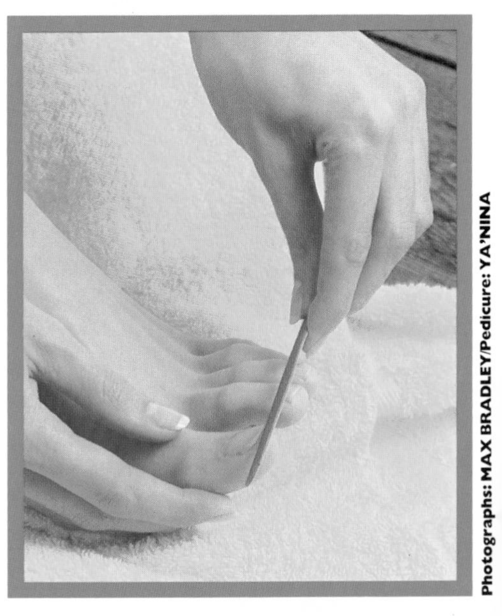

4 ▶ **Using an emery board, file nails smooth but don't try to shape them. Filing the sides can also lead to in-growing toe nails.**

Photographs: MAX BRADLEY/Pedicure: YA'NINA

PEDICURE POWER

Emery boards – *are the best file to use to get your nails smooth. Use the dark, rough side to make them shorter and the lighter side to smooth them.*
Nail clippers – *will cut a straight line across your nail to help prevent in-growing toe nails.*
Cuticle remover – *softens the cuticle making it easier to remove.*
Cuticle clippers – *to snip off obstinate bits of skin that won't come off any other way!*
Cuticle pusher – *to ease cuticles back once they've been softened.*
Toe separators – *hold toes apart.*
Hard skin remover – *use on ball of foot and heels.*
Orange sticks – *are indispensible for any pedicure. Use to clean under nail tips and cover with cotton wool to push back cuticles.*
Foot cream – *to soften dry skin and make your feet feel loved.*
Toe nail scissors – *shaped to make cutting toe nails easier.*
Foot file – *use after bathing to file off hard skin.*
Nail buffer – *to give a sheen to nails without varnish.*
Nail glosser – *file over nail surface to smooth out ridges.*

5 **Use an orange stick tipped with cotton wool to clean under your nails. Ease back the cuticles gently.**

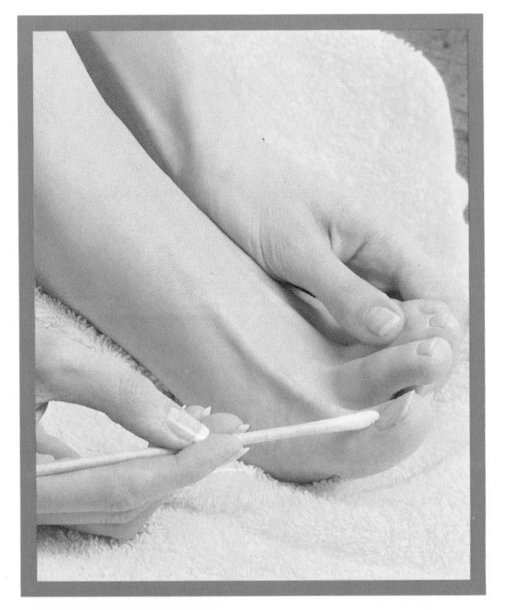

Wrap cotton wool around the end of an orange stick and dip in nail polish remover. Use this to clean up any varnish smudges around your nails.

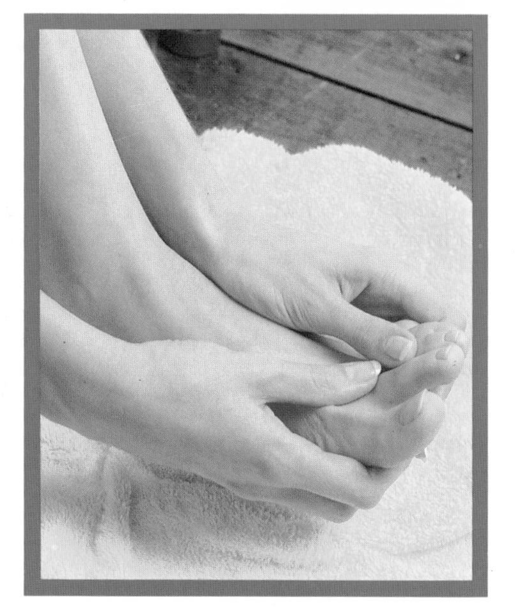

6 **Massage hand or body lotion into your feet and toe nails. Work upwards towards your ankles and calves.**

If you've got bad circulation in your feet try alternating between warm and cold footbaths to wake them up.

7 **Separate toes with a strip of cotton wool or special toe separators. Apply a base coat of varnish, followed by two thin coats of colour. Top with a layer of clear varnish for a no-chip finish.**

If you suffer from sweaty feet, rub them gently with surgical spirit and dust with foot powder.

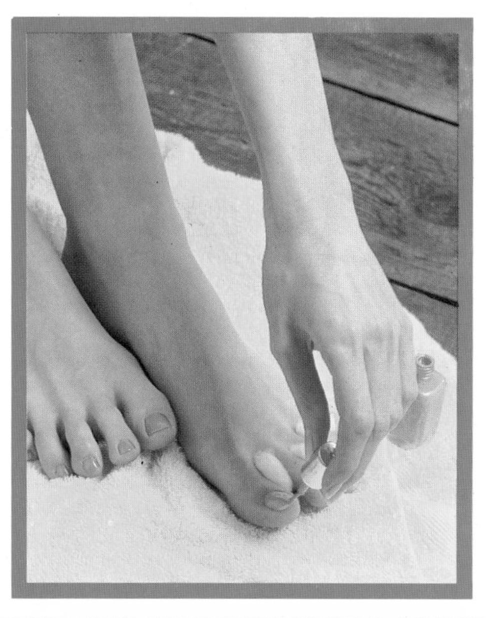

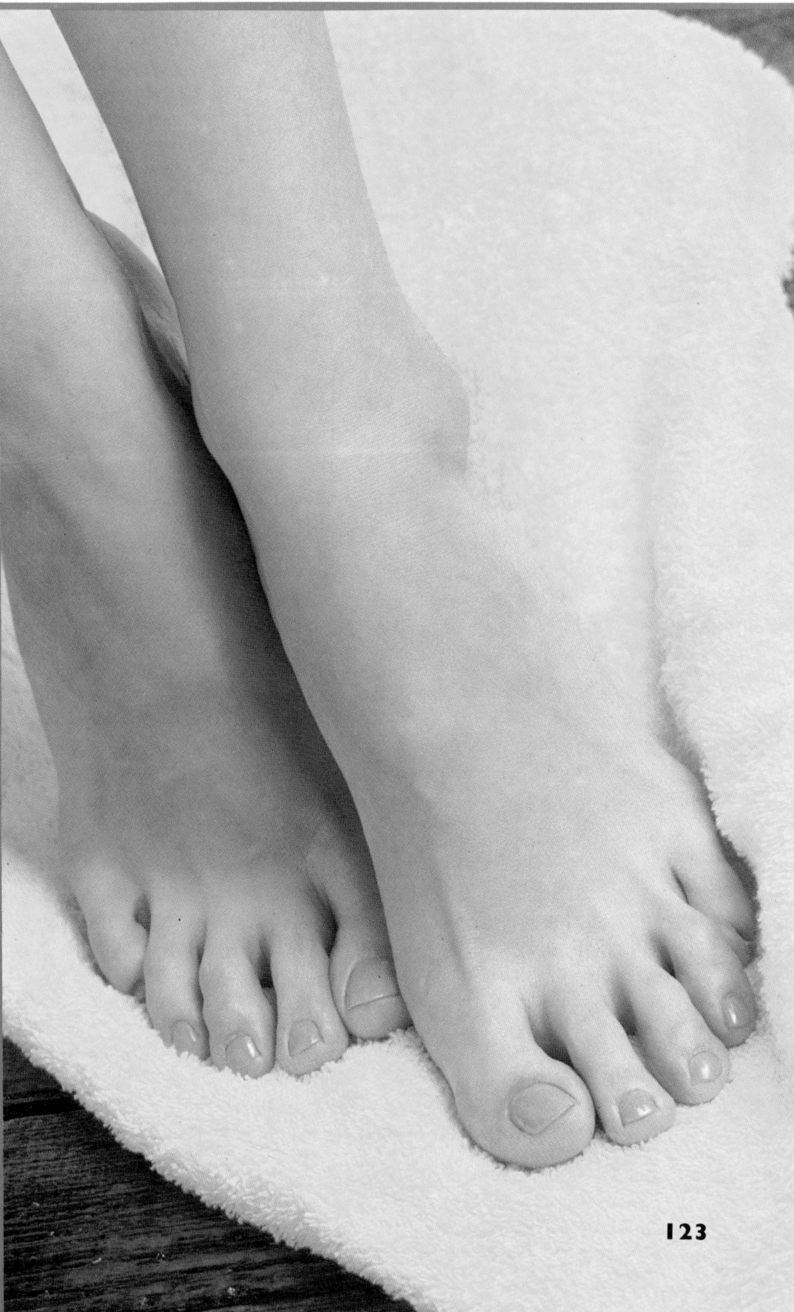

Pretty feet, polished and prepared to step out in style.

HOLDING BACK THE YEARS

Don't become a wrinkly before your time, start our anti-ageing action plan today. You'll stay looking younger – for longer!

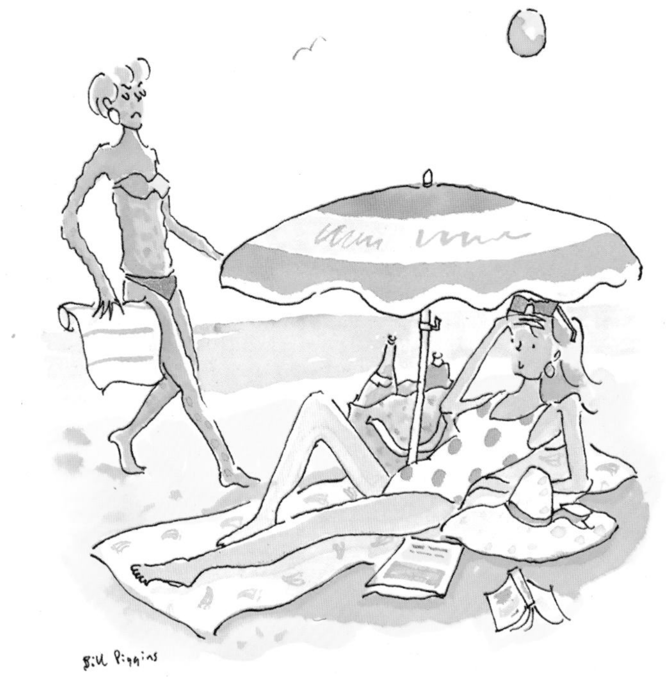

If you're the sort of person who likes to cram all you can into life and enjoy every minute of it, then you're probably doing more to ward off the ravages of old age than any anti-wrinkle creams will ever do. This is not to say you can neglect your skin but having a positive attitude to life will certainly help keep you healthy and your skin looking young.

If you're constantly fed up, unmotivated and generally down then this will begin to have a negative effect on your body. You'll begin to get wrinkles (frowning causes more wrinkles than smiling), bags under your eyes, dull skin and you'll be more likely to suffer from stress-related complaints like headaches and lack of energy.

POSITIVELY GREAT

The best way to grow old gracefully, is to start now by living life to the full. Work hard but make time for having fun and enjoying yourself. Surround yourself with people who have a positive effect on you – people you care about and who care about you.

It shouldn't involve any drastic changes, it's all a matter of common sense; getting enough rest, eating a balanced diet, exercising regularly and not drinking or smoking too much. And the earlier you start taking care of yourself the better.

SUN SENSE

The biggest single cause of your skin looking old before its time, is the sun. Dermatologists now agree that up to 70 per cent of what was previously thought of as being part of the natural ageing process is a result of sun damage.

Unfortunately, it's all too easy to forget just how strong the sun's rays can be and how necessary it is to protect your skin, at all times.

- Whenever you're out in strong sun, whether on the beach or in the back garden, always use a sunscreen of at least factor 10 on your face.

Check out the ranges specially for use on the face – they are less greasy and not so likely to give you spots. Most of them contain extra moisturisers too.

- Play safe and fake a healthy glow with a tinted moisturiser or a matt bronzing powder.
- Help protect your face by wearing a broad-brimmed hat.
- Don't forget to wear sunscreen on the backs of your hands and on your neck. Both are very susceptible to moisture loss and will be quick to wrinkle if unprotected.
- Choose a moisturiser with a sunscreen to wear every day.
- Remember, the sun's rays are at their strongest between 11 am and 3 pm. If you are out in the sun during this time, try and stay in the shade.

FACE SAVERS

A moisturiser is a must for all skin types. It stops the skin from drying out, protects it from the elements and helps to keep it soft and supple. If your skin is dry go for a cream moisturiser as they tend to be richer than lotions that are best suited to oily skins. Make sure you use moisturiser both night and morning, and don't forget to moisturise your neck too.

EYE OPENERS

You'll probably first notice your skin is beginning to age around your eyes. Lines appear here first because the skin is particularly thin and because we are constantly using the muscles around our eyes when we express ourselves. Smile and you can see why they're called laughter lines.

The skin around your eyes needs special care if you want to prevent your laughter lines turning into crow's feet! Ordinary moisturisers tend to be too heavy for the delicate eye area and many leave the skin looking puffy. Lighter eye creams are therefore well worth considering. Dot a little in a 'C' shape around your eye socket then very gently pat it into the skin. Be very careful when taking off your eye make-up as constant rubbing can make the skin sag.

PLAN FOR THE FUTURE

Follow our action plan for a healthier, more attractive you!

- A skin-friendly diet is well-balanced and rich in vitamins B (found in yeast), C and beta-carotene (fruit and vegetables) and E (wheatgerm oil).
- Limit the amount of time you spend in the sun and always use a high factor sunscreen.
- Take some sort of regular exercise, even if it's just a long, brisk walk. It'll increase the amount of oxygen going into your blood and boost your energy levels.
- Use a moisturiser every day to prevent your skin drying out. Dry skin is much more prone to wrinkles and will eventually look lined and leathery.
- Get enough sleep. If you're tired you'll look older.
- Cut down on alcohol and caffeine and cut out smoking. You'll look much better for it.

Illustration: BILL PIGGINS

The sun can be your skin's number one enemy, but with a sensible plan you'll get a gorgeous glow! Just follow our golden rules

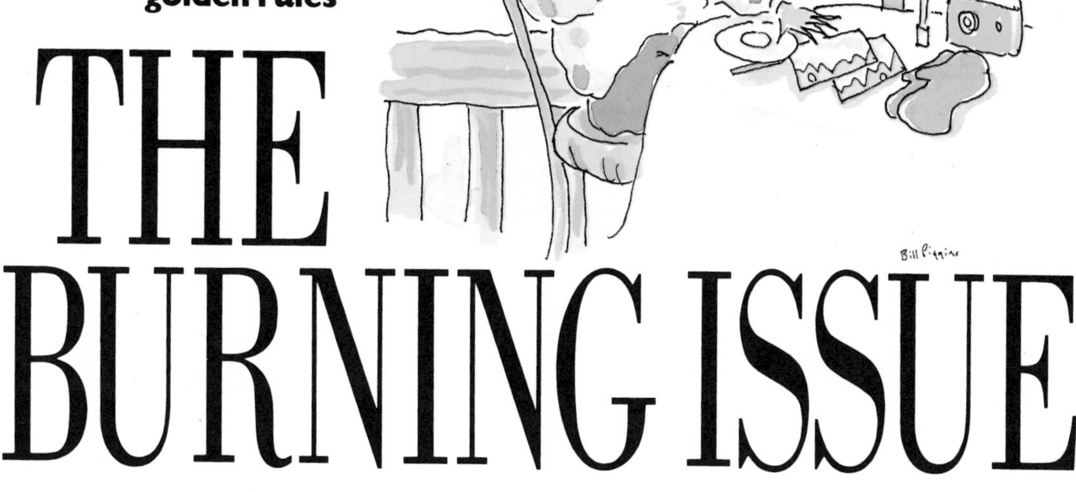

THE BURNING ISSUE

Most of us feel terrific with a tan. So if you've been browned off by all the reports saying stay out of the sun or your skin will suffer, then it's well worth remembering that the sun *can* be good for you too. Its rays clear bad skin and stimulate the production of vitamin D in the body – which is essential for good health.

A tan is just the skin's way of defending itself against the sun's potentially harmful rays. What happens is that melanin, the natural pigment found in the skin, forms a protective barrier by toughening the skin's surface.

RAY BANS

Sensible tanning is all about exposing your skin gradually to the sun, being aware of your skin type and understanding what the sun's rays actually do. The rays of the sun that tan and burn you are invisible to the naked eye and are known as ultra-violet (UV) rays. They come in three different lengths – A, B and C. About 80 per cent of the rays which reach your skin are UVA rays. These are the weakest but longest ones and penetrate furthest into the skin, reaching deep down and causing the skin to lose its elasticity and wrinkle. Their tanning effect is mild.

The other 20 per cent are UVB or burning rays. These mostly affect the top layer of the skin and are the ones that cause you to burn. In the long term they can cause skin cancers.

UVCs are the shortest rays, with a high concentration of energy, and potentially the most damaging. Fortunately, they are blocked out by the Earth's ozone layer hovering in the atmosphere, and don't reach your skin. But as this vital shield is being depleted, all ultra-violet radiation is now more powerful and damaging. For this reason, dermatologists advise using high sun protection factor creams and lotions at all times, especially in hot climates.

HOT SPOTS

When you're having fun it's easy to forget the damage that the sun can do to your skin. But certain factors can make all the difference to the intensity of UV rays.

- The sun is at its most intense at midday and at its strongest in midsummer – so these are the most dangerous times to be out.
- The nearer you are to the equator, the more powerful the sun is. And the higher up you go, the more intense the rays. A ski resort at 3,000 metres/9,400 feet exposes you to about double the amount of UV radiation that you would get at sea level.
- Snow reflects 85 per cent of the UV light which hits it and sand reflects about 25 per cent.
- Light buildings, garden furniture and pale pavements also reflect UV light – so you can get sunburnt walking around in built-up city streets!
- Swimming gives you absolutely no protection from the sun. UV rays can actually penetrate to a depth of several metres, so it can be dangerous to swim if you haven't got a water-resistant suntan lotion on. Re-apply it when you come out of the water.
- Glass blocks out UVB rays but not UVAs.
- The sun can pass through cloud. So don't be fooled and think that UV rays can't penetrate your skin on a dull day.

SAFETY IN NUMBERS

Avoiding the sun altogether isn't practical or necessary. You put your skin most at risk when you *burn*. So accept the fact that if you are fair-skinned and don't tan easily you'll need a sunblock or a high sun protection factor (an SPF of about 15) especially when the sun is hottest. Make sure you're aware of your skin's burning potential if you don't want to stay in the shade this summer.

SKIN TYPE	HOW SAFE ARE YOU?
I – You have pale blonde or red hair, light coloured eyes, pale skin and maybe masses of freckles.	You burn easily, go red rather than brown. Safe in the sun without protection for five minutes.
II – You have blonde or mousy hair and a fair complexion. Eyes of medium colour.	You burn easily, tan slowly. You're safe in the sun without protection for 10 minutes.
III – You have dark blonde or mousy brown hair, dark blue, hazel or light brown eyes and oily or combination skin.	You burn a little before tanning and are safe in the sun without protection for 15 minutes.
IV – You have Latin colouring – olive skin, dark eyes and hair.	You rarely burn and tan easily. Safe in the sun without protection for 20 minutes.
V – You are of Asian appearance – dark hair and eyes.	You rarely burn, tan deeply.
VI – You are of African appearance – dark hair and eyes.	You rarely burn, tan deeply.

Illustration: BILL PIGGINS

If you want to save your skin from the sun but still sport a stunning tan, just reach for the bottle and fake a golden glow

JOIN THE BROWNIES!

The days when a fake tan meant orange palms and streaky legs are over. The latest fake tanning products are quick and easy to use and will give you a bronzed skin that's sure to fool anyone!

There are lots of good reasons for faking a tan. We all know that too much sun can be damaging to our skin, so faking is the safest option. Fake tans are also handy if you can't get away to the sun, but still want to look as though you've been on holiday. And if you are heading for the beach, they'll save you the embarrassment of looking lily-white when everyone else is a lovely golden-brown. Once you've got a stunning tan, they can help prolong it by topping up fading colour, and for those with very fair skin that's prone to burning, faking it really is the only sensible pain-free alternative!

SMOOTH MOVES

To prevent streaks and a patchy finish, make sure your skin is super-smooth before putting on your fake tan.

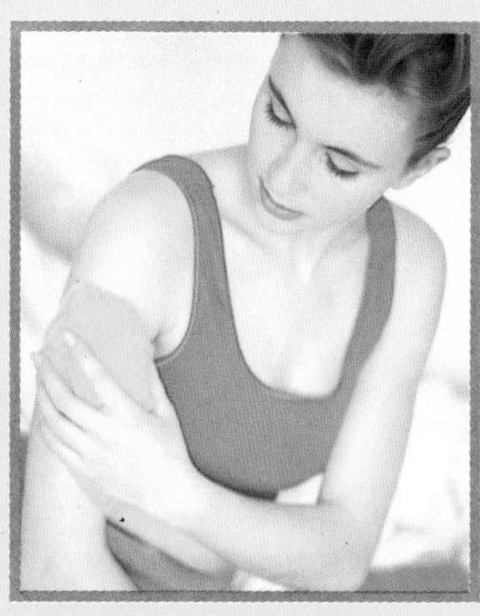

1 Rub off dead skin cells by putting a handful of salt onto a damp flannel and stroking upwards all over the skin.

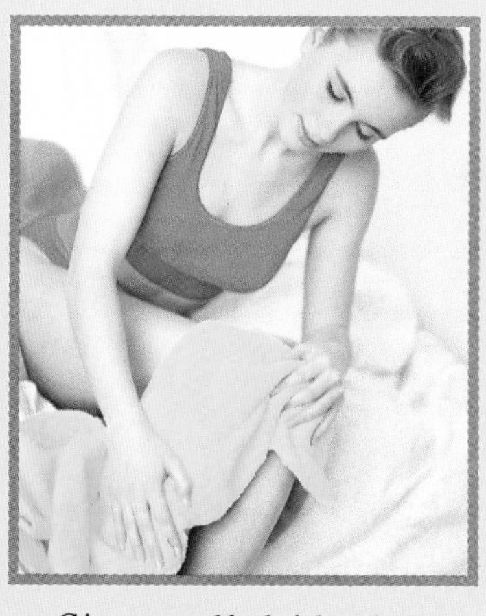

2 Give yourself a brisk rub down with a fluffy towel to remove any last traces of dry skin and improve skin tone.

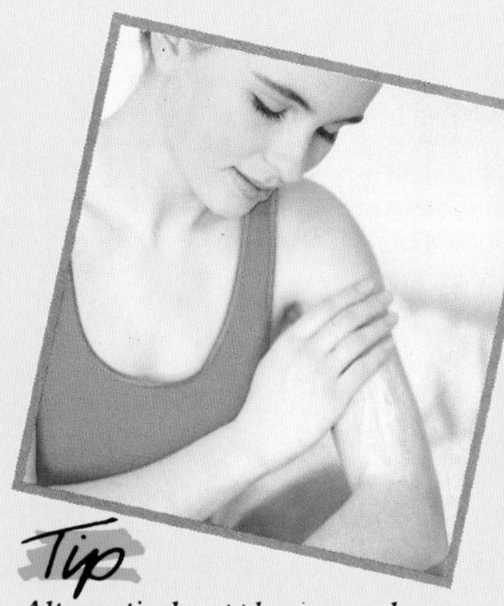

Tip
Alternatively, apply a granular body scrub with your fingertips or a loofah, using firm circular movements.

GOING FOR GOLD

A fake tan can't just be slapped on. The way you use it makes all the difference between streaky brown and beautifully bronzed skin!

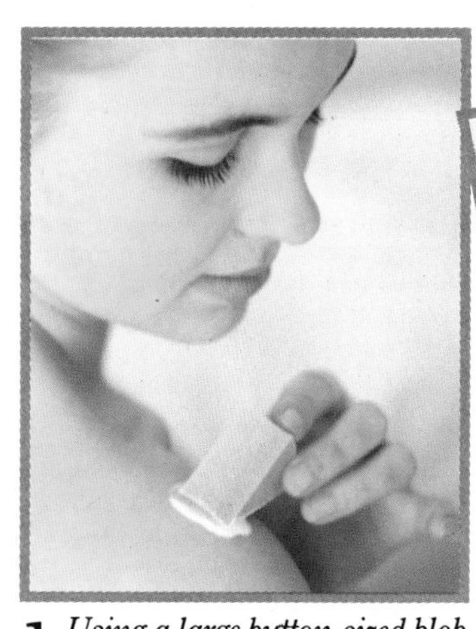

1 Using a large button-sized blob of tanning cream, smooth over clean, dry skin. Change direction as you go to avoid streaks.

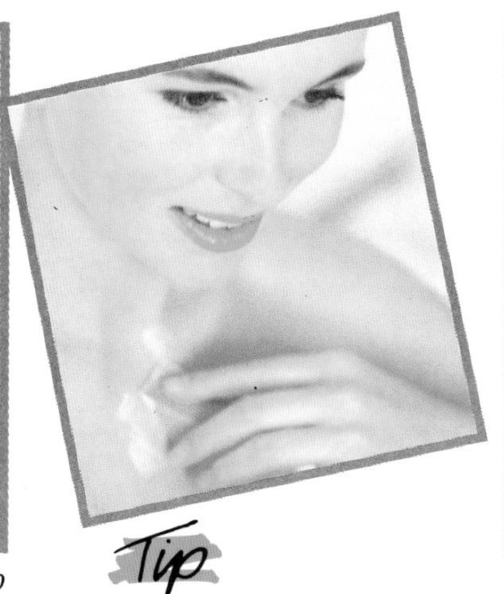

Tip
For even coverage and so that you don't get too much tan on your hands, use a small sponge to smooth it over your skin.

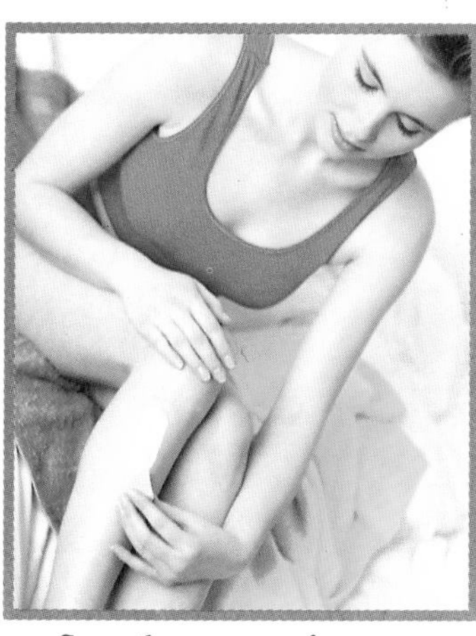

2 Smooth on cream from your neck down to your feet, leaving the joints until last.

Photographs: DAVID TODD/Hair and make-up: KAREN LOCKYER/Swimsuit: FREEMANS/Shorts: WAREHOUSE

HOW TANNERS WORK

Fake tans are available as creams, lotions or mousses. They're usually white, although mousse tends to be coloured which makes it easy to see where you've put it on.

The active ingredient in most fake tans is di-hydroxyacetate. This reacts with the protein in the surface cells of your skin and gradually turns them brown over a period of two to three hours. As tanners only affect the skin's surface layer, don't expect to go the same deep shade as you would in the sunshine.

A fake tan lasts for about a week and won't wash off. However, do remember that although your skin looks brown, your fake tan won't provide any protection at all from the sun, so make sure you use a sun screen as normal.

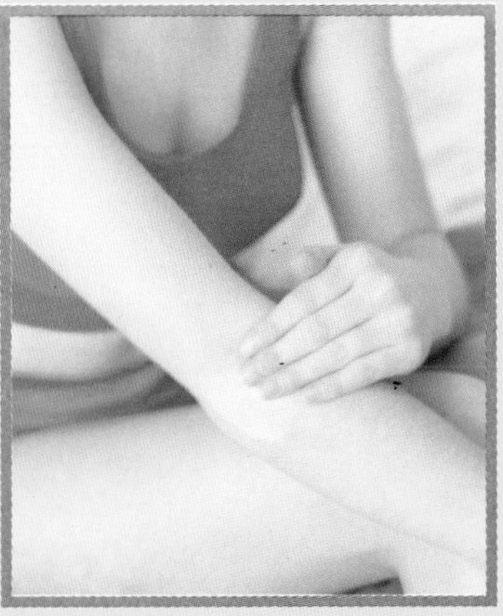

3 *Smooth some moisturiser over damp skin to help the tanner go on more evenly. Pay special attention to dry areas.*

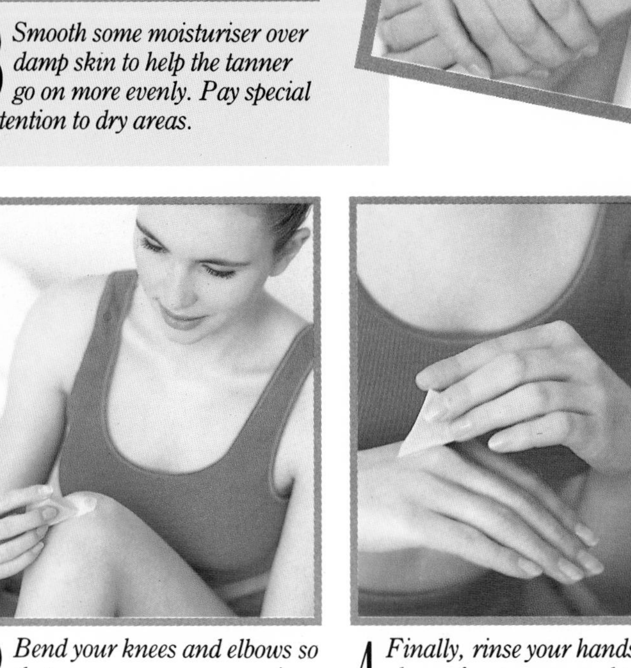

3 *Bend your knees and elbows so that you cover every crease in the skin.*

4 *Finally, rinse your hands clean of any cream and pat dry. Then use a sponge to cover each finger, avoiding nails as they stain easily.*

BROWNIE POINTS

- DO put on fake tan in a well-lit room – preferably natural daylight – so patchiness is easy to spot.
- DO remove unwanted hair from your legs at least 24 hours before to avoid irritation.
- DO allow at least half an hour to put the tan on and let it set.
- DO get a friend to help you with difficult-to-reach areas.
- DO use a full-length and hand mirror to check if you've put the colour on evenly.
- DO get rid of any streaky patches that develop by rubbing them with a body scrub or flannel.
- DON'T forget to read the manufacturer's instructions carefully – then follow them!
- DON'T use fake tan on your face. Use a tinted moisturiser or bronzing powder instead.
- DON'T use too much cream at one time. It's best to smooth on two thin coats for a convincing colour. Make sure you leave the first coat to develop before putting on the next.
- DON'T use fake tan just before bedtime or going out – the dye could stain the sheets, or worse, your best outfit!

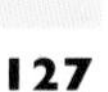

SUNBED SENSE

Yes, sunbed sessions can be good for your health and looks. Wise up to the health and beauty benefits and get an all-over glow, whatever the weather

KNOW YOUR SKIN
Before you rush off into the sun or hurry to your local sunbed salon, you should understand your skin and how and why it reacts to the sun. The colour of your skin comes from how much melanin it contains. We are all born with the same number of melanocytes (the special cells that produce melanin). Those of us with fair skin produce little melanin, olive complexions produce a greater amount, and those of us with black skins produce a great deal. Melanin acts as a natural sunscreen, it filters out the harmful rays of the sun so that they do not reach the deeper layers of your skin and cause damage. When your skin comes into contact with the sun, the melanocytes know that they need to produce more melanin and this is why your skin changes colour.

CHOOSING YOUR SUNBED
Basically sunbeds on the market fall into two main categories: low pressure and high pressure.

Low pressure sunbeds were the first to be introduced. They use long tubes of light – above and beneath you – to give off rays similar to those produced by the sun. These beds are the safest for paler skin. You should start off as you would in the sun with just a short exposure (maximum 20 minutes). Once you have built up to your sixth treatment (where the exposure now lasts 30 minutes) you should be ready to move on to a high pressure bed.

High pressure beds are a more recent innovation. Here the rays from the beds give a quicker, more concentrated tanning effect. The screens are located above you only. Originally produced for the treatment of skin disorders, the majority of the potentially damaging UVB rays are removed. These beds give a much faster result but are only suitable for you if you have a base tan, a dark complexion, if you tan easily and without any problem in the sun, or if you've recently followed a short tanning course on the low pressure beds.

Facial tanners – the rays here come from small screens so you get all the benefits of the high pressure sunbeds. Facial tanners can be a boon if you just want to concentrate on giving your face a healthy natural glow. They're quick too – each treatment lasts just 20 minutes. And there is an added bonus – many doctors recommend them for the treatment of acne. The initial treatment should consist of six sessions (one every other day) then keep up the improvement with a 'maintenance dose' of one treatment per week.

HIDDEN BENEFITS

- Sunbeds can help you if you are stressed – they're a great way to relax after a hard day's work.
- Sunbeds can improve certain skin conditions such as acne, greasy skin or psoriasis – but it's a good idea to ask your doctor's advice first.
- Sunbeds can be helpful if you suffer from SAD (Seasonal Affective Disorder), a condition where the sufferer's personality changes with the season when there is a lack of sunlight.

SAFE TANNING

Follow our DO's and DON'Ts for sunbed tanning and you'll be extra safe.

DO build up your colour gradually and allow your skin to get used to the rays.
DO wear protective goggles – they should be provided by the salon.
DO remove your contact lenses before tanning.
DO ensure that the timer is working properly and set it exactly before you start.
DO make sure that your sunbed is cleaned with a mild antiseptic spray before you use it.
DO moisturise your skin after each sunbed session.
DO ask your doctor's advice if you suffer from epilepsy, a heart condition, high or low blood pressure, allergies or are pregnant.
DON'T use perfume, cosmetics, or tanning products before using a sunbed.
DON'T use sunbeds for prolonged periods – they do dry out the skin.
DON'T use sunbeds if you have problems in the sun.
DON'T use sunbeds if you're taking antibiotics, tranquillisers or certain diuretics.
DON'T use sunbeds if there is a history of skin cancer in the family.
DON'T use facial tanners too often or you'll end up with wrinkles.

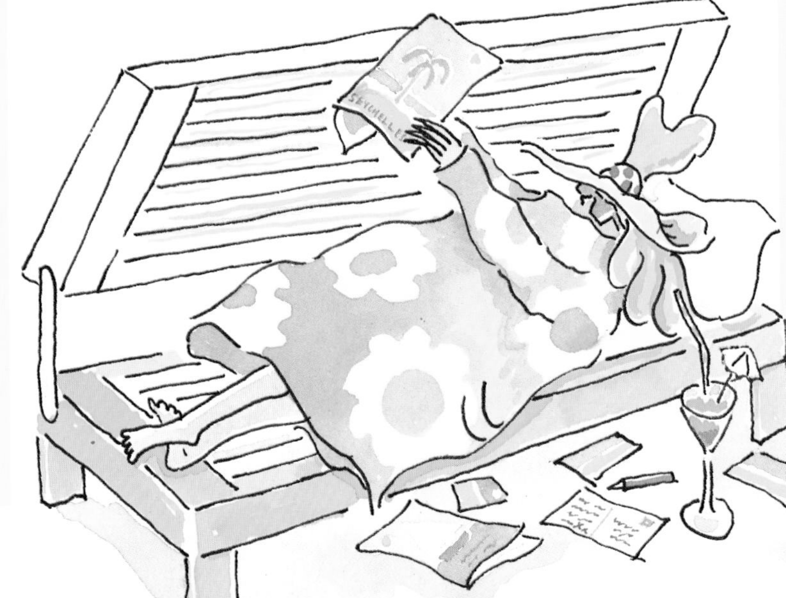

With thanks to BOB ELLIS of TANTALISE/Illustration: BILL PIGGINS

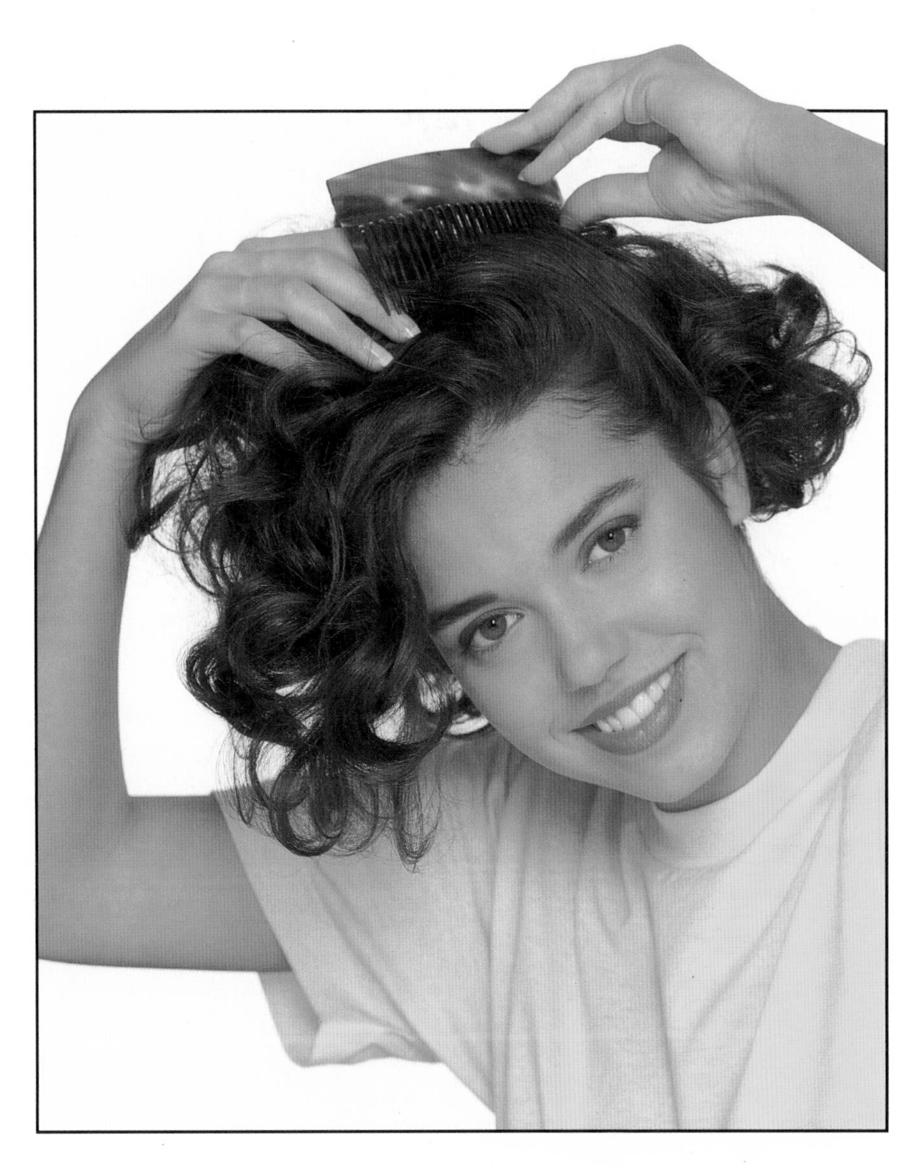

CHAPTER FIVE

Ways With Hair

HAIR NECESSITIES

Is mousse a mystery? Do hairdryers give you a headache? Here's a chance to brush up on hair essentials

COVERED ELASTIC BANDS

They're great if you wear your hair tied back a lot. Take them on holiday, comb a conditioner containing sunscreen through your hair. Plait your hair or just comb it off your face, then fix it with your covered elastic band. But, if you use them every day and pull your hair back tightly, you could actually do some damage to your hair.

Covered elastic bands are much kinder to your hair than rubber bands.

THE HAIRDRYER

One of the most useful basic hairdressing tools. Look for one that comes with different speed and heat settings and detachable nozzles (and, if possible, a diffuser attachment). Use your dryer on the warmer, faster setting for concentrated styling – like blow-drying a bob or a fringe straight and for blast-drying to help remove the moisture from your hair quickly. Use the diffuser attachment and the dryer on a cooler setting for scrunch-drying, to encourage your hair's natural wave or curl. Use the cool setting to 'fix' curls.

THE BRUSH

Choose a flat-backed brush with rounded bristles on a rubber base. You can use it for general styling and when blow-drying. A vent brush with holes that let hot air pass through while you're blow-drying is also useful. If you want waves or curls you need to buy a round bristle brush.

THE COMB

Everyone uses one, but in order to get the most from yours, buy a versatile wide-toothed comb. Use it to comb through conditioner and comb out wet hair, for making your partings or separating off sections of hair. It's also great for back-combing.

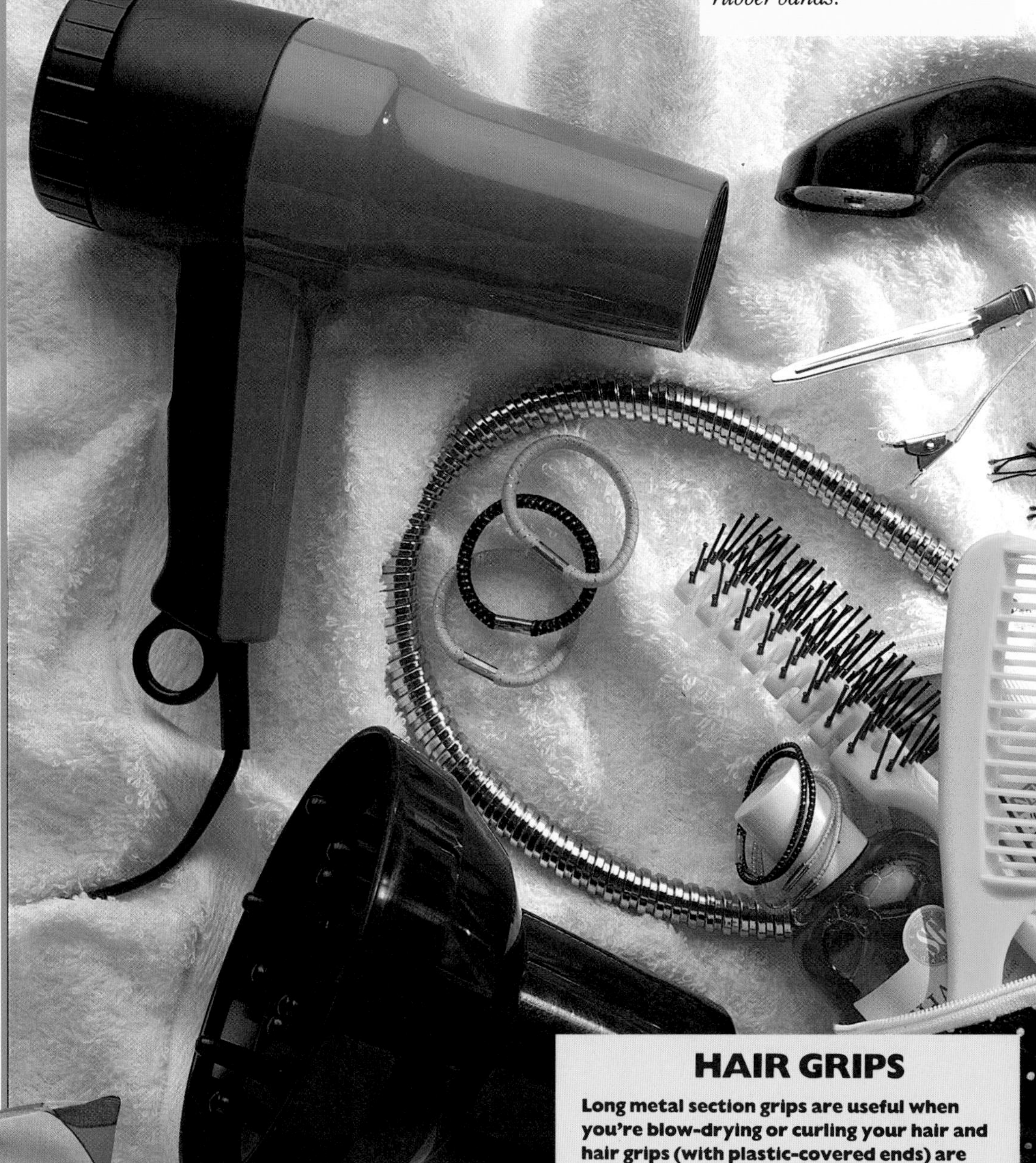

HAIR GRIPS

Long metal section grips are useful when you're blow-drying or curling your hair and hair grips (with plastic-covered ends) are good for creating pincurls. Or wear three or four decorated grips as a hair accessory.

SHOWER ATTACHMENT

It's a must for thoroughly rinsing yourself after a long soak in the bath, or for washing out colourant or shampoo and conditioner from your hair. If you use a cup or something similar to pour water over your hair, you probably won't be able to rinse it properly and you could end up with a sticky residue. This can cause your hair to look dull and flat. Not only that but hair that isn't well rinsed won't hold a style for very long.

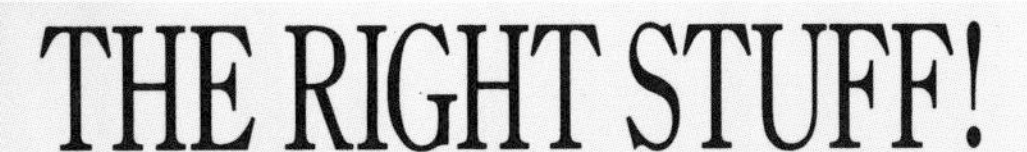

THE RIGHT STUFF!

Get set with the inside guide to the ultimate styling products.

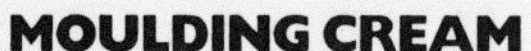

GEL

Just right for adding volume, root lift and definition to spiky styles, or to slick your hair back off your face. It suits all hair types and can be applied to wet or dry hair. Try a UV sun-screen gel if you spend time in the sun, or a wet-look formula for sleek styles. Gel brushes out easily, although a super-hold one may have to be washed out before you can put more on.

JOHN FRIEDA

MOULDING CREAM

With a consistency that's inbetween wax and gel it gives a slightly wet-look finish but a lasting hold. It's great for short, sleek styles and curly or spiky looks. Use it by rubbing a grape-sized blob into the palms of your hands and then working it through damp hair. Light moulding creams should brush out easily, but if you have a heavy one you might have to wash it out before using more.

You can also use it to tame frizzy or flyaway ends. Rub a pea-sized blob between your fingers, then work them down hair.

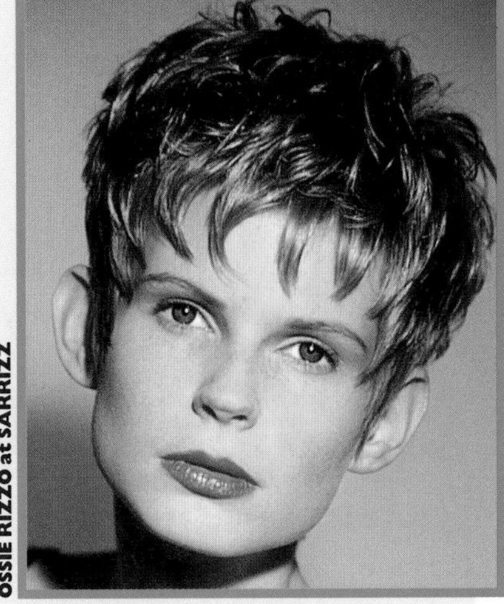

OSSIE RIZZO at SARRIZZ

GLAZE

A light, liquid gel in spray form which adds a glossy sheen to your hair. Glaze is good for slicking down ponytails or topknots when a bit of extra hold is called for and for scrunch-drying.

Glaze is not really suitable for very fine hair as it's a bit too heavy. To use, spritz a little into your palms, and work it through your damp hair. It doesn't brush out easily and needs to be washed out. To do this, massage a small blob of undiluted shampoo through your hair, then add water to build-up a lather. Rinse and repeat.

MOUSSE

This varies from natural to firm hold, depending on the look you want. As a guide, an egg-sized blob will be sufficient on short hair, an orange-sized blob on mid-length hair and a grapefruit-sized one on longer hair. To use it, squirt the foam into your palm and spread it over your palms. Work it into damp hair or scrunch it into dry, curly hair. You can use it several times before your hair needs to be washed. Many mousses also contain UV filters to protect your hair from the sun. Mousse isn't as good for very thick or wiry hair because it's too light.

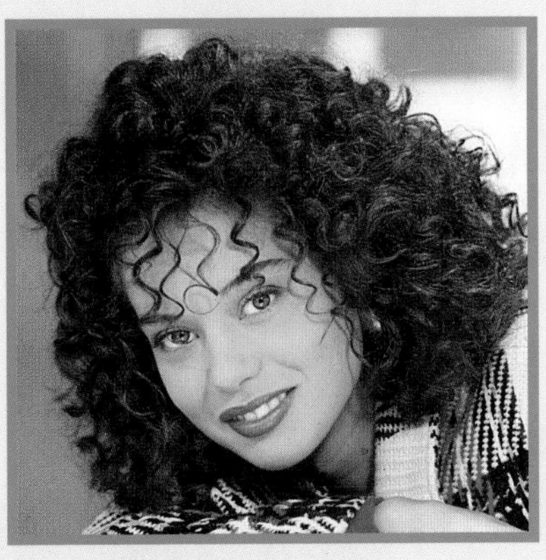

CLAIROL

CURL REVIVER

A spray that comes in a pump dispenser or an aerosol. Use it to inject new life into a flopping perm and to revive the volume of natural curls. Suits all types of curly hair. Spray on to damp or dry hair and scrunch it in. You can use it a few times before you have to wash your hair.

WAX

It's used to define curls and add a glossy finish to most styles. Wax is good for controlling frizzy curls. It's too heavy for very fine hair, but suits all other hair types. You only need a blob about the size of a thumbnail. Rub this between your palms and smooth through your dry hair. Hair must be shampooed to remove the wax.

FINISHING SPRAY

These spray-on mists hold your style and add gloss. They suit all hair types but can make fine hair look greasy. To use, shake the can, hold it about 25 cm/10 in away from your dry hair and spray. Brushes out easily.

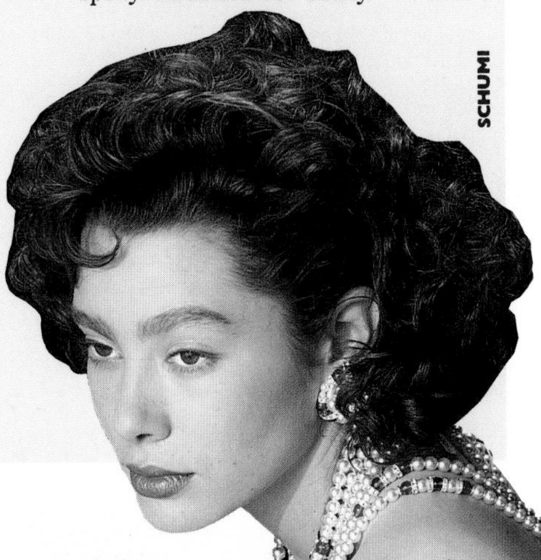

SCHUMI

Tip

Keep all your equipment in good working order for when you need it.

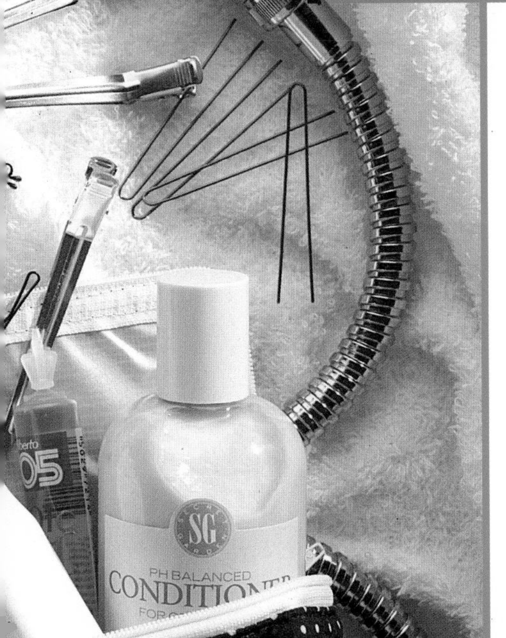

SHAMPOO AND CONDITIONER

Everyone's hair looks better when it's clean and well-conditioned. Choose a mild shampoo designed for frequent use since this should suit all hair types. Condition after each shampoo and use an intensive conditioning treatment (such as hot oil) once a month.

Photographs: ADRIAN TAYLOR

BRUSH WORK

Get a handle on our brilliant blow-drying advice! And fix a flat, floppy crop in a flash with the right brush. In short, you'll soon look stunning

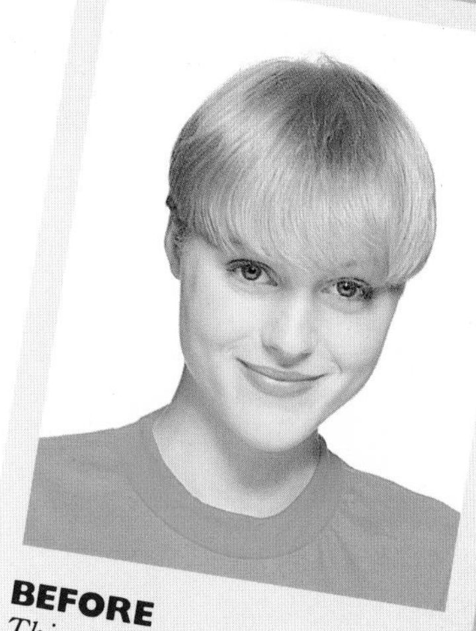

BEFORE
This short crop is well-shaped, but the hair looks a little flat and lifeless. Start with clean, dry hair.

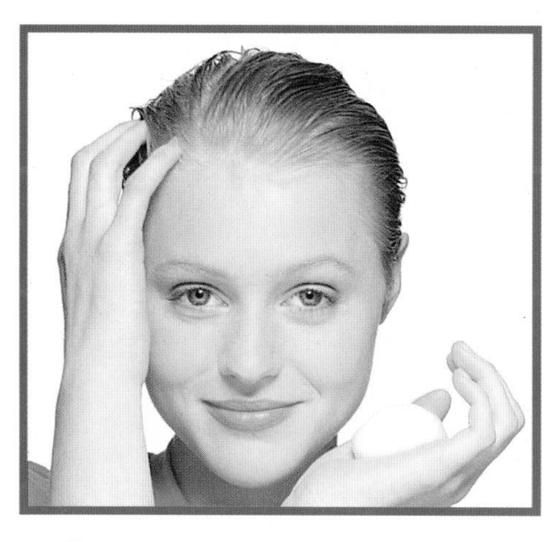

1 *Dampen your hair, squeeze a golf ball-sized blob of mousse onto your hand then work it quickly through your hair using your fingers.*

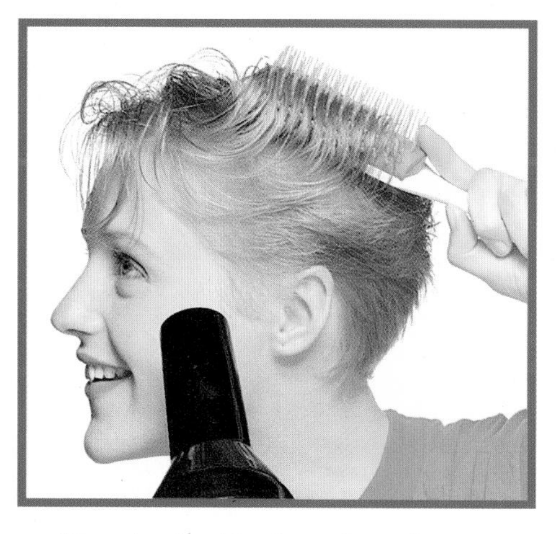

2 *Blow-dry the sides first using a flat-backed brush. Turn the brush upwards and outwards directing your hair off your face.*

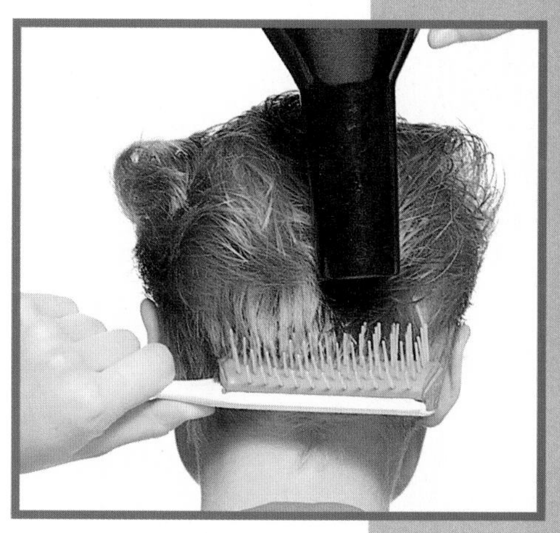

3 *Dry the back next, starting at the crown. Turn your hair under with the brush and direct your dryer's air jet downwards.*

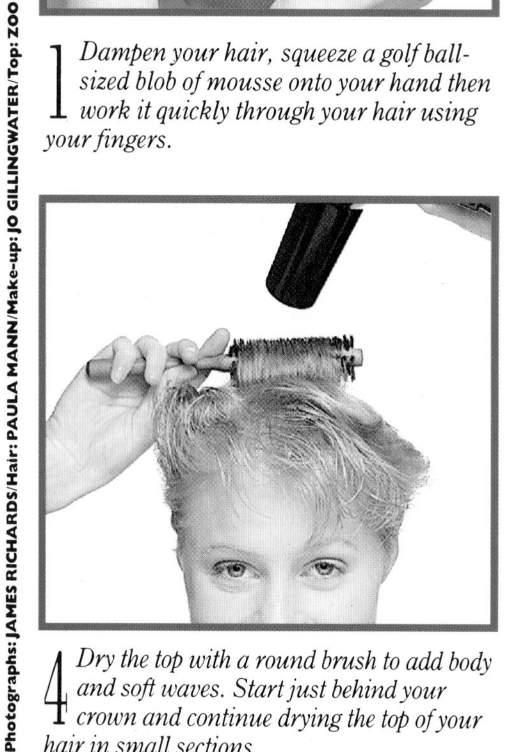

4 *Dry the top with a round brush to add body and soft waves. Start just behind your crown and continue drying the top of your hair in small sections.*

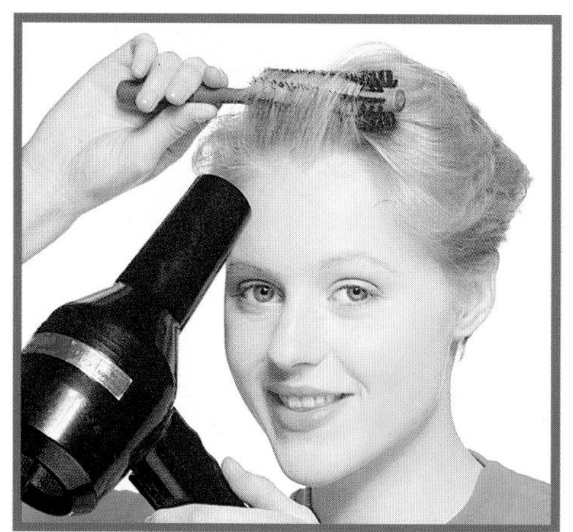

5 *Finish off with the front hair. Point the dryer at the roots to encourage volume and use the round brush to draw your hair back off your face.*

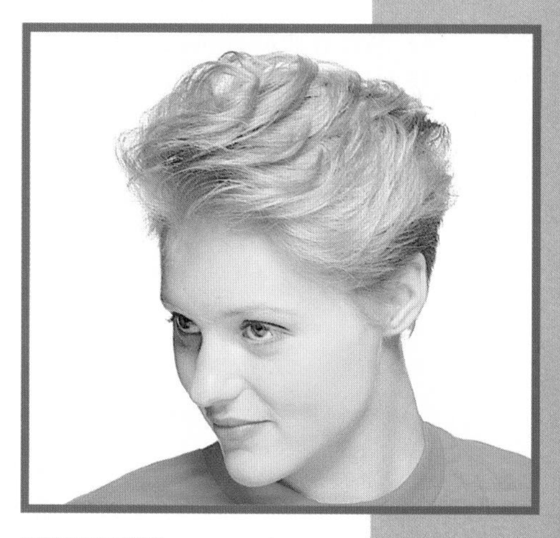

FINISHED
Fix with light coating of hairspray to hold the style in place all day long.

Photographs: JAMES RICHARDS/Hair: PAULA MANN/Make-up: JO GILLINGWATER/Top: ZOO

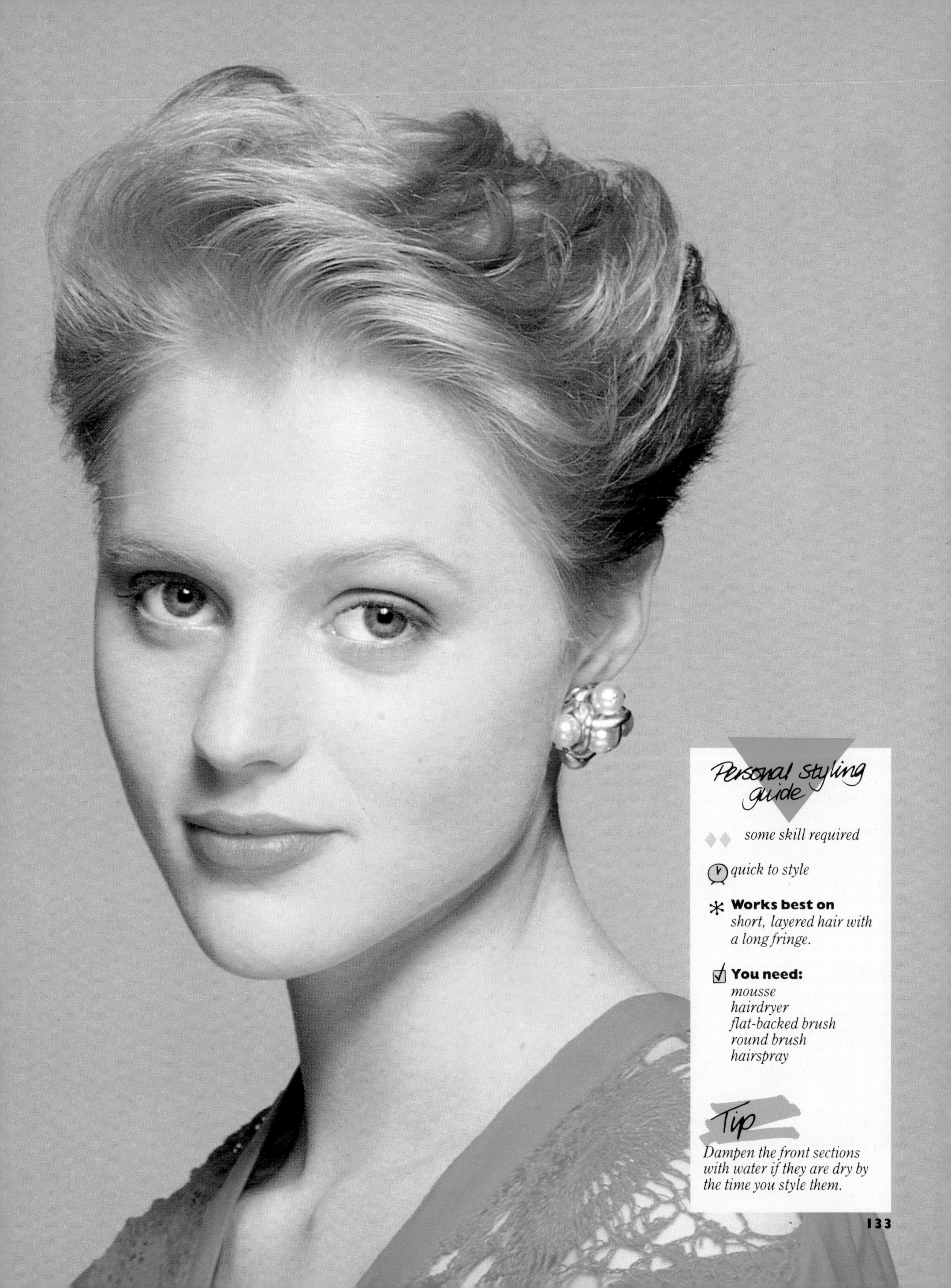
Personal styling guide
some skill required
quick to style
Works best on
short, layered hair with a long fringe.
You need:
mousse
hairdryer
flat-backed brush
round brush
hairspray
Tip
Dampen the front sections with water if they are dry by the time you style them.

LAYERED LOOKS

There's no need to let a layered cut limit you to one style. With our handy tips you can ring the changes and switch from sleek to tousled when you want

Unless your hair's cut in a bob or is all one length you've probably got layers. They're great for taking the weight out of long hair to give it more volume or for making thick hair more manageable. But sometimes having layers backfires and you're left feeling that your hair's always a mess. It's simple to put right though. If you wear your hair down learn how to scrunch-dry to give layers more body and shape. Or tie them away in a plait, a ponytail or even a topknot.

FRINGE BENEFITS

Growing out a layered fringe can be a nightmare. Here's how to keep it neat.

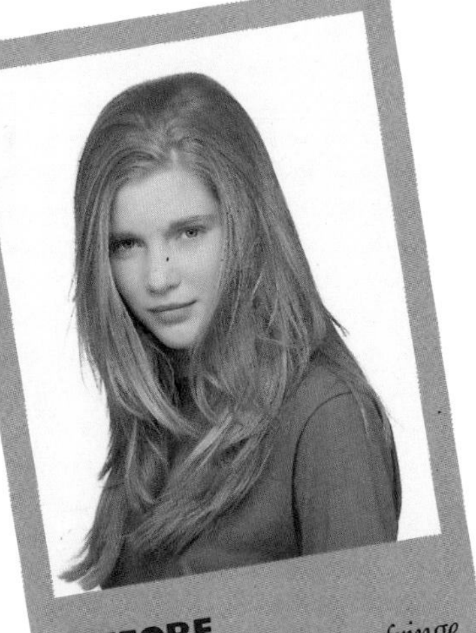

BEFORE
One-length hair with a fringe that's almost, but not quite, grown out.

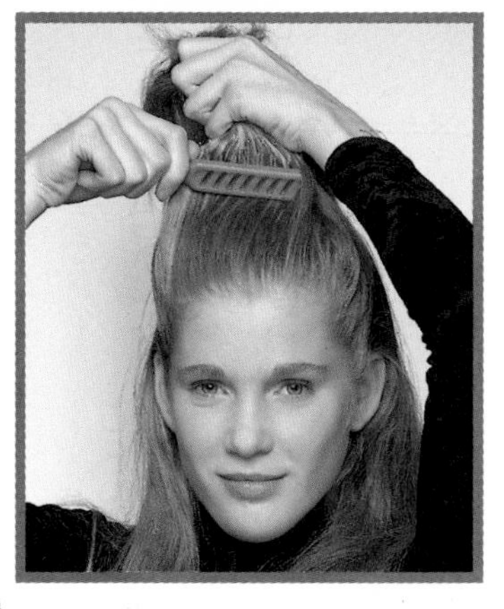

1 *To help minimise flyaway ends, squirt a brush with a little styling spray then brush the fringe hair up as if you were going to make a ponytail.*

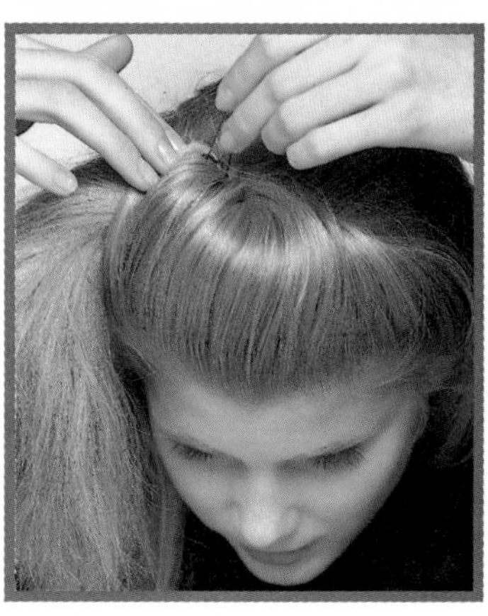

2 *Twist the section a couple of times and secure with a hairpin. Twist the length until it curls back and forms a roll. Tuck the ends under and pin.*

Watchpoint

Don't mix the fringe with longer hair. It's easier to twist hair if it's the same length.

Photographs: ANDY LANE/Hair: PENNY ATTWOOD
Make-up: LUCIE LLEWELLYN/Catsuit: SCRUFFS

HOT STUFF *Revive tired layers with heated rollers.*

BEFORE
Heat up your rollers before you start.

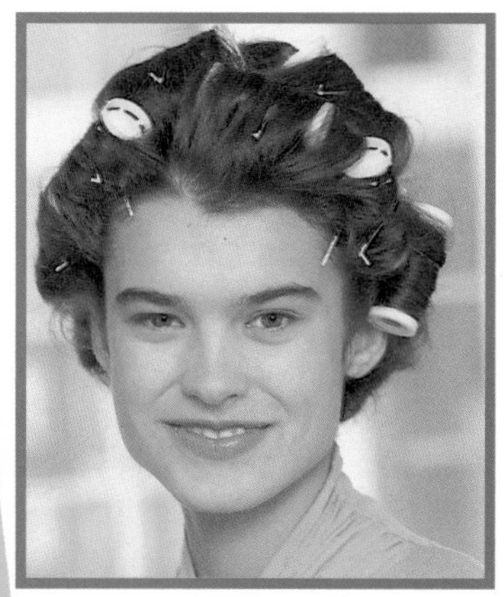

1 For big, loose curls to disguise uneven ends use large rollers and divide clean hair into 5 cm/ 2 in sections. Leave the rollers in for 10-15 minutes until cold.

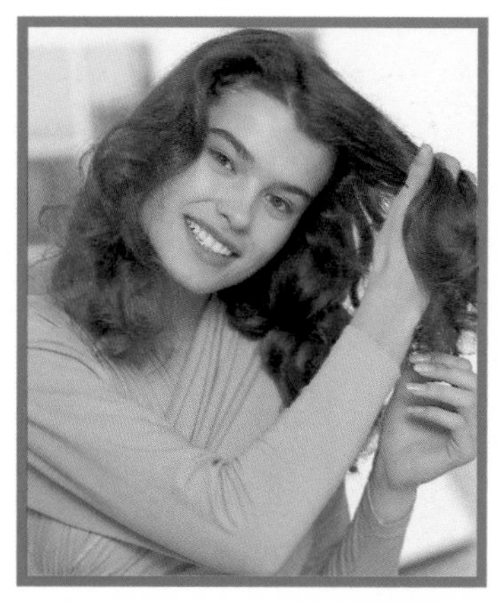

2 Take out the rollers and run your fingers from roots to the ends. Don't brush your hair as it may frizz.

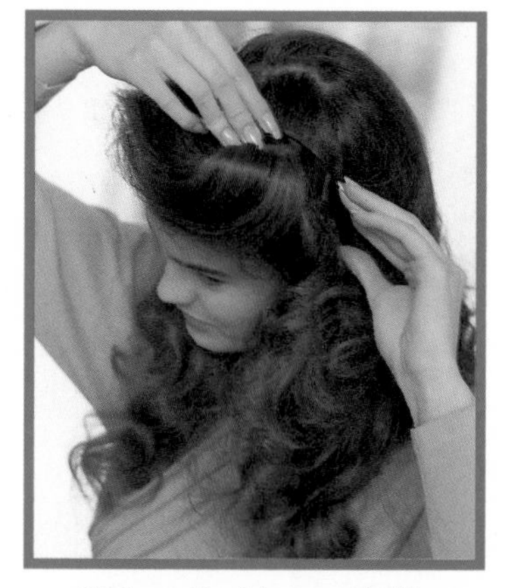

3 To keep the fringe and side layers out of your eyes, roll your hair back and secure with one comb for a side parting, or two for a middle parting.

ON THE WILD SIDE

Unleash layers and scrunch-dry for a full, frothy look.

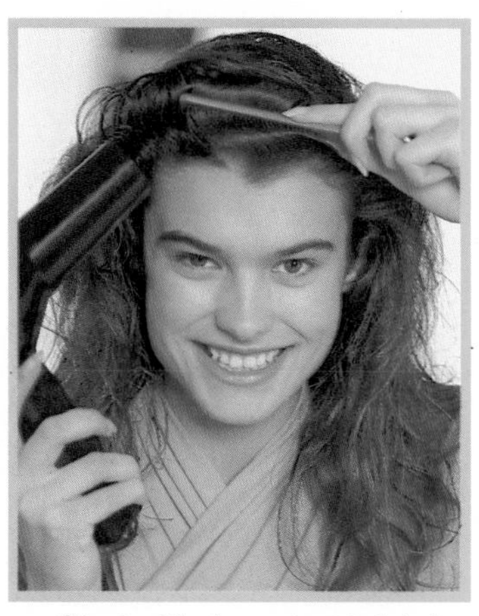

1 Start with clean, towel-dried hair and rub in an orange-sized blob of mousse. Using a comb to add height, dry layers at the roots away from your face.

If your hair is thick, the quickest way to reach the roots is to dry with your head tipped upside down.

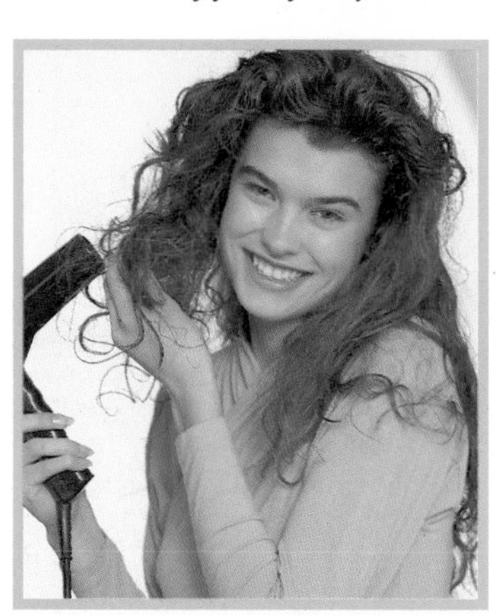

2 To build in lots of tousled volume scrunch-dry the mid-lengths and ends using your hands. Don't stop until your hair is completely dry.

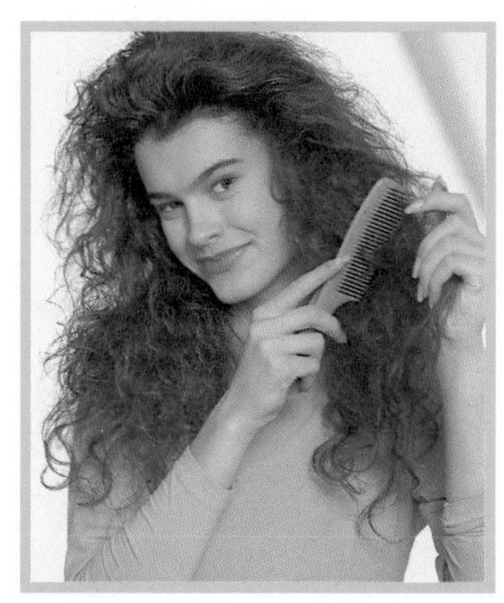

3 Using a wide-toothed comb gently back-comb through the lengths teasing the hair into shape with your fingers. Spritz with hairspray to set.

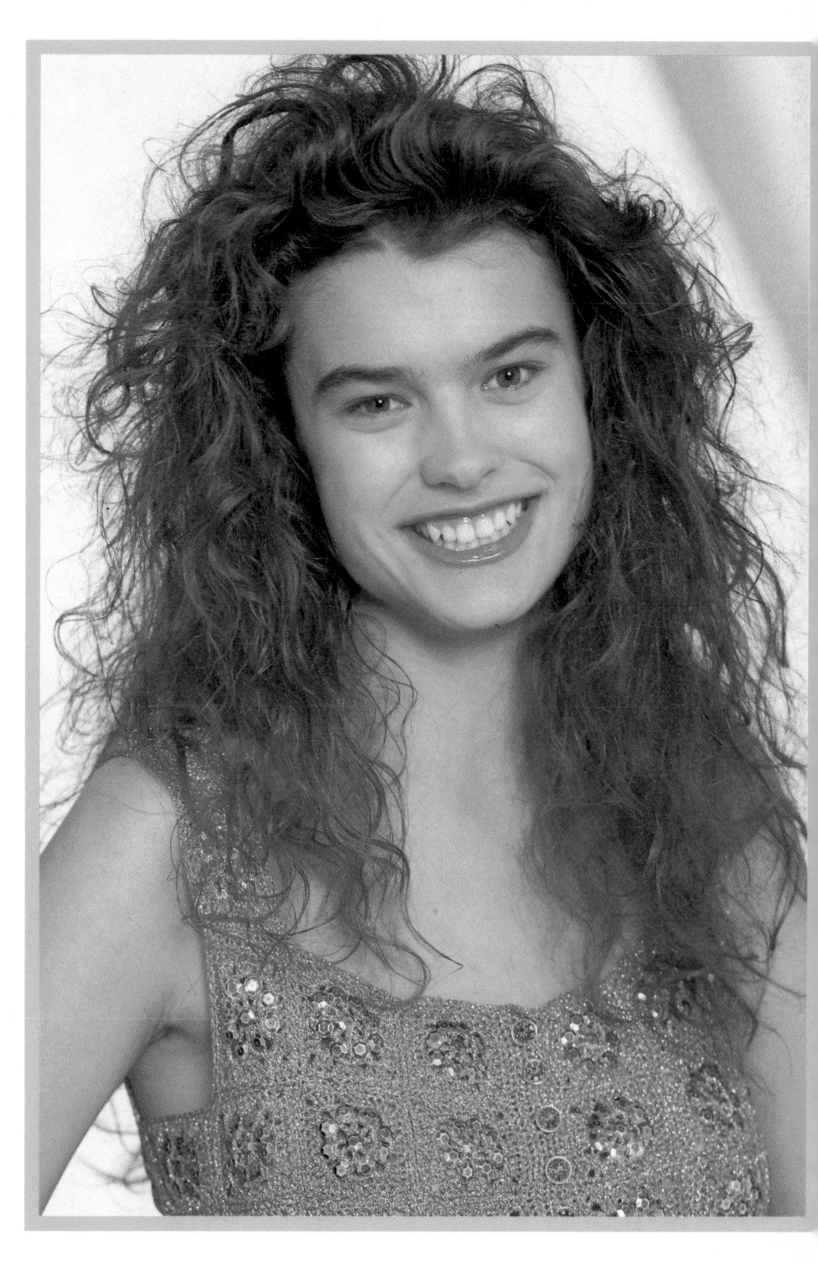

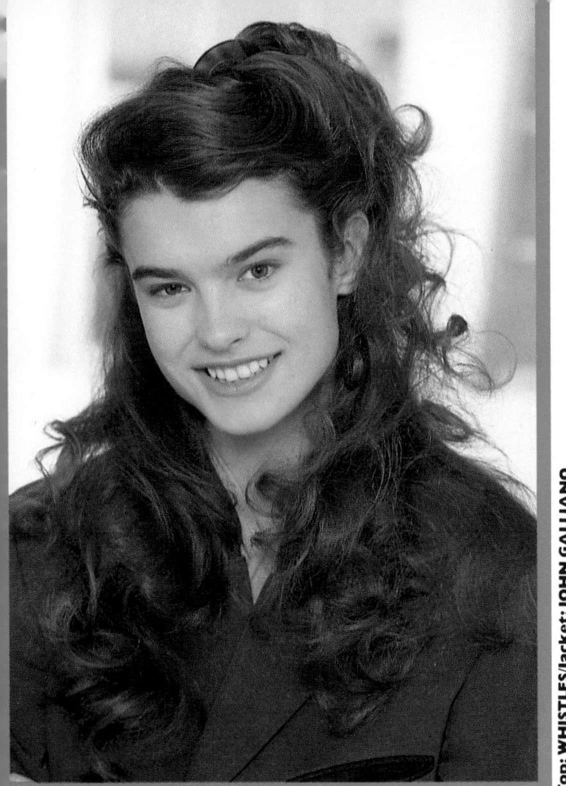

Top: WHISTLES/Jacket: JOHN GALLIANO

LIVEN UP LAYERS

- A layered cut can improve the look of your hair – fine hair can look thicker and thick hair looks less bulky. But just like any style you need to have your hair trimmed regularly to maintain the shape. Uneven ends do tend to stick out and look unsightly.
- If you're trying to put up layered hair neatly you'll find a tailcomb invaluable. Use the long end to tuck in any short strands of hair that keep falling out.
- If you want to wear your hair back but despair at taking in all the different lengths of hair, try a French plait for a neat solution. This style works well because the plaiting starts on top of your head and gathers in all the short layers from the front.
- Ponytails are often a problem because some of the layers are too short to tuck into the elastic band. For a neat alternative, make a French plait on the top of your head to gather up the short layers, fasten with a scrunchie then fluff out the lengths.
- To keep a layered fringe out of your eyes, take back your hair as if you were doing a pony-tail, then plait the top section as far as your nape. Secure with a scrunchie.
- If short layers stick out you can always smooth them down by running gel over them with your hands.
- To blow-dry layers smooth, use a small round brush and fit your dryer with a nozzle for concentrated heat without frizz.
- Wake up flat layers by lifting sections of hair and spritzing with styling spray close to the roots.
- Make the most of hair accessories to disguise untidy layers. Alice bands, bandanas, scarves, clips and slides will make your locks look neat and pretty.

PONYTAIL TACTICS

If layers fall out of a ponytail, do the twist to keep it neat.

Tip

If your hair is freshly washed, secure with a covered band first before you cover it with a decorative scrunchie.

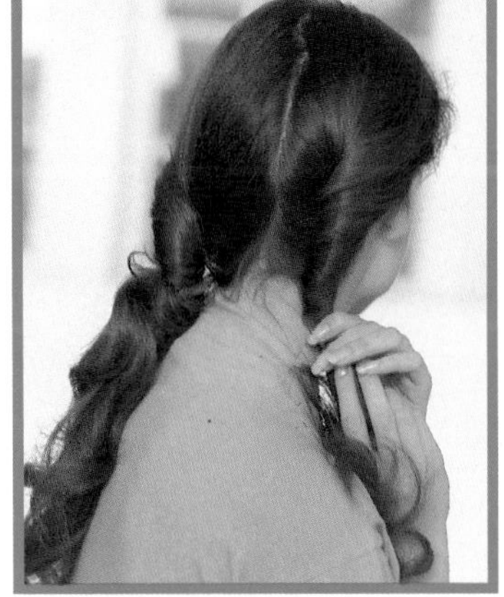

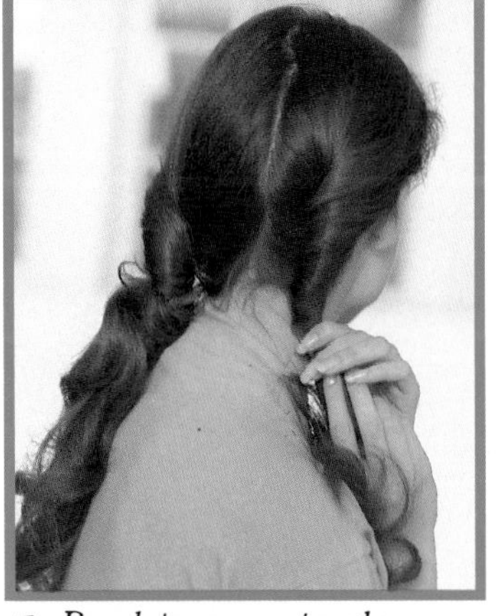

1 Brush to remove tangles. Make a centre parting and divide your hair into two bunches. Holding just above the nape, roll the bunches inwards.

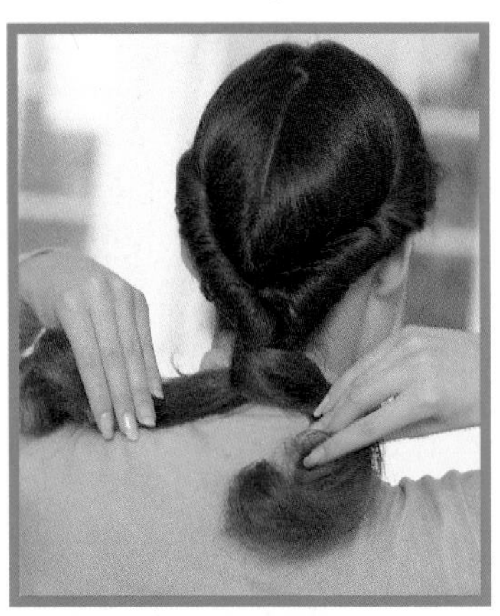

2 When both bunches are rolled as far as the nape, cross one over the other. Hold them tightly or they'll begin to unravel and short layers will fall out.

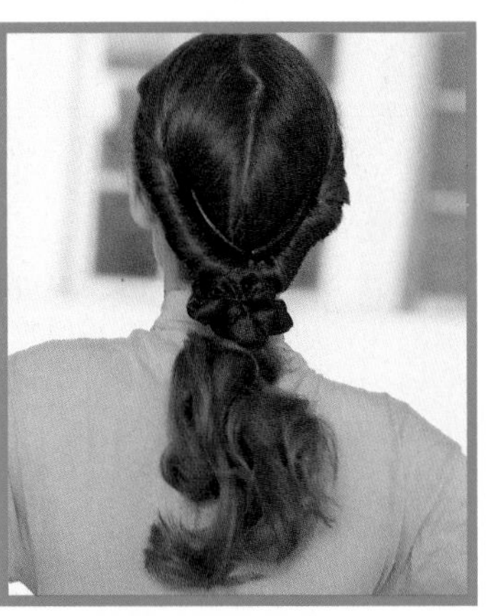

3 Hold the ponytail in place with a scrunchie. Wrap it around at least twice to make sure it holds the tail tightly.

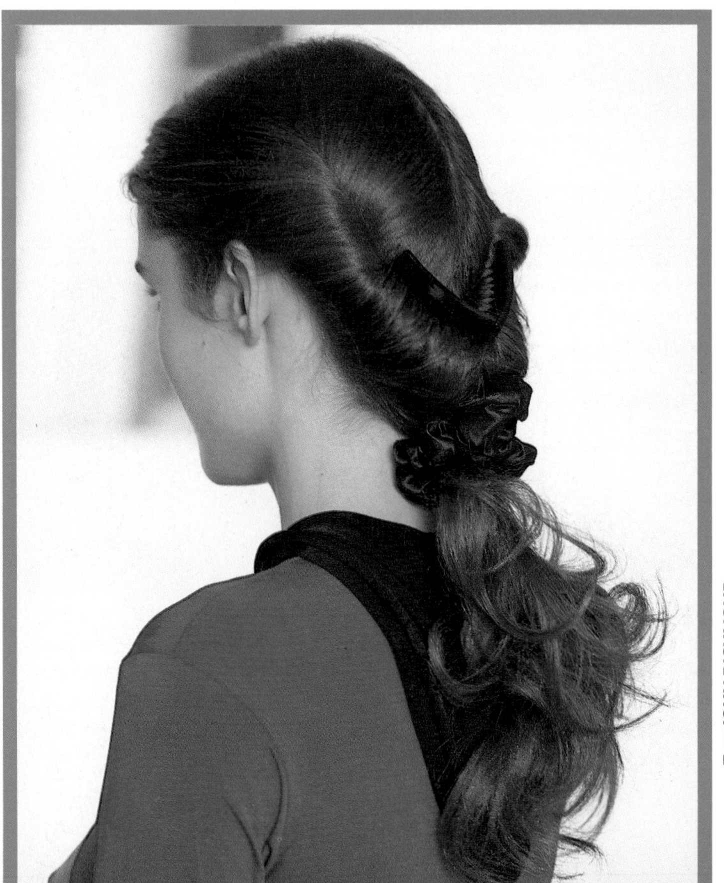

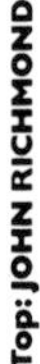

GOING STRAIGHT

There are lots of ways of making straight hair go curly, but it's harder to get curly locks to go straight. Here's how to use the latest straighteners to make smooth moves!

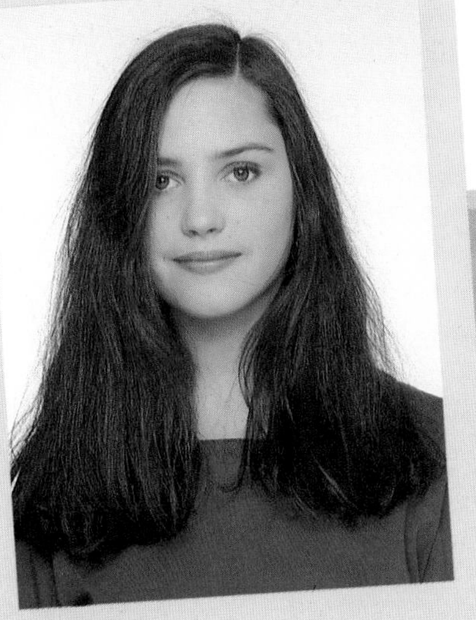

BEFORE
First dry hair thoroughly, then switch on straighteners to warm up.

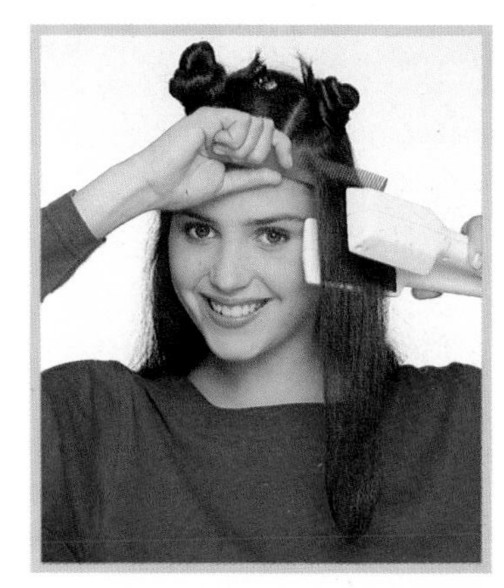

1 Section off the top of your hair, then lift a section away from your face with a comb. Clamp the straightener near the roots, then slide to the ends.

2 Work around your head, then pull down the top and straighten in the same way. When you've finished, spritz with hairspray and comb through.

FINISHED
A super-smooth, silky style with a rich sheen.

Watchpoint

Always ease straighteners down your hair in one smooth motion – if you stop and start you'll end up with kinks!

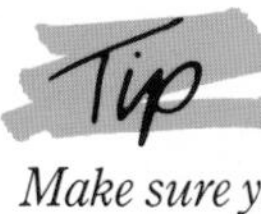
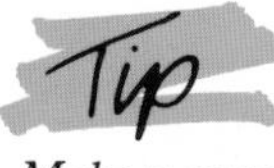

Tip

Make sure your hair is completely dry before using electric straighteners – wet hair will only sizzle and steam!

Photographs: MATTHEW SMITH/Hair: PENNY ATTWOOD/Make-up: YA'NINA/Jacket: JIGSAW

QUICK TIPS

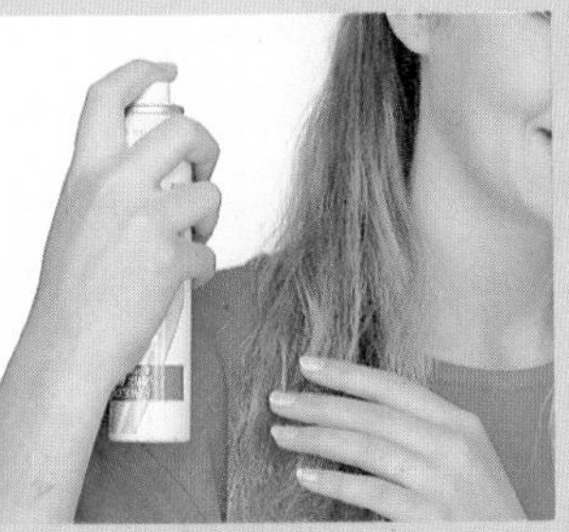

Spray on heat-styling lotion to protect your hair and add a little extra shine to the finished style.

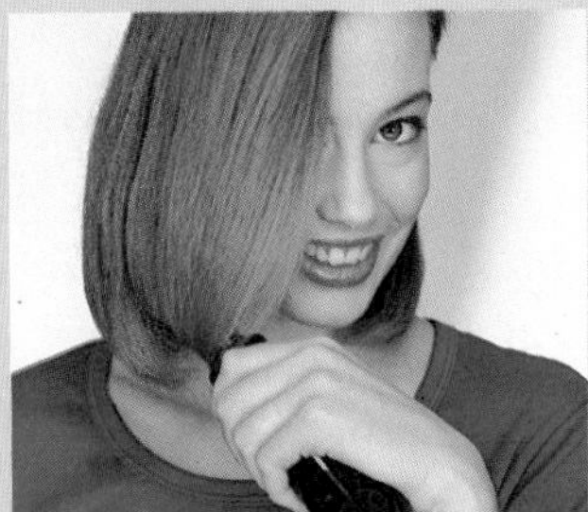

Use mini-straighteners to curve your hair under at the ends. They only take five seconds to work.

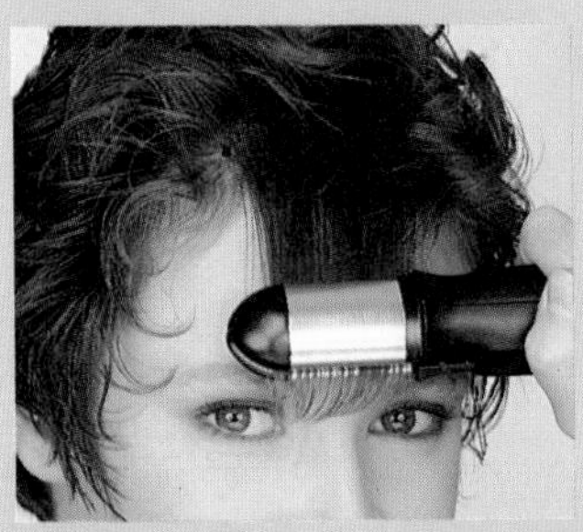

1 *To straighten a fringe, put the mini-straighteners close to the roots and slide them down the length.*

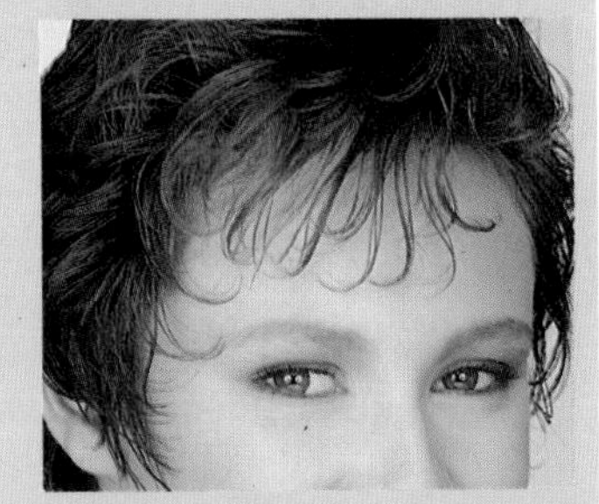

2 *Separate the fringe using a small amount of gel – this will create a softer frame for your face.*

TAMING LONG WAVES

Straighteners are an effective way of taming tousled curls so they can be incorporated into a smooth, upswept style. Large heated plates are best used here for speed and smoothness.

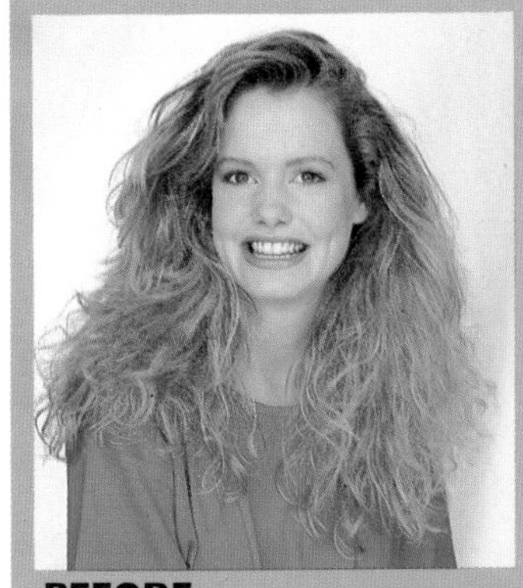

BEFORE
Begin with clean, dry hair. Brush out any tangles with a good brush.

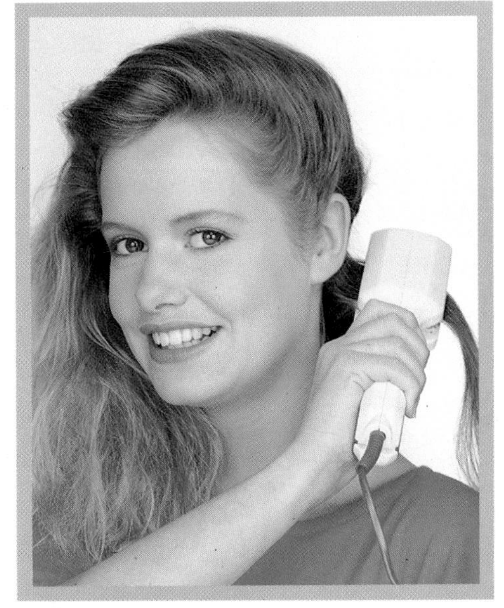

1 **Section the underneath of your hair and hold the full-size hair straightener close to the roots. Press it on firmly.**

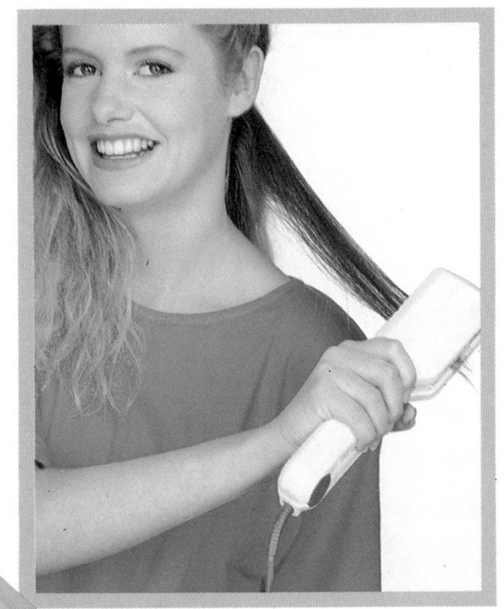

2 **Gradually slide the straightener down the length of your hair. Work over your whole head, straightening the hair section by section, until it is completely smooth.**

THE APPLIANCE OF SCIENCE
Most styling appliances are for creating curls and waves – but what about the occasions when you want to go sleek, smooth and sophisticated? Well, forget the brown paper-and-iron method granny would have favoured. The latest straightening appliances will control your tresses in next to no time.

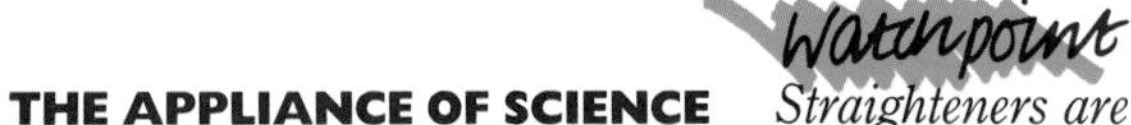

Watchpoint
Straighteners are great for special occasions but they are quite hard on your hair so shouldn't be relied on for regular use.

▲ MINI STRAIGHTENERS
Ultra-slim plates for root lift and adding the finishing touch to smooth styles. Ideal for fringes and ends.

▶ FULL-SIZE STRAIGHTENERS
Large size heated plates used to smooth out unwanted curl or frizz from bob-length to longer hair.

Black embroidered top: WAREHOUSE/Earrings and hair accessory: FENWICK/Photographs: ADRIAN BRADBURY
Hair: JENI/Make-up: JENNY NOLAN/Still life photographs: LEON

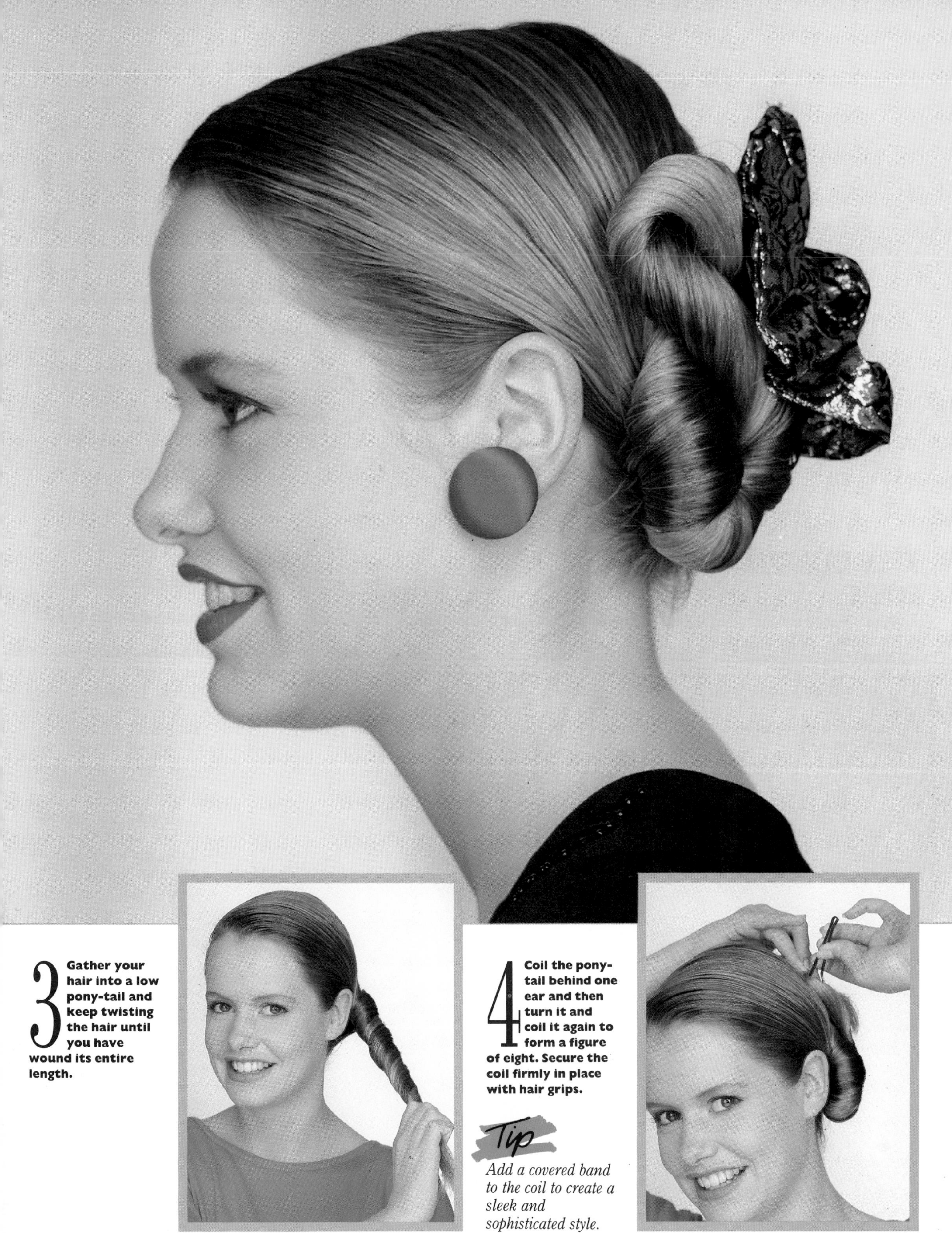

3 **Gather your hair into a low pony-tail and keep twisting the hair until you have wound its entire length.**

4 **Coil the pony-tail behind one ear and then turn it and coil it again to form a figure of eight. Secure the coil firmly in place with hair grips.**

Tip

Add a covered band to the coil to create a sleek and sophisticated style.

PROBLEM SOLVER

THIN HAIR

Thick, bouncy styles aren't an impossible dream if you have thin hair! You can't make more hair grow but you can make what you've got look thicker. So get ahead with this hair body-builder

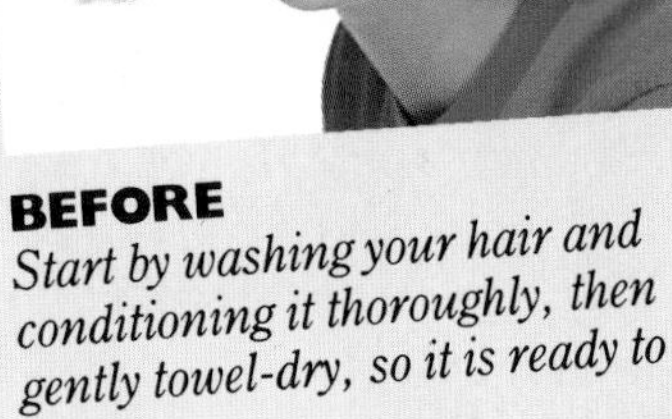

BEFORE
Start by washing your hair and conditioning it thoroughly, then gently towel-dry, so it is ready to be cut.

THE CUTTING EDGE

Thin hair looks its worst when worn in a badly shaped, growing-out or non-existent style. A short cut, such as a one-length bob, is full of the movement essential for creating an illusion of thickness, and it allows what volume there is in your hair to show.

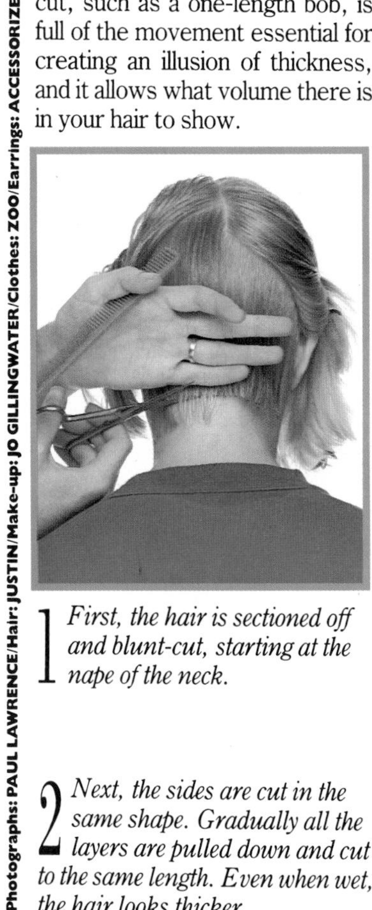

1 First, the hair is sectioned off and blunt-cut, starting at the nape of the neck.

2 Next, the sides are cut in the same shape. Gradually all the layers are pulled down and cut to the same length. Even when wet, the hair looks thicker.

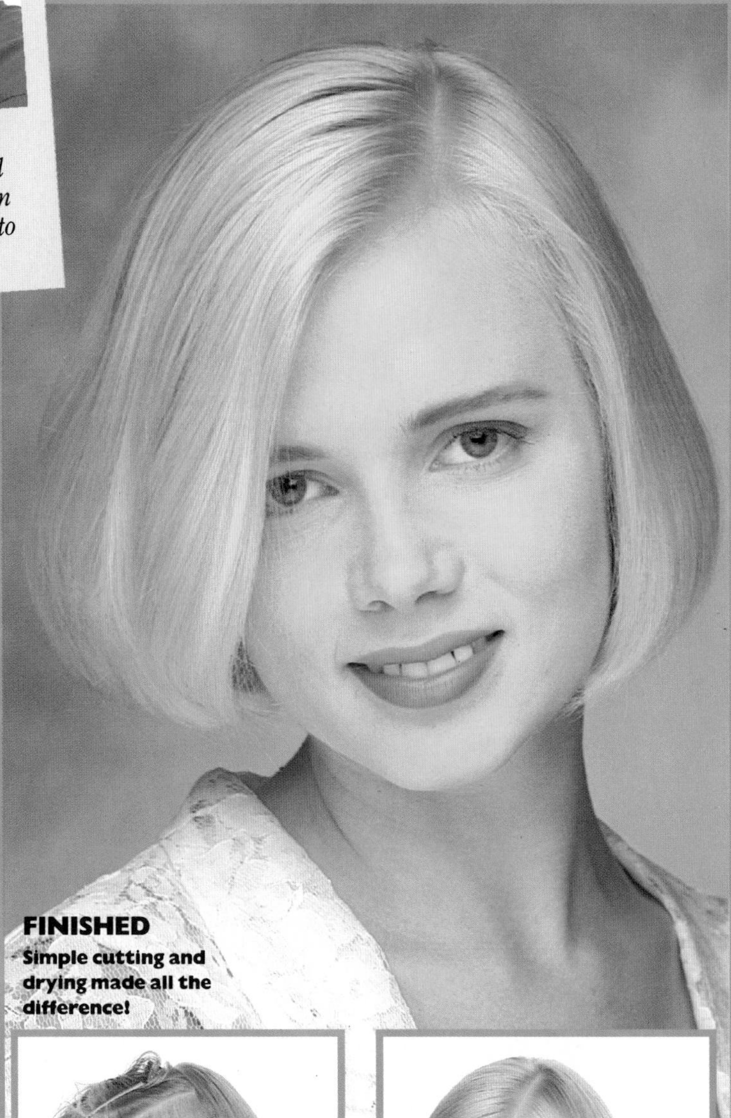

FINISHED
Simple cutting and drying made all the difference!

Thin hair is caused by having fewer follicles than normal and fine-textured hair. It's most common in fair-haired people and although there's nothing to worry about in health terms, it can be annoying if you want to try bouncy, voluminous styles. The hair tends to have flyaway ends and look limp too, and it's not unusual to see glimpses of scalp through it, most noticeably around the front hairline.

Fortunately, there's no need to hide your locks under a hat! With the right products and some nifty styling, you can pump up the volume. From the top here's how to give thin hair a boost.

3 Clever blow-drying can create volume and movement. Concentrate on getting lift around your hairline and parting. Work from underneath and blow-dry your hair on a low heat setting to prevent split ends. Using a flat-backed brush, pull it through your hair from roots to ends, lifting the layers away from your head to give root lift. Dry the ends under.

Photographs: PAUL LAWRENCE/Hair: JUSTIN/Make-up: JO GILLINGWATER/Clothes: ZOO/Earrings: ACCESSORIZE

TOP TRIO

Short hair's versatile and ever so quick to style! And here's the proof – three good-looking styles that can be yours in a matter of minutes

BEFORE
Make sure your hair is clean. Dampen it before you start.

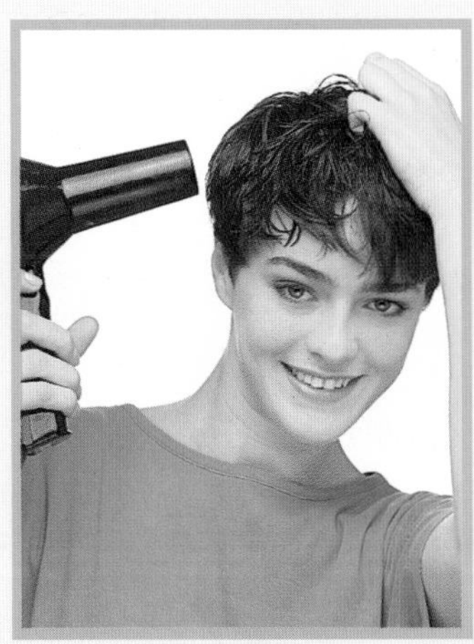

1 *Work a walnut-sized blob of mousse through the length of your hair from roots to ends and blast-dry.*

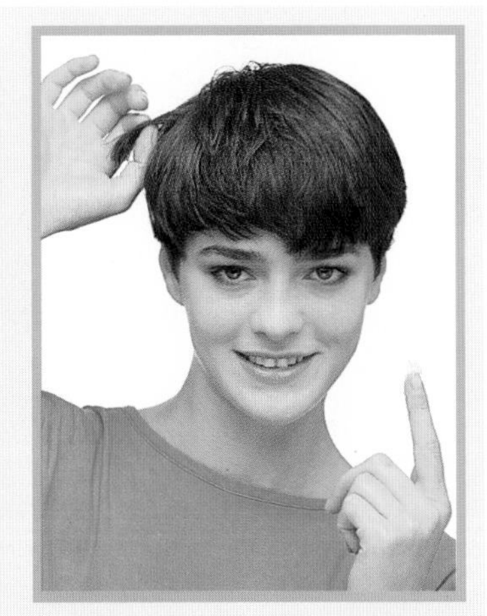

2 *Use a thumbnail-sized blob of wax to separate the ends of your hair. Pull them forwards on to your face.*

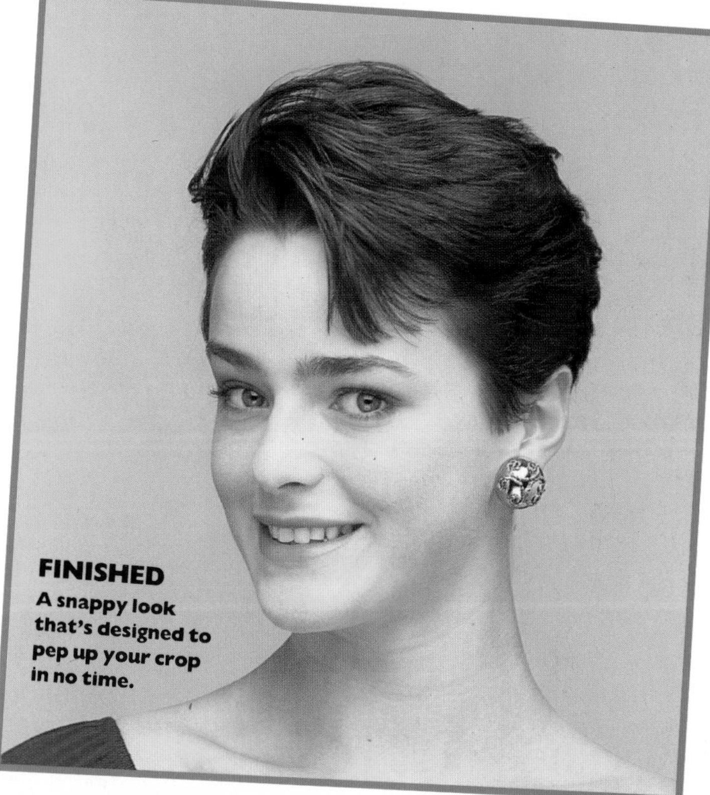

FINISHED
A snappy look that's designed to pep up your crop in no time.

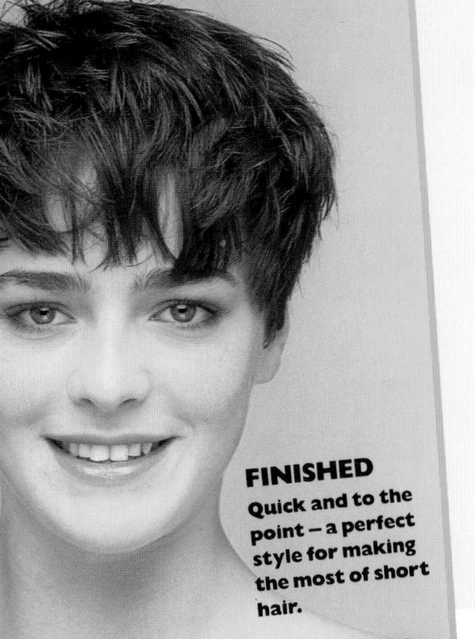

FINISHED
Quick and to the point – a perfect style for making the most of short hair.

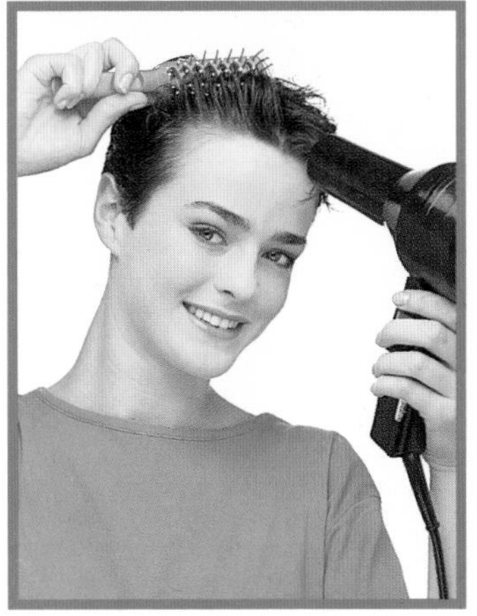

1 *Follow Step 1 as before, but blow-dry over to one side, using a vent brush.*

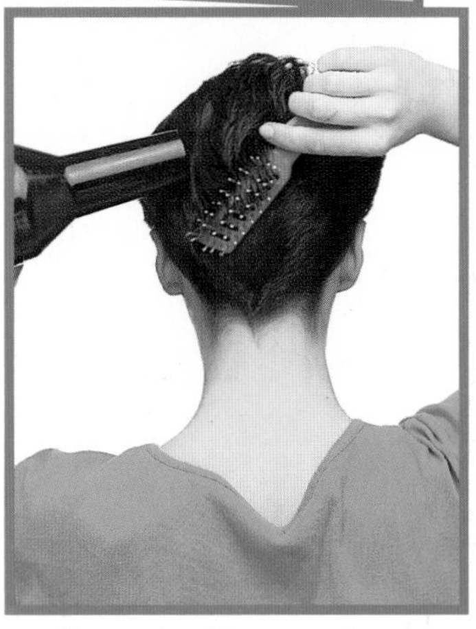

2 *Sweep the sides round so they meet at the back. Pull your fringe forwards above one eye.*

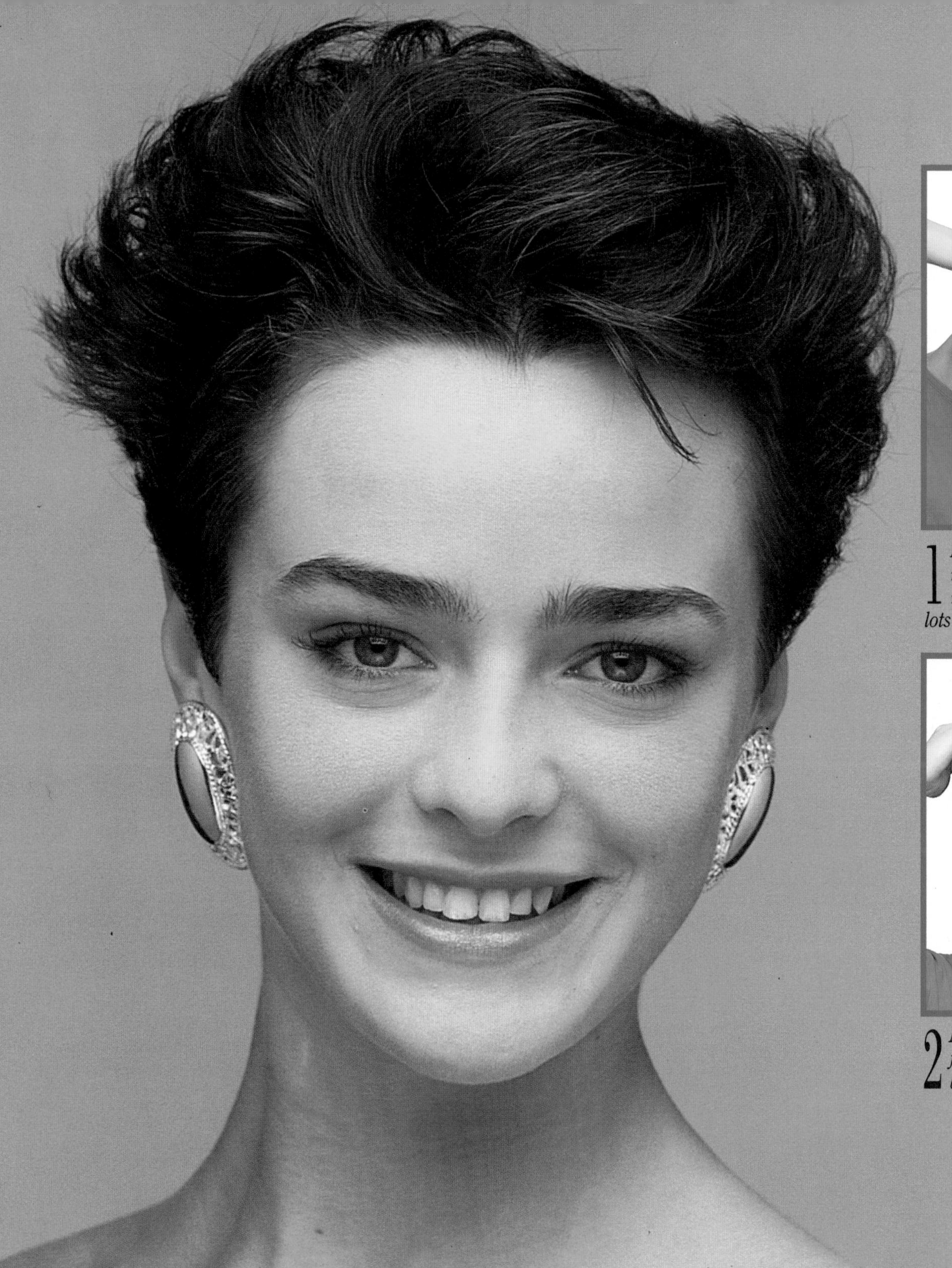

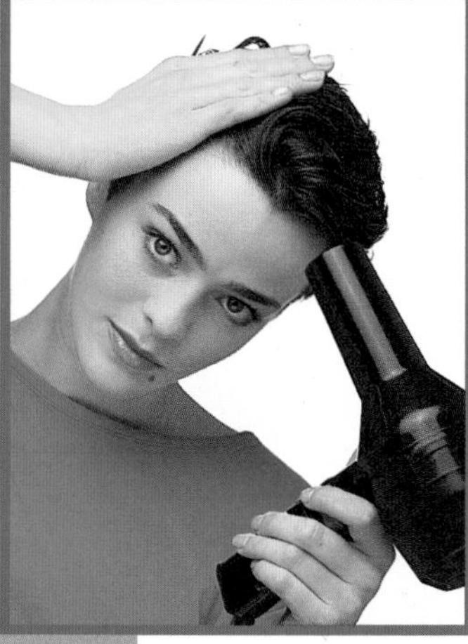

1 Follow Step 1 as before, but rotate your palm over your roots as you blow-dry to create lots of volume.

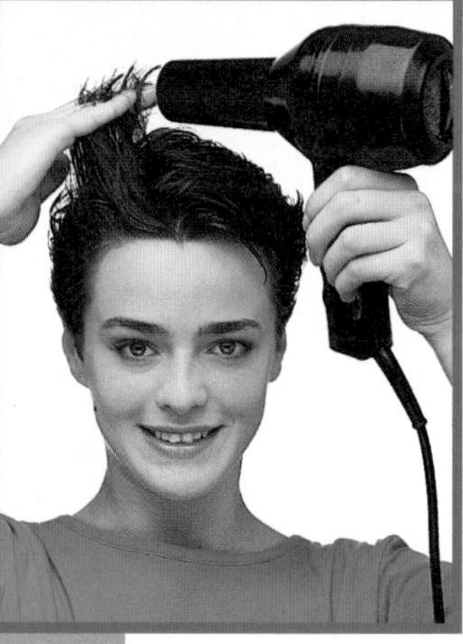

2 Next, lift your hair between your fingers to give even height and blow-dry away from your face.

Photographs: PAUL MITCHELL/Hair: PENNY ATTWOOD/Make-up: KAREN LOCKYER/Top: MARY QUANT/Earrings: ACCESSORIZE

FINISHED
Leave a strand to fall softly onto your forehead and there you have it – up and away to a glamorous night out.

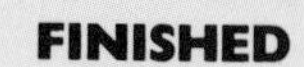

Personal styling guide

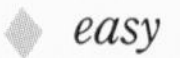

easy

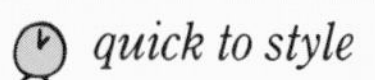

quick to style

Works best on
short, graduated cuts with layers of at least 7 cm/3 in on top of your head.

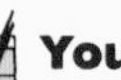

You need:
mousse
wax
hairdryer
vent brush

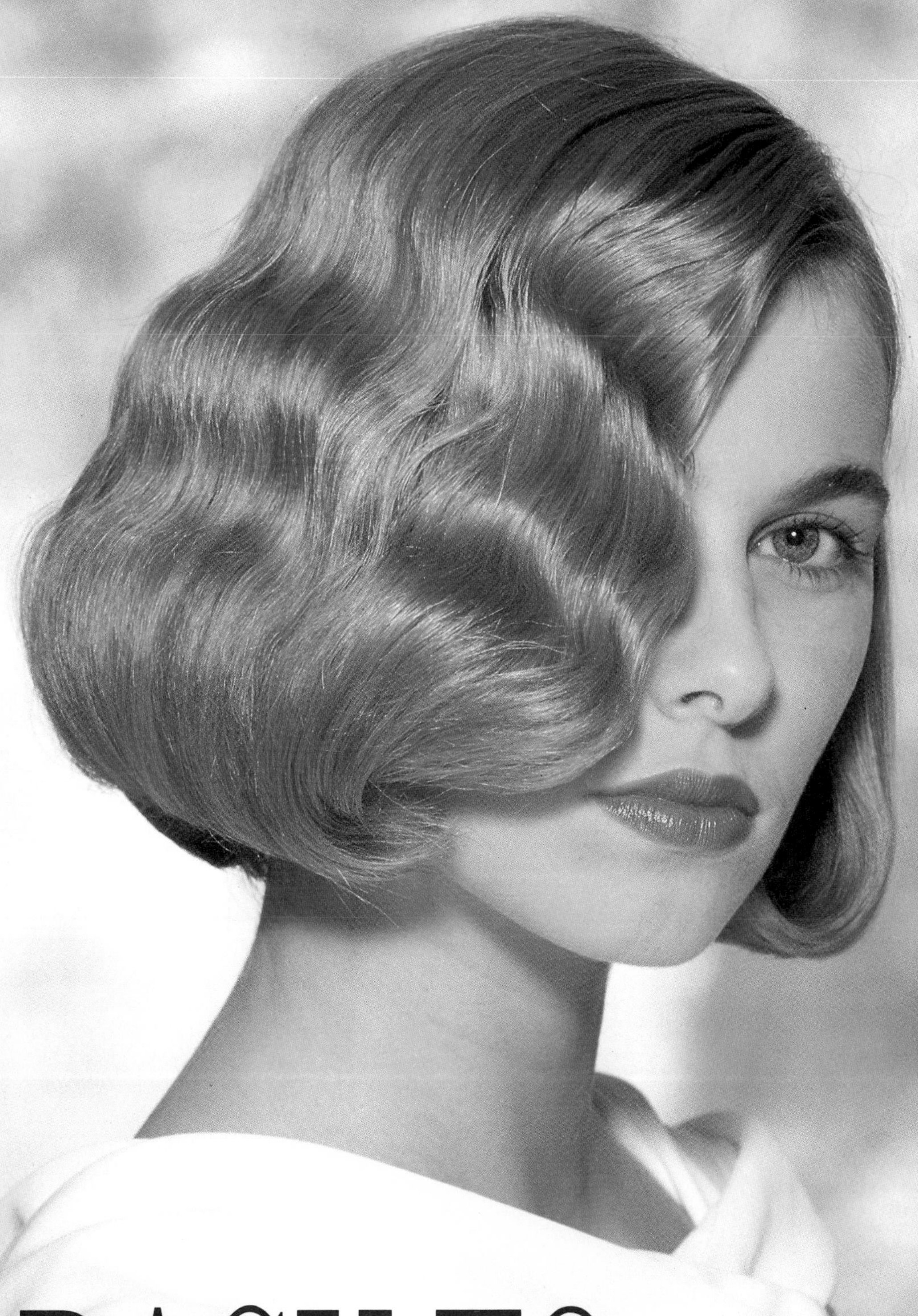

BACK TO THE FUTURE

For style to take you into the future with a flourish, try a touch of flashy French Marcel Waving

Marcel Waving is a styling technique which uses ordinary tongs to create glamorous waves in the hair. It first took shape in France in the late 1800s, but it wasn't until the 1920s that the style really hit the headlines when stars of the stage and high society set the trend that was to become so popular. Even those with the straightest of locks wanted – and could now have – that distinctive pattern of dips and crests.

With Marcel Waving back in vogue in the Nineties, why not learn how to do it yourself? Just take to your tongs and you'll quickly discover how to make great waves!

SUITS YOU!

Before you make for the waves check the list below to find out if Marcelling will be right for your kind of hair.

DO MARCEL:

- Hair that's below chin- to shoulder-level and is all one length. If it's longer, the weight will pull out the waves.
- Blonde hair – it's much easier to see the waves if they're on light-coloured hair.

DON'T MARCEL:

- If your hair has lots of split ends since you won't be able to achieve a really sleek finish. Get your hair trimmed to get rid of them first.
- Dry or damaged hair. You'll have to hold the tongs on your hair longer to set the waves in place and this can cause dry hair to break.

Photographs: SARAH HUTCHINGS/Hair: PENNY ATTWOOD/Make-up: ELLEN KRAMER/Clothes: HENNES/Jewellery: ADRIEN MANN

CREST OF A WAVE

Marcelling gives added interest to a straight bob and creates a head-turning look for evening.

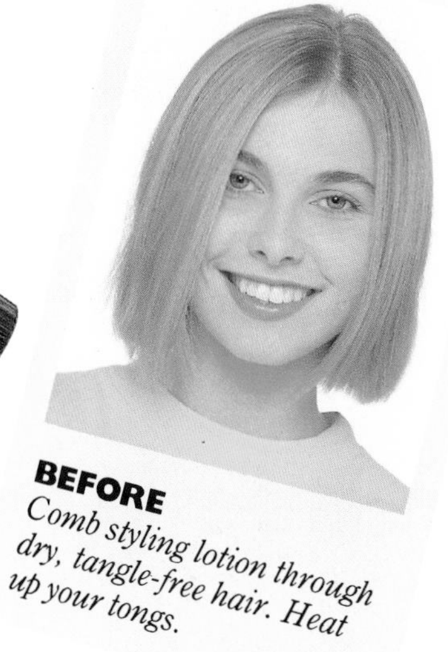

BEFORE
Comb styling lotion through dry, tangle-free hair. Heat up your tongs.

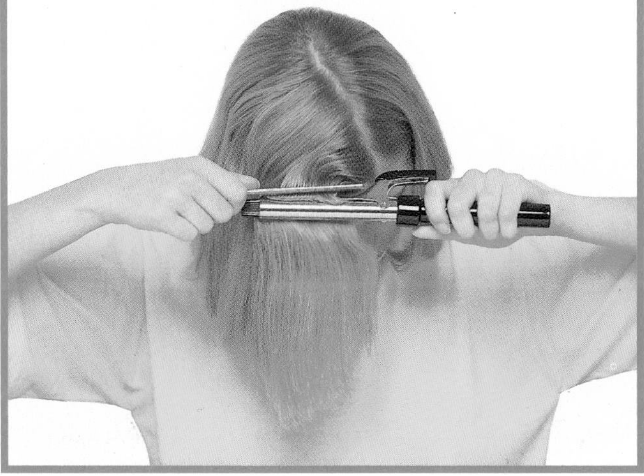

1 Make an off-centre parting using a tailcomb. Starting at the fuller side, take a 7.5 cm/3 in wide section at the front and lift with a comb. Slide the tongs through the hair, just below the comb, then twist them backwards and pull your hair in the opposite direction. Hold for a few seconds and release.

Finding it tricky? Get a friend to hold the comb while you tong.

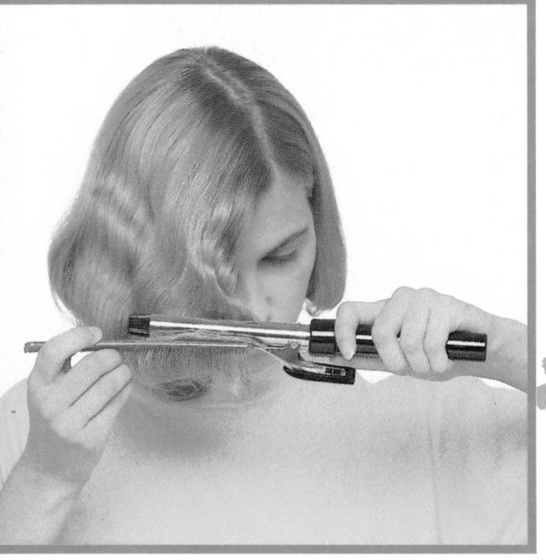

2 Moving down the section, place the comb on the crest of the previous wave and open the tongs. Repeat as before but this time pull the tongs and comb in the opposite direction to step 1.

Tip

On layered hair, only use Marcelling to give lift at the front.

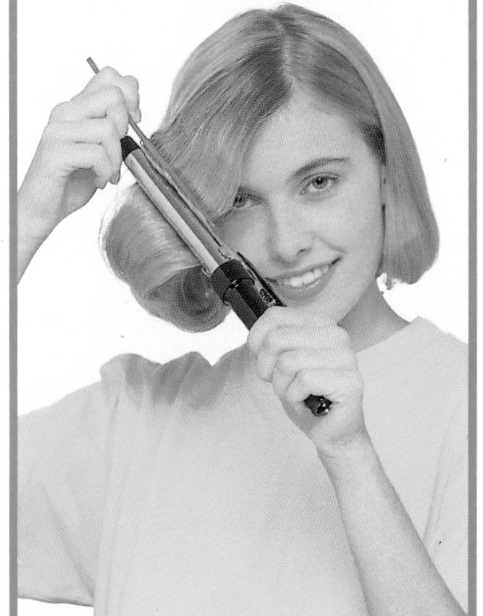

3 Continue making this pattern of dips and crests all the way down the hair length until you get to within 5 cm/2 in of the ends.

Give the waves added shine by spritzing hair with hair gloss instead of hairspray.

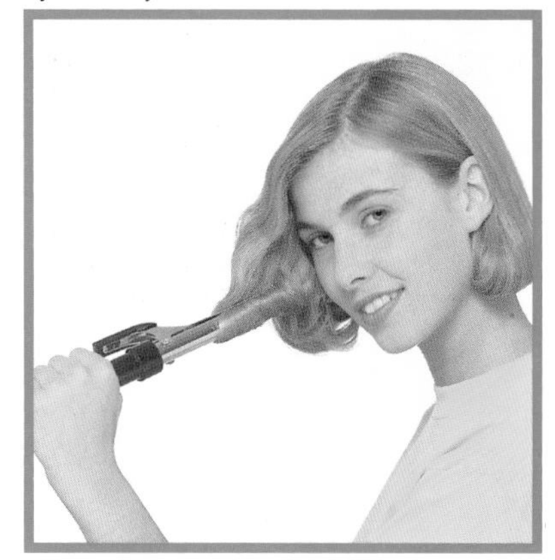

4 Use the tongs to curl the ends under. Then continue to wave the rest of your hair in the same way. Spritz the finished style with hairspray and use the back of the comb to gently smooth down any stray hairs.

THE WAVY LARK

Give a new twist to Marcel waving – use it on curly hair to give root lift at the front.

1 Lifting the front section of hair away from your face, slide the tongs through it, twisting them backwards towards your crown. Place the comb below the barrel and gently pull the comb and tongs in opposite directions. Hold for a few seconds then release.

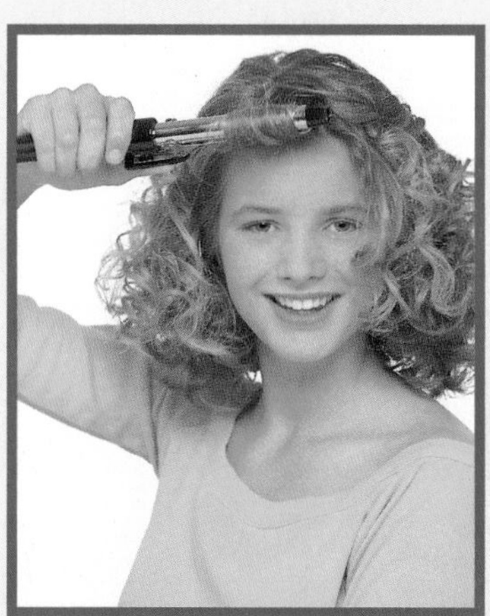

3 To achieve a neat finish, curl the ends of the hair upwards around the tongs.

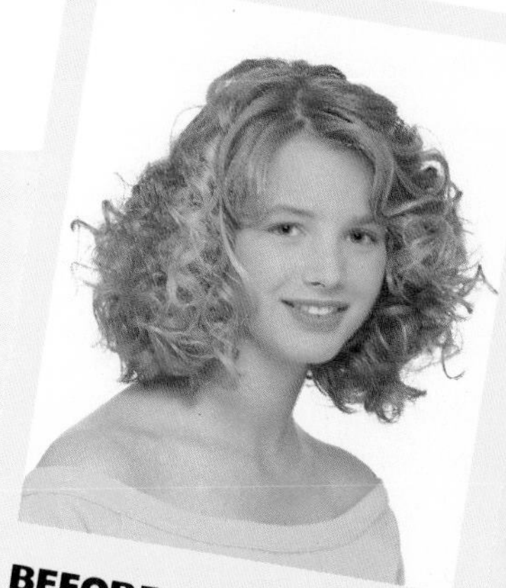

BEFORE

If your hair is lacking body or curl, scrunch-dry it first, or set it on heated bendy rollers to give it more bounce.

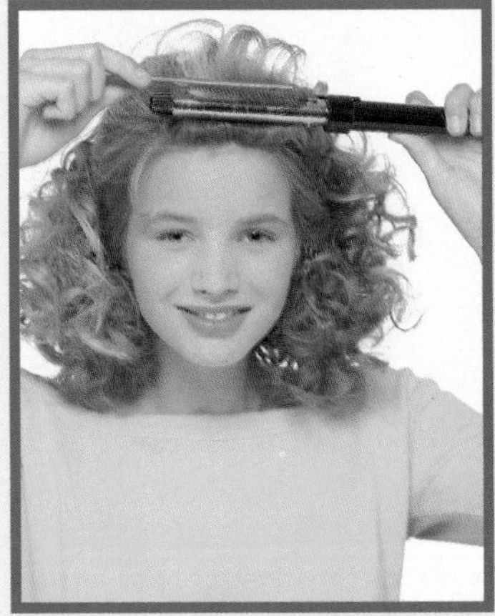

2 Open the tongs and close them on the crest you've just made. Now place the comb above the tongs then gently pull them both in the opposite direction to the previous wave you've made to create an 'S' shape.

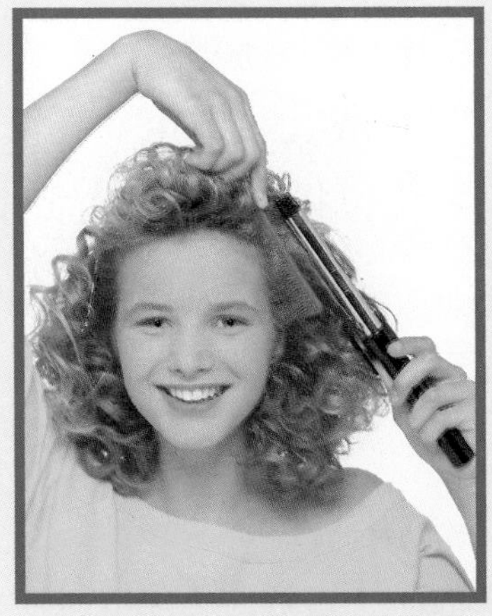

4 Continue waving the side sections around the hairline, but this time, keep the tongs almost vertical.

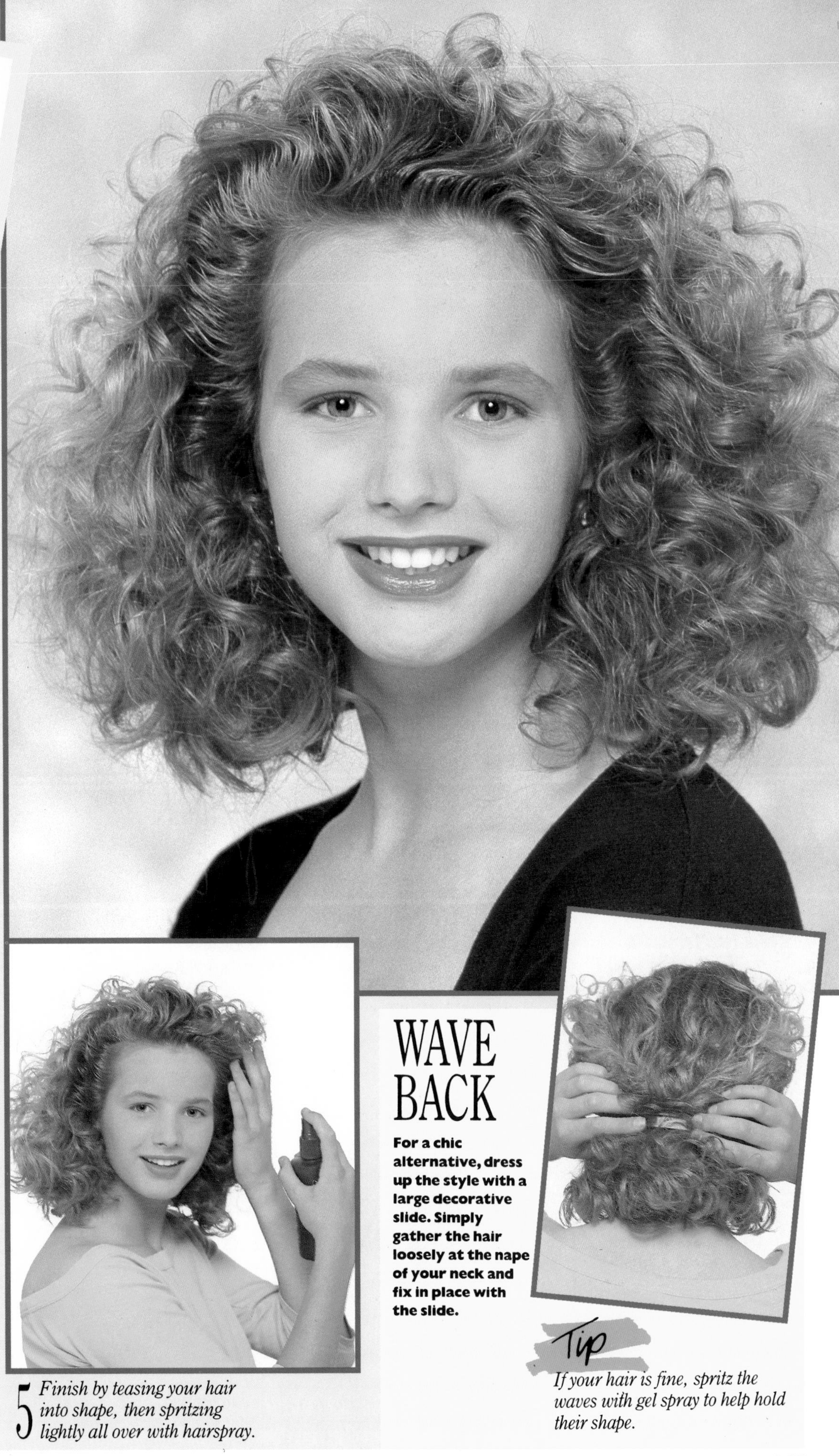

5 Finish by teasing your hair into shape, then spritzing lightly all over with hairspray.

WAVE BACK

For a chic alternative, dress up the style with a large decorative slide. Simply gather the hair loosely at the nape of your neck and fix in place with the slide.

Tip

If your hair is fine, spritz the waves with gel spray to help hold their shape.

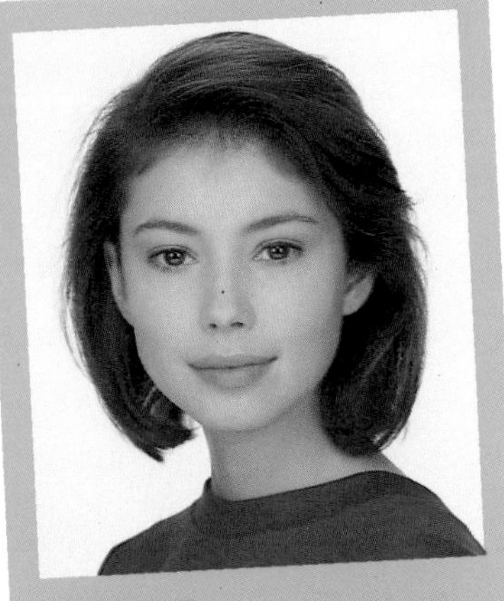

BEFORE
Work mousse through damp hair, rough-dry and you're ready to start curling.

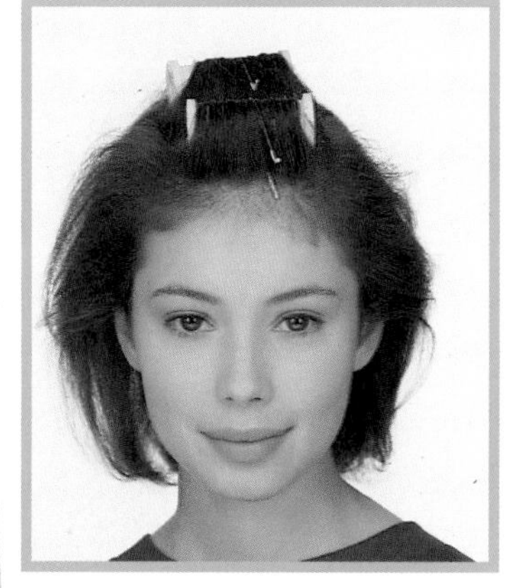

1 Section off the middle hair at the front. Wind backwards over medium-sized heated rollers working towards the crown.

ROLLER GIRL

Dust off those heated rollers and wind up with a luxurious crop of curls. You'll be switched on to great hair in a matter of moments!

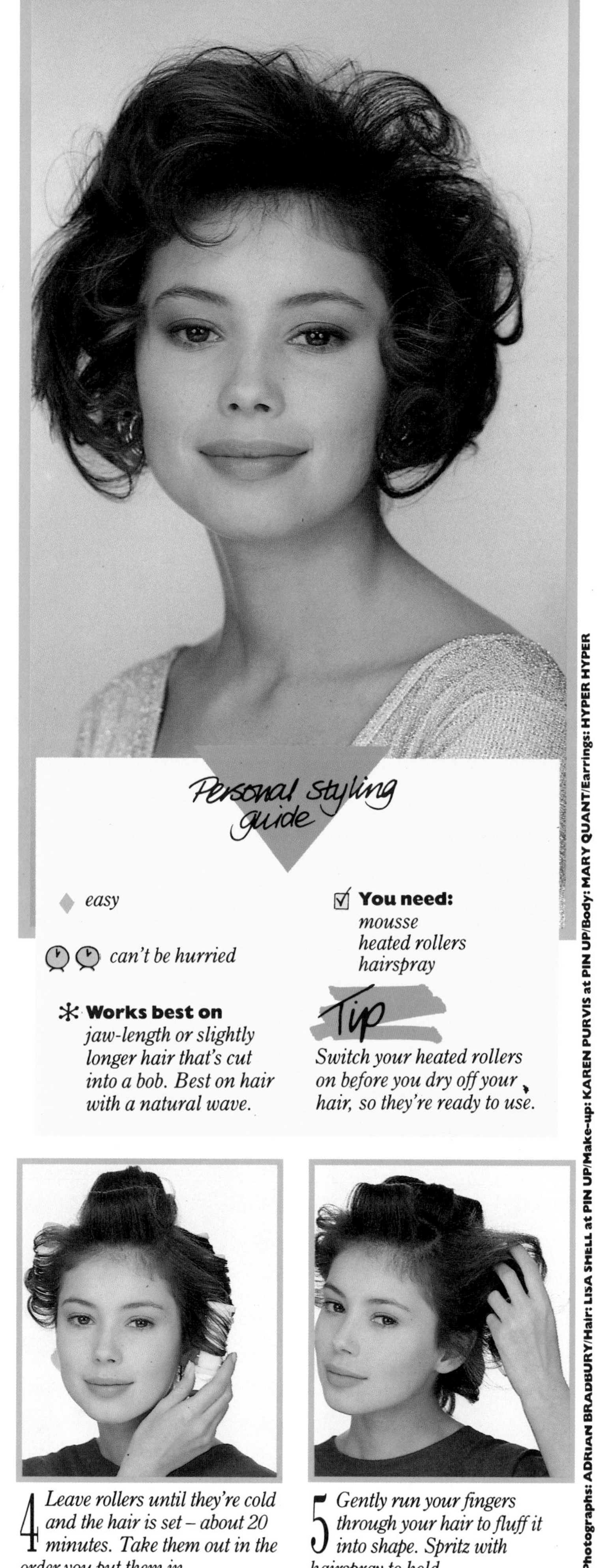

Photographs: ADRIAN BRADBURY/Hair: LISA SHELL at PIN UP/Make-up: KAREN PURVIS at PIN UP/Body: MARY QUANT/Earrings: HYPER HYPER

Personal styling guide

◆ *easy*

can't be hurried

Works best on
jaw-length or slightly longer hair that's cut into a bob. Best on hair with a natural wave.

You need:
mousse
heated rollers
hairspray

Tip
Switch your heated rollers on before you dry off your hair, so they're ready to use.

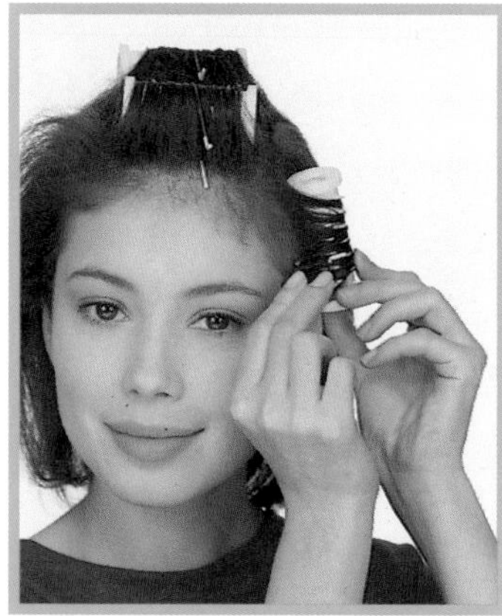

2 Next move on to the sides. Take vertical sections of hair and wind back over the rollers. Pin in position.

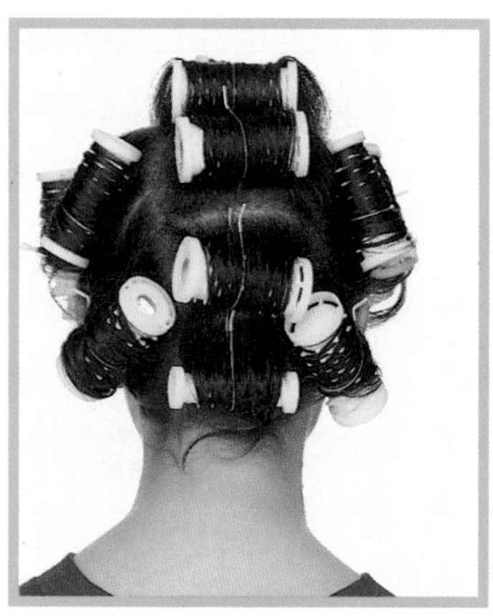

3 After you have completed the sides wind the back section in the same direction as the front.

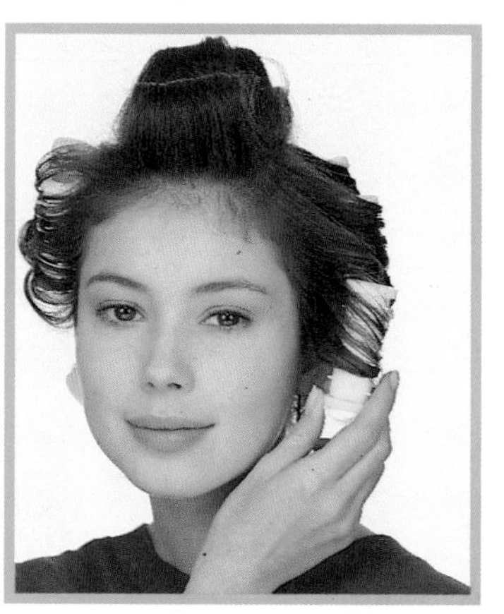

4 Leave rollers until they're cold and the hair is set – about 20 minutes. Take them out in the order you put them in.

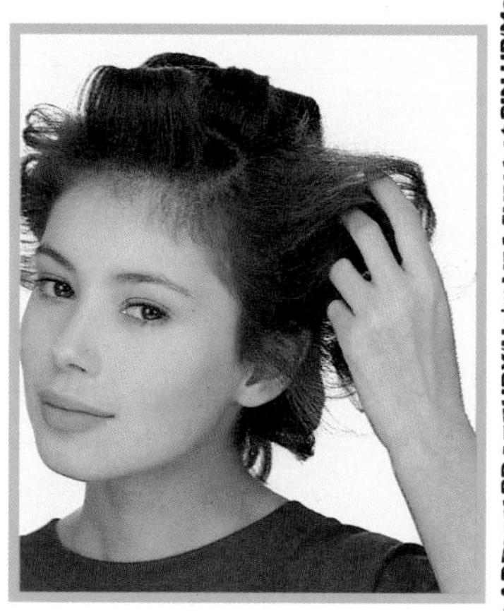

5 Gently run your fingers through your hair to fluff it into shape. Spritz with hairspray to hold.

Whether your hair's naturally curly, permed, Afro or just very thick, frizziness can be a problem, leaving it matted and unmanageable. However, with the right styling products and drying techniques, you can tame those tresses smooth and straight or bring out the curls for a head of hair that's fab – rather than frizzy.

WAVE IT!

Set tight curls on rollers to create cascading waves.

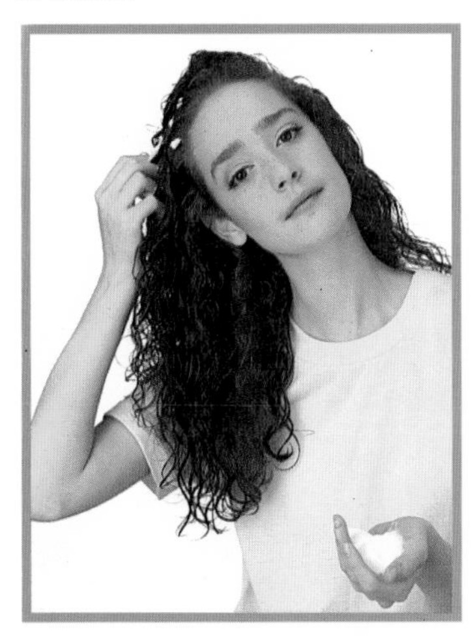

1 Start with freshly-washed, well-conditioned hair that's just damp. Comb through, then work in a grapefruit-sized blob of mousse.

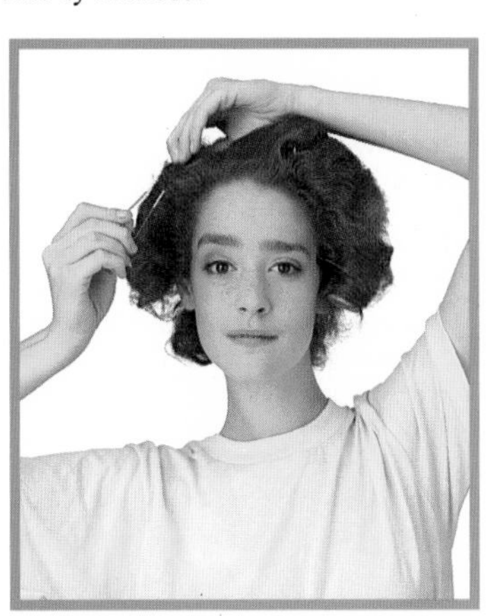

2 Divide hair into 5cm/2 in sections. Using large rollers, loosely wind up the hair and pin in place. Leave to dry before taking out the rollers.

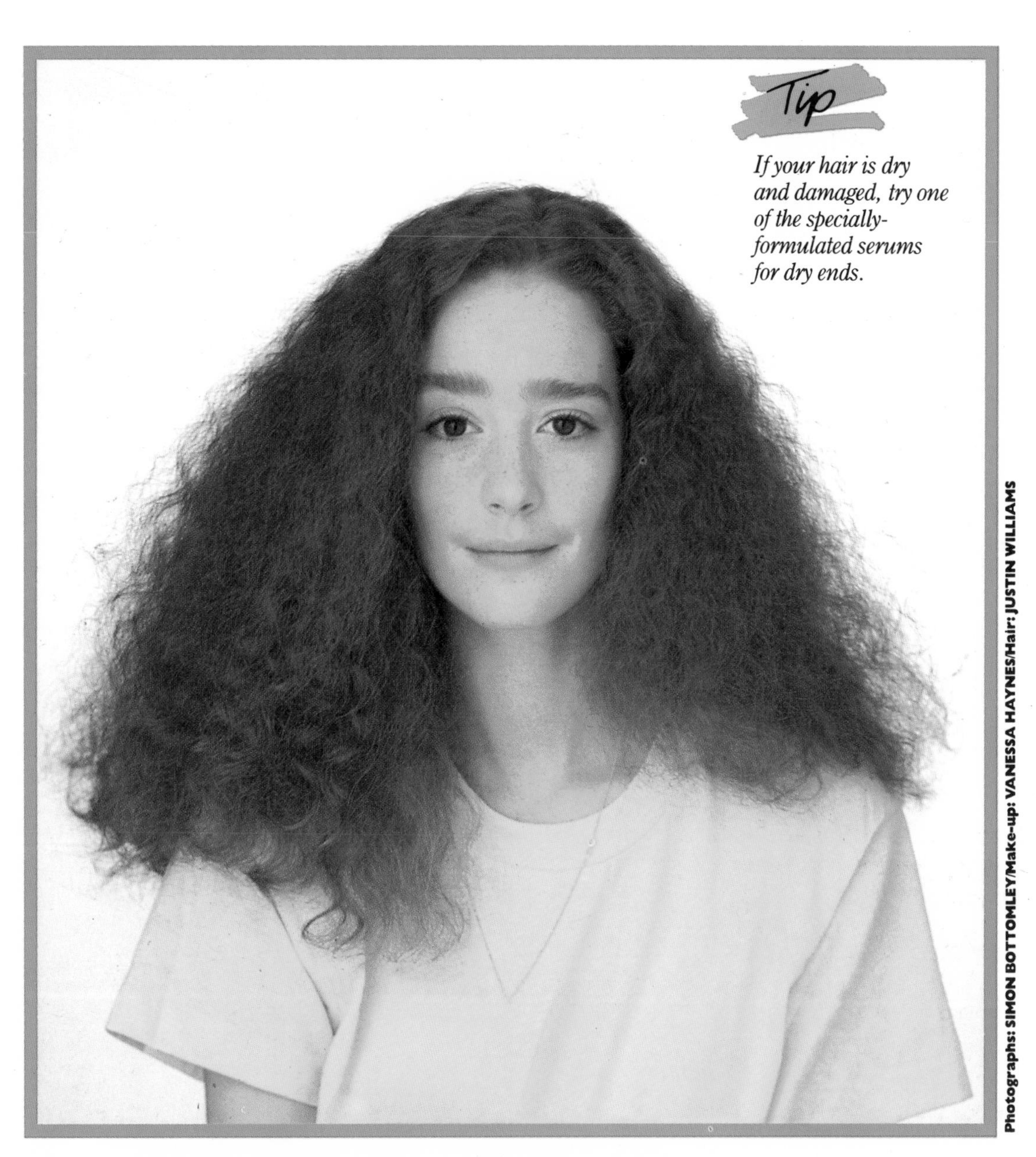

Tip

If your hair is dry and damaged, try one of the specially-formulated serums for dry ends.

Photographs: SIMON BOTTOMLEY/Make-up: VANESSA HAYNES/Hair: JUSTIN WILLIAMS

FRIZZY HAIR

'My hair is naturally wavy. And no matter what I try to do to it, it always seems to end up looking dry and tangled – especially when I blow-dry. Is there anything I can do to get rid of the frizzies?'

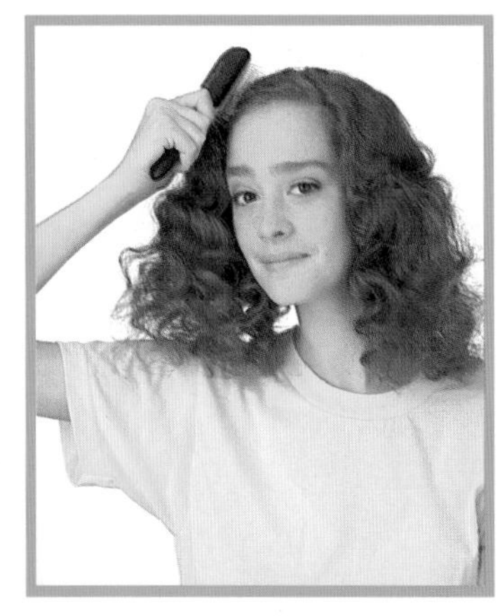

3 *Take the rollers out carefully. Brush your hair through with a flat-backed brush to smooth the curls into soft waves.*

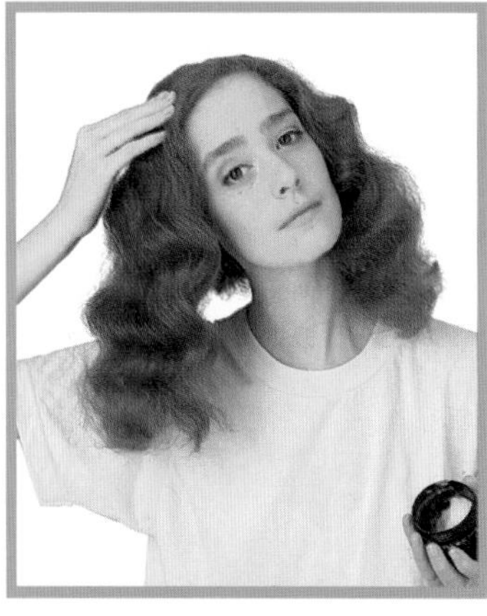

4 *Finish the style by smoothing over a thumbnail-sized blob of wax to prevent static and flyaway ends.*

SCRUNCH IT!

Soften curls with the right styling products.

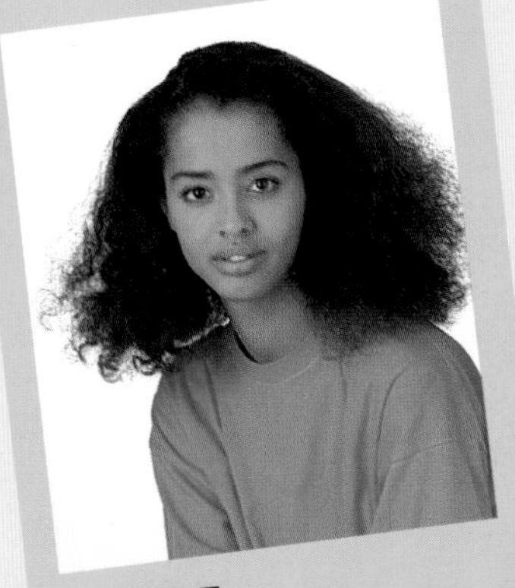

BEFORE
Rub conditioner into the ends of freshly-washed, damp hair.

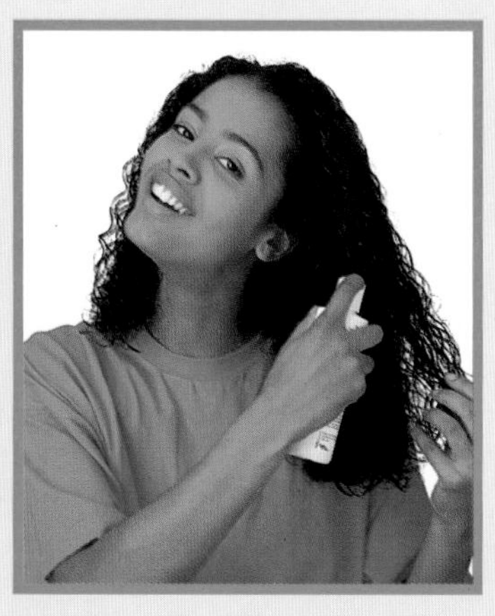

1 *Spritz hair lightly with spray-on gel to help define the curls and hold their shape.*

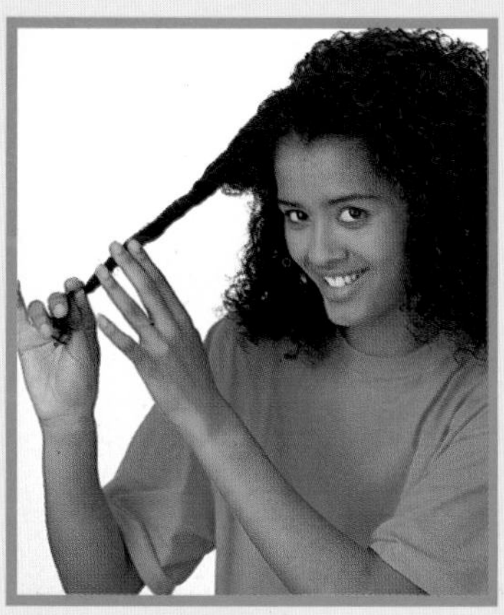

3 *Take large sections of hair and twist each one into a spiral. Rub a thumbnail-sized blob of wax between your palms, then run your waxed palms down the twists.*

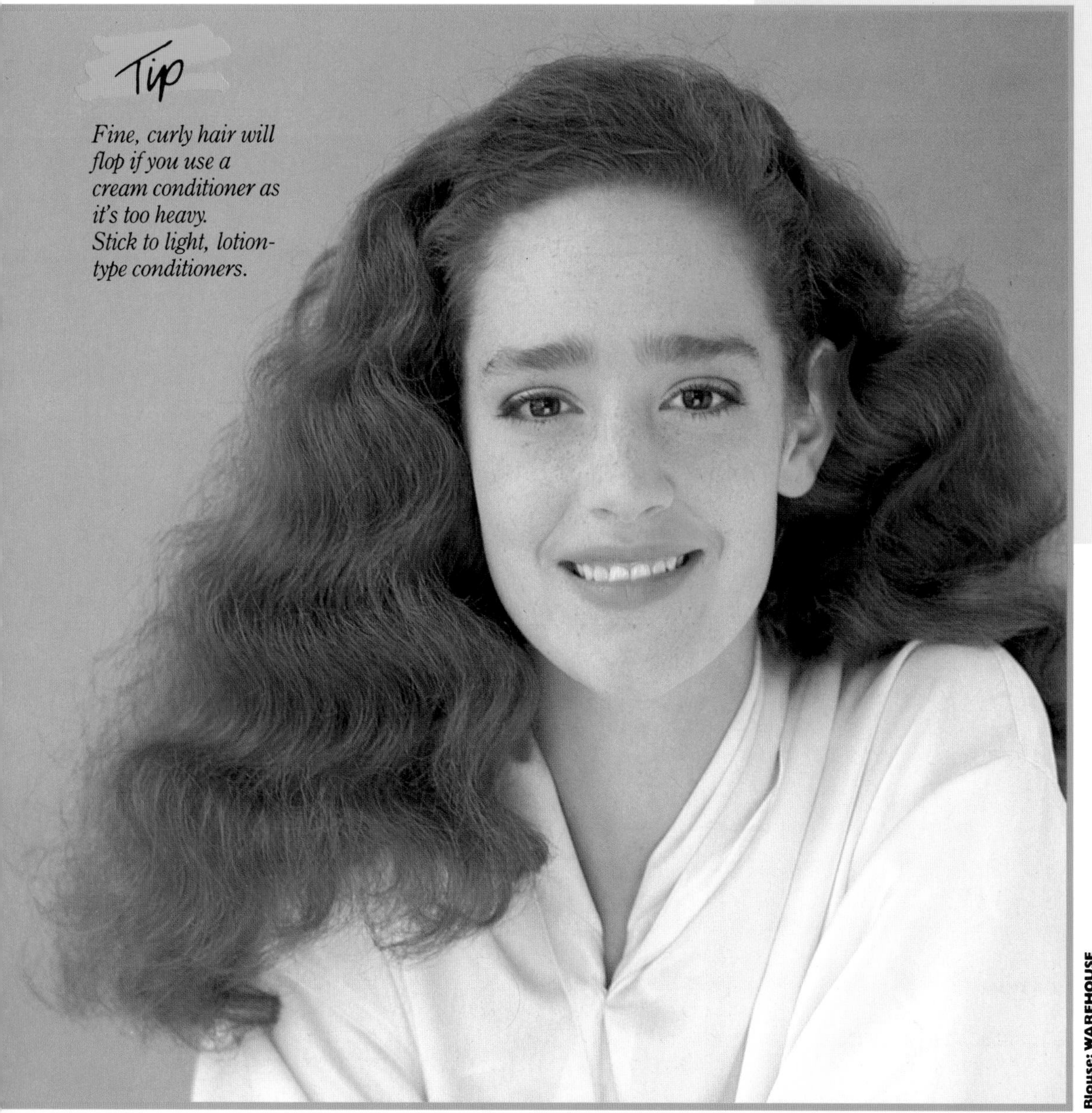

Tip

Fine, curly hair will flop if you use a cream conditioner as it's too heavy. Stick to light, lotion-type conditioners.

Blouse: WAREHOUSE

FRIZZ FIXES

- **Look out for mild shampoos suitable for dry, frizzy, coarse or curly hair as they are less likely to strip the hair of its natural oils.**
- **Condition curly hair regularly. Rub a marble-sized blob of conditioner between your palms and run through the ends of freshly-washed hair – don't rinse out – then blow-dry into style.**
- **Use a wide-toothed or Afro comb as they're much kinder to curls.**
- **Comb curly hair when wet, not dry, as you'll tug and stretch the hair as you pull the comb or brush through it.**

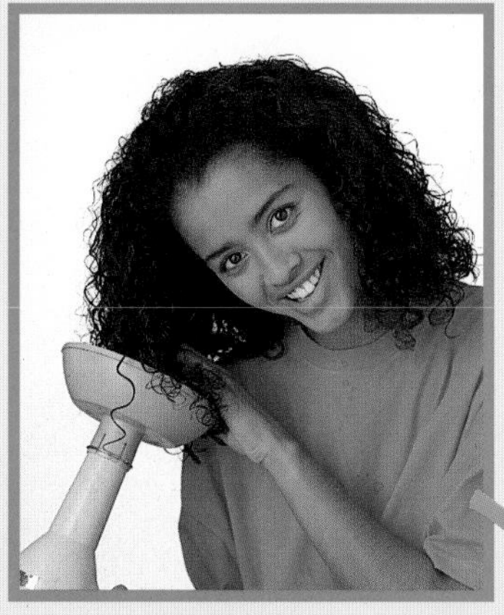

2 *Scrunch-dry hair using a diffuser attachment on your dryer until the hair is just slightly damp.*

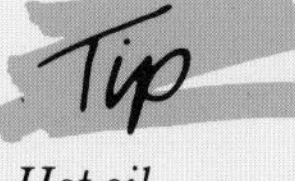

Hot oil treatments are great for coarse-textured and Afro hair. Try one once a month to help keep your hair in tip-top condition.

Watchpoint

Damp weather can make hair frizz even more, so when it rains take cover under a hat!

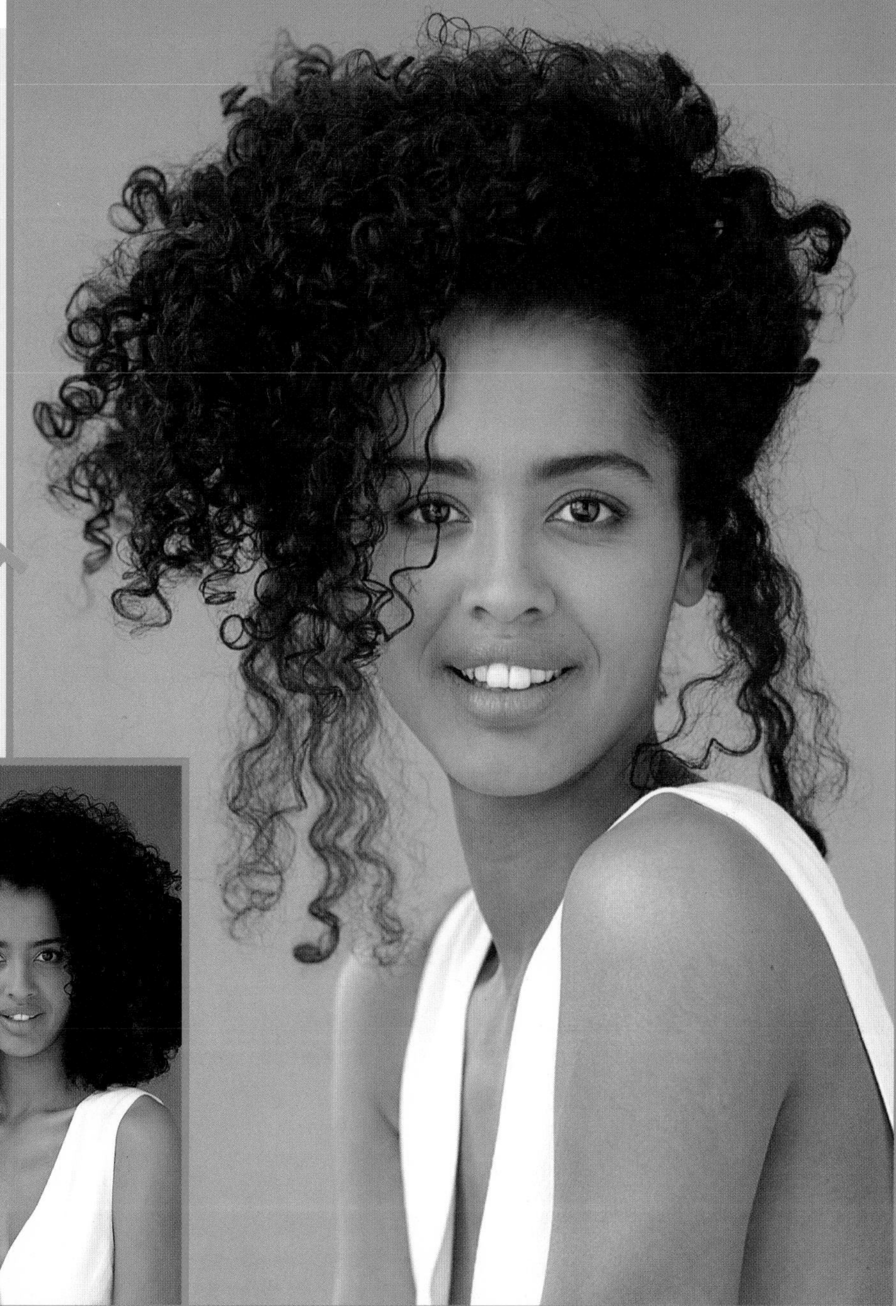

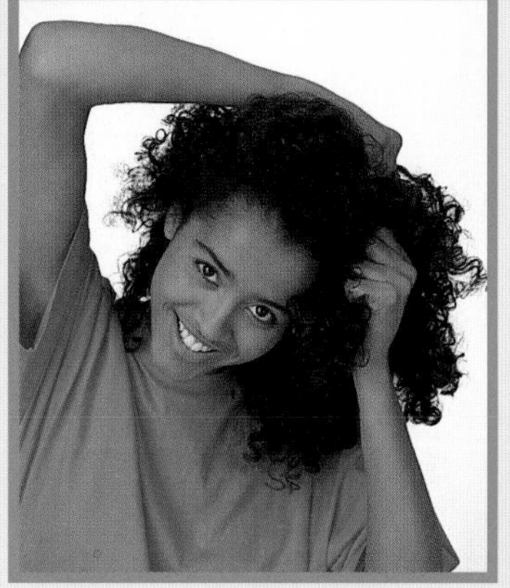

4 *When you've waxed all your hair, tip your head to one side and ruffle the roots with your fingers to loosen the style.*

Dress: WAREHOUSE

- **Occasionally let your hair dry naturally to help prevent it from drying out.**
- **Don't blow-dry Afro hair – it will frizz even more.**
- **Always take small sections of hair and dry each one by directing the hairdryer's nozzle downwards from the roots – if you don't do this, your hair will tangle.**
- **Spritz each section of hair lightly with a waterspray if it's already dry by the time you're ready to blow-dry. This will help prevent static.**
- **Smooth a thumbnail-sized blob of wax or gel over dry hair to help control it.**

GOING STRAIGHT

Smooth those frizzies with a professional blow-dry or straighteners.

To vary the style, hold the front of your hair back with a hairband.

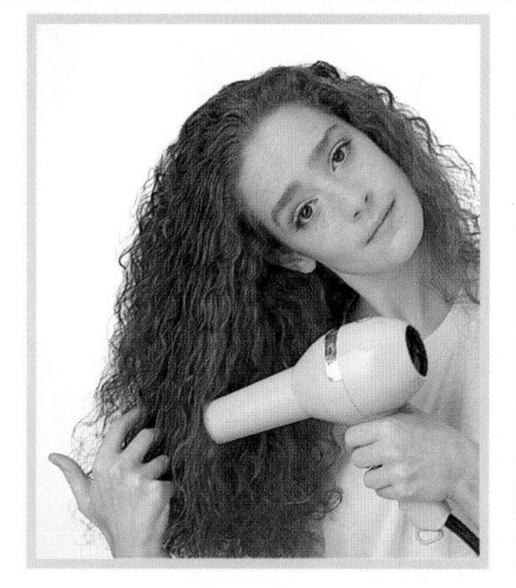

1 *Spritz freshly-washed, damp hair with styling spray. Blow-dry until just slightly damp, raking your fingers through it as you blow-dry to separate the curls.*

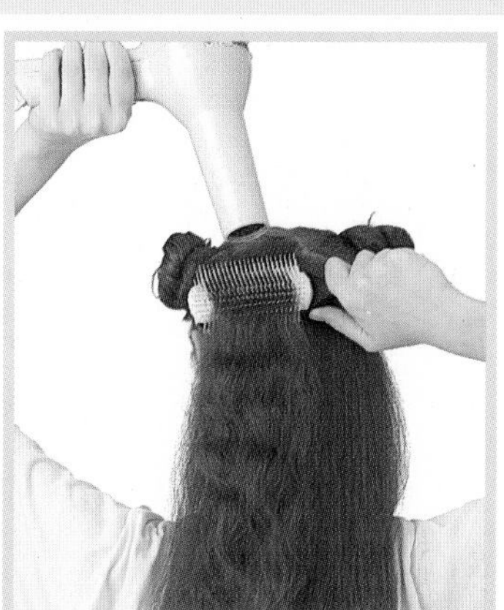

2 *Starting at the back, separate out a 5 cm/2 in wide section of hair. Using a flat-backed brush, take it down the hair, following with your hairdryer. Work round your whole head.*

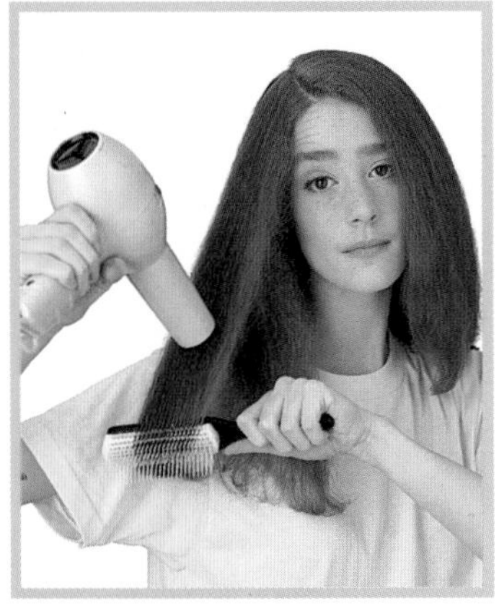

3 *Make a side parting then blow-dry the ends of your hair under. Blow-drying could be enough to straighten your hair, if not, follow steps 4 and 5.*

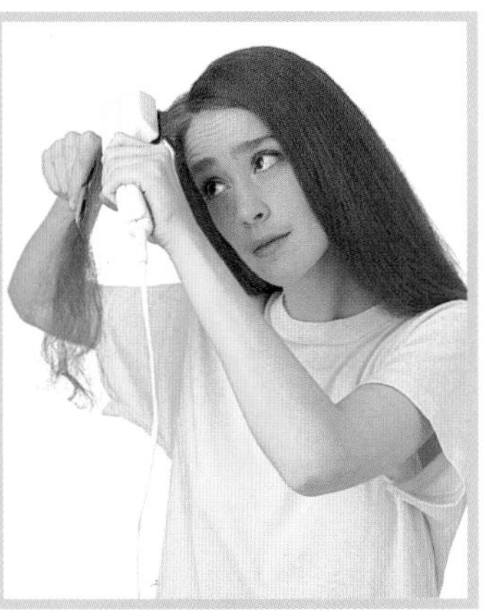

4 *Take 2.5 cm/1 in wide sections of hair and clamp between hot straighteners. Pull the hair through smoothly.*

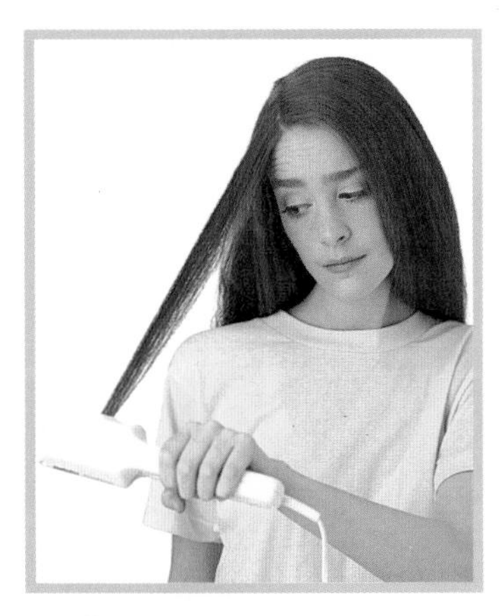

5 *Continue to use the straighteners all over your head, pulling the hair through from the roots to the ends.*

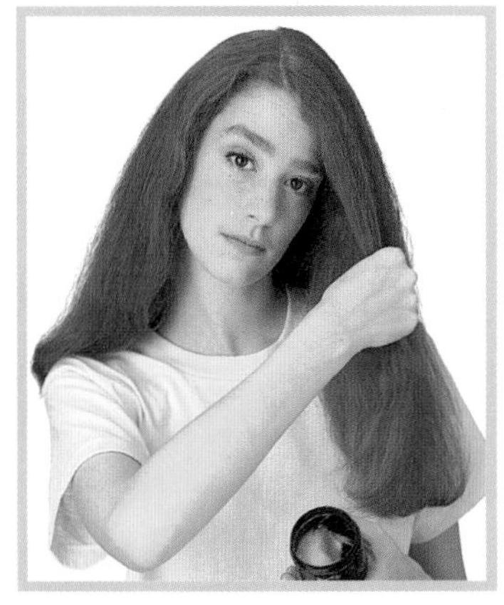

6 *Smooth any flyaway ends by rubbing a thumbnail-sized blob of wax between your fingers then run them over your hair.*

Top: PINEAPPLE

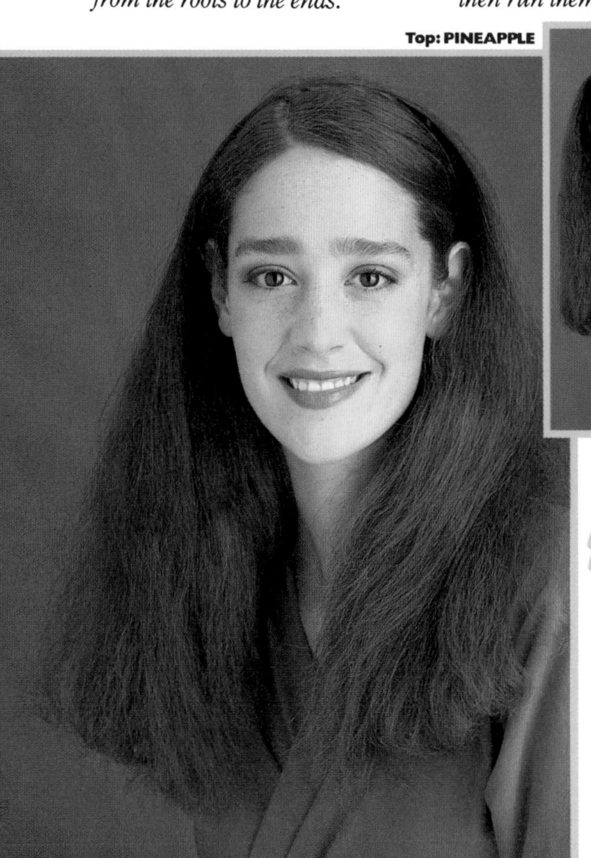

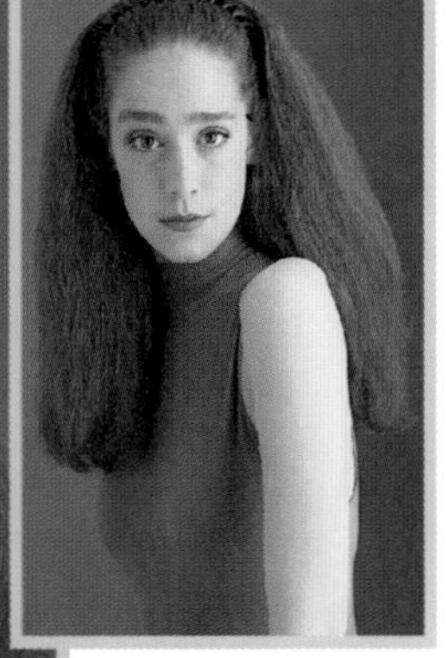

Salon secrets

It's essential to keep a tight, even grip on your hair as you blow-dry, to make it smooth.

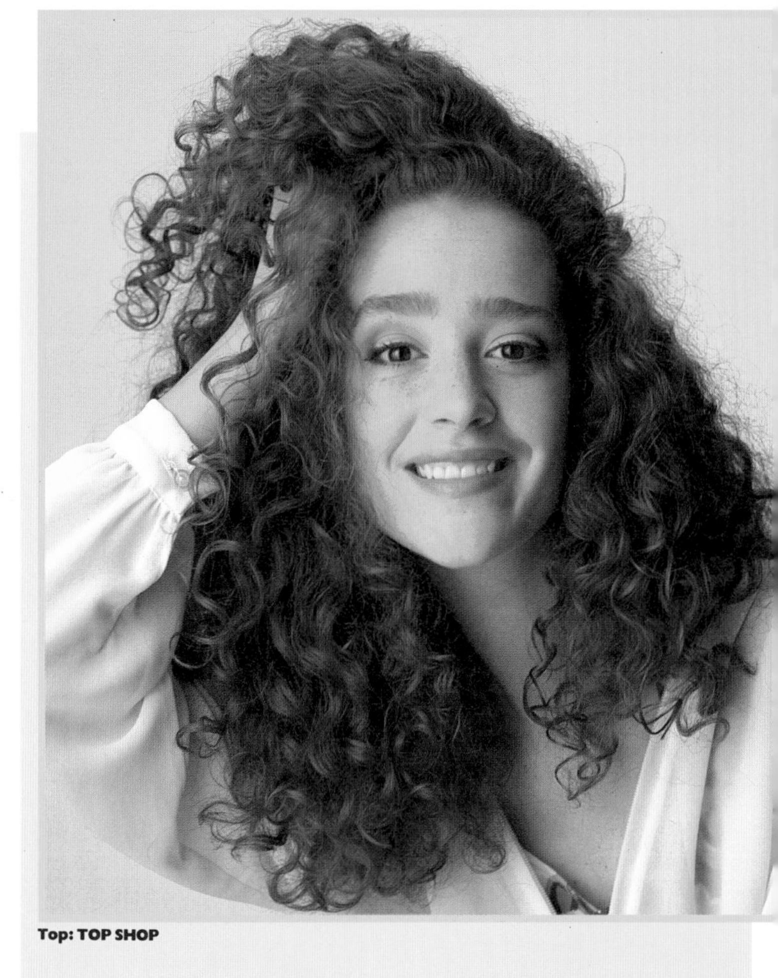

Top: TOP SHOP

NICE 'N' NATURAL

Too much heat can cause your hair to tangle, so leave it to drip dry once in a while.

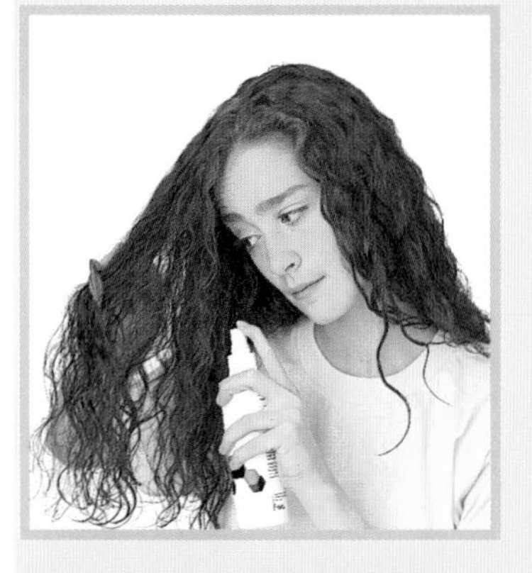

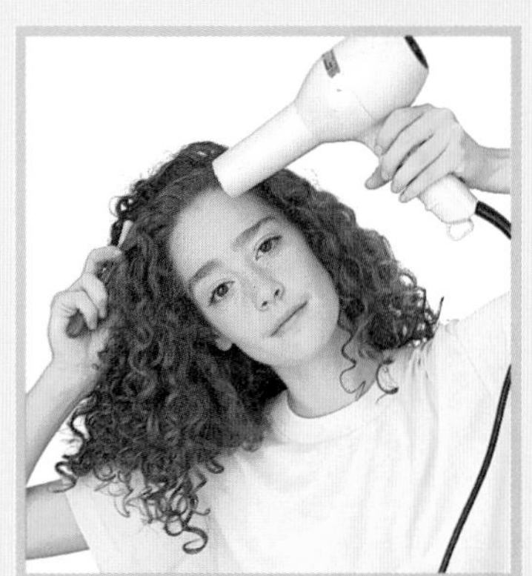

1 **Wash hair with a mild shampoo and spray with a generous amount of styling spray or conditioner – don't rinse it out. Comb the hair from roots to ends.**

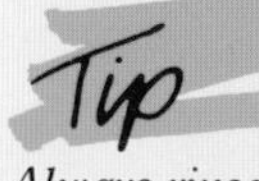

Tip

Always rinse hair thoroughly. Any residue of shampoo will cause curls to flop.

2 **Let your hair dry naturally. Once dry, add height to the front of your hair by smoothing an egg-sized blob of mousse all around the hairline. Lift the front of your hair with a wide-toothed comb then push it slightly forwards. Leaving the comb in position, direct the nozzle of your hairdryer onto it until the hair has set in a wave.**

DRY RUN

Do you want great looking hair without the bother of tugging and teasing it with a brush and comb? Try one, or more, of our four fab methods that let your fingers do the styling!

PALMISTRY

Hands up if you want to add body and bounce? It's easy with palm drying – all you have to do is rub gently . . .

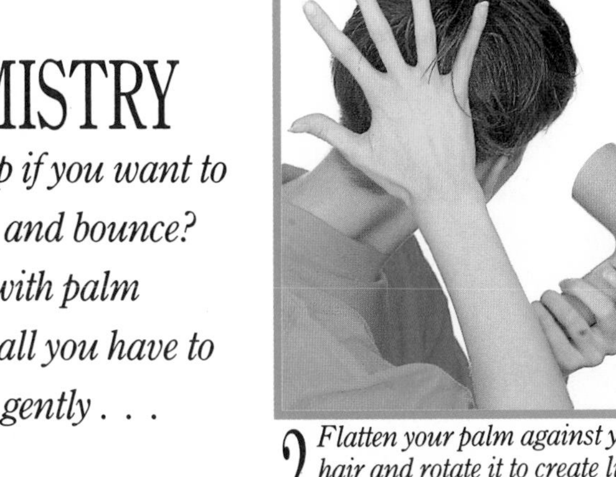

Tip

If you want to create lift as well as volume, use a firm-hold mousse.

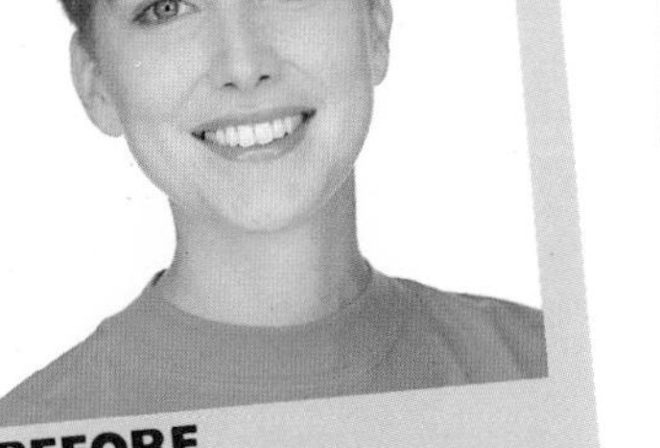

BEFORE
This drying method will give lift to your hair if it's short. But begin by washing, conditioning and towel-drying your hair thoroughly.

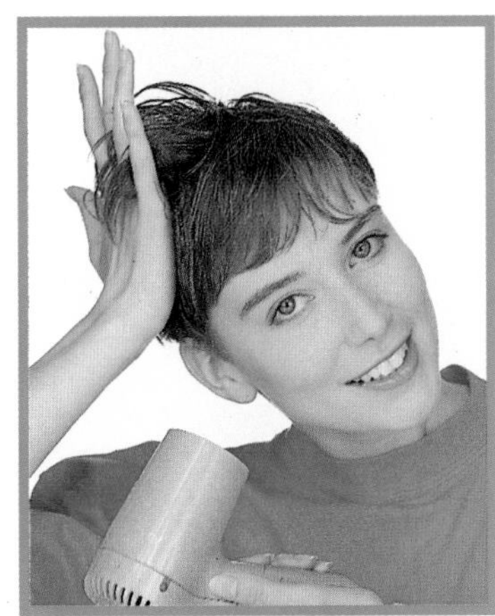

1 *Work an egg-sized blob of mousse through your damp hair from roots to ends and begin blow-drying.*

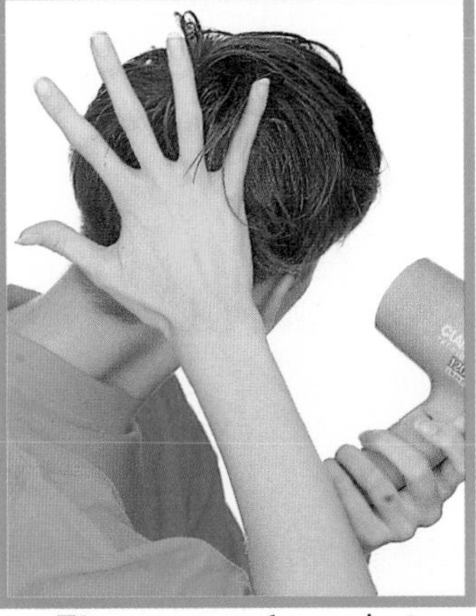

2 *Flatten your palm against your hair and rotate it to create lift, as you blow-dry.*

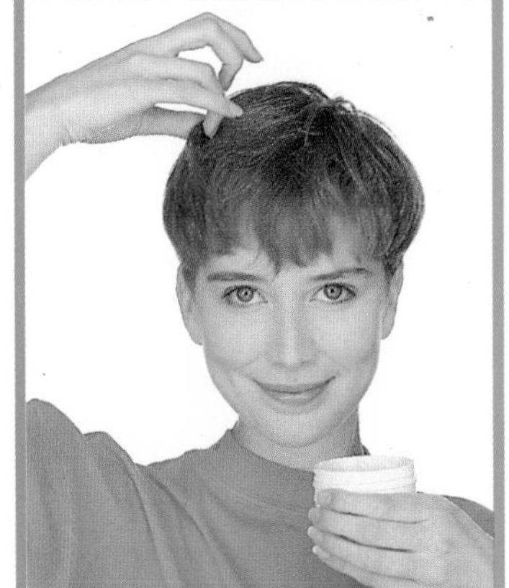

3 *When hair is dry, rub a thumbnail-sized blob of wax between your fingers and tease the top strands for added texture.*

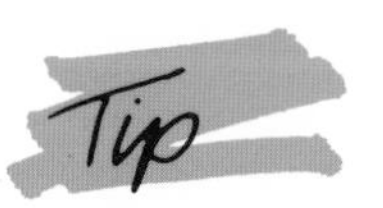

Tip

This technique can work on longer hair too, if you want to add volume and height.

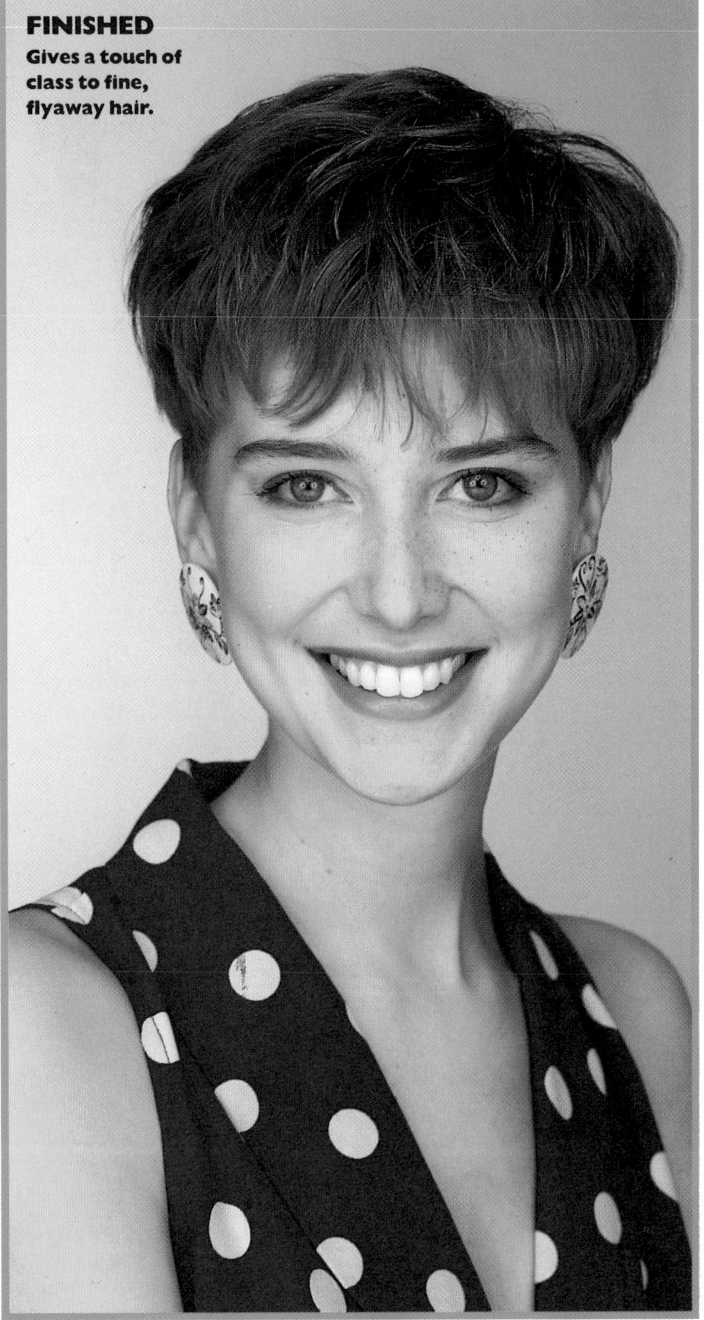

FINISHED
Gives a touch of class to fine, flyaway hair.

Top: ZOO/Earrings: ACCESSORIZE

CIRCULAR DRYING

A speedy method that's guaranteed to add body to shiny, well cut hair. You'll need two clean towels.

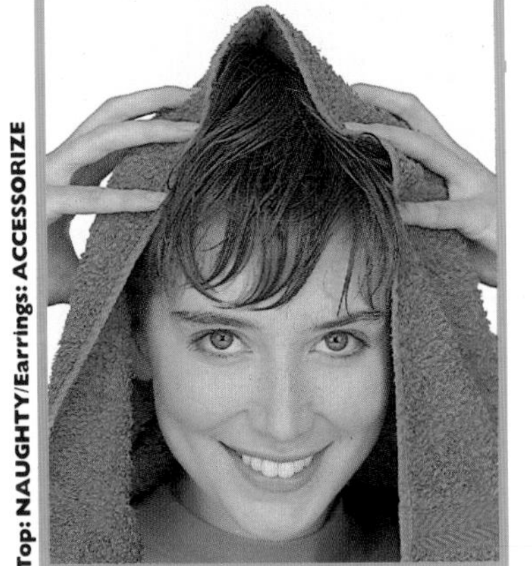

Top: NAUGHTY/Earrings: ACCESSORIZE

1 *First wash your hair then towel-dry gently to remove the excess moisture.*

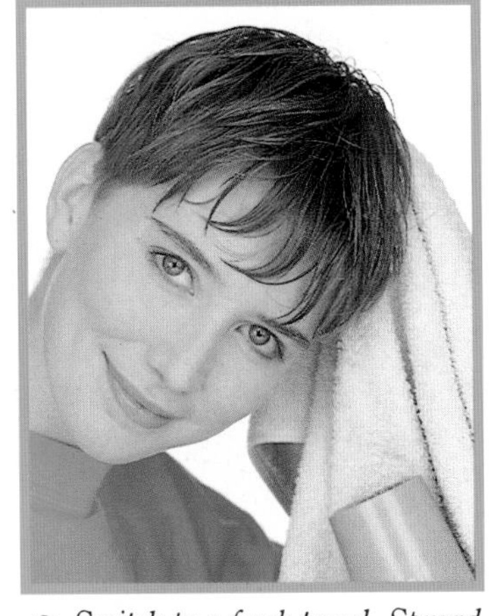

2 *Switch to a fresh towel. Spread it over your flat palm and rub over your head in a circular movement as you blast-dry.*

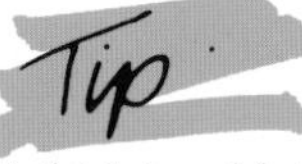

A thick towel helps speed up the drying process. Use different parts of the towel so that it doesn't get too wet and stop working!

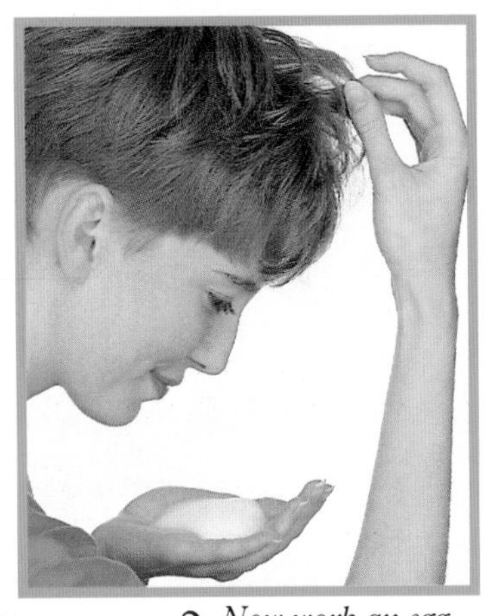

3 *Now work an egg-sized blob of mousse from roots to ends to create extra volume and hold.*

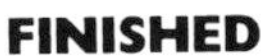

FINISHED

Soft layers give added height and shape.

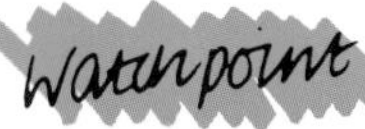

Add the mousse after you have dried your hair so that the towel doesn't absorb it.

HANDY HINTS

- Keep nails short or you could scratch your scalp while finger styling.
- Partially dry longer hair before finger-drying to prevent your hair flopping quickly.
- For extra volume and root lift, tip your head forwards as you style.
- For a tousled look, try finger-drying your hair in all directions.
- Revive lifeless curls by spritzing your hair with water, then scrunch-dry small handfuls to put back the bounce.
- Create instant lift on fine, floppy layers by holding small sections at a 90° angle to your head, then spritzing the roots with firm-hold spray.
- If you are trying to create ringlets; don't worry if they unwind as you dry them – they'll still make waves!
- Don't forget that the warmth from your hands will help to dry short, layered styles.
- Towel-dry your hair thoroughly before rubbing on a setting product, otherwise it'll be diluted and won't hold your style.
- For extra texture on short, layered hair, rub a thumbnail-sized blob of wax over the palms and slowly work it through the layers as you style and dry your hair.
- Use your fingers as a comb and rake them through the finished style to shape it.

DIGITAL DISPLAY

Use your fingers to create volume and curl. It's especially good when you're growing out layers.

FINGER DRYING

Here's how to coax flat, straight hair into a full bouncy look.

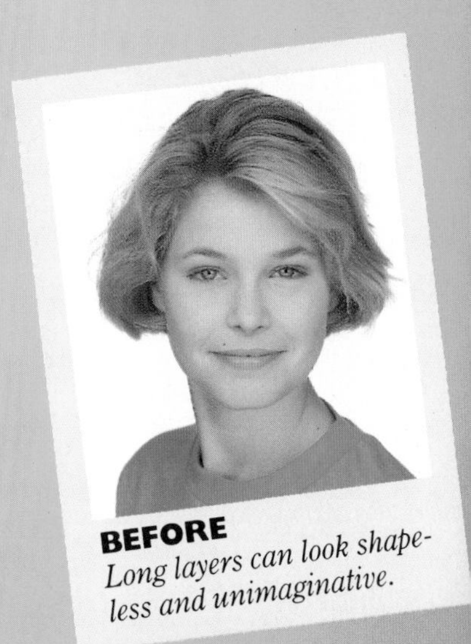

BEFORE

Long layers can look shapeless and unimaginative.

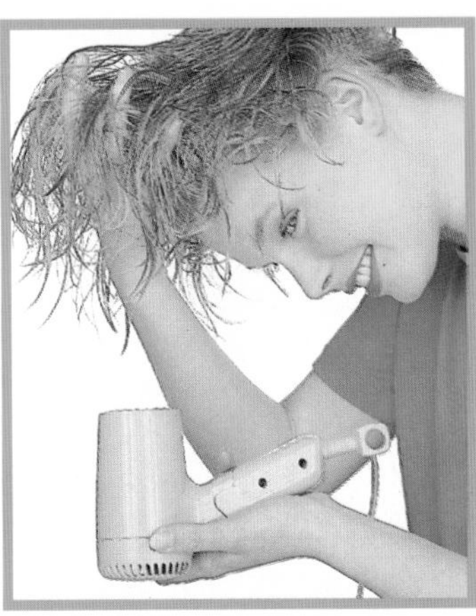

1 *Wash and towel-dry your hair then blast-dry from underneath. Spread your fingers and comb them upwards to create lift.*

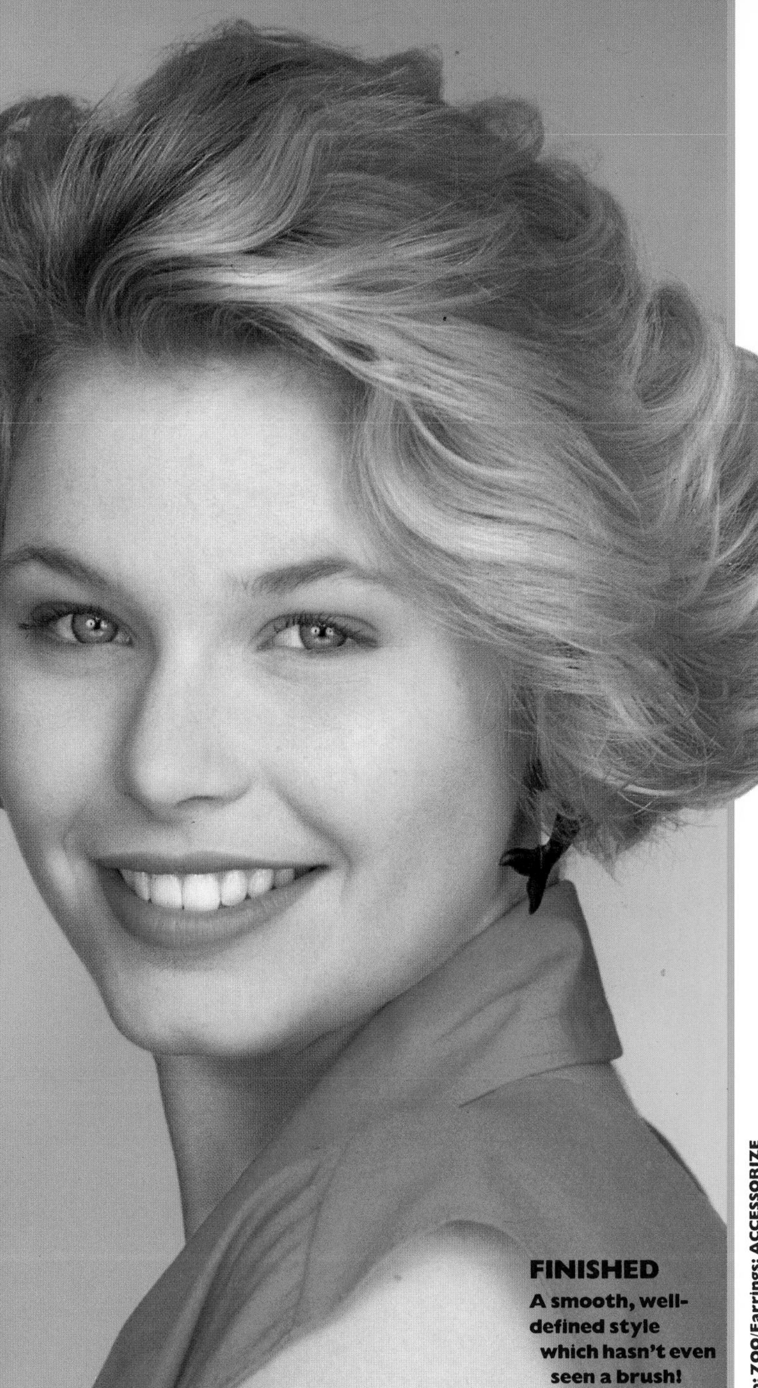

FINISHED
A smooth, well-defined style which hasn't even seen a brush!

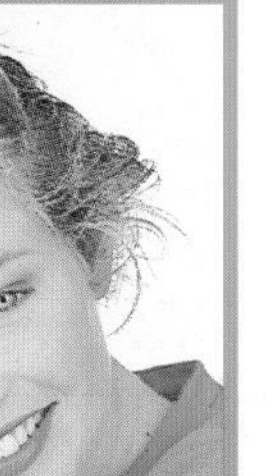

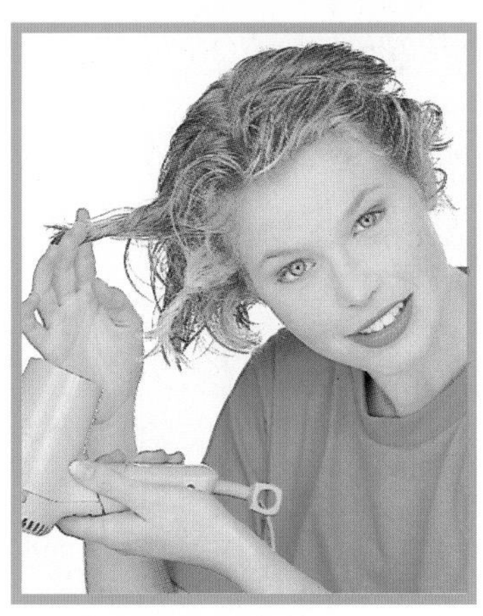

2 *Work an egg-sized blob of mousse through your hair from roots to ends.*

3 *Twist 2.5 cm/1 in sections of your hair then blow-dry each one upwards and back. Then run fingers through to style.*

Top: ZOO/Earrings: ACCESSORIZE

SCRUB DRYING

This is similar to 'scrunching' but you rub your hair very quickly with your palms.

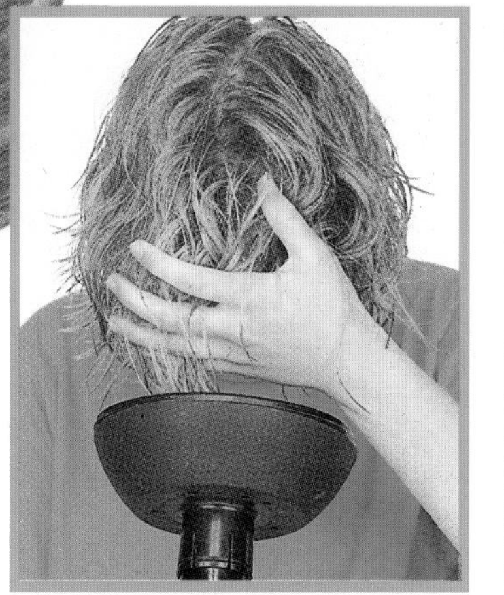

1 *Work an egg-sized blob of mousse into your damp roots. Take handfuls of hair and rub them quickly while blast-drying with a diffuser.*

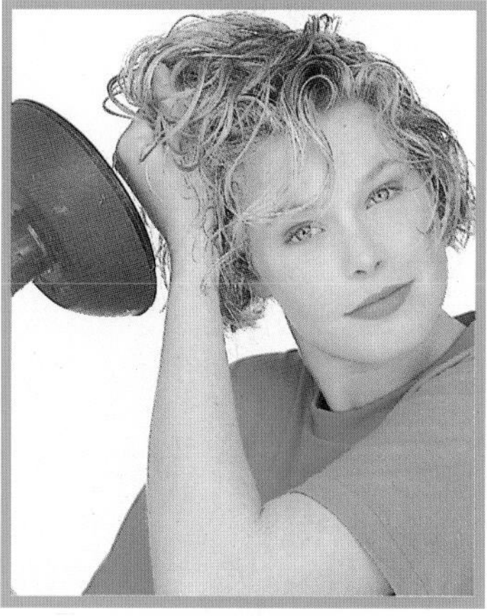

2 *Move at random over your head to ensure that you don't create partings.*

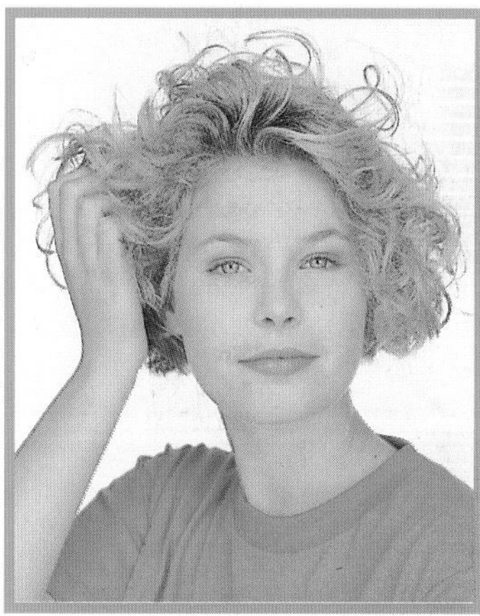

3 *Define the curls by working in a thumbnail-sized blob of wax and scrunching up the ends.*

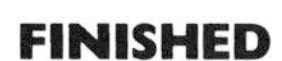

FINISHED
Wear your hair loose and tousled or swept back in a wide band.

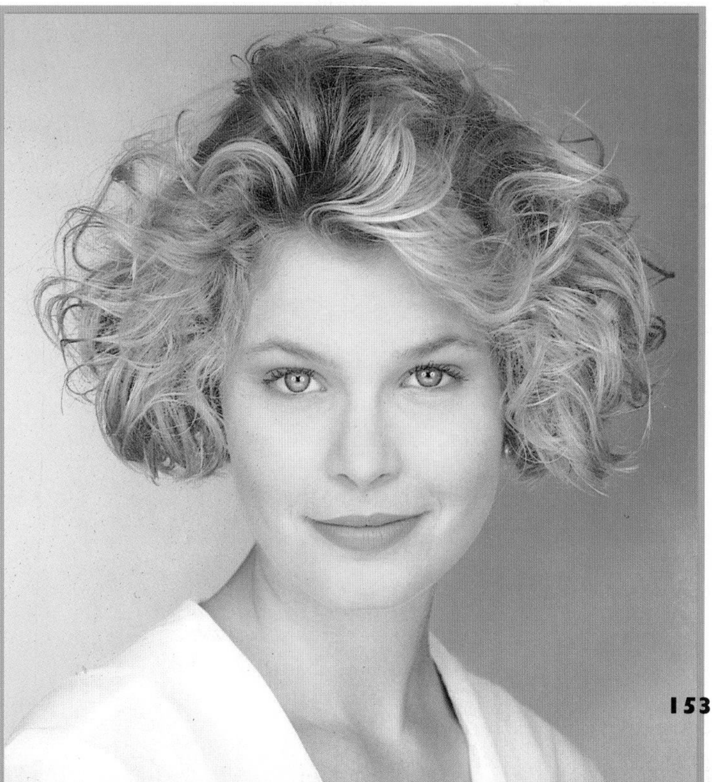

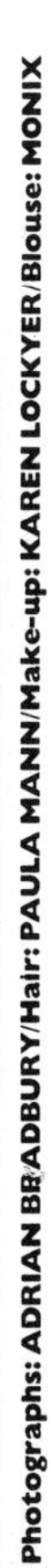

Photographs: ADRIAN BRADBURY/Hair: PAULA MANN/Make-up: KAREN LOCKYER/Blouse: MONIX

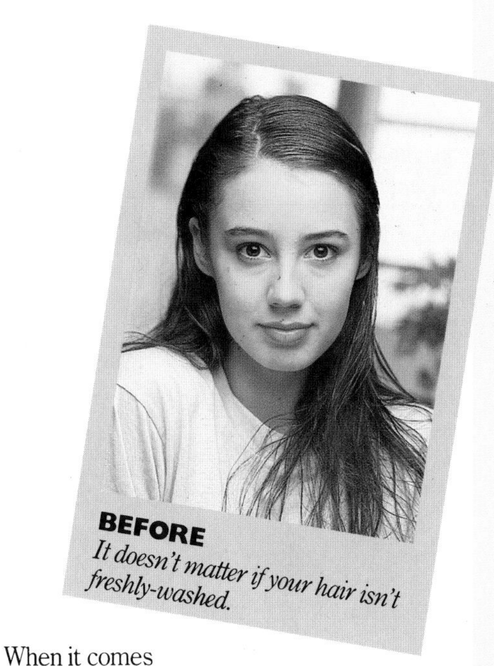

BEFORE
It doesn't matter if your hair isn't freshly-washed.

ON THE DARK SIDE

Browned off with your hair? Don't stay in the shade out-shine everyone by making the most of your dark locks

When it comes to desirable hair colours, being a brunette often comes pretty low down on the list. Everyone wants to be a bubbly blonde or a vivacious red head, and being brown-haired is often considered boring! Funny, when you realise that some of the most celebrated beauties are brunettes!

So, instead of reaching for the bottle of peroxide, make the most of what you've got and bring out the shine and condition – and prove that brown *is* beautiful!

SHINING EXAMPLES

Healthy hair has the best shine of all. This is because the cuticle (outer layer) on strong hair lies flat, creating a surface which readily reflects light. Therefore:

- **Trim ends every six weeks.**
- **If your hair needs a conditioning boost to help bring back the shine, reach for a deep conditioning hair pack.**
- **Always condition the ends of long hair after shampooing.**
- **Natural shine enhancers include beer and vinegar. Make a weak solution of one part vinegar or beer to eight parts water and use it as the final rinse.**
- **Temporary hair colourants can condition your hair as they colour. The shade of your hair will only vary very slightly, for example, adding a more reddish or chocolate tinge but the healthy shine will show.**

COLOUR CAPERS

Dark hair is more difficult to colour to more than a few shades because it doesn't take colour as well as fair hair.

- When using permanent colours, choose carefully from shades ranging from black to deep red, but expect the result to be fairly subtle.
- Highlighting can look artificial on dark-haired people, unless you like the salt and pepper look it creates. Instead, try lowlighting and add some warm reddish tones – it's the best way to brighten dark hair. Very fine lowlights in several subtle shades look great and you won't have to worry about unsightly roots showing. For a special night out, try a bright paint-on colour to contrast with your dark hair. Try mixing hair gel with gold coloured glitter and paint it on to your hair.

GLOSSY TOP

Gel can show off the shine on dark hair as well as emphasising a sculptured style.

1 *Comb a pea-sized blob of gel through the roots of your hair, then spread it over crown.*

Wearing an outfit with a tight neckline? Get dressed before styling your hair to stop the gel from marking your clothes.

2 *Gather hair into a ponytail. Fix with a covered elastic band. Wrap section of hair around band to cover. Pin.*

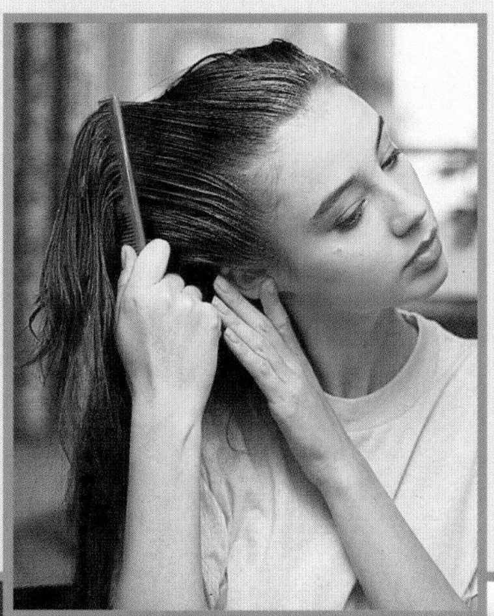

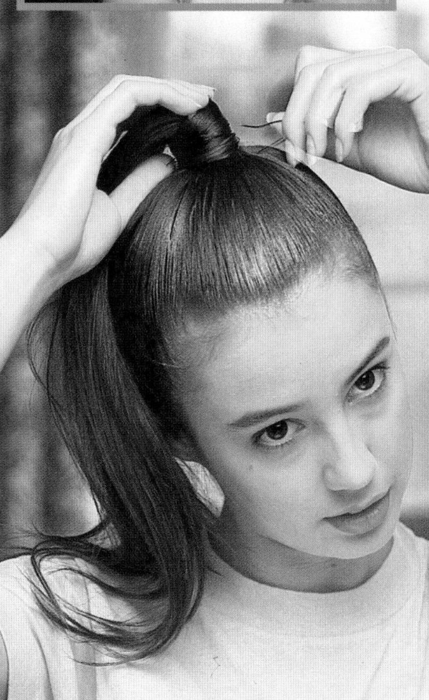

Dress: MARY QUANT

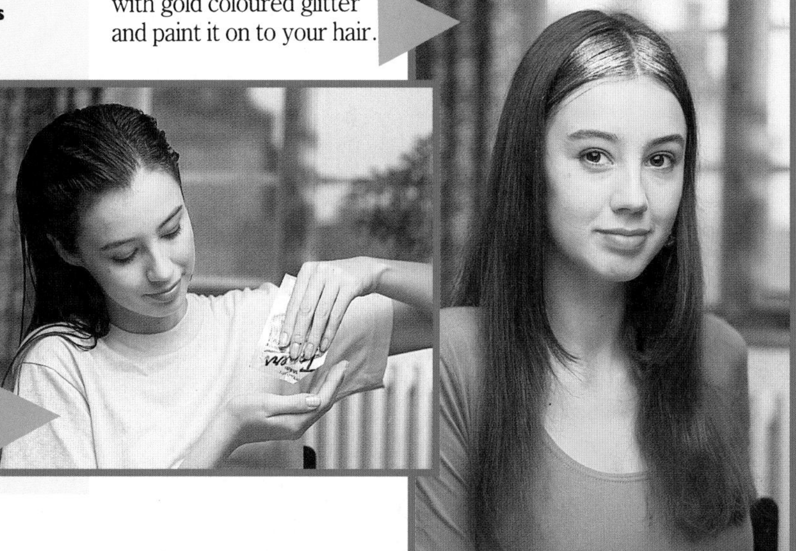

3 *Take a 2.5 cm/1 in section and comb a smidgen of gel along the length. Make a loop with it and pin to the base of the ponytail. Continue until all of the ponytail has been gelled, looped and pinned on top of your head.*

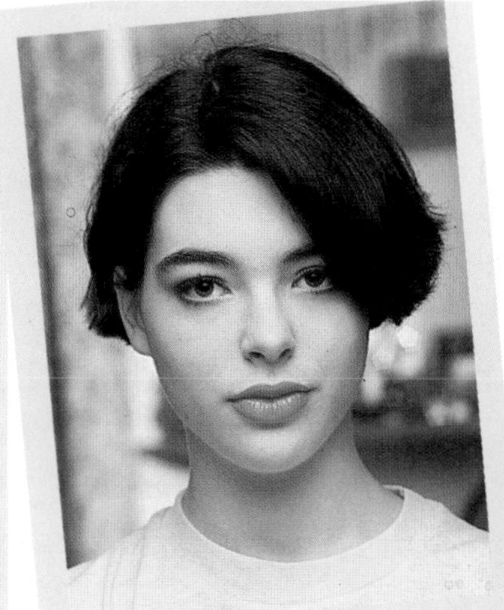

BEFORE
Hair is freshly-washed and then gently towel-dried.

DRYING FOR SHINE

You can improve the shine of dark hair simply by drying it carefully.

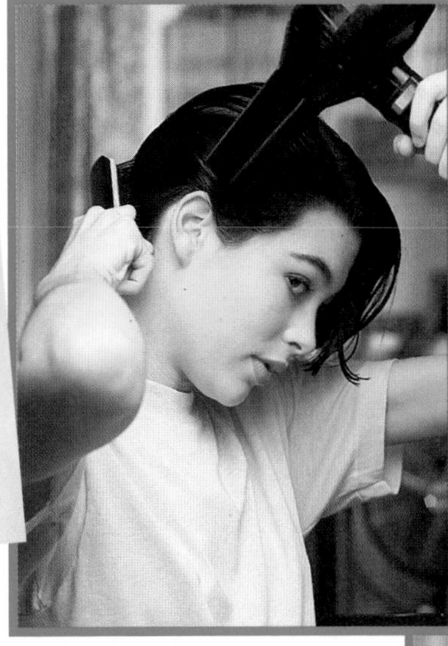

1 *Use a rubber-backed brush to smooth the hair gently but firmly as you dry. Dry the underneath layers first.*

2 *Brush hair down from roots to ends, following with the air jet as you dry the sides. This will flatten the cuticles and create maximum shine.*

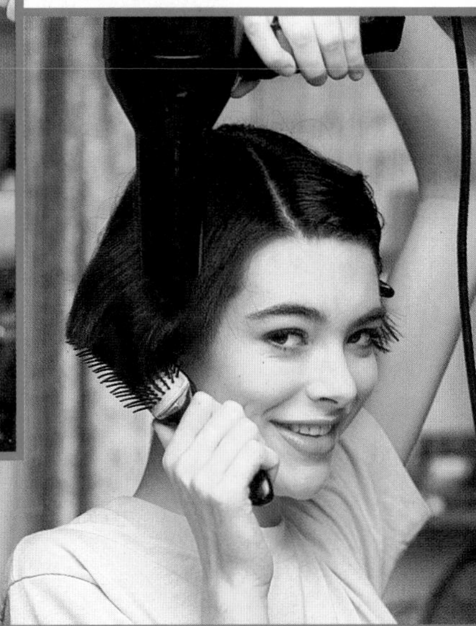

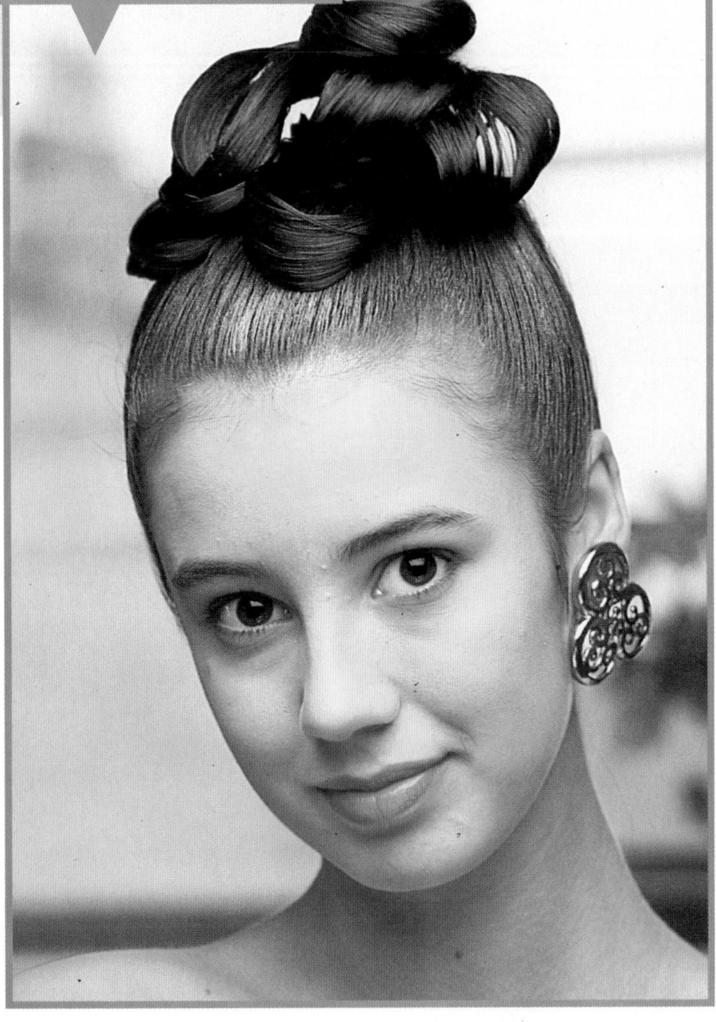

SMOOTH MOVES

Create lift at the front of your hair with a comb for a more sophisticated look.

Wet-look gel can be used on towel-dried or dry hair.

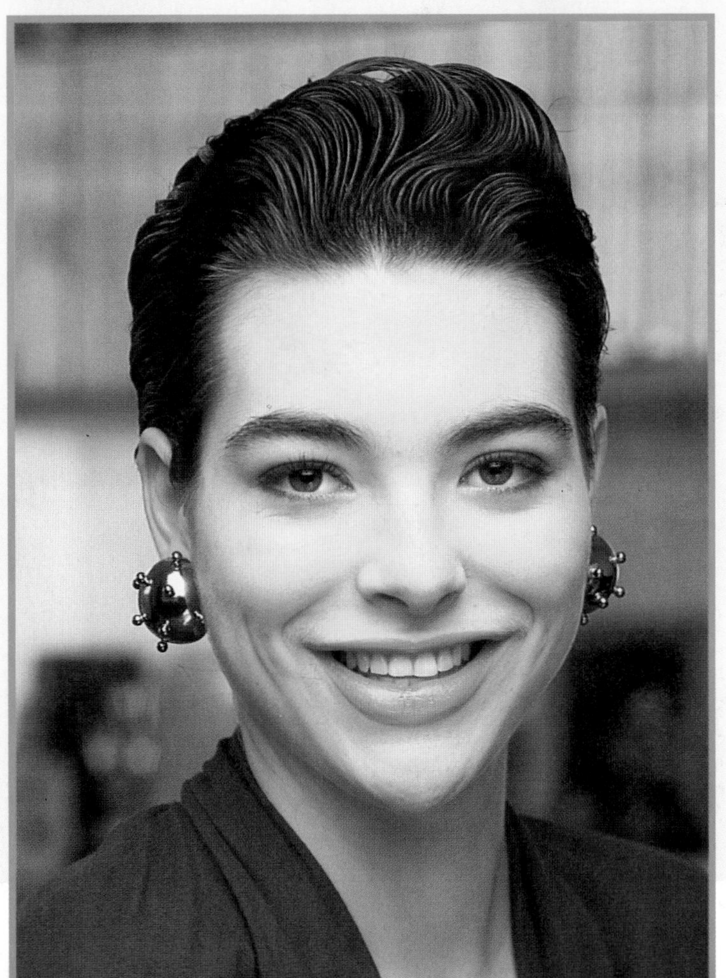

Photographs: PAUL MITCHELL/Hair: PENNY ATTWOOD/Make-up: KARIN DARNELL
Colour: SILVIKRIN Shaders and Toners/Earrings: ACCESSORIZE

Top: HENNES

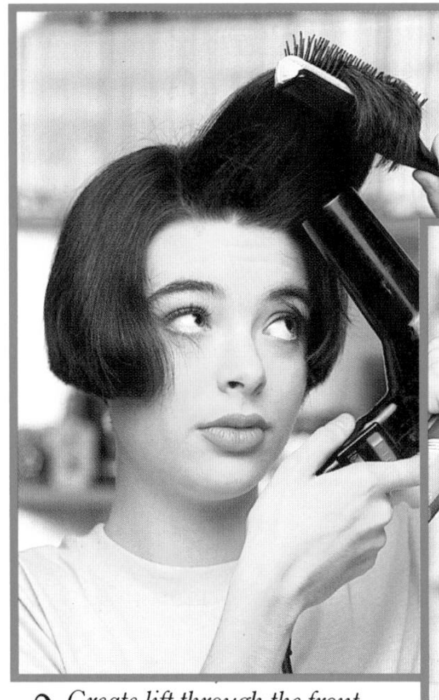

3 *Create lift through the front section by pointing the dryer up into your roots.*

Tip

For a glossy finish, spritz hair with spray-on shine. It produces a mist of oil to make your hair gleam!

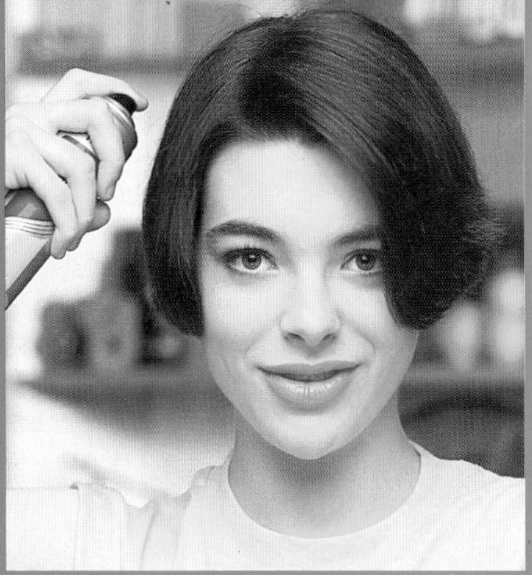

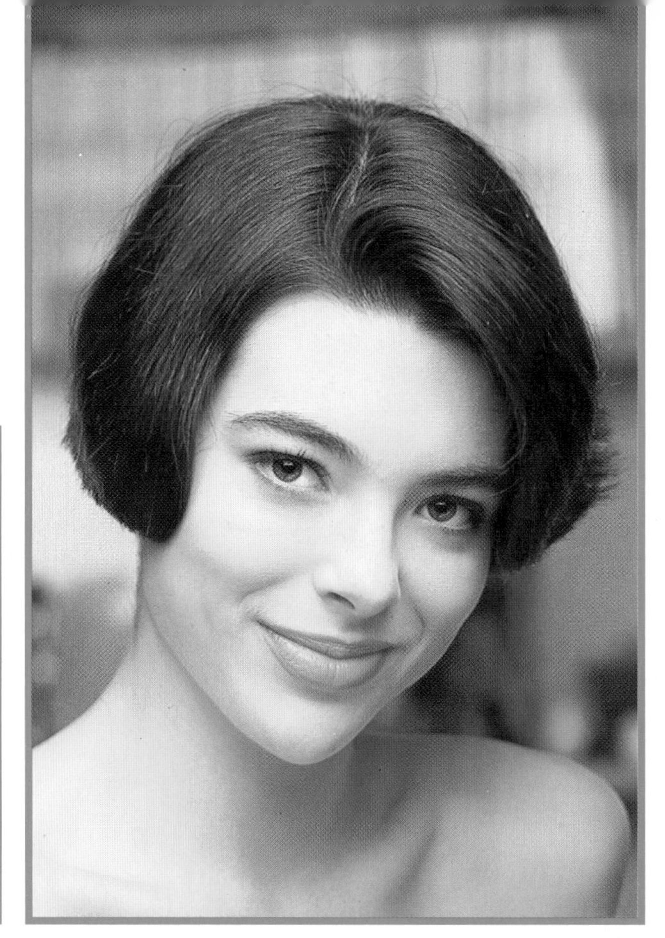

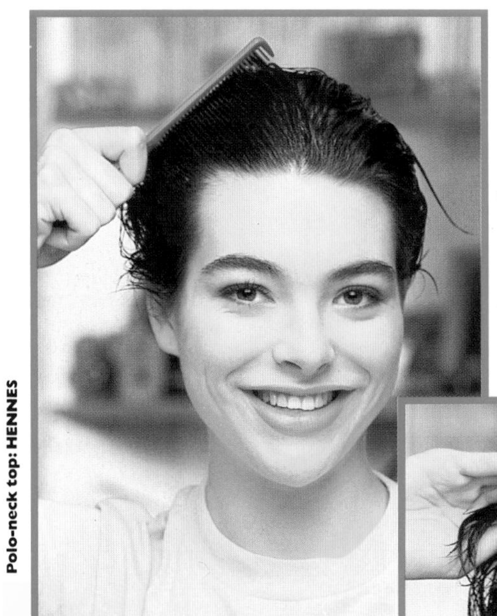

Polo-neck top: HENNES

Tip

Unless you're going to pin up your hair don't use wet-look gel on hair that's longer than shoulder-length! It'll just make your hair look lank and unattractively greasy.

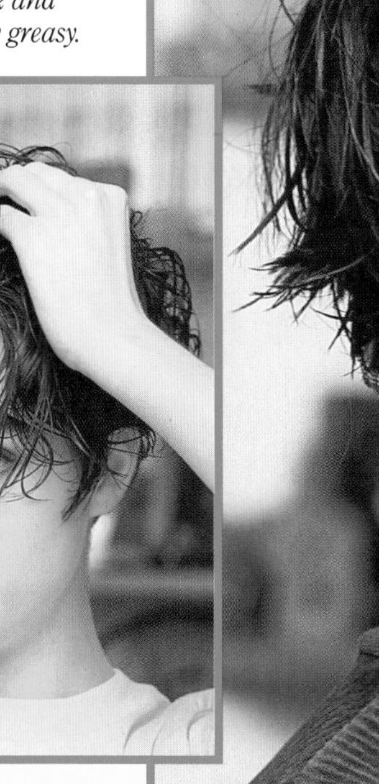

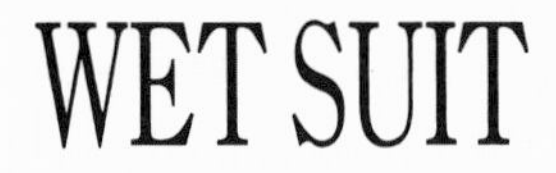

WET SUIT

For really super shiny dark locks, try styling your hair with wet-look gel.

1 *Comb a walnut-sized blob of wet-look gel through your hair so that it is completely coated.*

2 *For a tousled look, run your fingers through the length, then position into place.*

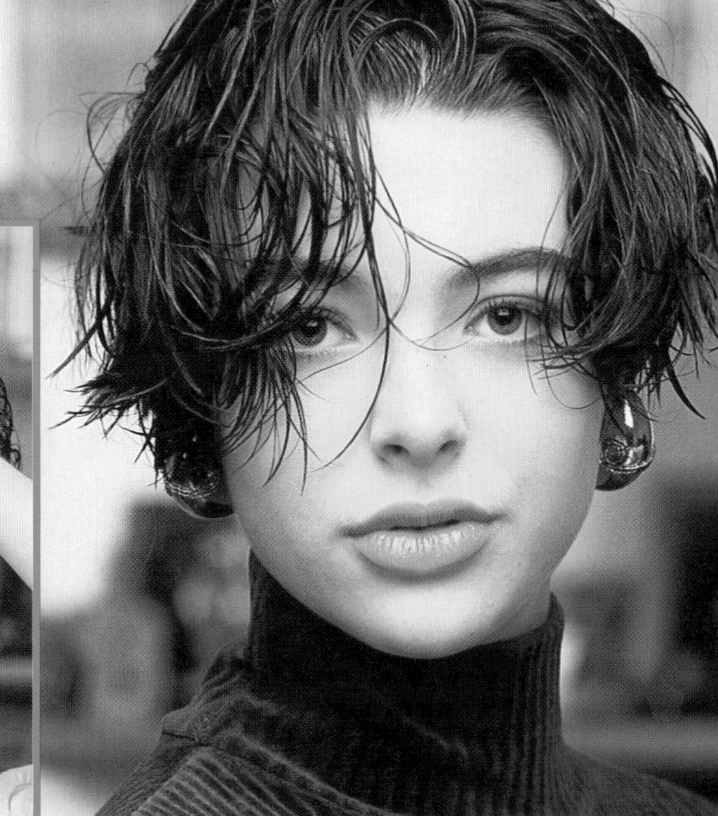

COARSE HAIR

'My hair is really coarse and wiry. It always looks dull and frizzy and it's difficult to style. Please can you help me to get it into shape?'

Coarse hair *does* feel thick and wiry compared with normal or fine hair. (Run a coarse hair between your thumb and forefinger and you'll see what we mean!). And it often looks dull since it produces less natural oil than other hair types. It also has less natural elasticity, making it particularly susceptible to breaking if it isn't handled correctly. However, with plenty of conditioning and careful styling, coarse hair can look absolutely great, (it's naturally thick and generally has plenty of body to hold a style). So get going with our five-step guide and you'll soon be on course for gorgeous-looking hair!

Tip

Leave your hair for 24 hours after washing before attempting a particularly difficult style.

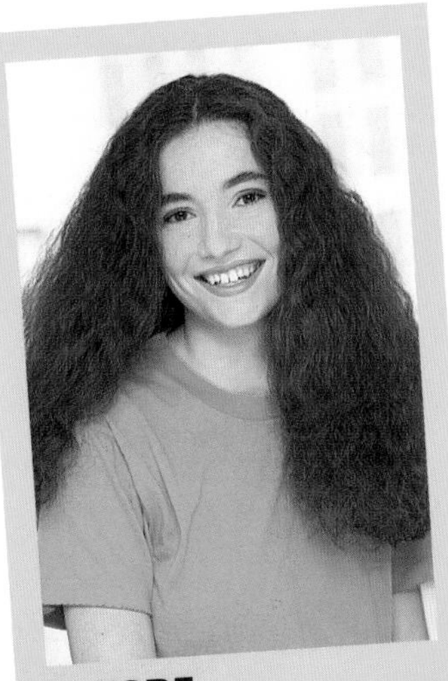

BEFORE
Hair is long and wiry as well as split at the ends.

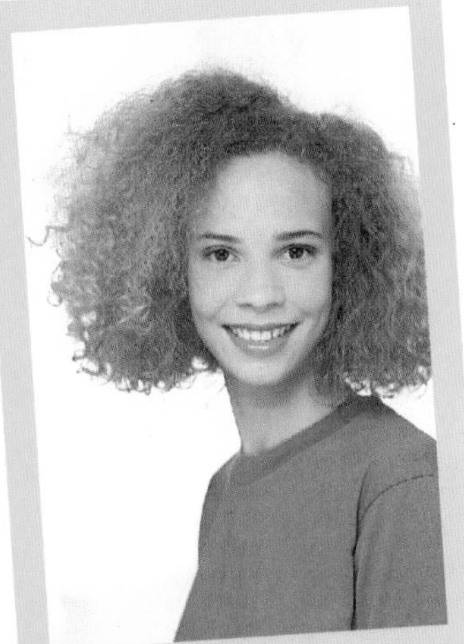

BEFORE
Afro hair tends to be coarse, but it can still look fabulous!

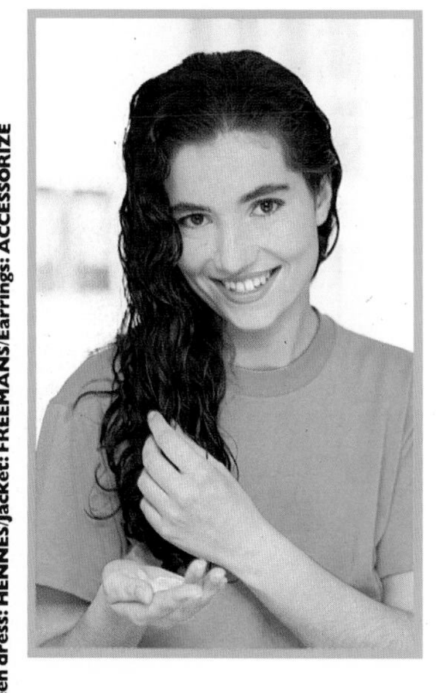

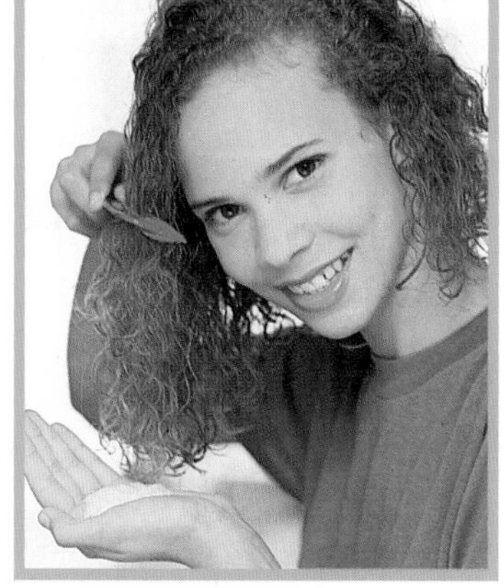

COMB IN CONDITIONER

Coarse hair needs lots of protection to prevent it being damaged. After shampooing apply a no-rinse or very light conditioner to the length of your hair as usual, but don't wash it away. The conditioner will provide a protective layer for your hair.

Don't brush coarse hair as you will make it more frizzy, instead use a wide-toothed comb.

Wet hair is very vulnerable to damage so treat it with extreme care. To remove tangles, work conditioner through the length with your fingers and then very gently follow through with a wide-toothed comb. Start combing your hair in small sections – the ends first, then the middle section and then finally comb the length of the hair, from roots to ends.

SHINE ON

Add a healthy gleam to coarse brown hair with a vinegar rinse. After shampooing, shake vinegar all through your hair, then rinse it away with plenty of warm water. It's an old-fashioned remedy that never fails – the acidity of the vinegar restores the acid balance to your hair after using an alkaline shampoo.

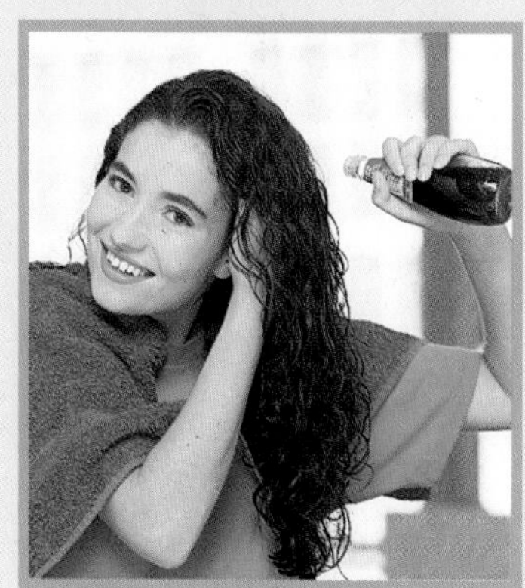

Wax works wonders – adding gloss and protecting your hair. Simply coat your fingertips in wax, then tease the dry curls around your fingers.

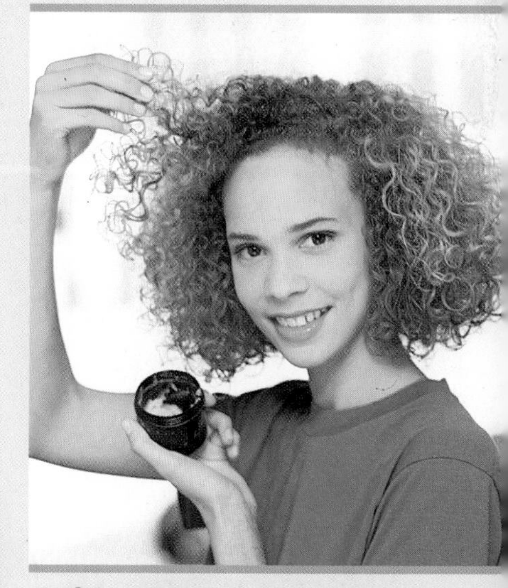

▲ *Other shine enhancers include such deep-action hair 'perks' as raw egg (rinse off with tepid water, not hot, so it doesn't scramble!), spray-on glossers, and conditioning serums.*

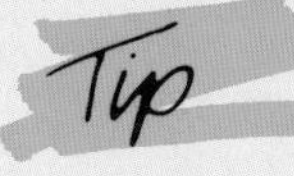

For gentle, soft control, melt the wax in the warmth of your hands before styling.

Print top: FREEMANS/Polo neck: WAREHOUSE/Green dress: HENNES/Jacket: FREEMANS/Earrings: ACCESSORIZE

AT THE CONTROLS

One plus point with coarse hair is that it generally holds a hairstyle well. Heated rollers are good for taming and setting it in the way you want it to fall, although to minimise damage they shouldn't be used too often. If you do need to use styling products for more holding power, try spray gel or a firm-hold hairspray. You can aim these exactly where you want and coat your hair evenly. Use gel on wet or dry hair and hairspray only on dry hair.

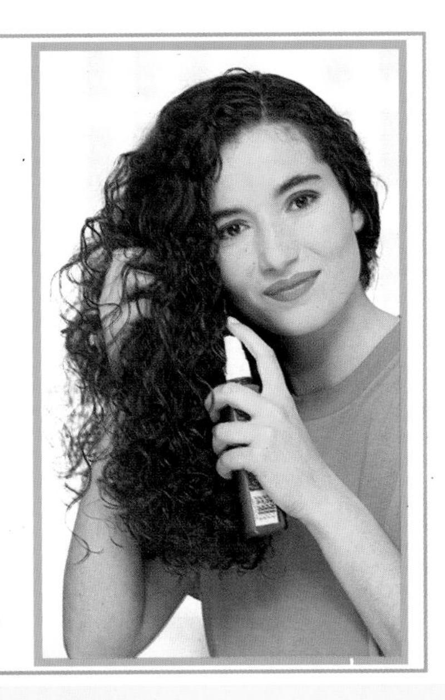

DRY MEASURES

Coarse hair is easily damaged so keep the use of heated appliances to a minimum.

Hair that is allowed to dry naturally lies flatter at the roots than if it is blow-dried, so it looks smoother. To speed up the drying process, towel-dry your hair, squeezing it gently until it is just damp to the touch. Then leave it alone until it is completely dry.

If you want to emphasise the curls in coarse hair and reduce frizziness, use a diffuser dryer on a low heat setting. First, work a large amount of mousse through towel-dried damp hair. Coarse hair is very absorbent so you will need to use plenty – short hair: egg-sized blob; medium hair: orange-sized blob; long hair: grapefruit-sized blob.

Put your hair inside the diffuser and switch your dryer to a cool heat setting. Work all over your hair until it is completely dry. And don't be tempted to turn up the heat to speed up the drying process.

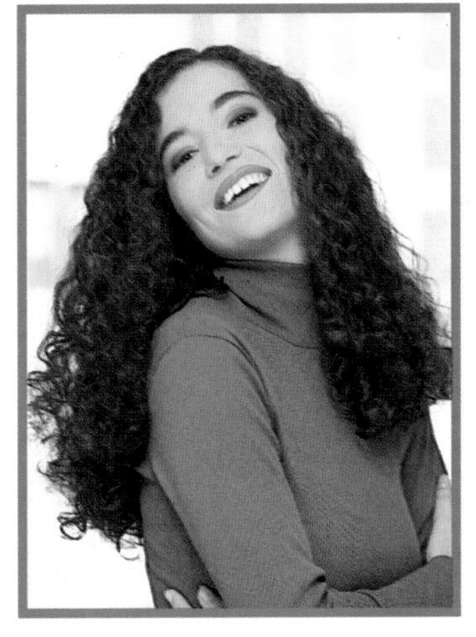

GETTING ON COURSE

- DO use water-soluble styling products, so you can wash them out of your hair.
- DON'T try to brush them out.
- DO choose products for Afro or thick hair, and pick conditioners formulated to untangle your hair.
- DON'T wash your hair every day – it will only make it even more frizzy.
- DO use a diffuser dryer on a cool setting to dry your hair, or allow it to dry naturally.
- DON'T blast-dry your hair.
- DO use a wide-toothed comb – but keep combing to a minimum.
- DON'T back-comb your hair.
- DO leave your hair to dry naturally if you want flatter, smoother-looking hair.
- DON'T sleep on your hair when it is wet – it'll knot and go frizzy.
- DO curl your hair using pincurls and rag rolling.
- DON'T use heated appliances more than once a week.

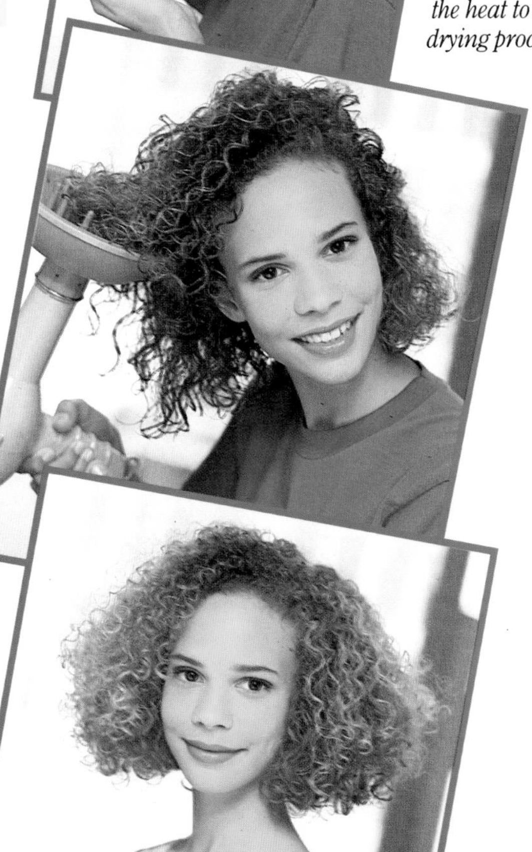

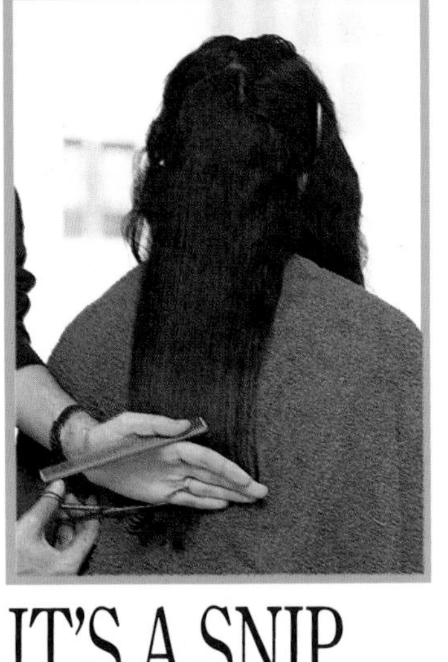

IT'S A SNIP

Damaged ends make hair look frizzy and dull and the only way to be rid of them is with regular trims. Ask your hairdresser to create a blunt cut with a straight edge so your hair has a solid appearance that makes the most of its natural thickness. Avoid long layers as they will only emphasise the volume and unruly look of your hair. Aim to have about 2.5 cm/1 in of hair cut off about every six to eight weeks.

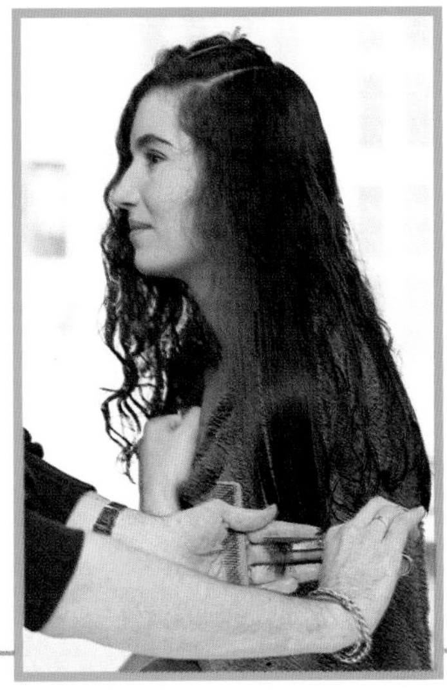

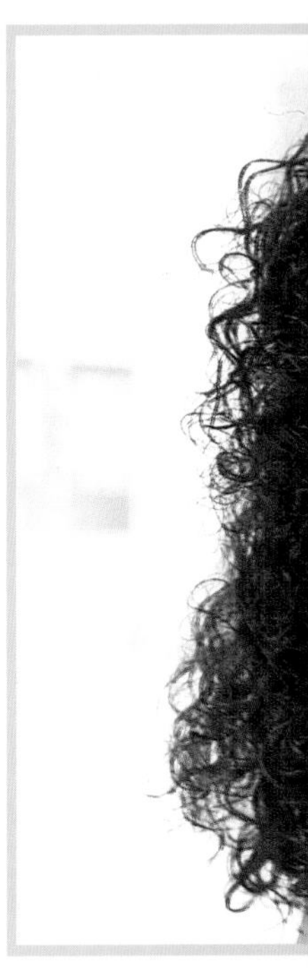

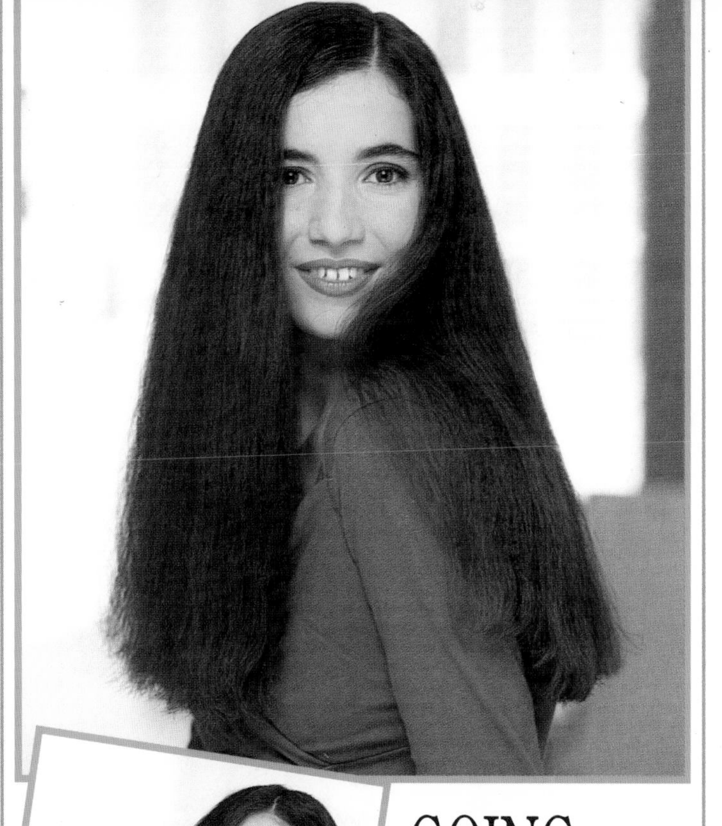

GOING STRAIGHT

▲ *Straight hair looks smoother and finer than curly hair so this style is a good way to hide coarseness. And it's nice to know you can switch to a sleeker look when you feel like it! The secret is straightening irons. Use on dry hair and work on small sections – around 7 cm/3 in wide – to make sure your hair is smooth and even. Slide the iron down each section in one movement to avoid kinks.*

CURL OPTION

Make the most of the body and curl in coarse hair! First, define your curls by spritzing them with wet-look spray gel. Then sweep one side section up and pin it so that the hair cascades down the other side of your head. The combination of natural lift at the roots, volume, and shiny, bouncy curls is sure to turn heads!

Watchpoint

If your hair's very thick, don't attempt to pin it all on top of your head as it may dwarf your face and make you look unbalanced.

AFRO HAIR

This hair type may be coarse, but it's extremely versatile because of its thickness. Learn how to control your curls and then be creative!

PARTY TIME

A style for special evenings out. First use plenty of mousse and diffuser-dry your hair. Smooth it all into a ponytail and fasten on top of your head with a covered elastic band. Rub wax between your palms and spread it onto your fingers, then arrange the curls over to one side. The hair should fall over one eye.

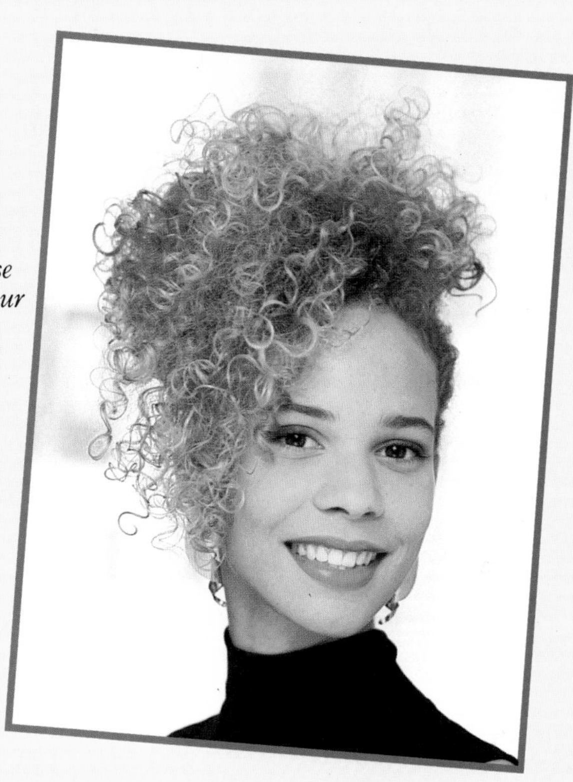

WILD SIDE

It's fashionable to emphasise the movement in Afro hair, so pump up the volume! Massage in an orange-sized blob of mousse and then diffuser-dry hair. Coat your fingers in fridge-cooled wax and tease the curls around your face upwards and outwards. Spritz with hairspray to hold.

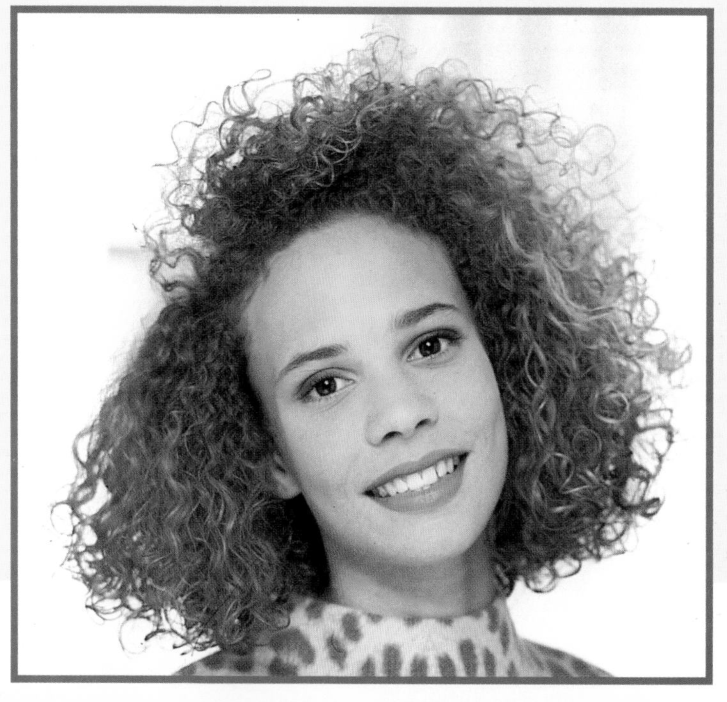

Don't be dull – be at the forefront of fashion with these stunning styles for layered or blunt-cut long hair. Go 4 it!

TIMES THE STYLE

Variety is the spice of life! And when you've got lovely long hair it seems a pity not to make the most of it and experiment. So If you're keen to try different styles without having your hair cut, you can create some stunning looks in a matter of minutes with clever drying and styling using tongs and rollers.

Since long hair is very versatile, why not try a different look to suit every occasion? Plait it and preen it, wear it up, loose or curly, and get a long way ahead with our great looks from one cut. We're sure you'll be longing to try them!

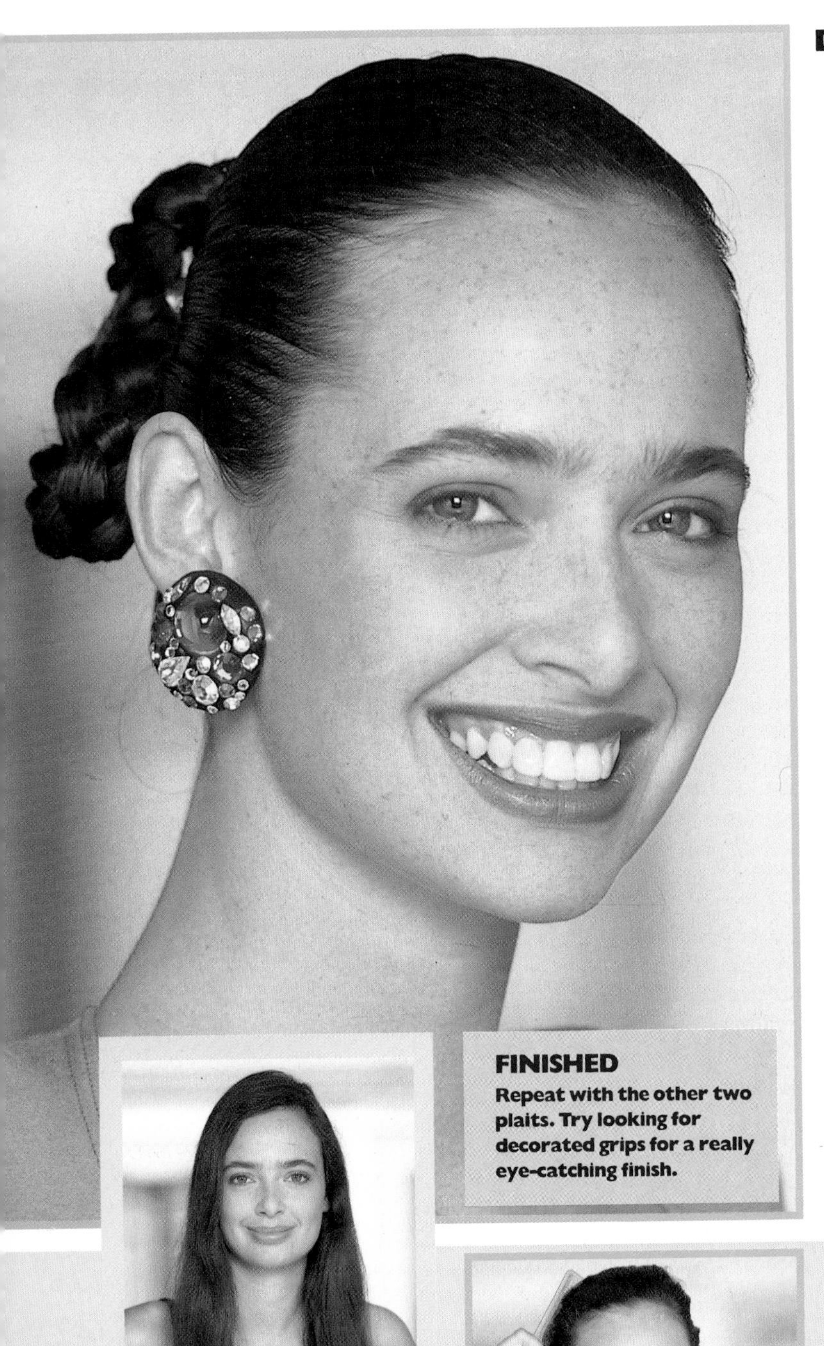

FINISHED
Repeat with the other two plaits. Try looking for decorated grips for a really eye-catching finish.

BRAID WINNER

For evening elegance, opt for a twisted topknot

BEFORE
Hair should be clean and completely dry.

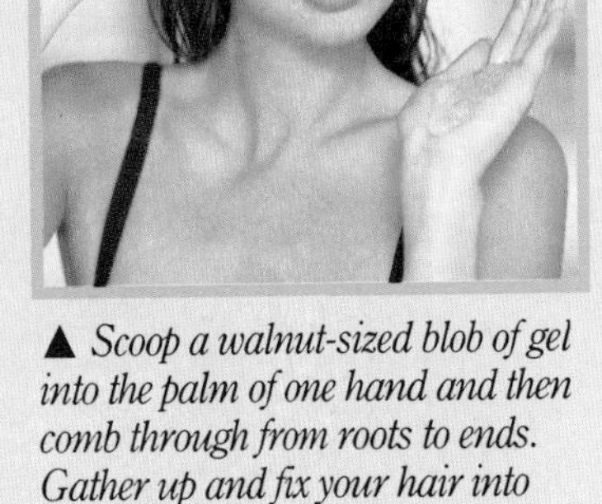

▲ *Scoop a walnut-sized blob of gel into the palm of one hand and then comb through from roots to ends. Gather up and fix your hair into a ponytail, then divide it into three sections.* ▶

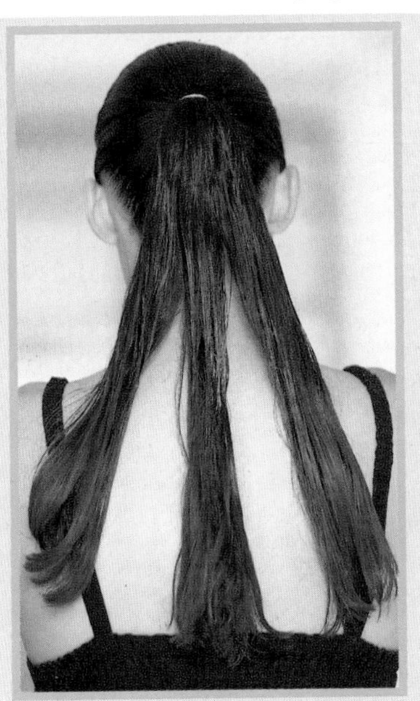

▼ *Plait each section. Fix ends with a covered elastic band then wind metallic thread round. Take one plait and wind around the base of the ponytail. Pin with hair grips.*

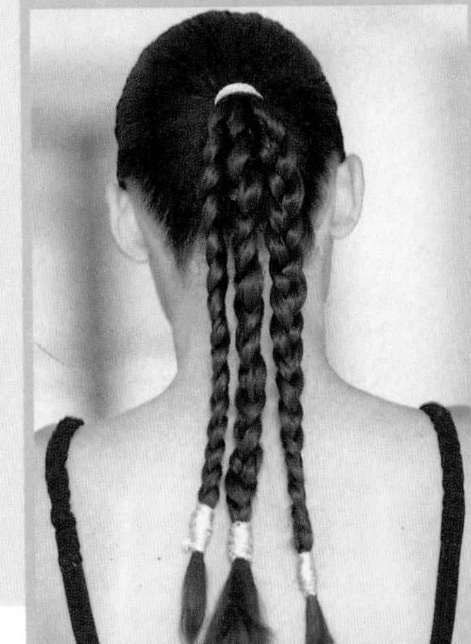

PARTY CURL **Curl up and be the mane attraction!**

▲ *Plug in your bendy rollers to heat them up. Rough-dry your hair, combing the layers with your fingers.*

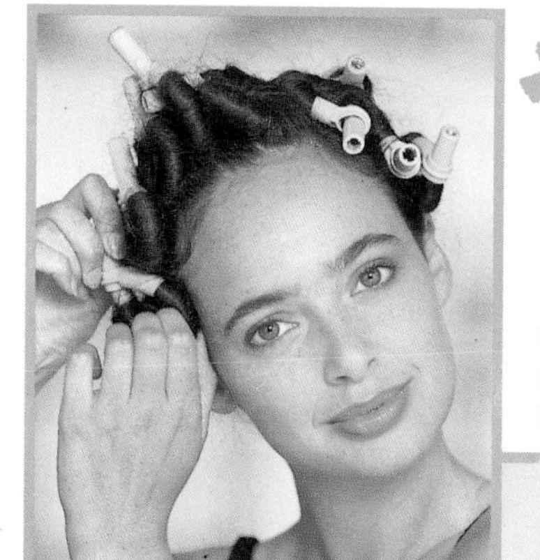

▲ *Starting at the front, take small sections of hair and wind each one evenly along the rollers.*

Tip

Time on your hands? Use cold bendies and wind them up into damp hair, then leave in overnight.

▼ *Unwind the rollers when they're cold. Then rub a thumbnail-sized blob of wax through the curls to give them a sheen.*

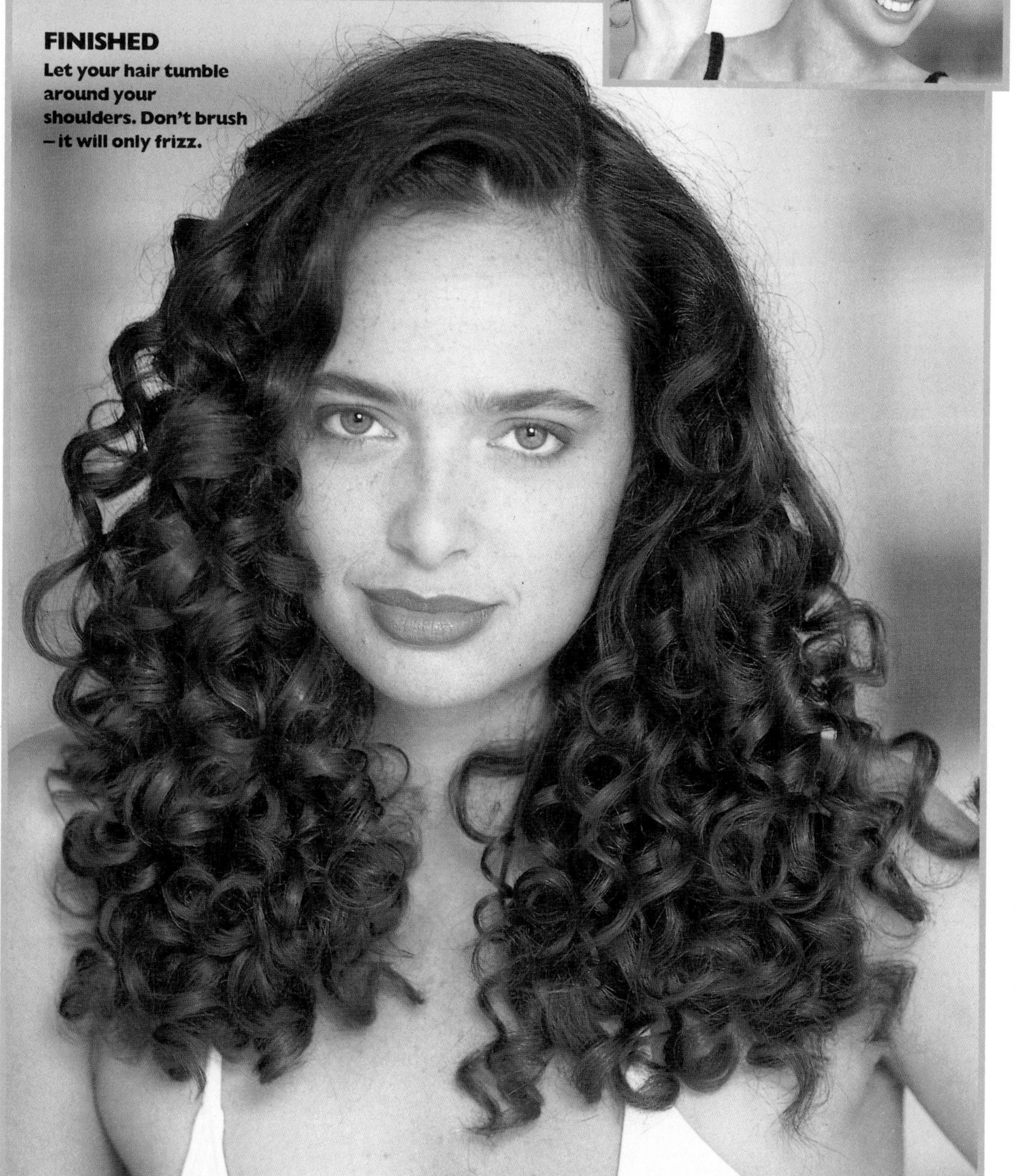

FINISHED
Let your hair tumble around your shoulders. Don't brush – it will only frizz.

MAKE WAVES

A casual look with body

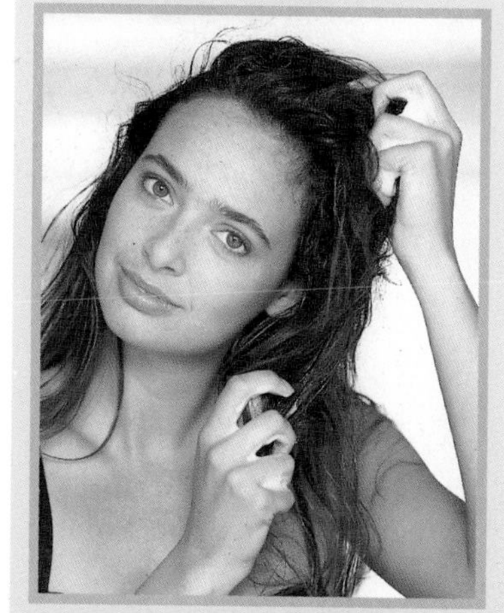

▲ *Plug in your heated rollers. Squirt a grapefruit-sized blob of mousse on to your palms and smooth it through the length of your hair from roots to ends.*

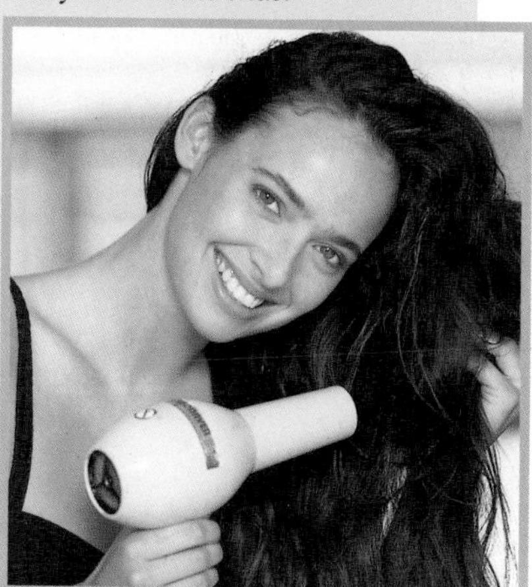

▲ *Roughly blow-dry your hair. When it's dry, wind it up on large heated rollers to create soft, bouncy waves. Wind the rollers away from your hairline.*

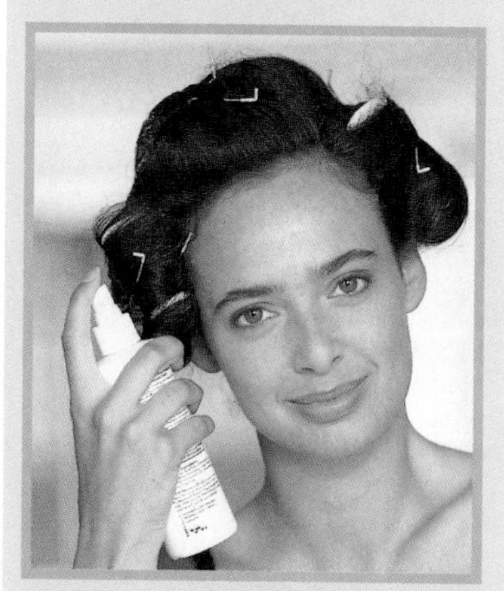

▲ *When you've wound them all up, spritz your hair lightly with hairspray. As soon as the rollers are cool remove them, starting with the roller that you put in first.*

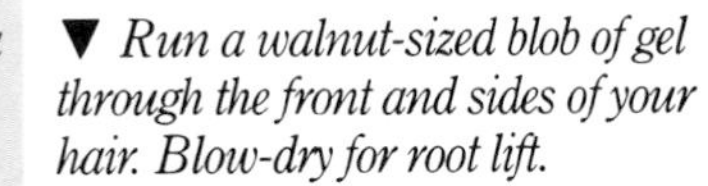

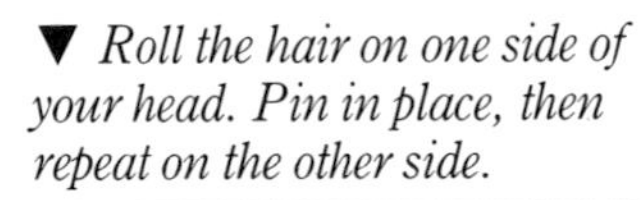

▼ *Brush your hair through using a flat-backed brush to soften and separate the curls. Spritz with spray.*

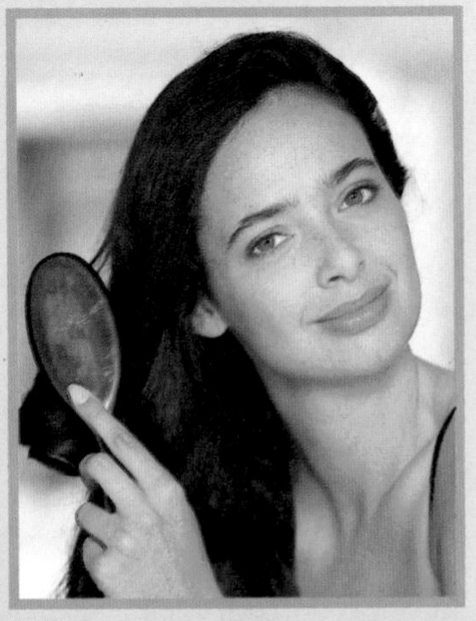

▼ *Run a walnut-sized blob of gel through the front and sides of your hair. Blow-dry for root lift.*

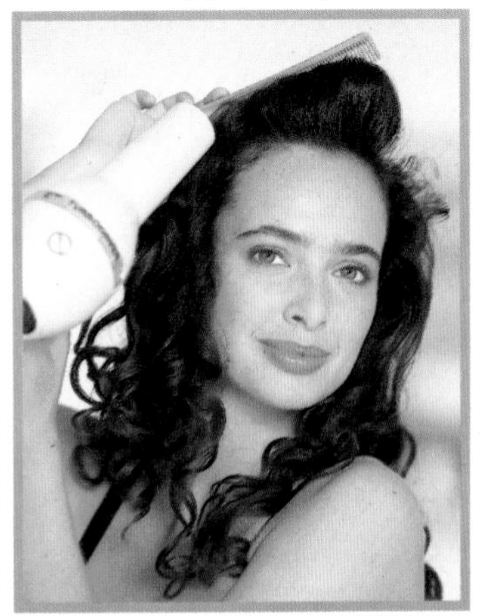

▼ *Roll the hair on one side of your head. Pin in place, then repeat on the other side.*

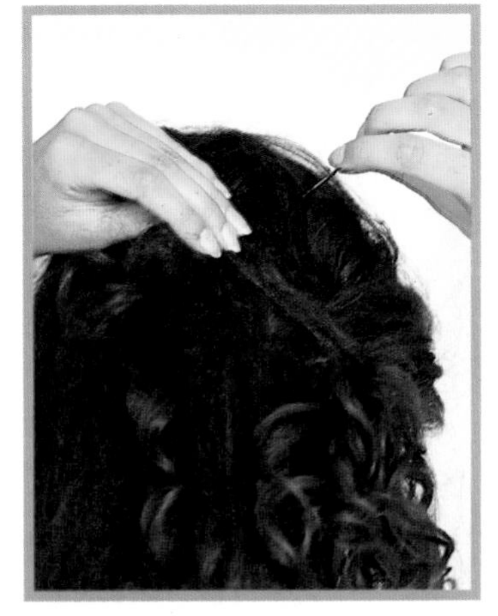

▼ *Push two combs into your hair to hide the hairpins. They will hold the style in place.*

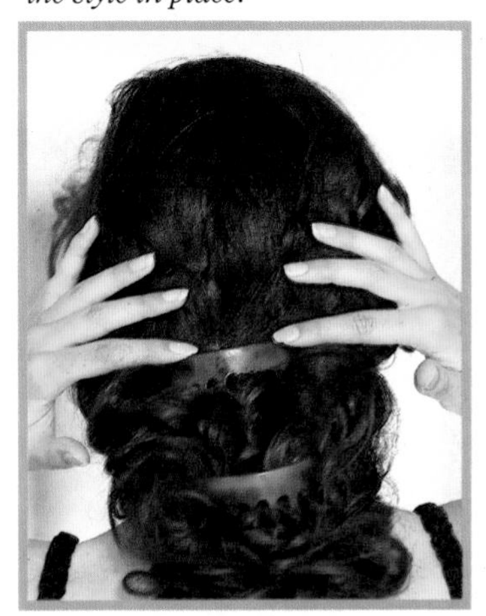

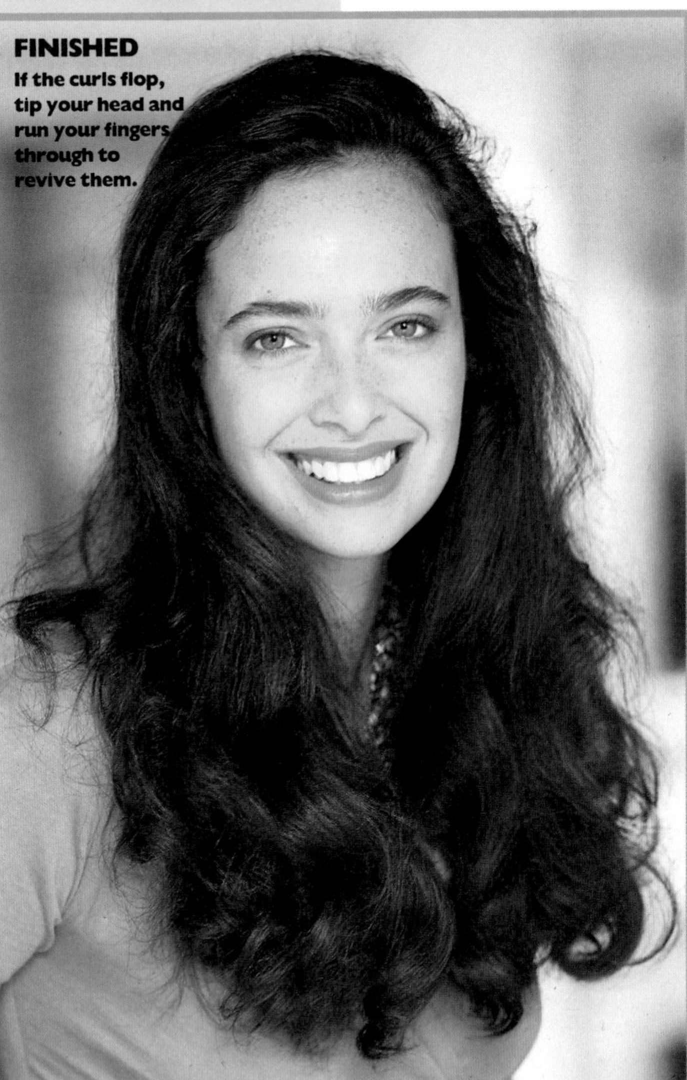

FINISHED

If the curls flop, tip your head and run your fingers through to revive them.

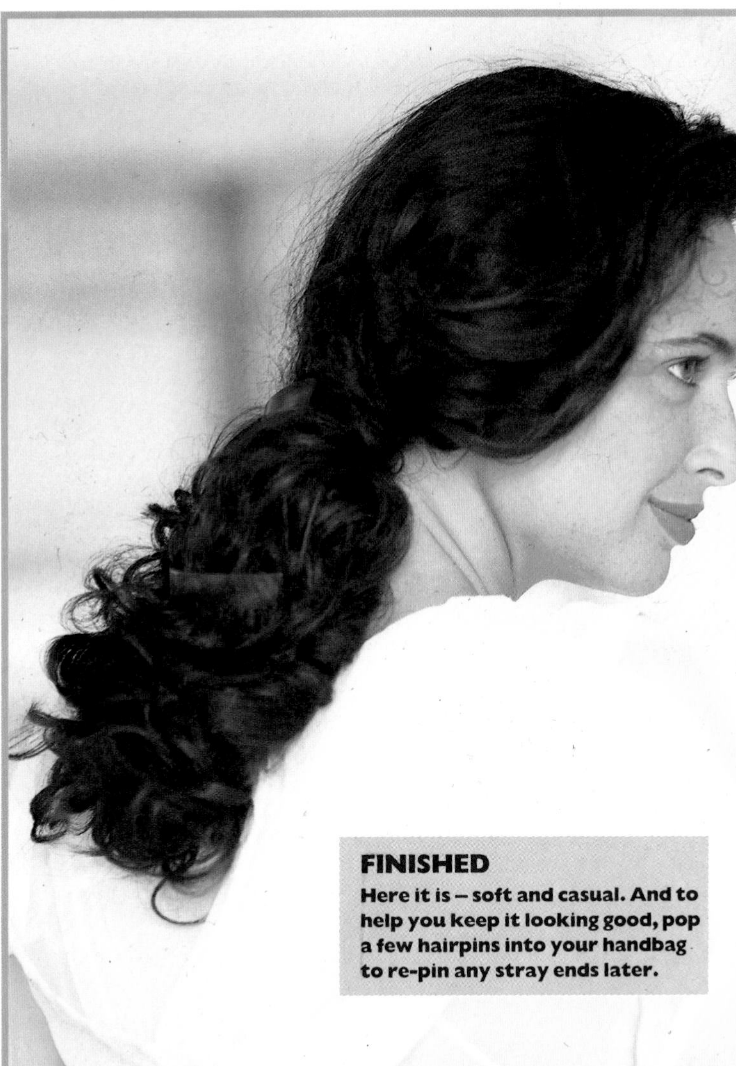

FINISHED

Here it is – soft and casual. And to help you keep it looking good, pop a few hairpins into your handbag to re-pin any stray ends later.

ALL CHANGE!

Get all tressed up with a quick and easy style switch:

- **CHIGNON: Brush your hair back, then pin some hair grips in a criss-cross pattern from just left of the centre back. Start at the nape and work towards the crown. Roll the remaining length of hair back on itself so that it covers the grips. Next, push in some hairpins along the length of the roll to fix it tightly to your head.**
- **PLAIT TAILS: Divide your hair into three and French plait it until you reach the nape. Fix the plait with a covered elastic band or scrunchie, leaving the remaining hair loose. Or plait along the length and then fix.**
- **TOP TRICKS: Gather hair into a high ponytail and hold it with a covered elastic band. Twist the length around its base to make a bun and fix it with pins.**
- **Or separate the length of hair into three and plait each one. Hold them all together with a covered elastic band and a really brightly coloured scrunchie.**
- **Divide the ponytail into six and roll each one around your index finger to make a loop. Pin to your head with grips.**

Photographs: NICK COLE/Hair: JUSTIN/Make-up: JO McKENNA/Lavender top: PINEAPPLE/Lilac top: TOP SHOP/White top: PINEAPPLE/Black top: WAREHOUSE/White blouse: PINEAPPLE/Jewellery: BOND

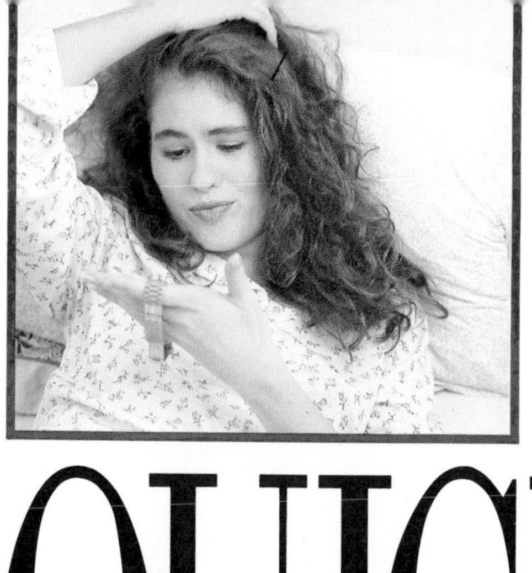

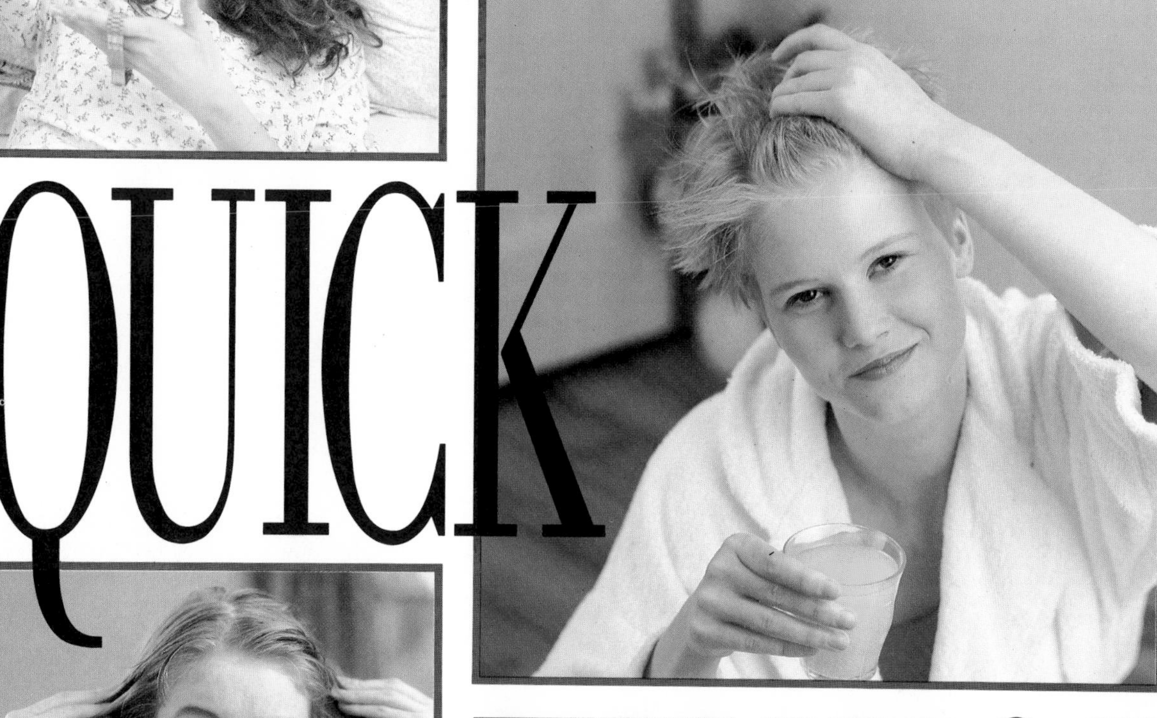

QUICK FIXES

Don't panic if you wake up late and your hair's flat and dull. Try one of our revivers to put life back into your locks no matter what length they are. Adapt them to suit your hair when you need to look great – fast!

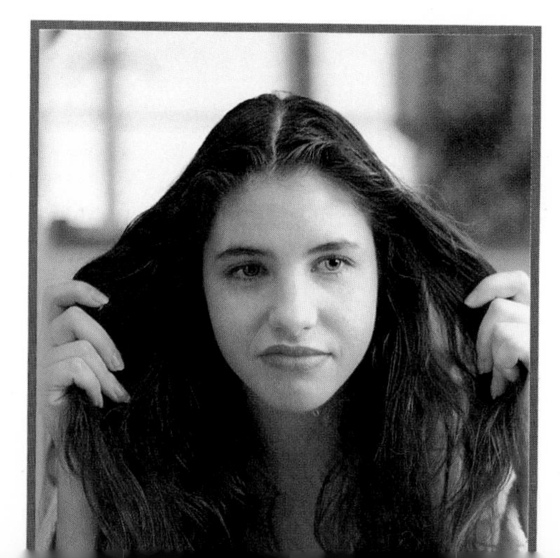

No matter how cleverly your hair is cut or permed it's sure to need fixing at some time during the day to keep it looking its best. Now it's no problem, even if your styling kit is at home and you're at work as there are simple steps you can take to revive those flagging locks. The trick with quick fixes is to keep your hair style as simple and as fuss-free as you possibly can.

Then there are those odd occasions when you're in a hurry and haven't had time to wash your hair or you have to go to a glamorous function when you're feeling and looking a lot less than lovely. But all it takes is a few spare minutes and just a little know-how and you can be transformed from a greaseball to the belle of the ball!

QUICK TIPS

- Make sure combs and brushes are clean so that they don't transfer more dirt onto your hair. And avoid touching your hair during the day or you'll only make it dirtier.
- Never brush frizzy curls. Instead, use a wide-tooth Afro comb to avoid making more frizzies!
- Nip to the office loo before you leave work, dampen your hair in the sink and then use the hot air hand-dryer for some quick scrunch drying!
- Keep your style simple because over-handling will make it oilier and flatter.
- Keep mousse, gel or wax to a minimum when hair is due for a wash because any excess will attract dirt and make hair even greasier.
- Remember, even if you're in a rush, take time to apply a little light make-up. Lipstick is particularly useful for brightening up your face and focusing attention away from dirty or lank hair.

Photographs: PAUL MITCHELL/Hair: SHAUN GLOAG at ARTISTIC LICENCE/Make up: LIZZIE COURT at PIN-UP

GREASE BALL!

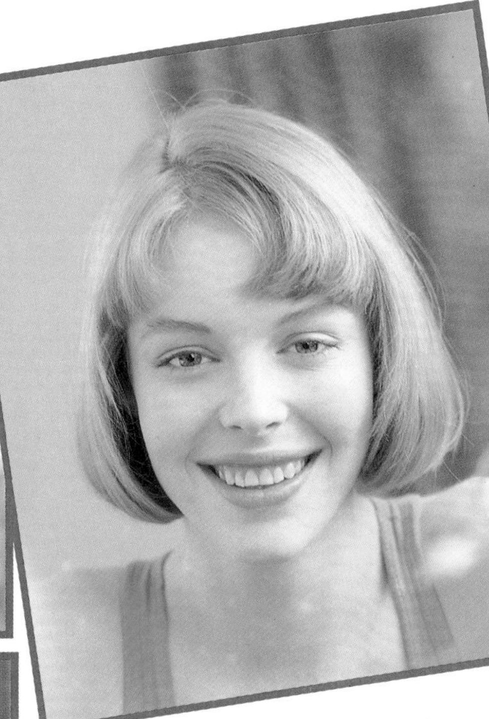

DAY INTO NIGHT

Blouse: FRENCH CONNECTION/Earrings: FENWICK

CURL REVITALISER

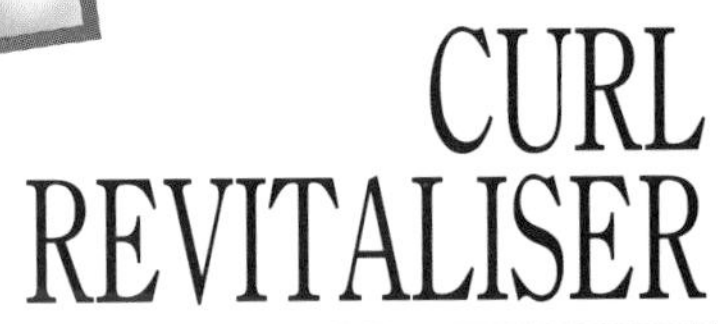

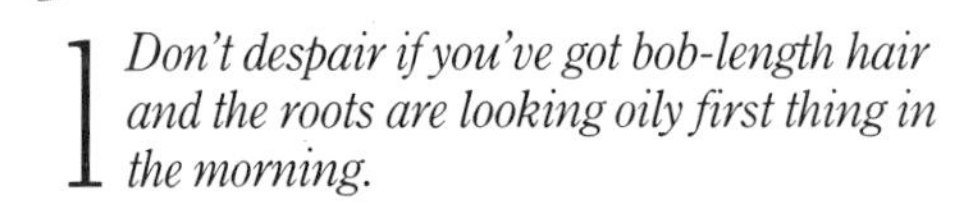

1 *Don't despair if you've got bob-length hair and the roots are looking oily first thing in the morning.*

2 *Try shaking a little talcum powder along your parting, and then brush it out thoroughly.*

3 *The talcum powder will absorb most of the oil from your hair, leaving it looking, and feeling, very much cleaner for the rest of the day.*

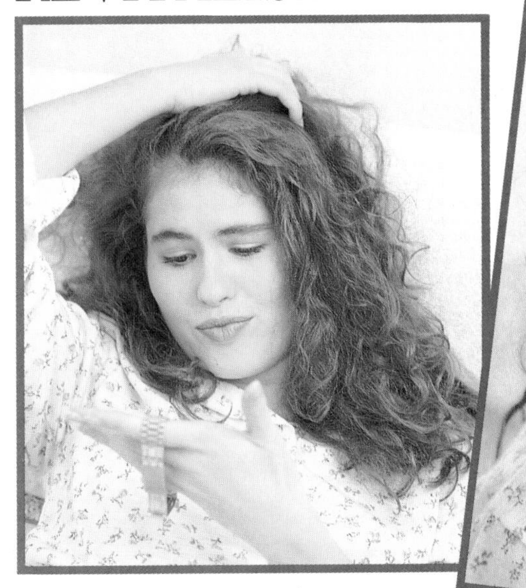

A LITTLE LIFT

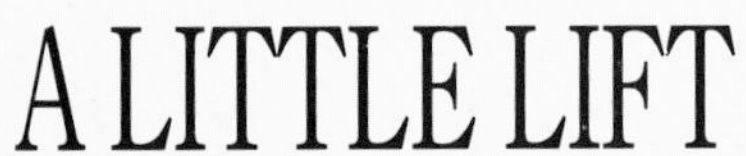

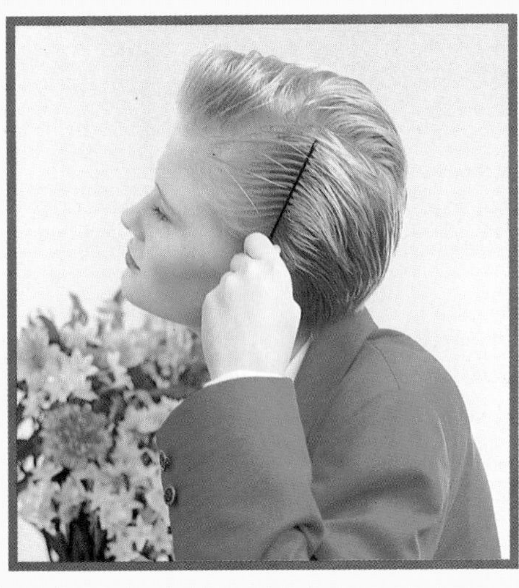

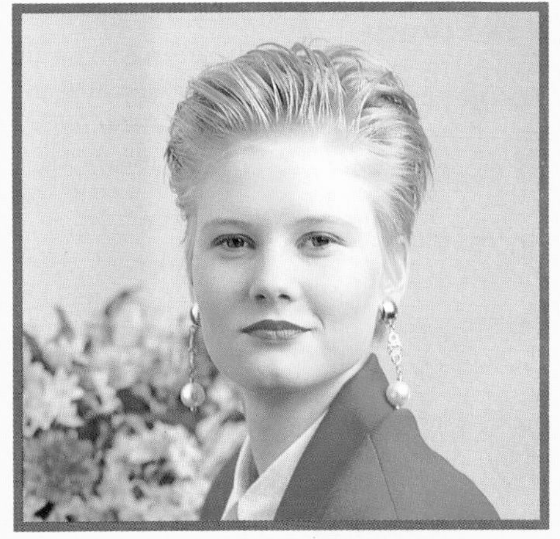

When short, layered hair is in need of a lift before a night out, comb a thumbnail-sized blob of wax right through to create texture and height, and to hide oily roots!

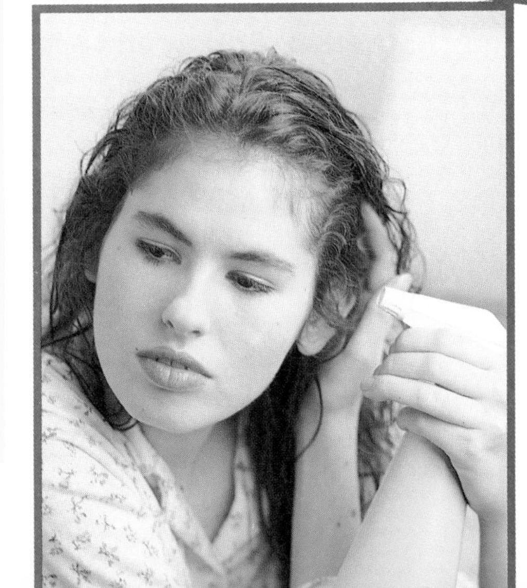

Dressing gown: MARKS & SPENCER/Jacket and Blouse: FRENCH CONNECTION/Earrings: NADIA MINKOFF at EDMONDS

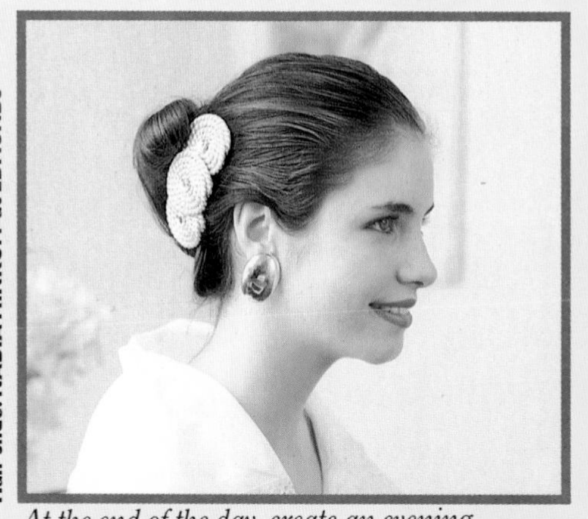

Hair slide: NADIA MINKOFF at EDMONDS

At the end of the day, create an evening look by rolling your hair into a smooth, sophisticated French pleat. Add a decorative hair slide for an eye-catching finishing touch that will focus attention away from not-so-clean hair.

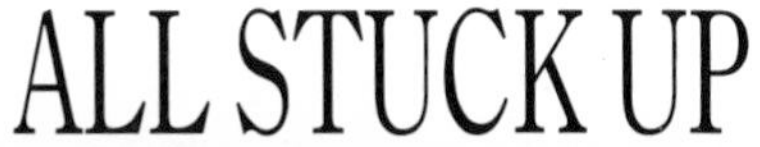

ALL STUCK UP

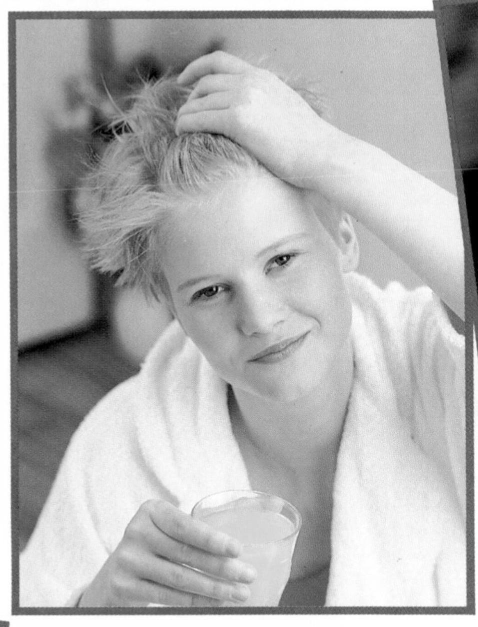

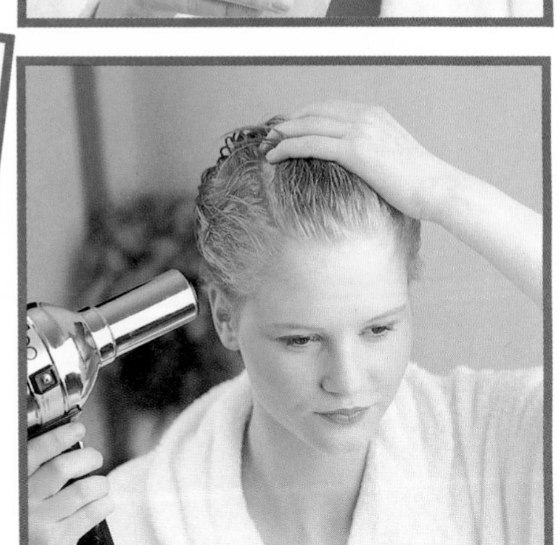

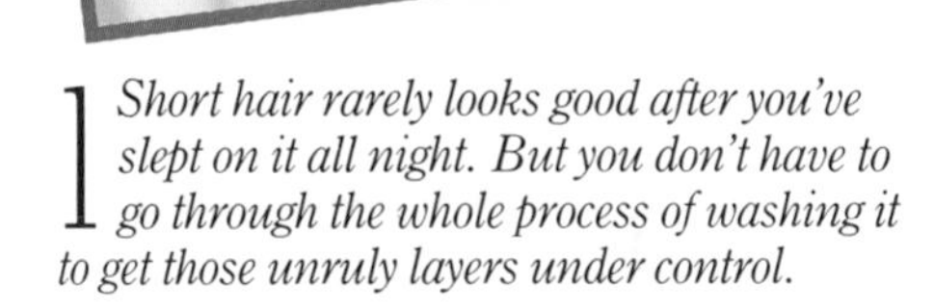

1 *Short hair rarely looks good after you've slept on it all night. But you don't have to go through the whole process of washing it to get those unruly layers under control.*

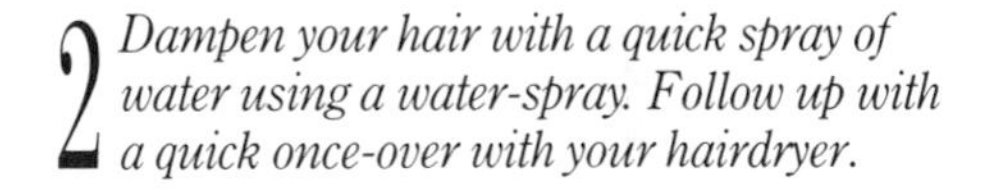

2 *Dampen your hair with a quick spray of water using a water-spray. Follow up with a quick once-over with your hairdryer.*

3 *Work a small blob of gel through your hair, then mould your hair into shape with your fingers.*

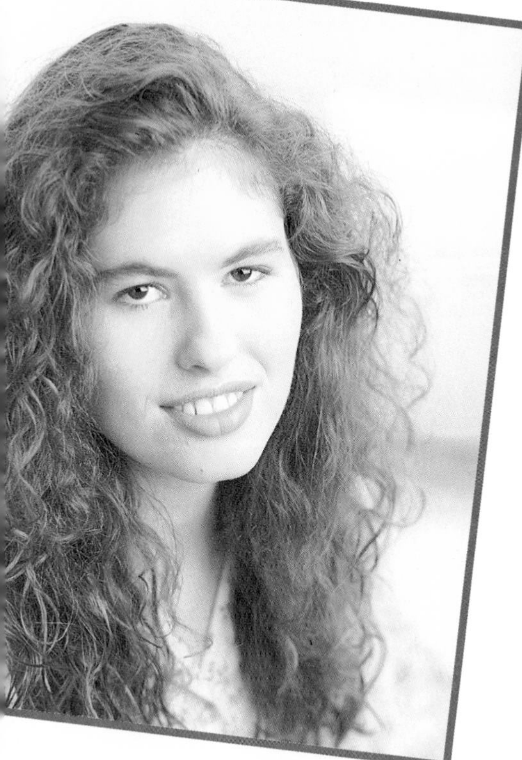

1 *The day that you wake up late is sure to be the day that your curly perm gets an attack of the frizzies!*

2 *Put the curl back in by lightly damping your hair all over with a water-spray.*

3 *Leave it to dry naturally, work in a little mousse and you'll be frizz-free before you've finished eating your breakfast!*

INSTANT STYLE

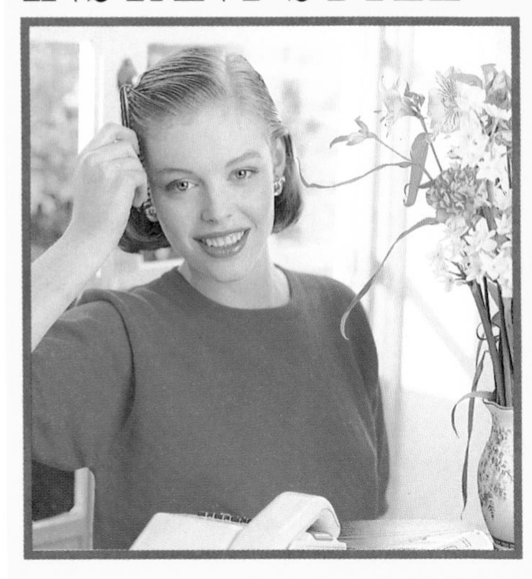

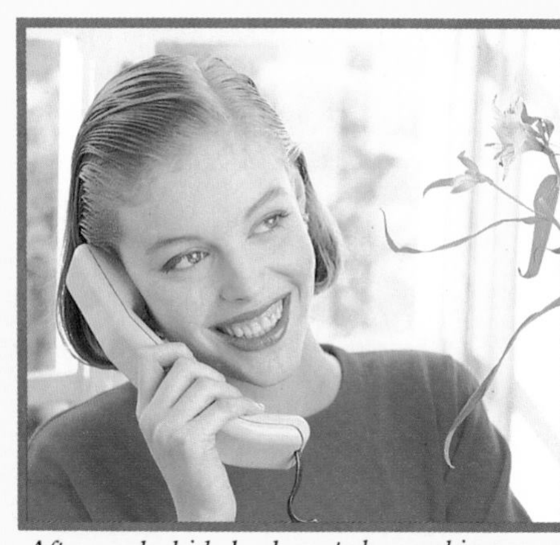

After work, hide lank roots by combing a pea-sized blob of gel through your hair. You can then smooth the roots back into a sleek style, leaving the ends loose. No one need ever know that you're due for a hair-wash.

Body: KNICKERBOX/Sweater: FRENCH CONNECTION/Pyjamas: DAMART

FULL HAIR AHEAD!

You don't have to be a punk to benefit from back-combing! Head for the heights with our hair raising styles

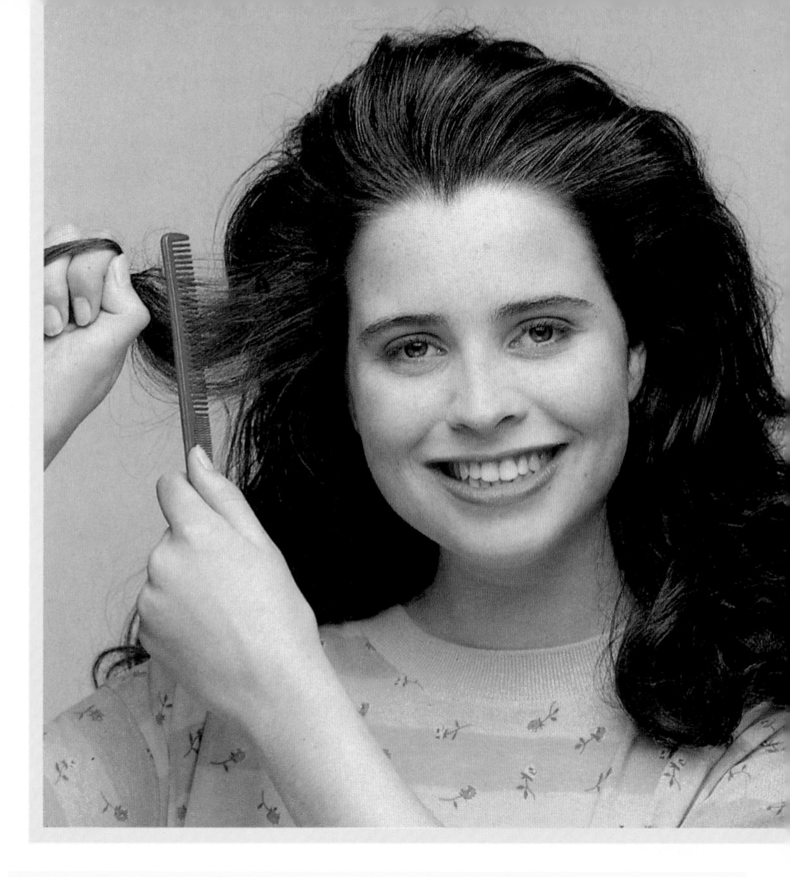

The most trendy looks around benefit from the extra support that back-combing brings – especially on fine hair that tends to flop out of style quickly.

To back-comb, all you need to do is comb your hair from the ends towards the roots. Each stroke temporarily raises the cuticle on your hair shaft so that the hairs become locked together. It's the opposite of combing your hair from root to ends for smoothness! For best results, use a narrow-toothed comb if you want to create support, and then change to a wide-toothed comb to give more volume.

Separate 2.5 cm/1 in sections and work from a quarter of the way along the length back to the roots to create support, or just through the ends of longer one length hair for volume. Work along the whole length of a section for a really big or tall style or to fix short hair.

Back-brushing curls will soften and separate them. Use a rubber-backed brush with rounded bristles so you don't snag or tear your hair.

Work quickly through your hair, holding each section at a 90° angle to your head as you back-comb or brush for an even result.

ANY QUESTIONS?

Q Will back-combing harm my hair?

A No, not as long as you make sure that you brush it out very carefully afterwards.

Q I'm growing out a perm and it's left me with straight roots and curly ends. How can I perk it up?

A Back-comb the roots to give them some body. But beware of back-combing permed dry ends because they have a tendency to knot easily.

Q Which styling products help keep back-combed hair in place?

A Products that dry on your hair – mousse, hairspray and setting lotion – provide excellent back-up support. Use gel and wax only on the tips of your hair as they can smooth it out.

Q Does back-combing cause split ends?

A No, but always use a plastic comb and make sure all the teeth are intact.

PUMP UP THE VOLUME

Back-combing gives long hair a lift. It even works on very fine hair.

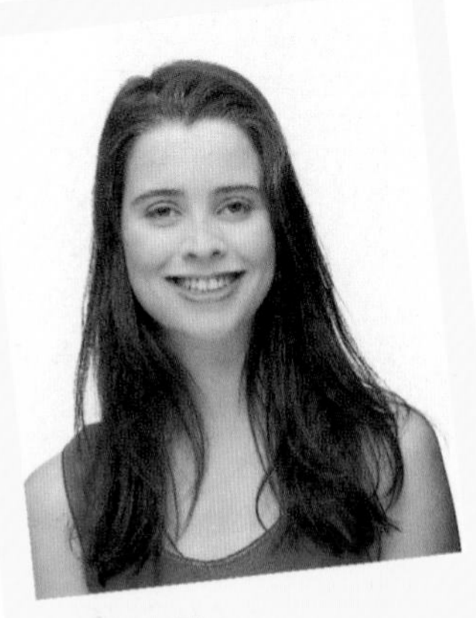

BEFORE
Dampen your hair with a spritz of water.

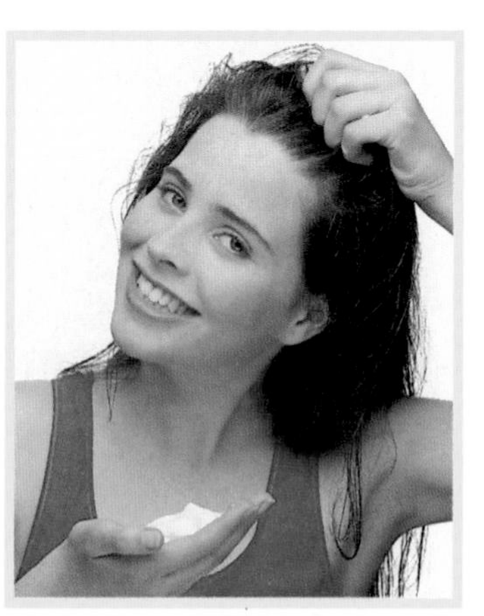

1 *Take an orange-sized blob of mousse and work right through from roots to ends.*

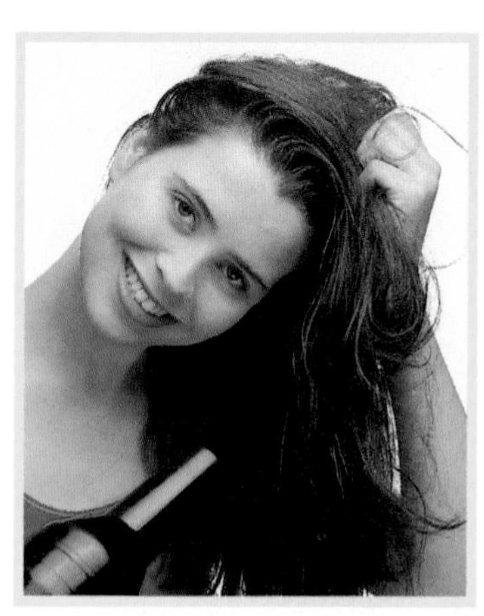

2 *Blast dry your hair thoroughly. If you leave any dampness, you will lose some of the support given by back-combing.*

Photographs: PAUL MITCHELL/Hair: PENNY ATTWOOD/Make-up: KAREN LOCKYER/Vest top: KNICKERBOX
Striped T-shirt, striped blouse: THE GAP/Printed top: HENNES/Earrings: ACCESSORIZE

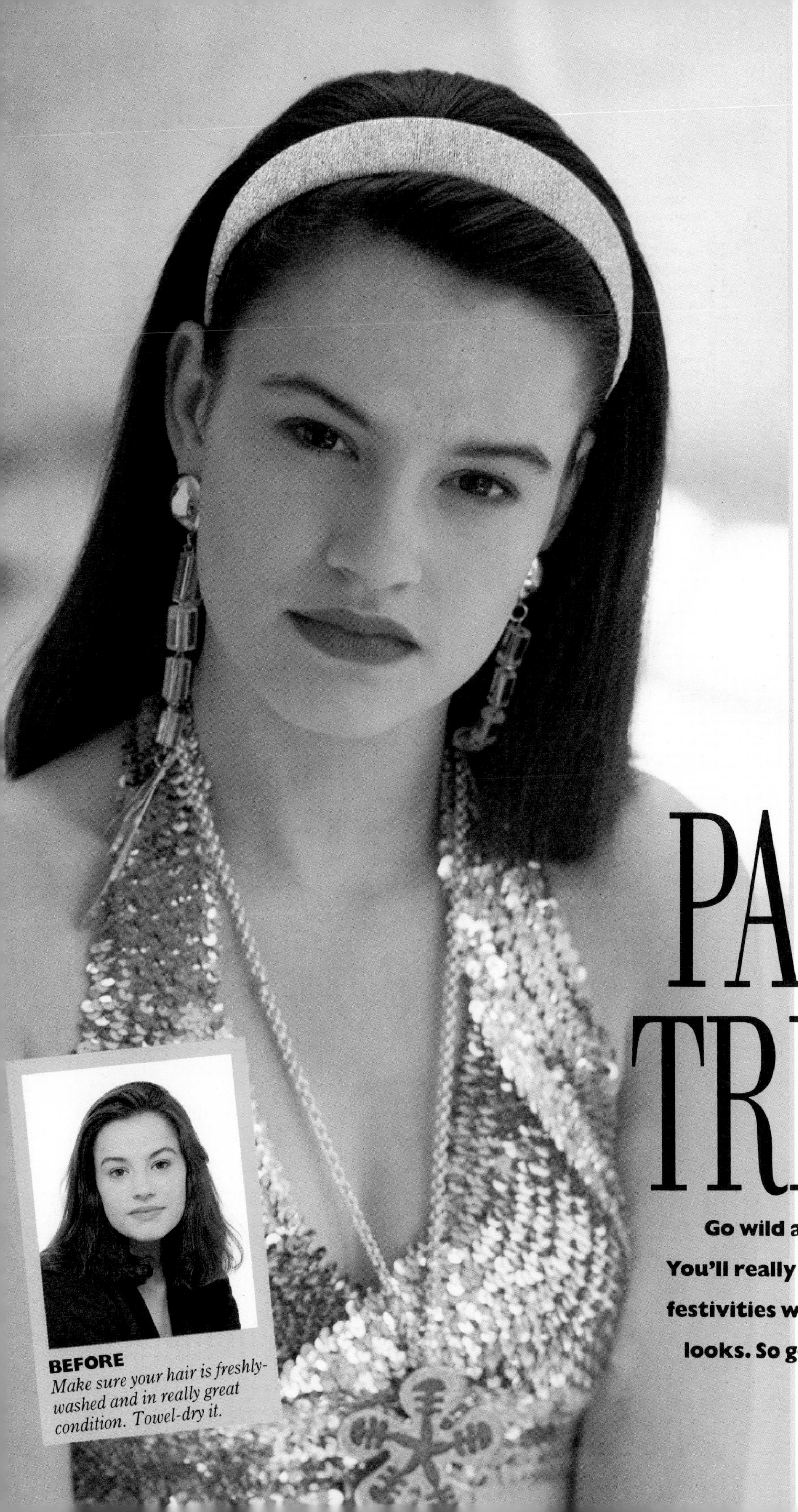

IT'S THE TOPS

◀ **For new age glamour, wear a silver Alice band to sleek back your hair. Try wrapping a velvet or tortoiseshell hair band with silver crochet thread for cost-effective chic. Blow-dry your hair smooth, rub in a thumbnail-sized blob of wax from your front hairline backwards. Hold your fringe down with grips, if necessary and cover them with the hair band.**

You've bought the frock, perfected your make-up, but have you given your hair enough thought? An extra-special style can make all the difference to your party look, so it's worth trying out a few different ideas during the run-up to the big night. Whatever you do, don't leave your hair to the last minute!

So get in the mood and get noticed – by trying these stunning party toppers.

PARTY TRICKS

Go wild and get ready to party! You'll really enjoy all the fun of the festivities with our glam and glitzy looks. So get out and celebrate in sensational style

BEFORE

Make sure your hair is freshly-washed and in really great condition. Towel-dry it.

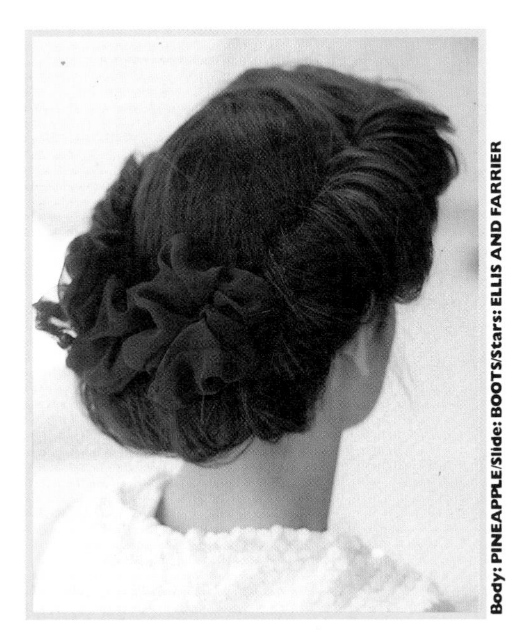

Body: PINEAPPLE/Slide: BOOTS/Stars: ELLIS AND FARRIER

ROLL UP

◀ **Flaunt your face when you give your hair an instant lift with this scooped up style. Gently roll your hair back from your face pinning with hair grips along the roll. Next, roll the hair up at the nape of your neck. Pin a few navy or black velvet or brightly coloured scrunchies along the back to liven up the look and hide the edge of the hair grips.**

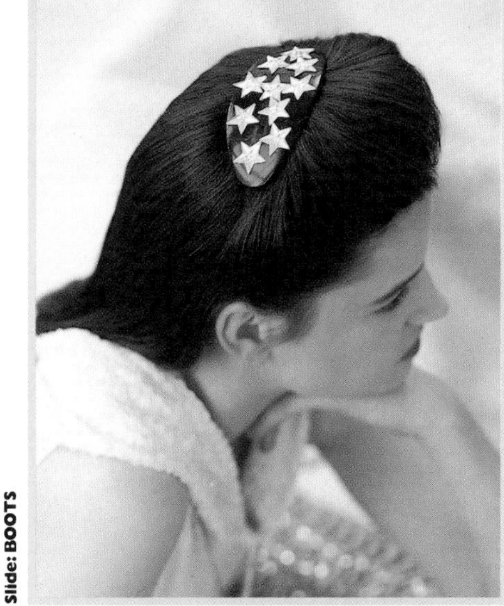

Slide: BOOTS

STAR TURN

◀ **A star-studded slide will put you at the top of the bill. Choose a wide tortoiseshell or dark coloured hair slide and cover it with stick-on stars. Blow-dry your hair smooth then divide it into two sections by parting across the head from ear to ear. Lift up the front section and create a small quiff at the hair line. Pin the hair to your head with the hair slide. Comb hair for a smooth finish.**

EAR EAR

◀ **Use glitzy clip-on earrings instead of a hairslide. Blow-dry your hair, then smooth over a thumbnail-sized blob of wax to add shine. Take the side section back above your ear and pin with a hair grip. Clip the earrings – the bigger the better – on top of the grip for instant glitz!**

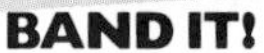

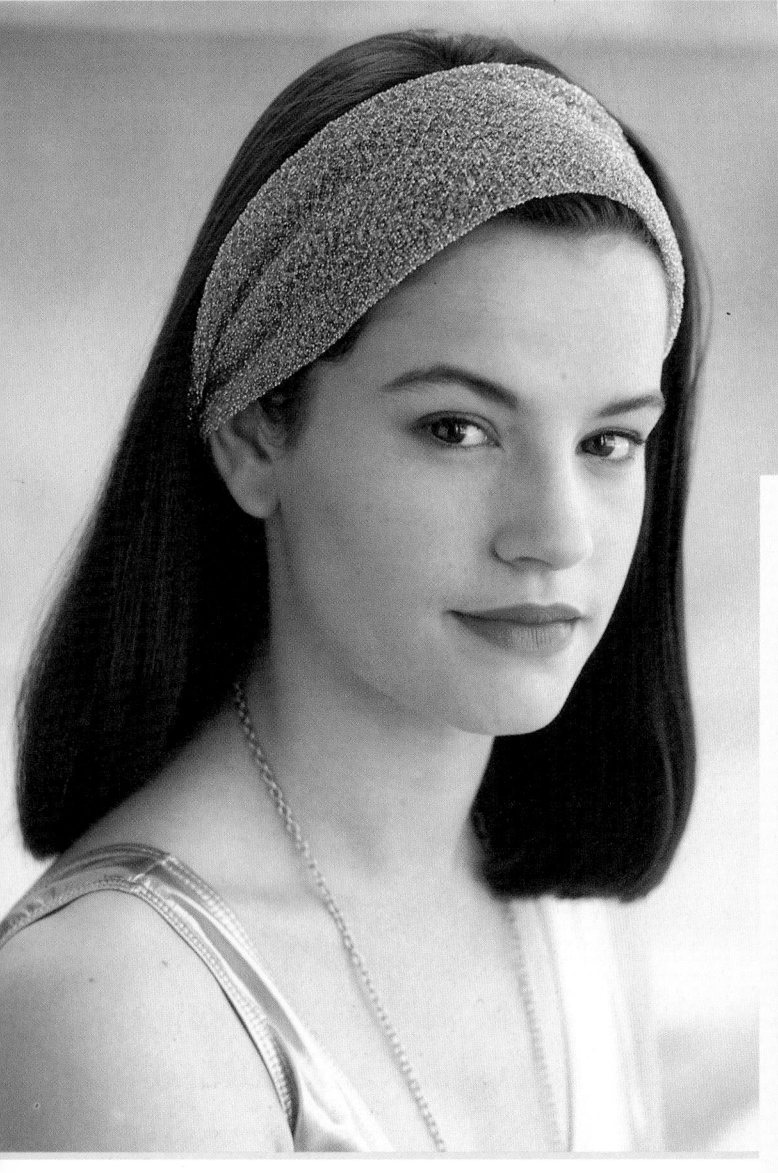

BAND IT!

◀ **Wide, elasticated hair bands are THE ultimate hair accessory. So add a touch of evening glitz with a Lurex one. (Make your own from a length of Lurex fabric if you can't find one.) Blow-dry your hair smooth and spritz with hairspray. Pull your hair band over your head, then back up to the hair line.**

TWILIGHT TIME

Afro hair is high on style with these party pieces.

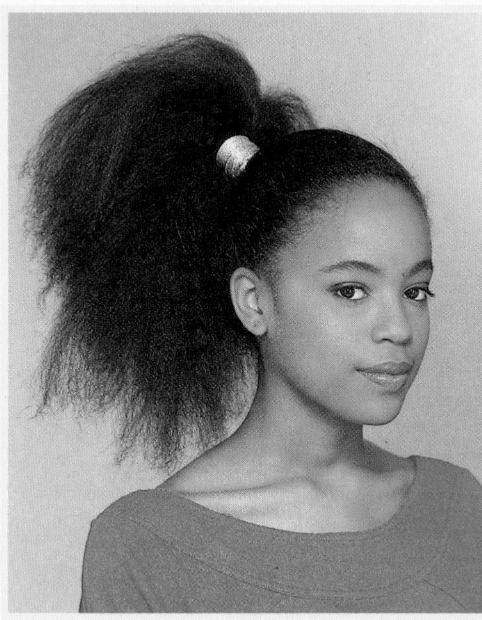

QUICK SILVER

◀ Brush back your hair on to the crown of your head. Pull it slightly to one side and fix it in a ponytail with a covered elastic band. Take a length of silver crochet thread and bind it from the root of the ponytail upwards for about 2.5 cm/1 in, to hide the covered elastic band. Fluff out the ends of your hair to finish the style.

BEFORE

Hair doesn't need to be freshly-washed for these particular styles.

BACK SLIDING

▶ **Roll the sides of your hair back from the hair line to the nape and pin. Hold both rolls temporarily in place with a section clip. Divide the remaining hair into three. Take the first section, twist it tightly until it coils back on itself, then pin it at the nape. Repeat with the other sections. Finally, replace the clip with a decorative slide.**

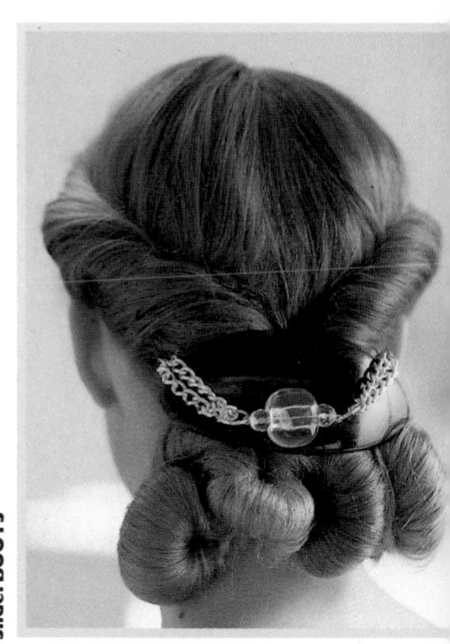

Slide: BOOTS

PLAIT TRICKS

◀ **A pretty plait woven from the side of your head is stunning and sophisticated – great for hair when it needs a wash but there just isn't time. Divide your hair into three 5 cm/2 in wide strands above one ear. Plait the hair across your head, taking in strands as you go, then plait the length of hair and fix with a covered elastic band. Finally, bind the ends of the plait together with a beaded tassel or a curtain tassel.**

Top: KNICKERBOX

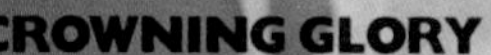

CROWNING GLORY

Start above one ear with three 5 cm/2 in sections of hair and plait across the top of your head and then down the length of your hair. Wind the plait on to the top of your head Heidi-style. Decorate it with beads or pearls. Use fine hairpins to pin the string of pearls along where the plait meets the crown of your head.

Blouse: PINEAPPLE

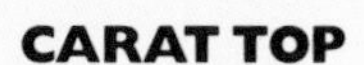

CARAT TOP

◀ Scoop your hair up into a ponytail, fix with a covered elastic band and bind with gold braid. Divide the ponytail into six equal sections. Plait each one tying and binding the ends with gold braid, then wind it around the base of the ponytail and pin in place. A real golden great!

BEEHIVE YOURSELF!

▶ If you've got Afro hair a beehive can be yours in minutes. Gather your hair up on to the crown, grasp it firmly at the ends and wind the hair towards the crown keeping the height in front. Pin with hair grips and smooth the front with a thumbnail-sized blob of wax.

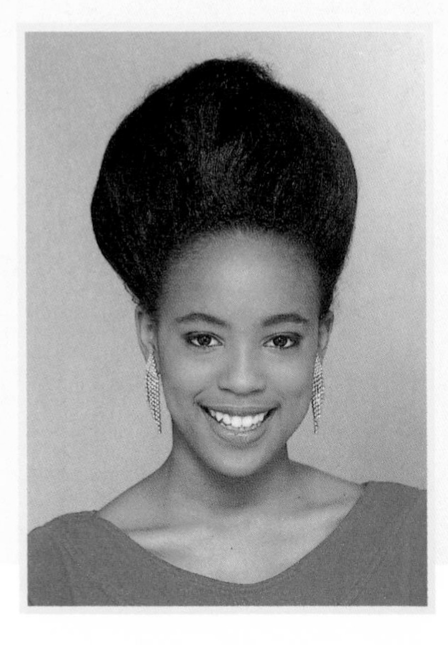

Photographs: NICK COLE/Hair: JUSTIN WILLIAMS/Dress: KAREN BOYD
Earrings: WRIGHT and TEAGUE

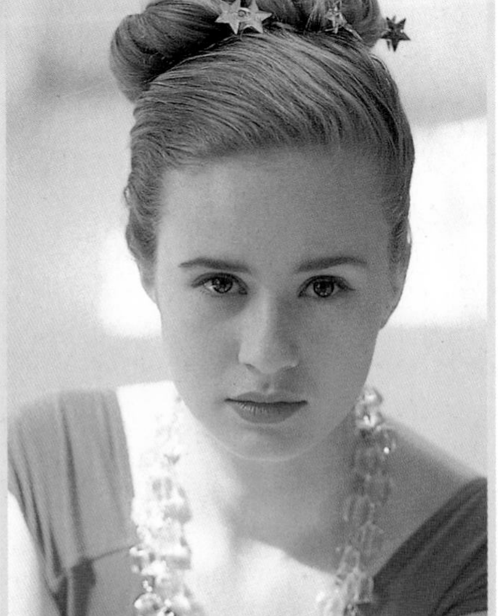

Top: PINEAPPLE

SHINE ALL NIGHT!

▲ **Pretty star decorations add a sparkle to a topknot. Gather your hair into an off-centre ponytail and fix with a covered elastic band. Divide the ponytail into three, then take each section and twist until it coils back on itself. Pin to your crown. Thread fine hairpins through some sequinned stars and pin them on.**

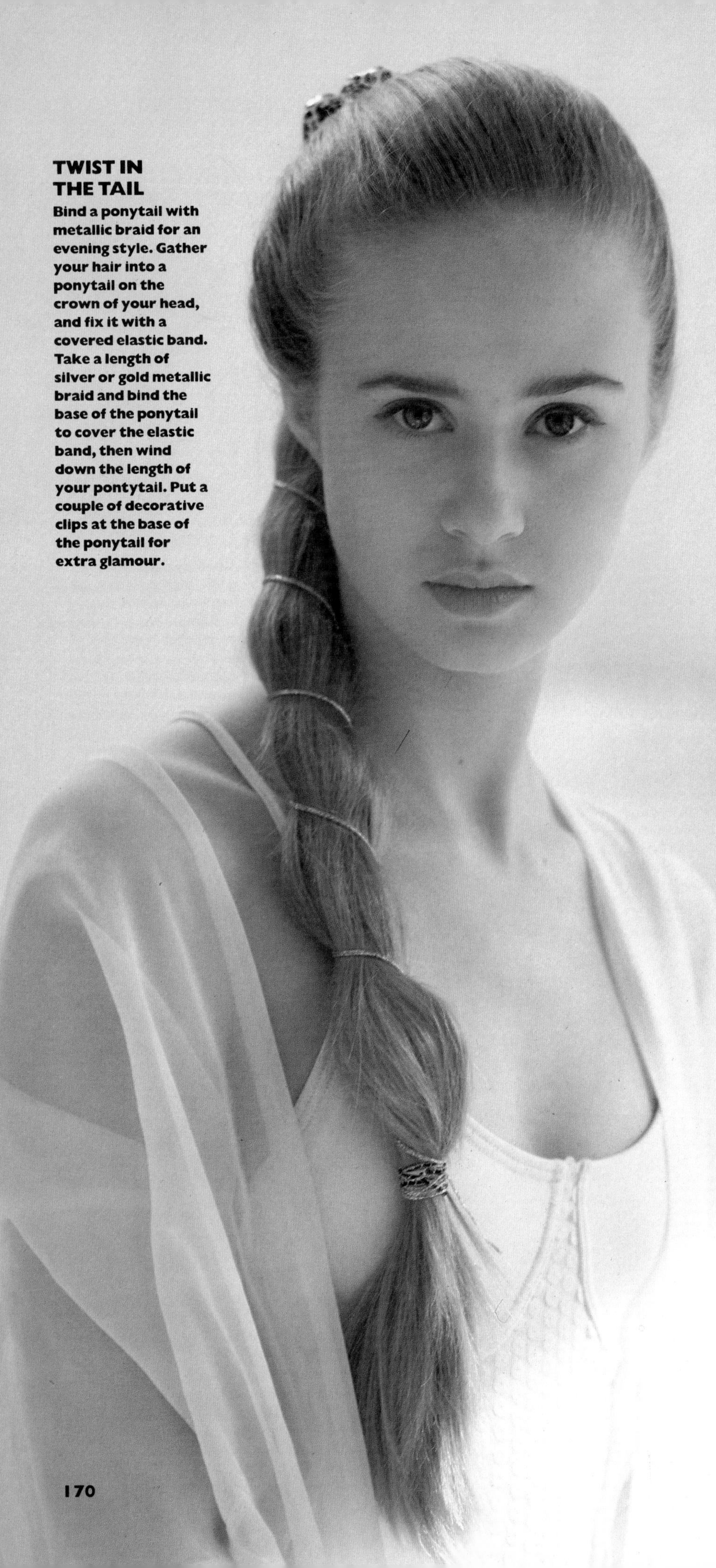

TWIST IN THE TAIL

Bind a ponytail with metallic braid for an evening style. Gather your hair into a ponytail on the crown of your head, and fix it with a covered elastic band. Take a length of silver or gold metallic braid and bind the base of the ponytail to cover the elastic band, then wind down the length of your pontytail. Put a couple of decorative clips at the base of the ponytail for extra glamour.

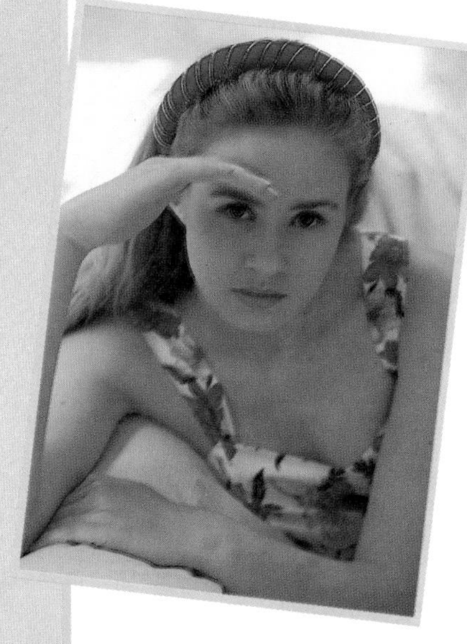

LET YOUR HAIR DOWN

▲ Leave your hair loose and flowing to show off its tip-top condition and shine. Hold it back with a pretty velvet hair band decorated with gold or silver thread. Smooth a thumbnail-sized blob of wax through your hair to give it extra shine.

10 ALTERNATIVE PARTY THEMES

1 Colours – wear all gold or pink clothes with matching hair streaks and make-up.
2 Hats – wear customised bowlers or boaters.
3 Come as you are – in your gardening clothes, your tracksuit or your old pyjamas!
4 Decades – wear styles from the Forties, Fifties or Sixties.
5 Lookalikes – copy the styles of Madonna or Prince. Or go as your favourite film star or a member of the Royal family.
6 Town names – wrap up in a big towel and clutch a scrubbing brush for Bath. For Wellington, wear a pair of green wellies!
7 Disguises – wear wigs, false noses and glasses or funny masks.
8 TV or radio programmes – a character from EastEnders, The Archers or Neighbours.
9 Tight 'n' Bright – wear mini skirts, boob tubes, masses of body glitter and fluorescent make-up.
10 Whodunnit – turn detective for the evening and solve the clues to a staged set-up.

Photographs: SIMON BOTTOMLEY/Hair: DENISE/Make-up: JOANNE HARBER/Floral body: KNICKERBOX/White body and blouse: PINEAPPLE

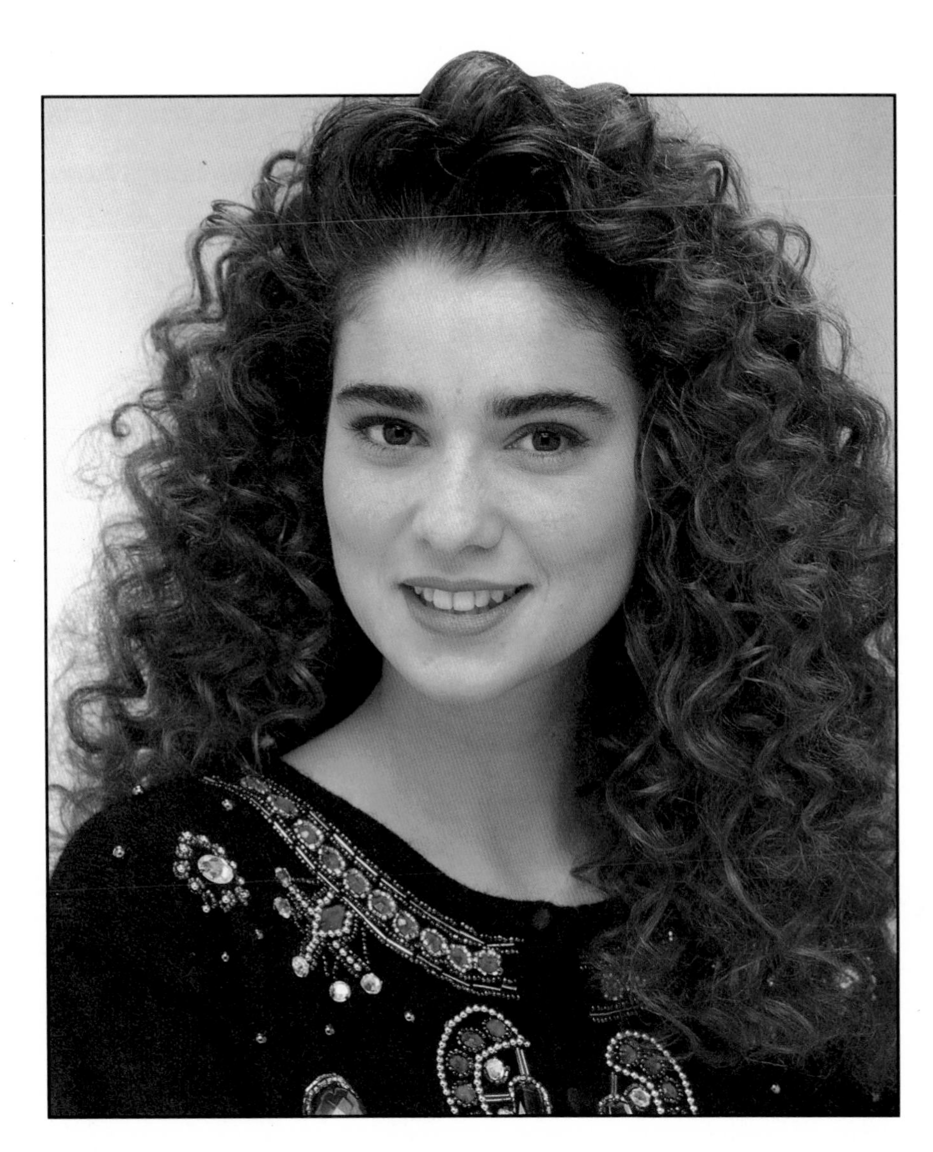

CHAPTER SIX

The Healthy Hair File

DID YOU KNOW?

You may be great at tonging or blow-drying, but how much do you really know about hair? We've got facts that'll make your hair curl and heads turn. So hair's how to amaze your friends

1 All the hair follicles you're ever going to have are formed before you are born, even if they're not activated until you're in your teens.

2 Next time you're called a big head, remember that the scalp covers an area of approximately 800 sq cm/130 sq in!

3 If your boyfriend is worried that his hair is starting to drop out, he's not alone! One in five men start to thin or develop a receding hairline before they're 20 and many are very bald by the time they're 30.

4 If you look at individual hairs under a microscope, the magnified cross-section of an average straight hair looks round, a curly hair tends to be oval, whereas an Afro hair is kidney-shaped and flat on one side.

5 'Virgin hair' is the term used by hairdressers to describe hair which hasn't previously been chemically-processed in any way, or in the case of black hair, hasn't been relaxed or straightened.

6 Most people have about 100,000 hairs on their head. Redheads have the thickest hair with the fewest strands (90,000); brunettes come somewhere in the middle, followed by blondes who have the finest hair with the most strands (up to 140,000).

7 The hair shaft is composed of 70 to 80 percent protein (keratin); three to six percent oils; one percent colouring pigment; 12 to 15 percent moisture, plus traces of minerals and carbohydrates.

8 Next time the sink's full of hair after you've shampooing – don't panic. On average, you lose 100 hairs a day.

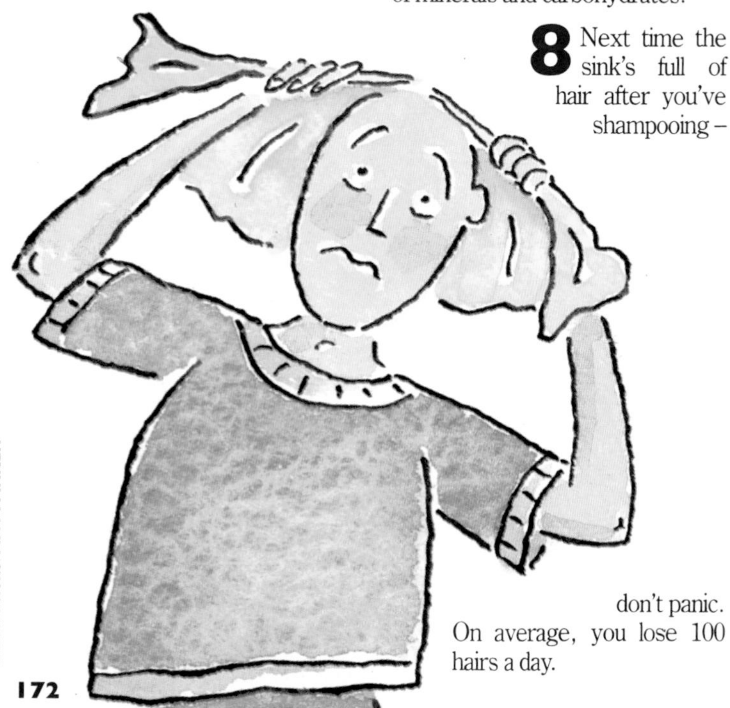

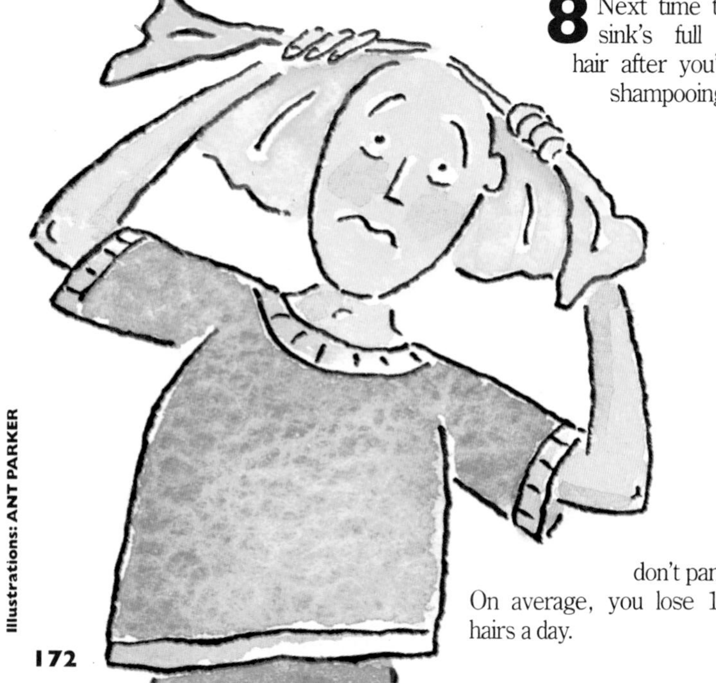

9 The living part of the hair follicle is connected by nerve fibres, so movement of the hair in the follicle is felt – for example when you pluck your eyebrows. When a hair leaves the follicle and emerges on to the surface of the scalp, it no longer receives nourishment and is, to all intents and purposes, dead. This is the reason why you can burn it with chemicals and tongs and not feel a thing!

10 Although limp, lank and dull hair is generally the result of illness or a bad diet, it isn't entirely due to the fact that you haven't been eating your greens. Nourishment of the hair follicles comes pretty low on the body's list of priorities when it's trying to fight off infection, so the blood supply is diverted to vital organs instead.

11 The hair grows about 1.25 cm/½ in a month. It grows more in warmer weather and less as you get older.

12 Contrary to popular belief hair does not continue to grow after you've died.

13 Hair is a very strong substance and is also very elastic. In tip-top condition, it can resist a pull of about 200 g/8 oz and stretches by about one-fifth of its normal length before breaking.

14 There are three distinct phases in the life of your hair: the growing period, known as anagen; the resting phase, telogen; and the shedding period, catagen. Although this cycle varies from person to person, normally about 86 percent of scalp follicles are in anagen while the remaining 14 percent are in telogen and catagen.

15 It is possible to lose up to 30,000 hairs in the two or three months after pregnancy. This is caused by the increase of certain hormones during pregnancy, which settle down once the baby is born.

16 In 1949, it was reported that an Indian monk had hair 7.92 m/26 ft in length.

Illustrations: ANT PARKER

17 If you don't like your hair, you could try hiding it under a – very expensive – hat! The highest price ever paid for a hat is $66,000 by a New York museum for a fifteenth-century ceremonial frog helmet!

18 On average, the lifespan of a woman's hair is a quarter longer than a man's.

19 The average lifespan of a hair is anything from two to six years.

20 The average length a human hair grows to within its life if left uncut, is anything from 55-70 cm/22-28 in. Hair that is more than 90 cm/3 ft long is quite rare.

21 Tearing your hair out is actually a recognised medical condition. It mainly affects teenage girls, menopausal women and highly-stressed people. Someone who quite literally tears their hair out is called trichotillomanic.

22 Grey hair doesn't really exist. The overall impression of greyness is given by a mixture of pure white hairs containing no pigment and the remaining strands of pigmented hair. A hair shaft is either pigmented or it is colourless – not a combination of the two.

23 Wigs never seem to go out of fashion! Solid silver and gold wigs have been found in many of the tombs of the Pharaohs, while wigs made from human hair, wool and palm-leaf fibre were normal daytime wear for the ordinary Egyptian.

24 Curly hair is genetically determined and occurs as a result of uneven cell division around the diameter of the growing hair – one side grows more quickly, causing a bend in the shaft.

25 Wearing your hair scraped back, for example in a ponytail or braid can lead to a condition known as traction alopecia. This is when the hair starts snapping off around the hairline.

26 Hair cells can roughly reflect the levels – both good and bad – of minerals in the body, and can be a guide to your health. Deficiency levels of lead and aluminium can leave you feeling run down, while zinc deficiency can result in poor skin and slow growth.

27 Your hair colour is determined by your genes, which are responsible for the pigment granules that make up your hair shade. The colour comes from red, yellow and black pigments but the mix and ratio is uniquely yours.

28 The chemical acidity or alkalinity of your hair is measured on the pH scale. Neutral is seven, while numbers above seven indicate alkalinity and numbers below seven, acidity. The pH of your hair is between 4.5 and 5.5, making it acidic. Therefore, although it sounds harsh, an acid wave perm is actually kinder than other types because it won't upset your hair's balance.

29 One of the first thing a man notices about you is apparently your . . . hair! A fab cut is definitely your best beauty asset and rates higher than your eyes, boobs, legs or bottom in man appeal.

30 If you suffer from an eating disorder such as anorexia or bulimia – your hair may begin to fall out.

31 In the last 20 years or so there has been a big increase in the number of women losing their hair. It is claimed that this is happening because as more women take on high-powered jobs (and experience higher levels of stress), they produce the male hormone androgen – and begin to lose hair in a way that has previously only affected men.

32 A big proportion of us are actually allergic to dairy products without realising it. One of the effects of the allergy is a flaky scalp – so if you suffer from this, cut down on milk, butter and cheese.

33 Most of us actually lose more hair than usual in the autumn. This is known as seasonal hair loss and is nothing to worry about.

34 Hair is a very hard-wearing substance and there are many instances of it having survived centuries without rotting. In the British Museum's Egyptian Room a body dating back 4,000 years, which had been dried and preserved by the desert sands, can be found with strands of perfectly preserved hair still on the skull.

35 Throughout history hair has been seen as a symbol of sexuality and to have it cut off was thought to 'desexualise' women. So-called witches were punished by having their hair cut off, as were prisoners. Similarly, it is traditional for nuns to cover their hair (and in some cases shave their heads) as a symbol of their chastity.

36 Afro hair is very porous all over, whereas European hair is usually only porous at the ends.

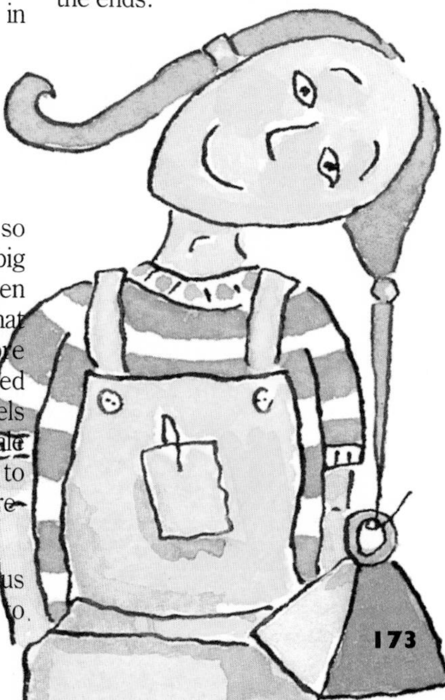

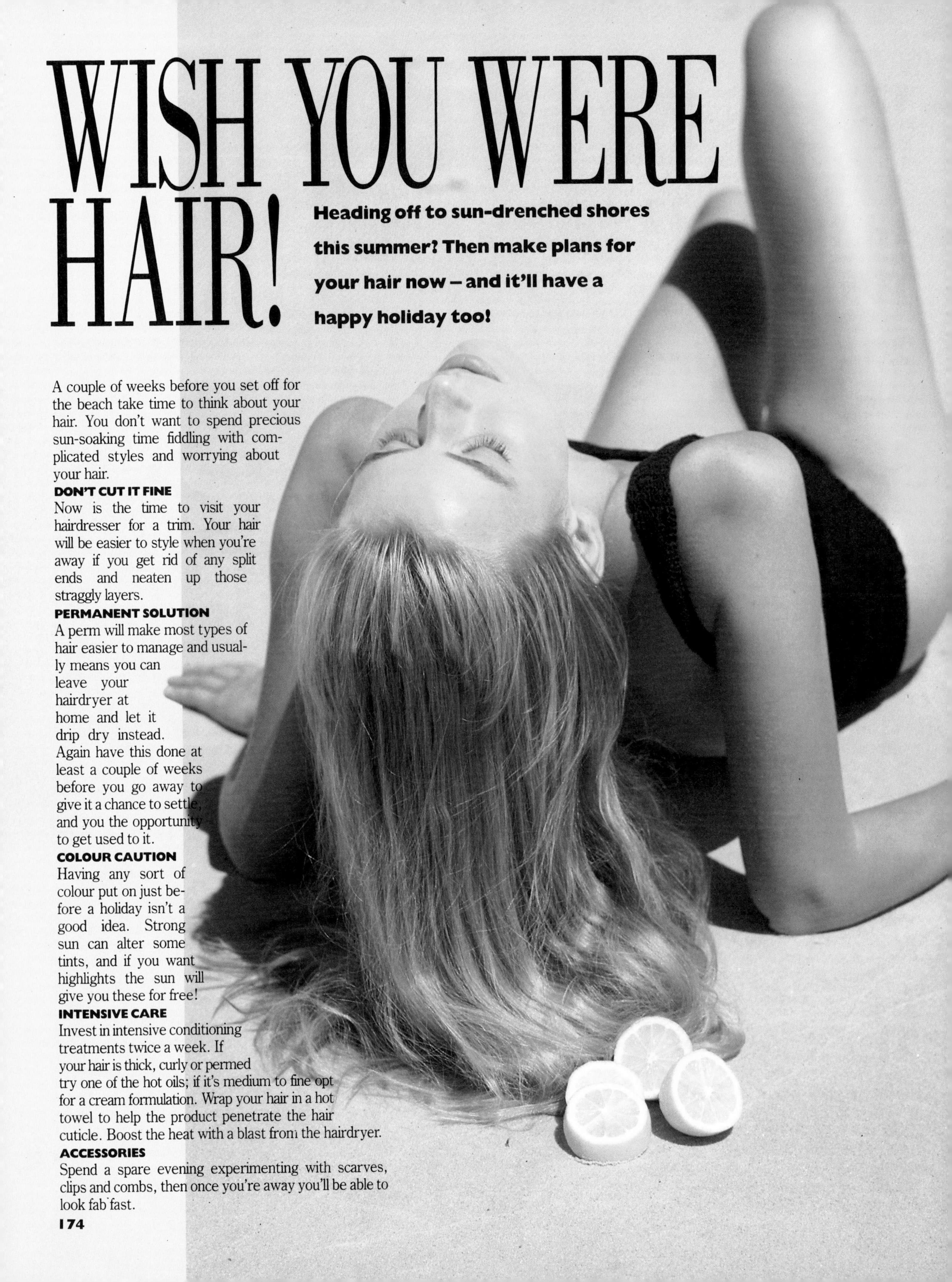

WISH YOU WERE HAIR!

Heading off to sun-drenched shores this summer? Then make plans for your hair now – and it'll have a happy holiday too!

A couple of weeks before you set off for the beach take time to think about your hair. You don't want to spend precious sun-soaking time fiddling with complicated styles and worrying about your hair.

DON'T CUT IT FINE

Now is the time to visit your hairdresser for a trim. Your hair will be easier to style when you're away if you get rid of any split ends and neaten up those straggly layers.

PERMANENT SOLUTION

A perm will make most types of hair easier to manage and usually means you can leave your hairdryer at home and let it drip dry instead. Again have this done at least a couple of weeks before you go away to give it a chance to settle, and you the opportunity to get used to it.

COLOUR CAUTION

Having any sort of colour put on just before a holiday isn't a good idea. Strong sun can alter some tints, and if you want highlights the sun will give you these for free!

INTENSIVE CARE

Invest in intensive conditioning treatments twice a week. If your hair is thick, curly or permed try one of the hot oils; if it's medium to fine opt for a cream formulation. Wrap your hair in a hot towel to help the product penetrate the hair cuticle. Boost the heat with a blast from the hairdryer.

ACCESSORIES

Spend a spare evening experimenting with scarves, clips and combs, then once you're away you'll be able to look fab fast.

WATERWAYS

● You may not wash your hair every day at home but it's a good idea to wash your hair more regularly on holiday to get rid of sand, sea and suntan lotion. Use a frequent wash shampoo and complementary conditioner that will be gentle on your hair.
● Always try to rinse your hair in fresh water immediately after you've been swimming. Chlorine and salt water are both very dehydrating if left to dry in your hair.
● If your hair is highlighted or bleached always rinse out chlorine as soon as you can. The copper present in the water to prevent algae can react with the chemicals and turn your hair a delicate shade of green!
● Water babies should watch out for the new anti-chlorine shampoos which are now available. They neutralise the smell as well as cleaning your hair. Use them as an all over body wash and they'll rinse out your swimsuit too.
● Keep your hair out of the water altogether by wearing a bright swimming cap. Wear goggles to match and you'll look impressively sporty!

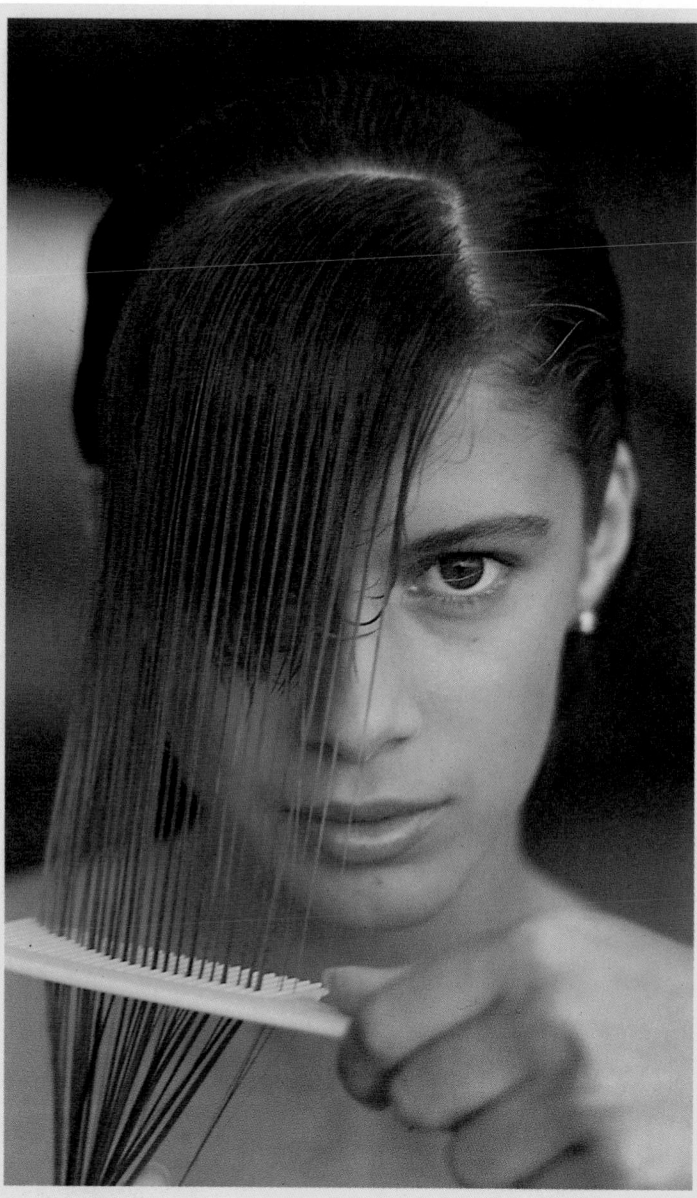

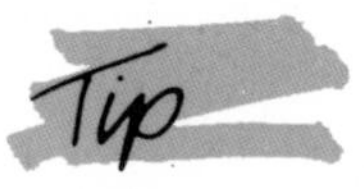

A change in humidity can give natural curls and perms an attack of the frizzies. Calm them down by scrunching mousse into the ends.

▼ Add some natural highlights by squeezing a little lemon juice onto a comb and running this through your hair. But only do it once! Any more will damage your hair and may turn it a brassy colour.

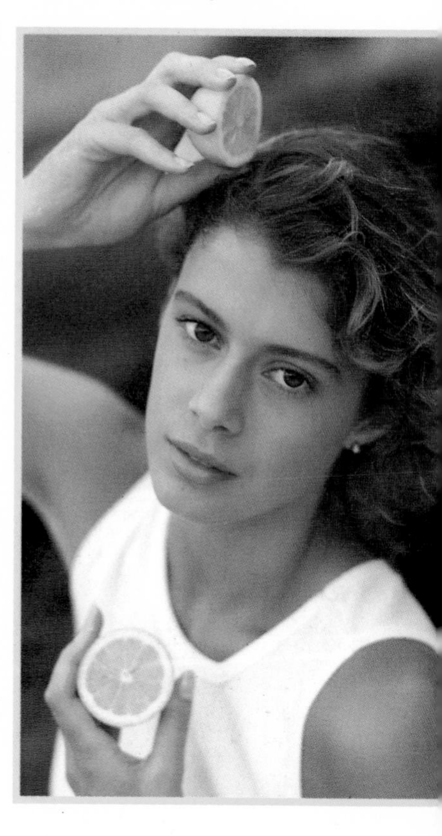

ON GUARD

You wouldn't dream of sunbathing without using some sort of protection from the burning rays of the sun and the same should apply to your hair. Because it's 'dead' you don't feel any pain while it's burning, but it happens all the same. Strong sun will dry up the natural oils leaving it lack-lustre, and even frizzy. The more dehydrated your hair becomes the more likely it is to split.

Sun damage is a very common problem and can take months of trimming and conditioning treatments to correct. Yet a few preventative measures are all that are needed to keep your hair in tip-top condition.

Every time you slap on the sun cream, use a hair protector too. These contain UV filters – just like skin protection products – as well as conditioners to keep hair feeling soft and looking shiny. They also help to keep colour-treated hair the shade you originally intended and stop it turning brassy in the sun.

Hair protectors come in several different formulas:

Gels: easy to use and give a sleek, wet look. Especially good on short hair.

Sprays: available in two types. Invisible spray screen that protects the hair without having any holding power and protective spray that also acts like a normal-hold hairspray.

Creams: these offer a much lighter hold than gel protectors and won't leave your hair feeling sticky or greasy.

If you forget to pack a sunscreen, comb conditioner through your hair. Use a wide-toothed comb and leave it on while you sunbathe – it's not ideal but it's a lot better than nothing at all.

Remember that all protection products need to be re-applied every time you've been for a swim or shower.

Whether you go for a conditioner or protective sun shield, it's best to use a cream or gel rather than oil – otherwise your hair will fry!

HOT STUFF

Don't waste valuable case space with lots of heavy electrical applices, take mini travel-sized versions instead. Hairdryers, heated rollers and styling tongs are all available in small sizes. There's even a hairdryer that doubles as a travel iron which works on all but the heaviest fabrics. All of these appliances are multi-voltage but do pack an adaptor as sockets vary around the world.

If you have to rely on heated styling tools to get your hair

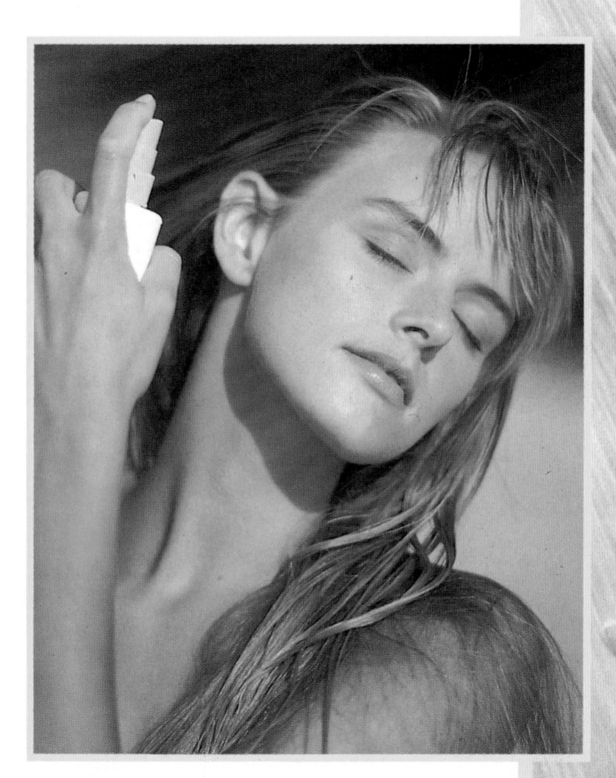

▲ **Another way to lighten your hair under the sun is with a blonding spray. These are activated by heat so work with a hairdryer or the sun's rays. Again they should be used sparingly as the results can be unpredictable.**

► **Freshen up with a shower after a dip. No showers on the beach? Take a bottle of water to splash on.**

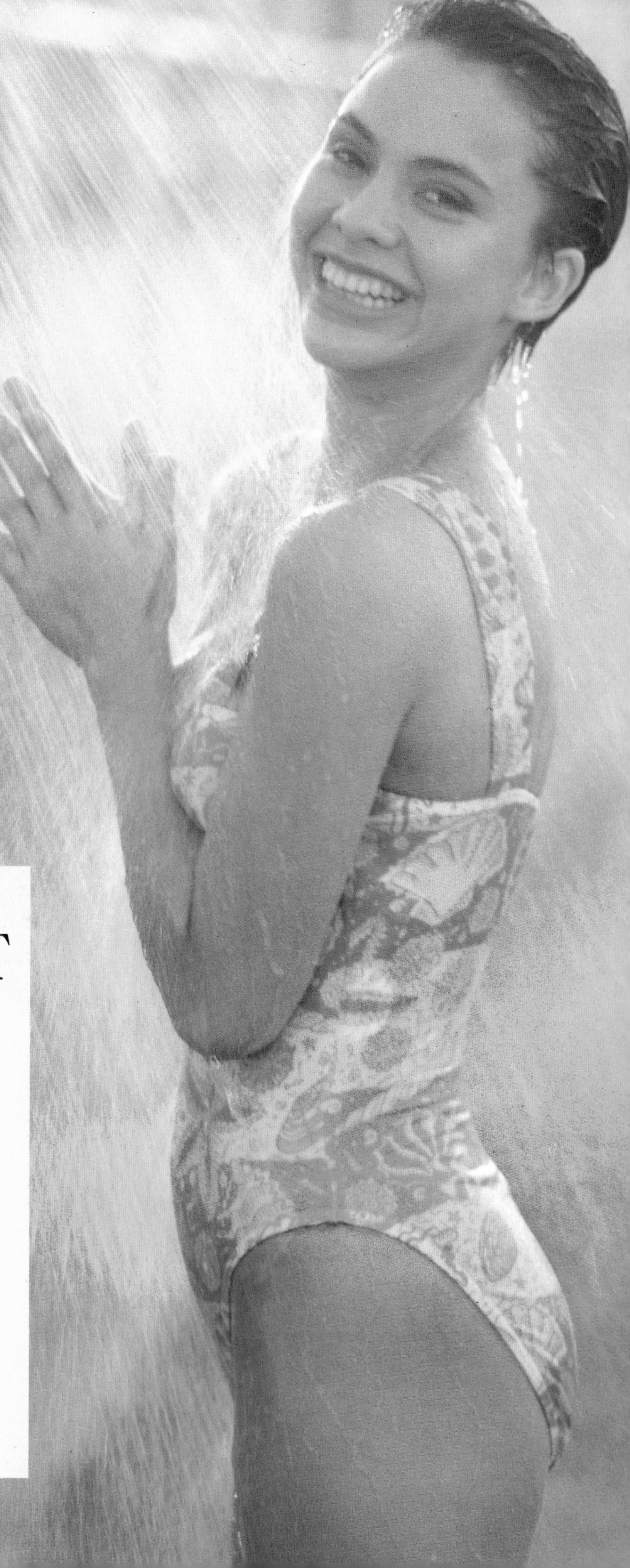

If you're away for a couple of weeks treat your hair to an intensive re-moisturising treatment on holiday.

looking good then maybe it's time to consider a less fussy style. For example, if heated rollers are the only way to build volume into your limp locks, a body perm could solve all your problems. Electrical appliances are fine to use occasionally but they may damage your hair if used every day.

If you can't bear to part with your rollers or hot brush, check out non-heated bendy rollers which will give much the same results. They take longer to work but they're kinder to your hair.

Make sure you buy everything your hair needs before you go away. You'll pay double the price for that can of firm-hold mousse in many tourist hot spots.

HOLIDAY CHECKLIST

ESSENTIALS

- ☐ **shampoo**
- ☐ **conditioner**
- ☐ **sunscreen**
- ☐ **wide-toothed comb**
- ☐ **scarf/hat**
- ☐ **assorted accessories**

OPTIONAL EXTRAS

- ☐ **hairdryer**
- ☐ **socket adaptor**
- ☐ **brush**
- ☐ **bendy rollers**
- ☐ **styling appliances**
- ☐ **mousse**
- ☐ **gel**
- ☐ **hairspray**
- ☐ **wax**

DRIP DRY HAIR

Give your hair a holiday from your hairdryer and leave it at home. Letting your hair dry naturally is good for it and is easier than you might think.

- Wrap your head in a big towel, turban-style, to blot up excess water. Leave this on for five minutes then ease out any tangles with a comb.
- Squirt an egg-sized blob of mousse onto your palms, then smooth over the surface of damp hair. This will help prevent static and flyaway ends.
- To build body into layered cuts, work mousse into the roots with your fingers. For waves and curls, set your hair on bendy rollers in 5 cm/2 in sections. Leave in until they are completely dry then style using your fingers.
- Speed up drying time by continually running your fingers through the length of your hair, lifting it away from your head as you do so. Even long hair will be dry in 15-20 minutes – even though your arms might ache!
- Don't bake your hair dry by lying in the sun. Go for a walk instead and let the breeze gently blow it dry.
- Plait long hair just before you go to bed and in the morning when you unplait it, you'll find a mass of rippling waves.

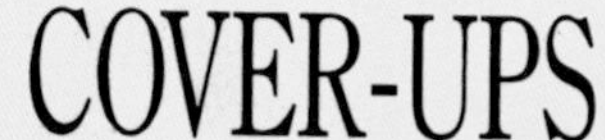

COVER-UPS

Foolproof ways to keep your hair healthy in the sun.

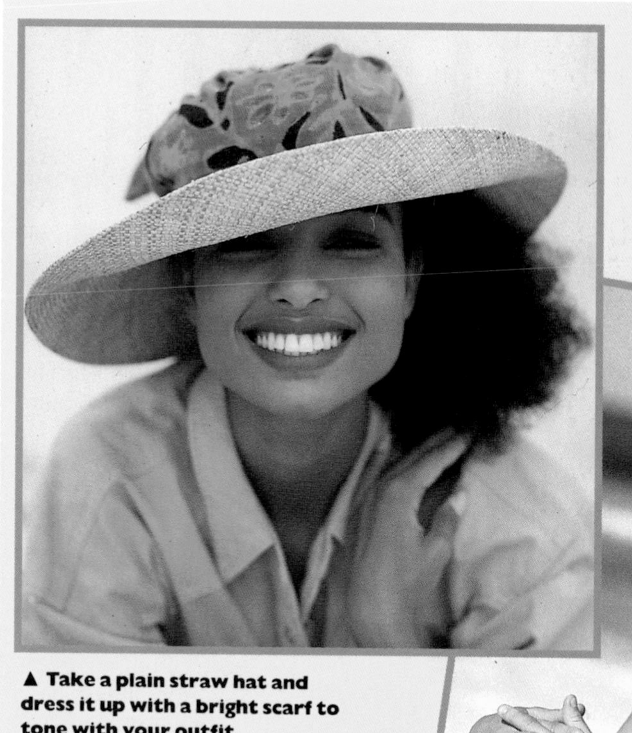

▲ Take a plain straw hat and dress it up with a bright scarf to tone with your outfit.

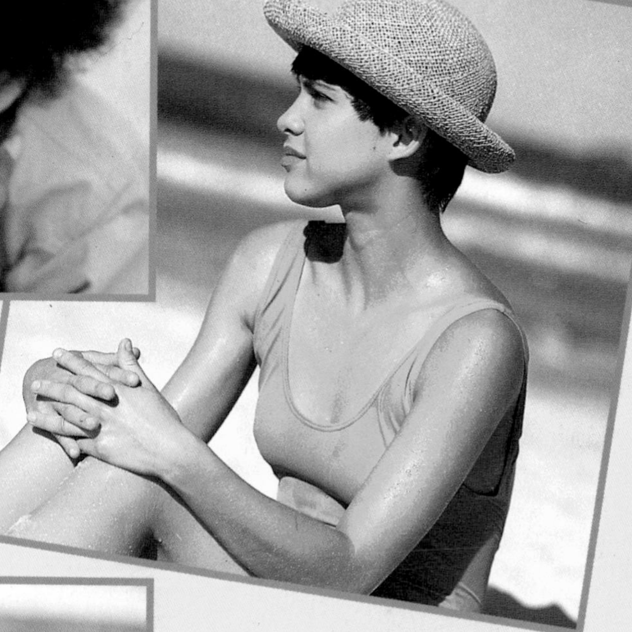

▼ Wear a natural straw hat to cover up when you laze on the beach.

▼ If your skin has a tendency to burn easily, choose a wide-brimmed hat to protect face and shoulders.

◄ Tie a scarf at the back or the front of your hair in a big bow – it'll help you keep your cool.

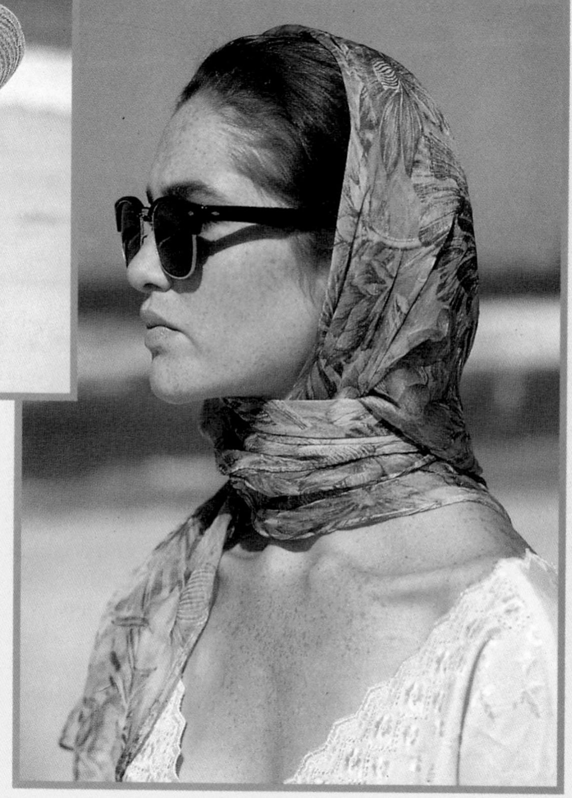

► Wrap a scarf over your hair then around your neck Grace Kelly-style for instant sleek chic.

Photographs: DIDIER DE FEYS/Black swimsuit: HENNES/Blue print swimsuit: NEXT DIRECTORY/Straw hat: FRENCH CONNECTION/Shirt: PEPE/ Straw boater: C&A/Swimsuit: PINK SODA/Wide-brimmed straw hat: THE HAT SHOP/Leotard: PINEAPPLE/Red scarf: FENWICK/Top: NAF NAF/Flowered scarf: FENWICK

HAIR DIET

If your hair's looking a lot less than healthy, it's worth taking a close look at your diet. Find out which types of food actually help your hair – after all, you are what you eat!

Your hair acts as a mirror reflecting the general state of your health. So if you have been ill, under stress, crash dieting, eating badly, or if you are pregnant or take the contraceptive Pill – these are all likely to take their toll on your hair.

You cannot change your hair's natural texture and the rate at which it grows by what you eat, but you can improve on what nature has given you by eating the right foods. A well-balanced diet should provide all your essential vitamins and minerals, but if you know your diet is erratic, try taking supplements.

For healthy hair (and good health generally) you need to eat a diet that also gives you protein, carbohydrates, fats, fibre, vitamins and minerals in the right quantities.

Liver remains one of the best things that you can eat for beautiful glossy hair. This is because it contains large amounts of vitamin A (essential for the proper functioning of the hair's sebaceous glands), zinc and B vitamins – all of which are very important for keeping the hair in really tip-top condition.

VEGETABLE MATTERS

For those who are vegetarian or don't like red meat, it's essential that the same vitamins and minerals are found in other foods.

Choose from eggs, potatoes, carrots, cabbage, citrus fruits, wholegrain cereals, wholegrain breads, pulses, spinach, nuts and oily fish.

But most importantly, enjoy your food – eating your way towards healthy hair shouldn't be a form of torture!

FOOD FOR THOUGHT

A healthy hair diet is pretty much common sense. For instance, those suffering from greasy hair should avoid eating greasy and fatty foods.

Similarly, having got your hair into a good state avoid alcohol and caffeine if you want to keep it in peak condition. No one should need reminding of the harmful effects caused by smoking, but if you must puff, at least take a multi-vitamin supplement to make up for the variety of vitamins that are destroyed by cigarettes.

It's not necessary to give up everything that's enjoyable, just cut down. Substitute herbal teas for tea and coffee and always add mineral water to alcohol, or opt for one of the many flavoured, bottled waters instead.

PUT IT RIGHT

PROBLEM	POSSIBLE CAUSE	WHAT TO EAT
Greasy Hair	*Over-active hormones/ eating too much fatty food.*	*Avoid all greasy food and grill or bake instead of frying. Eat plenty of fresh fruit and vegetables.*
Dry hair	*Over-use of heated hair appliances/not taking enough B vitamins.*	*Eat foods rich in B vitamins – wholemeal bread, brown rice, pulses, liver, bananas, nuts and oily fish.*
Dull hair	*Ill health/over-use of styling products like gel or wax/the Pill/ medication prescribed by doctor/smoking.*	*Choose foods rich in minerals – green vegetables, avocados, nuts, lentils, wholegrain cereals, shrimps, oily fish and milk.*
Dandruff/ Flaky scalp	*Stress/ill health/ build up of styling products on hair.*	*Cut down on dairy products – they can aggravate dandruff. Choose other foods rich in vitamin A – carrots, root vegetables, apricots, liver and fish.*

Illustration: BILL PIGGINS

DRY HAIR REPAIR

Is your hair so dry and damaged that the ends are breaking and it feels like straw? If so, don't despair, just follow our comprehensive conditioning guide

Hands up if you've been abusing your hair! You might have been doing it without even realising as there are a great many things that affect the condition of your hair. Check our list of hair tortures to find out why your locks are looking lack-lustre. Once you know where you're going wrong you can change your haircare routine to put back the shine. Whatever your hair type or problem there's a conditioning treatment to suit you.

CAUSE & EFFECT

If your hair is dry all over and you know you've not been treating it badly, then the cause is most likely to be a hormonal one where your body just doesn't supply enough natural oils to the hair. If the problem is very bad it may be worth asking your GP to refer you to a trichologist for specialist advice. The likeliest causes of dry hair are external factors: what you put on it, how you dry it and whether it's been chemically treated with a colour or a perm. But do remember, having dry hair doesn't necessarily mean it's dry all over. A very common complaint, especially for anyone with long hair, is an oily scalp and dry ends. Still, whatever your problem, you can help put the life back into your locks with our straightforward conditioning advice.

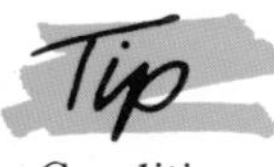

Conditioner can't mend split ends. The only way to get rid of them is to cut them off.

Conditioning Action Plan

Hair type	Every wash	Once a month	Products	Recipes
Greasy scalp with dry ends	*Cream or lotion conditioner on ends*	*Intensive conditioner with added heat*	*Dry ends cream*	*Yoghurt & egg conditioner*
Dry scalp with overall dry hair	*Cream conditioner all over*	*Hot oil massaged into scalp*	*Spray-on conditioner*	*Avocado & egg conditioner*
Over-processed hair	*Basic conditioner for chemically-treated hair*	*Hot protein treatment or henna wax*	*Restructurant lotion*	*Cocoa butter conditioner*
Flyaway hair	*Light lotion conditioner*	*Heavy cream conditioner*	*Rosemary oil*	*Yoghurt & egg conditioner*

WHAT MAKES HAIR DRY?

- Over perming.
- Too much chemical colouring.
- Over use of heated styling appliances.
- Brushing or combing your hair too roughly.
- Too much sun.
- Swimming in chlorinated or sea water without rinsing.
- Using too strong hairsprays and setting aids.

HOW CONDITIONER WORKS

Every hair on your head is covered in a series of overlapping scales. If your hair is in good condition the scales lie flat and smooth, light is easily reflected and the hair looks shiny.

If you treat your hair roughly these scales become ragged and your hair will look dull. Conditioner will help to flatten and smooth the hair surface and can go some way towards putting back lost natural oils.

BASIC CONDITIONING

This is everyday conditioning that you should do every time you shampoo. See our chart to find out which formulation best suits your hair. If you feel basic conditioning is all your hair needs, then follow the steps below.

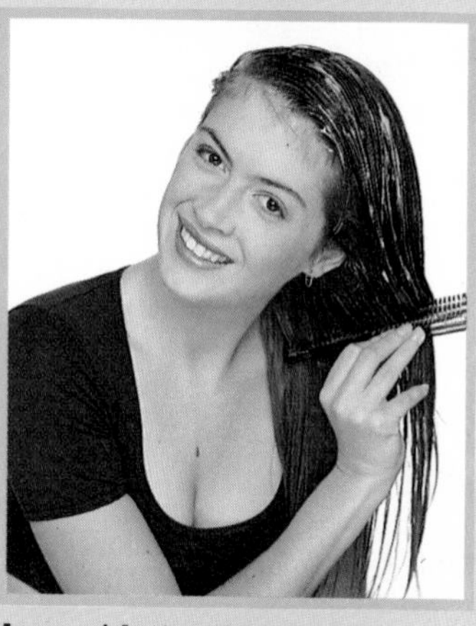

Use a wide-toothed comb to spread conditioner through your hair. If your scalp is oily, work in from the mid-lengths to the ends only.

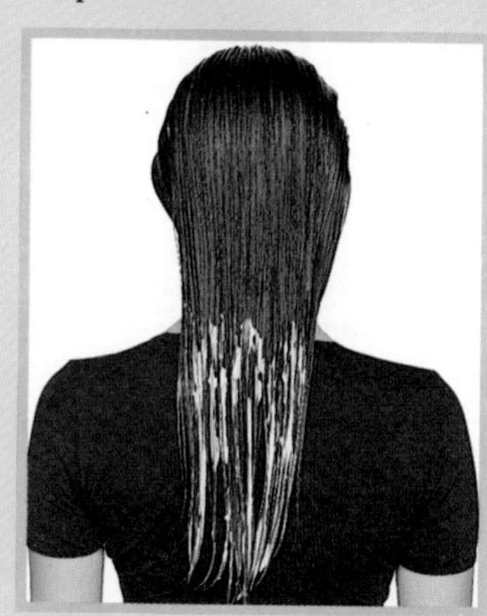

Long hair probably only needs intensive conditioning from mid-length to the ends – choose a dry ends cream and leave it on for 5-10 minutes.

Photographs: LIZ MCAULAY/Hair: LUKE at CAREY, TEMPLE MCADAM/Make-up: KARIN DARNELL/Black top: PINEAPPLE

DEEP HEAT

Intensive or deep-conditioning treatments have a slightly stronger action than basic conditioners, and can be used once a week on hair in poor condition or once a month for a general shine boost. These types of conditioners are available in cream, wax or oil formulations.

Using heat with a conditioning treatment will intensify the result. Wrap your hair in cling film and keep it warm with a hairdryer. This keeps the heat in and helps the conditioner do its job better.

CREAM CONDITIONER

Badly damaged hair can be restored by regular – about once a month – cream conditioning treatments. These are sometimes known as protein conditioners. Stand a sachet of cream conditioner in tap-hot water for a few minutes. Massage from your scalp to the ends of your hair, then comb the warm conditioner into your hair. Leave it for 10-15 minutes and keep it wrapped up in hot damp towels.

Alternatively, you can wrap a towel around your head while you're in the bath and let the heat rising from the steamy bathwater keep your hair warm.

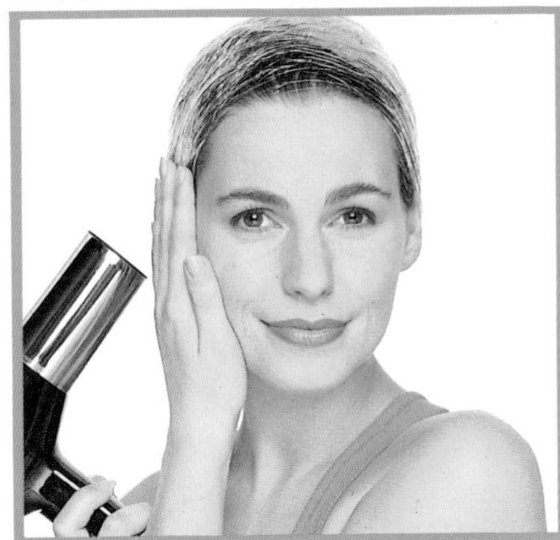

After washing, towel-dry your hair and comb a cream conditioner through from the roots to the ends. Smooth long hair onto the top of your head and wrap in cling film or kitchen foil. Set your hairdryer on low and dry over the cling film for two to three minutes. Unwrap your hair then rinse out the conditioner thoroughly.

SEALING WAX

Treatment wax is extremely good for dry and damaged hair. The heat makes the wax runnier, helping it coat each hair with a fine waxy layer. This helps correct dryness by sealing in the hair's natural moisture and protects your hair from the elements. The wax also smooths down the cuticles on each hair and leaves your hair looking thicker and shiny. You can be fairly generous with the amount you use – start with a good handful – as whatever your hair doesn't need will be rinsed off. Work in after shampooing and towel-drying, then wrap your hair in hot towels or cling film to keep it warm so that the wax can work more effectively. Leave on for at least half an hour and rinse off thoroughly with warm water using a shower attachment. Finish with a rinse of cool water to give your hair an extra shine.

AFRO HAIR

This is often very dry and coarse in texture so it needs lots of careful conditioning. The problem is caused by the difficulty natural oils produced at the scalp have in travelling down the curls – they usually only manage to get halfway so the ends in particular remain very dry and often look frizzy. Treat Afro hair like over-processed hair with a rich, effective conditioner.

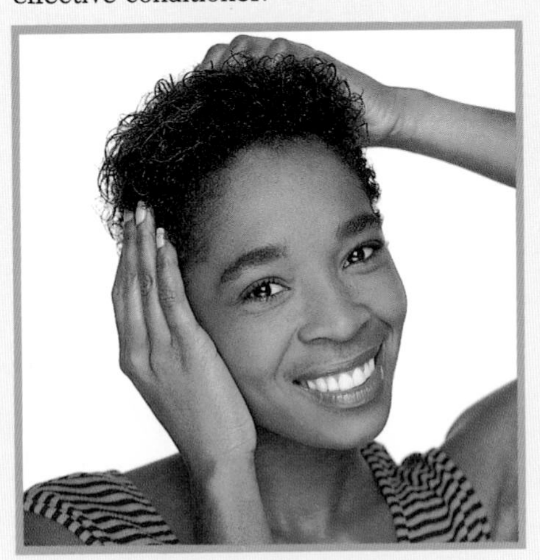

Oil treatments are especially beneficial to Afro hair. Give your scalp a treat at the same time by massaging thoroughly with oil then smoothing through to the ends with your fingers.

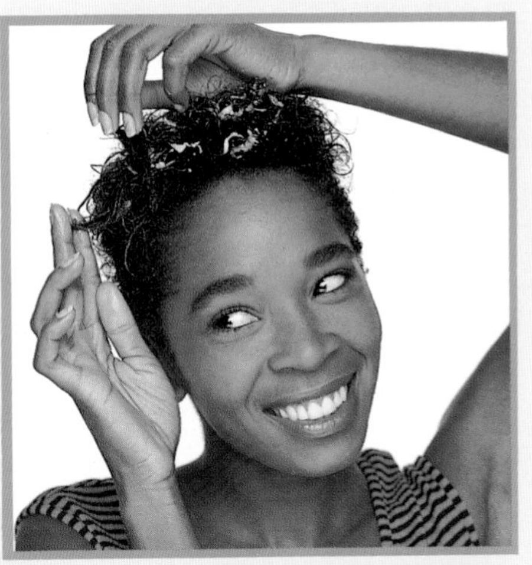

Dry ends cream will help tame Afro hair. Twist it into the ends and then leave for 10-20 minutes. Wrap hot towels around your head if you've time, then shampoo off with a gentle or frequent-use shampoo and rinse your hair thoroughly with warm (not hot) water.

Watchpoint

Although you may think Afro hair looks coarse and strong, the individual hairs are actually finer than Caucasian hair – it's the curl that makes them appear thick. The hair can be very brittle after relaxing or straightening, so take extra care when conditioning.

NATURAL REMEDIES

Yoghurt & egg conditioner – *for oily or flyaway hair.* After shampooing, whisk together 5 tbls natural yoghurt and 1 egg and massage into the scalp. Leave on your hair for a few minutes then rinse out thoroughly.

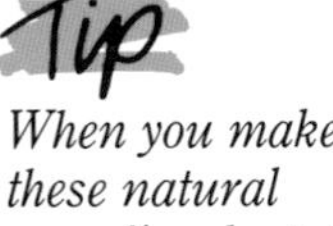

When you make these natural remedies, keep them in the fridge and use up within two days.

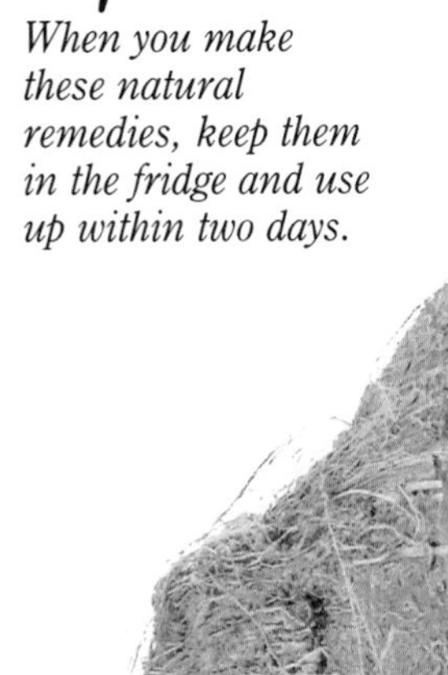

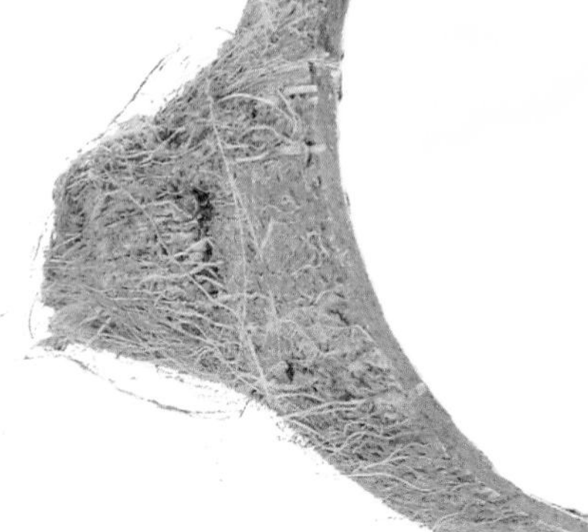

Wrapping your head in a warm towel or one that's been wrung out in hot water is a way of intensifying the effects of a deep conditioner.

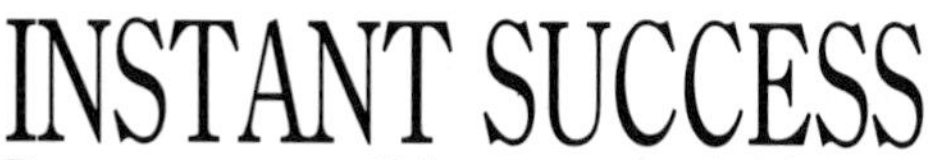

INSTANT SUCCESS

Put spray-on conditioner on towel-dried hair before styling and don't wash it out. It's ideal as a quick pick-me-up for your hair when time is short. In between shampoos use on dry hair for a shine boost, concentrating the conditioner on the damaged parts of your hair. For an instant healthy sheen, use a spray-on shine product on freshly washed and styled hair. These aren't really conditioners in the traditional sense, but take the form of a very light oil in a spray.

Always be sparing with your spray conditioner, especially if your hair has a tendency to be lank or greasy.

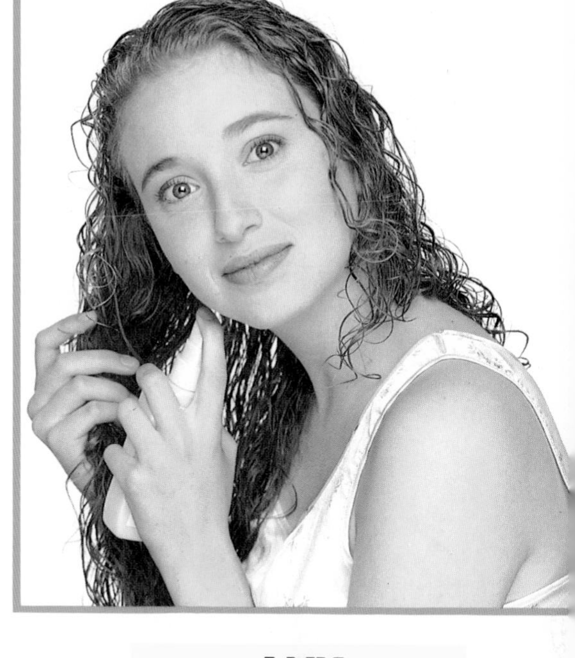

Avocado & egg conditioner – *for dry hair.*
Blend together 2 tbls avocado oil, 1 tbls castor oil and 1 egg. Massage into your hair then comb through. Wrap your head in a warm towel and leave for 30 minutes. Shampoo and rinse with warm water.

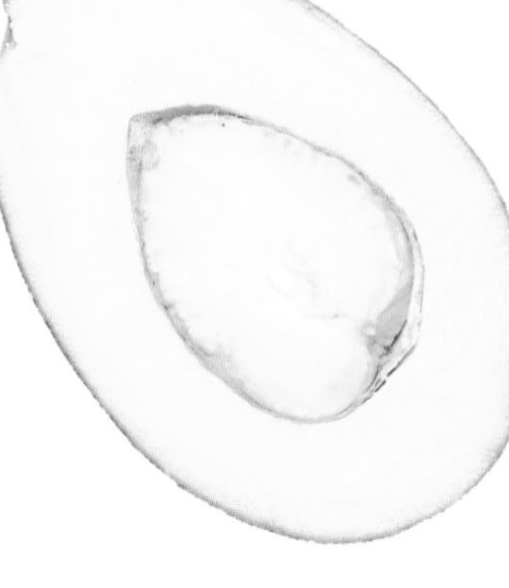

Egg & coconut oil conditioner – *for all hair types.*
Heat 2 tbls coconut oil. Then add 1 beaten egg and 1 tbls vinegar. Massage it into your hair while still warm. Keep your hair covered for 30 minutes with a steaming towel, then shampoo and rinse.

Tip

Adding a few drops of rosemary or lavender oil to your hairbrush before brushing your hair will add gloss and help to prevent static.

Cocoa butter protector – *this protects your hair while you are in the sun. It's also good as a conditioner for chemically treated and Afro hair.*
Melt 1 tbls cocoa butter, 1 tbls lanolin (both available at the chemist counter) and 4 tbls olive oil in a double boiler and beat together when melted. Add 1 tbls water to 3 tbls mixture before putting on your hair. Shampoo off when you've finished sunbathing.

LAST-MINUTE RECIPES

- **Any leftover home-made mayonnaise makes a good hair conditioner.**
- **A liquidised avocado massaged into your hair works well as a conditioner.**
- **Use the yolk of an egg for a quick protein treatment.**

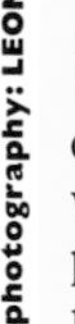

ANY QUESTIONS?

Q My hair is quite oily but the ends are dry and splitting. Why is this?

A You're probably using too many heated appliances such as curling tongs, hot brushes or heated rollers on your hair. Save them for occasional use only. Use a lower setting on your dryer too and let your hair dry naturally as often as possible.

Q Can you over-condition your hair?

A Yes, if you don't rinse it out thoroughly. You can use conditioners on your hair every day, but failure to rinse well will make your hair look lank and heavy.

Q I'm going on a beach holiday soon and I always find that when I'm away my hair gets very dry. What can I do to prevent this?

A Slick your hair back with a special suncare hair conditioner or wear a hat when you're in the sun to prevent it drying out. Always rinse sea water out after swimming as the salt will dry your hair.

Pink top: PINEAPPLE/Pink and white vest top: NEXT

THINK YOU'VE GOT DANDRUFF?

People know less about dandruff than almost any other hair problem. But the good news is that 95% of all people who think they've got it, haven't. Our expert explains...

WHAT IS DANDRUFF?

Real dandruff is a medical condition where the skin's cells are over-produced and it is always accompanied by irritation. It results from a disturbance of your normal bodily function and comes in two different forms: dry and greasy.

Dry dandruff looks whiter than greasy; if it's greasy the flakes will look yellowish and may have an unpleasant smell.

Many things cause dandruff, such as worry, stress and a bad diet. You usually develop dry dandruff in cold weather, and greasy dandruff when it's warm. If you really have got dandruff (and remember that most people who think they have, haven't), the bad news is that it's not curable. But the symptoms (flaky bits and irritation) are easily dealt with and can be kept permanently under control.

DRY SCALPS

The scalp is like a loaf of bread. The two top layers form a crust, and flaky bits of skin break off just like crumbs. When most people see flaky specks of skin, they automatically assume they've got dandruff. But if you think you've got dandruff, you're more likely to be suffering from a dry scalp, and dry skin conditions are quite easy to cure. Most people who think they've got dandruff are in fact experiencing a normal, and healthy, process. The cells in your body are continuously replacing themselves, and they shed dead cells in the process.

You've probably read about this exfoliation process happening to the skin on your face. Well, it happens all over your body – including your scalp. In normal conditions, you won't notice the process at all, but as with dry skin on your face, it does show up if your scalp is dry.

WHAT IS THE CAUSE OF A DRY SCALP?

Sometimes people suffer from a dry and flaky scalp when they're not eating properly, or when they use hair styling products in the wrong way, or choose ones that aren't suitable.

If you use a lot of styling products, like gel, mousse or spray and you don't wash them out properly, that could cause a build-up of dried product and loose bits of skin.

Regular, careful washing, an improvement in diet and oil-based conditioning treatments should clear a dry skin condition in a matter of weeks. Just follow our PUT IT RIGHT plan and you can't go wrong!

You can catch dandruff from other people's brushes and combs. MYTH

FACT Dandruff is not contagious. It's a condition that comes from within your body, which means it's impossible to catch from someone's comb.

Washing hair too often makes flaky scalps worse. MYTH

FACT Provided you use the right shampoo and rinse your hair thoroughly, washing won't worsen your condition – it'll probably help it. Choose a gentle, mild shampoo without any chemical additives – dandruff shampoos contain harsh minerals and chemicals and can often worsen the condition not improve it. Use cool water for your final rinse.

A good scrub will get rid of the flakes. MYTH

FACT Even though it's good to wash your hair often, it's vital to shampoo it very gently. If you do have dandruff it means that your scalp is irritated and very sensitive. What it needs is delicate handling, using mild, frequent-wash products that will soothe.

Children are more likely to get dandruff than adults. MYTH

FACT You're more likely to have dandruff in your early twenties, than at any other time in your life. In fact, children very rarely suffer from the condition at all.

PUT IT RIGHT

DRY SCALPS

●Don't scratch, rub or comb your hair vigorously. Be sure to wash out styling products the day you use them. Avoid using harsh products on your hair.

●Use a mild shampoo and wash your hair at least three times a week.

●Only shampoo once and massage it into your scalp. Don't leave the lather on your hair for long.

●Rinse your hair VERY thoroughly.

Follow the tips above for 28 days and if your scalp is still flaky or irritated you could have dandruff. (Consult your doctor to find out.) There are no miracle cures, but these things may help:

●Use a dandruff shampoo that contains tar, zinc, pyriothine or selenium sulphide twice a week.

●Use a nettle rinse to stop the itching. Put a handful of nettles in 300ml/½ pt of boiling water and leave to cool for 10 minutes. Strain and add a dash of vinegar or cider vinegar to the water. Use this as a rinse.

●Cut down on cheese and dairy foods. Tuck into fresh fruit and vegetables.

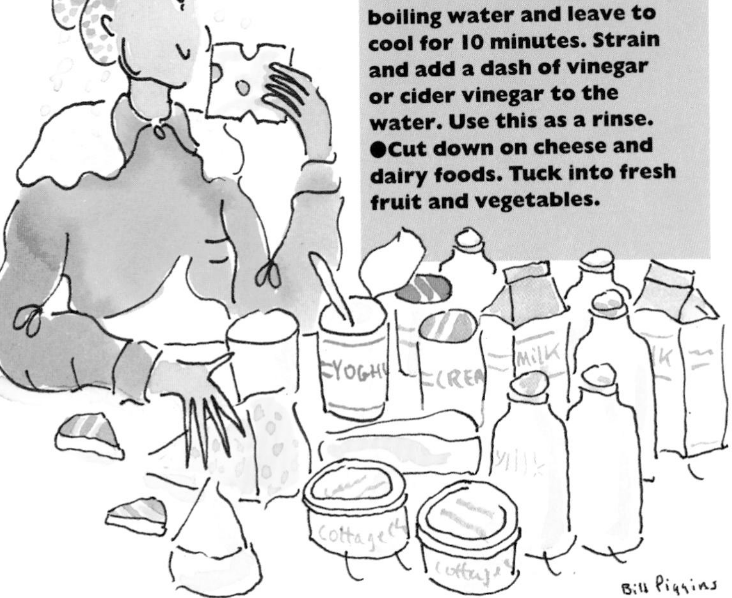

Illustration by BILL PIGGINS

HAIROBICS

Believe it or not you can actually improve the condition of your hair through exercise. So shape up and get your hair working out for a change

Regular exercise doesn't just benefit your body and mind. In fact, by stimulating the blood supply, which carries vital nutrients to your scalp, you'll also help to promote healthy new hair growth. And the better the condition of the hair coming out of the follicles, the more able your hair will be to withstand the stresses and strains of its everyday life. You'll also find that reducing stress and muscle stiffness benefits your hair by improving your general health. So give lacklustre locks a treat with our hairobics routine beginning with a good warm up.

CIRCULAR SOOTHER

Benefit: Relaxes muscles in the neck and eases tension.

► To help increase the blood circulation in your neck, sit up straight, gently drop your head onto your chest and relax the muscles in your shoulders. Slowly lift your head up and make a semicircle from shoulder to shoulder first looking to your left and then to your right. Repeat in each direction ten times.

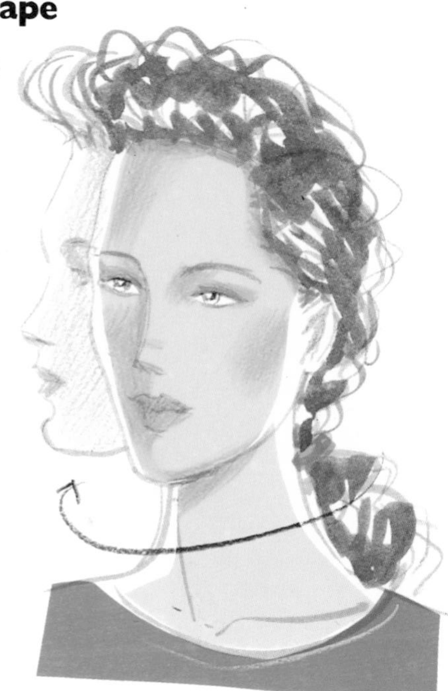

SHOULDER SHRUG

Benefit: Reduces stiffness at the base of the neck.

◄ This is another way to ease tension build-up in your neck. Kneel on the floor, sitting back on your heels. Put your hands on your waist and shrug your shoulders up and down, then backwards and forwards. Repeat 25 times. Make exaggerated circles with your elbows five times to relax every part of your shoulders too.

WARM UP

◄ Before you take part in any kind of exercise routine it's a good idea to warm up. Start off by doing some simple twists, bends and stretches. Then gently jog on the spot for a couple of minutes, arms by your sides. Then raise your knees up as high as possible and land lightly on your feet. Keep your breathing regular and even – when concentrating on exercise it's easy to forget!

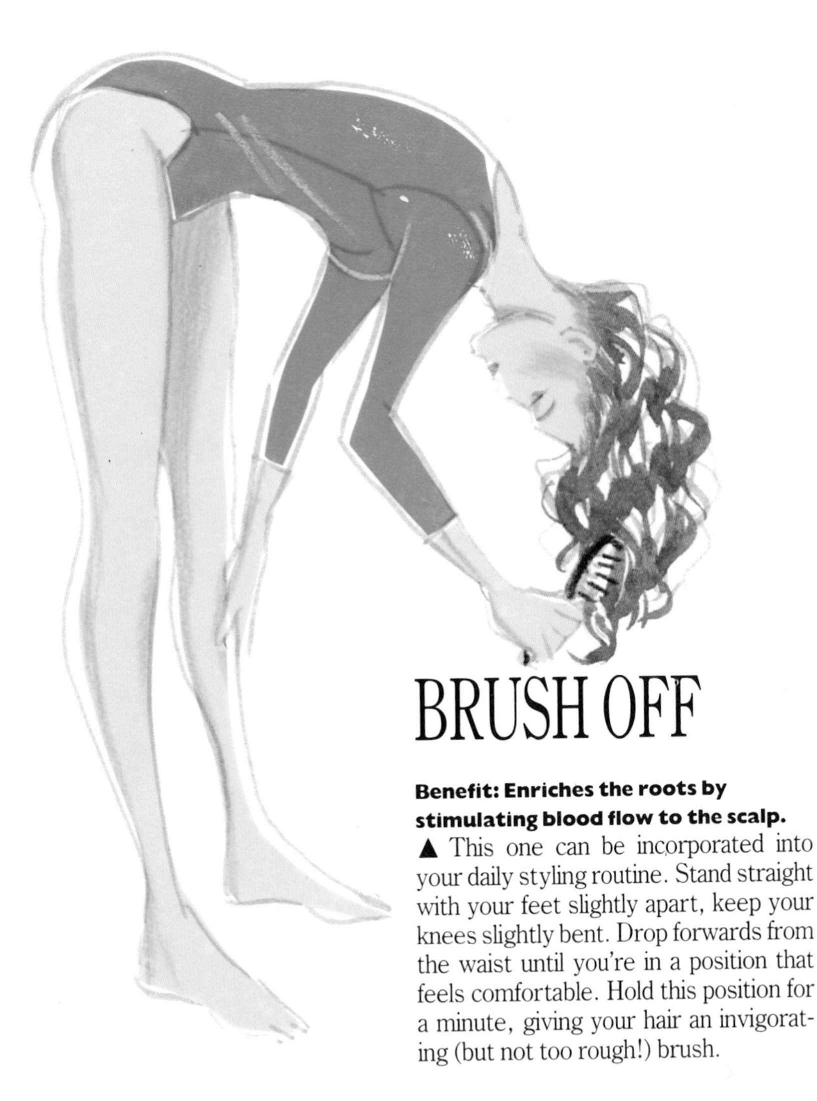

BRUSH OFF

Benefit: Enriches the roots by stimulating blood flow to the scalp.
▲ This one can be incorporated into your daily styling routine. Stand straight with your feet slightly apart, keep your knees slightly bent. Drop forwards from the waist until you're in a position that feels comfortable. Hold this position for a minute, giving your hair an invigorating (but not too rough!) brush.

MASSAGE MESSAGE

Benefit: Reduces tension in your neck and your shoulders.
► There's no better way for relieving tension in your neck and shoulders than by having a soothing massage. Get someone to gently knead away aches and pains at the end of a long, hard day. Sit or lie down comfortably during the massage with your eyes closed. Try to empty your mind of everything other than feeling relaxed, and put some soothing music on.

Try both of these techniques in turn for instant stress relief:

- Use a deep, kneading movement with the fingertips and the palms of the hands, making sure the hands stay relaxed.
- Make a rhythmical drumming movement with the fingertips over tense areas, but keep the touch light.

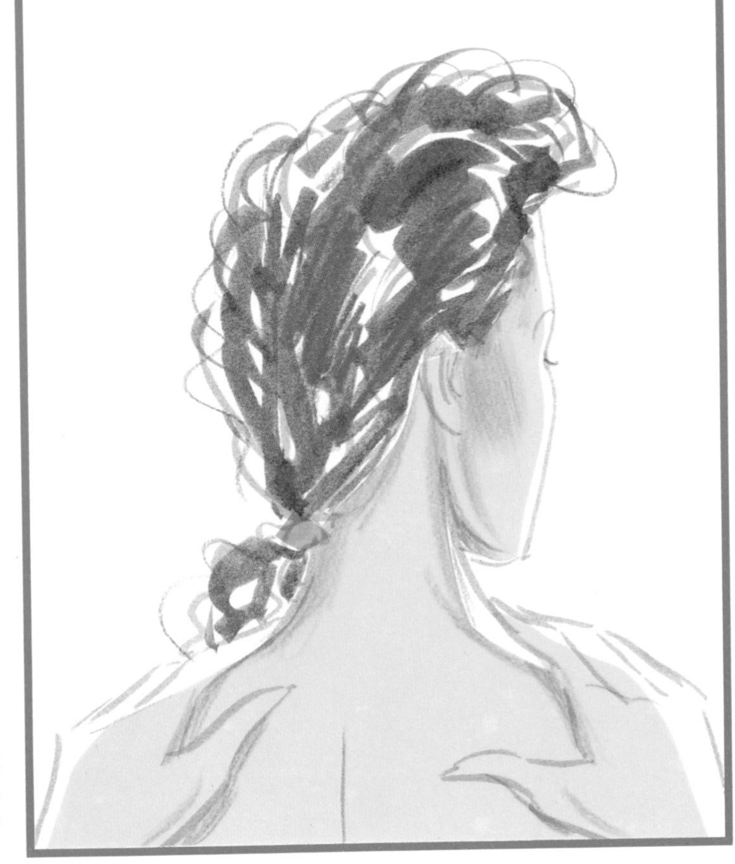

HEADS DOWN

Benefit: Improves circulation which in turn nourishes roots.
▲ For maximum effect with the minimum amount of effort sit on a chair and lower your head between your knees. Once you feel comfortable, and your back isn't strained, put your hands on your knees and hold this position for two to five minutes.

To prevent hands dragging on the skin, put a little baby oil or aromatherapy oil on your fingertips before you begin for a smooth massage.

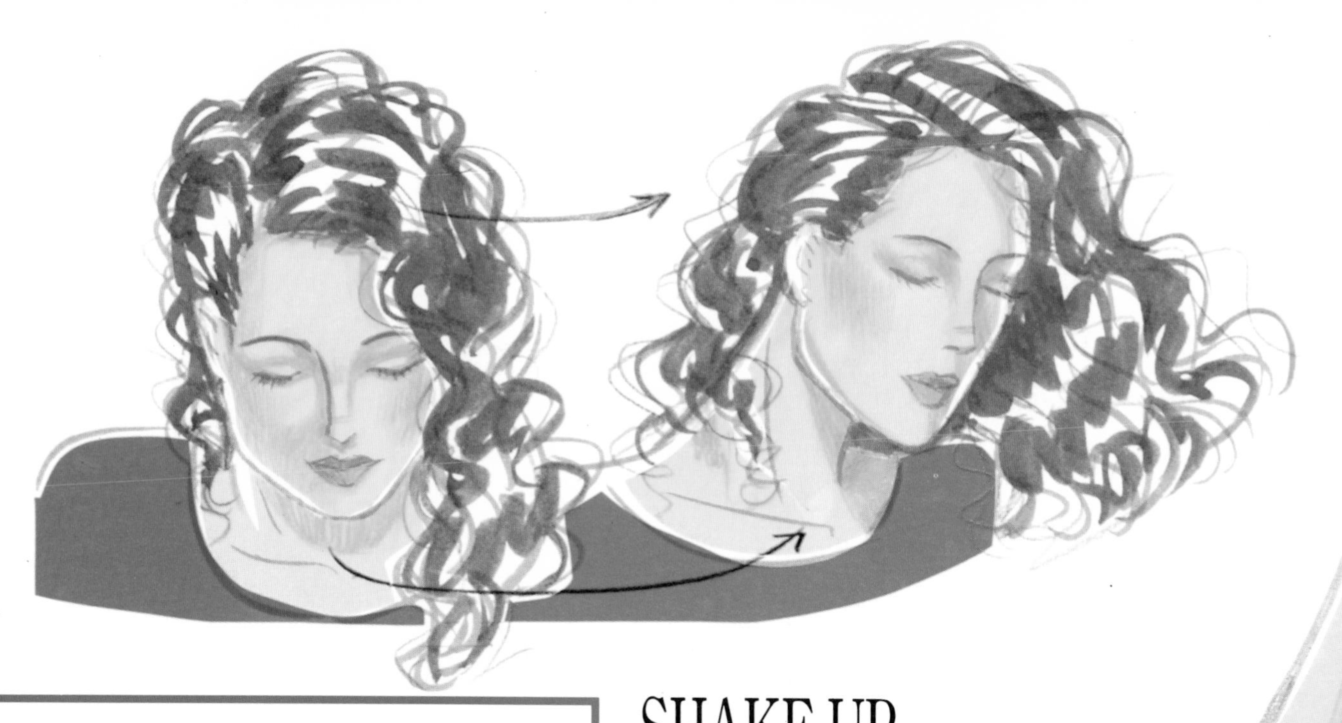

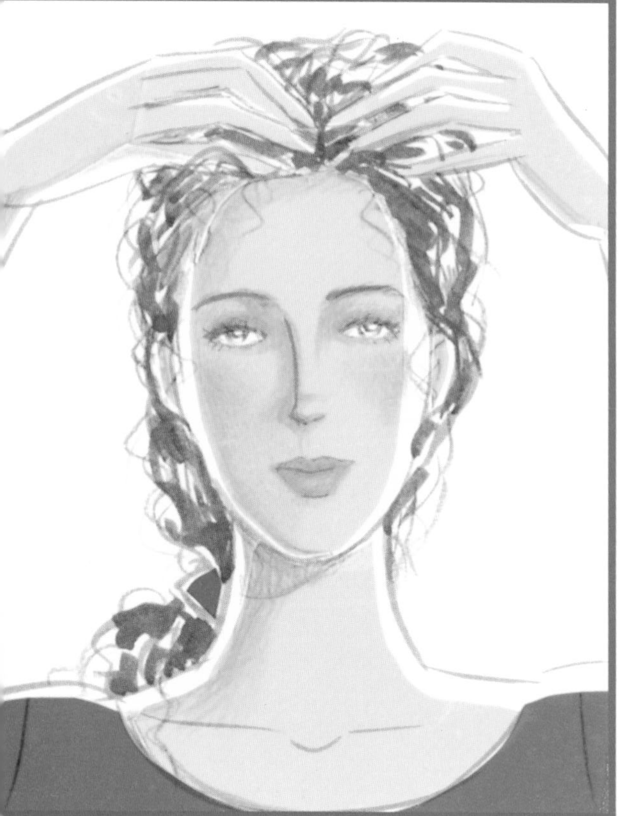

SCALP STIMULATOR

Benefit: Encourages the flow of oxygen and blood to the hair follicles.

▲ Tension in your scalp can lead to dull, lifeless hair. Whenever you feel nervous or uptight give your scalp a quick massage. Start at the front of the head by pressing your fingertips firmly against your scalp. Move the scalp gently back, forwards and in a series of circles but don't actually move your fingers. Repeat the process all over your head. Alternatively, you can incorporate the massage into your shampoo routine.

SHAKE UP

Benefit: Loosens stiff, tense neck muscles.

▲ To get your hair glowing, give your head a gentle shake then sit straight, shoulders back, and slowly tilt your head as far as you can from side to side. Take care not to make any sudden, jerky movements. Repeat ten times, then relax. Now tip your head slowly back until you're looking at the ceiling, bring your chin slowly down to rest on your chest. Repeat ten times.

HEAD FIRST

Benefit: Quickly sends blood to your scalp.

► A minute spent standing on your head should get you tingling all over. Put a cushion on the floor about one foot away from a wall. Swing your legs up against the wall to help you balance and use both hands to support you.

Watchpoint

Stop exercising immediately if you begin to feel dizzy, light-headed or any muscles start to feel strained.

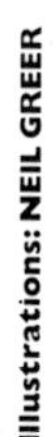

HEAD DOCTOR

Don't worry about a scalp or hair problem – just head down to your nearest trichologist and quickly get to the root cause . . .

A trichologist is to your hair and scalp, what a chiropodist is to your feet. In other words, someone who specialises in the scientific study and treatment of hair and scalp problems. Many people are unaware of the benefits of trichology. This could be because hair/scalp problems don't actually cause physical pain and are often perceived as cosmetic complaints. But a trichologist can help and the prescribed treatment may be something as simple as making adjustments to your diet or the products you're using on your hair.

HAIR SAY

Finding a reputable trichologist isn't always easy. Ideally your doctor should be able to recommend a good one. But if you have no personal knowledge of where to go, be on your guard for someone who promises a free (and generally extremely quick) initial consultation and then tries to sell you all manner of fancy lotions and potions.

A reputable trichologist will ask you to pay for the initial diagnosis, but should then take up to an hour and a half to examine you and note the details of your lifestyle, diet, family history, medical history and what products you use on your hair. This information is vital because it can pinpoint whether your complaint is the result of illness, stress, poor diet, or even pregnancy.

If your problem can be treated by counselling, or changing your diet or haircare habits, the trichologist probably won't book you in for any more visits and that means that you pay for *one* only.

COMMON SENSE CARE

In a way, good trichology is as much about common sense practices as it is anything else. For instance, following the most basic haircare habits like keeping your hair clean (a flaky scalp is very often caused by nothing more than a build-up of dead skin cells or styling products and these can quite simply be washed and rinsed away); not using heated styling appliances on your hair too often (these can make the hair brittle so it just snaps off); and of course keeping healthy and eating sensibly. A trichologist can tell by looking at your hair whether you've been crash dieting, missing meals, or if you're anorexic.

HAIR TODAY . . .

In the past few years, despite the fact that most of us have become aware of the value of eating well and looking after ourselves, trichologists have reported more young career women suffering from hair loss. It is the most common complaint they are asked to deal with and is the result, they argue, of women having to cope with more stress and responsibility in their lives. This has led to an increase of the production of the male hormone androgen in the female body, so women are starting to lose their hair in a way that has previously only affected men. Most female hair loss (unless it is an inherited characteristic) is temporary. It could be that you've been working hard, skipping meals and are now slightly anaemic. Alternatively it could be depression or stress that is causing your hair to drop out. Whatever it is, the trichologist will prescribe the most effective treatment and, all being well, you'll have a full head of hair again in about three months.

HAIR SCARES

Some top hairdressing salons actually employ a trichologist, who is consulted if the salon is in any doubt about perming or colouring hair that's in poor condition. But there aren't many of these salons and it's a sad fact that there are unscrupulous people who'll go ahead with a perm without checking what sort of state the hair's in. So you could end up with damaged hair. If the salon is uncooperative and refuses to do anything about putting your hair right, then make an appointment to see a good trichologist and explain what has happened. Your hair and scalp will be closely examined, the details of the damage noted and photographs taken too. The trichologist will then advise you if you have sufficient grounds to sue.

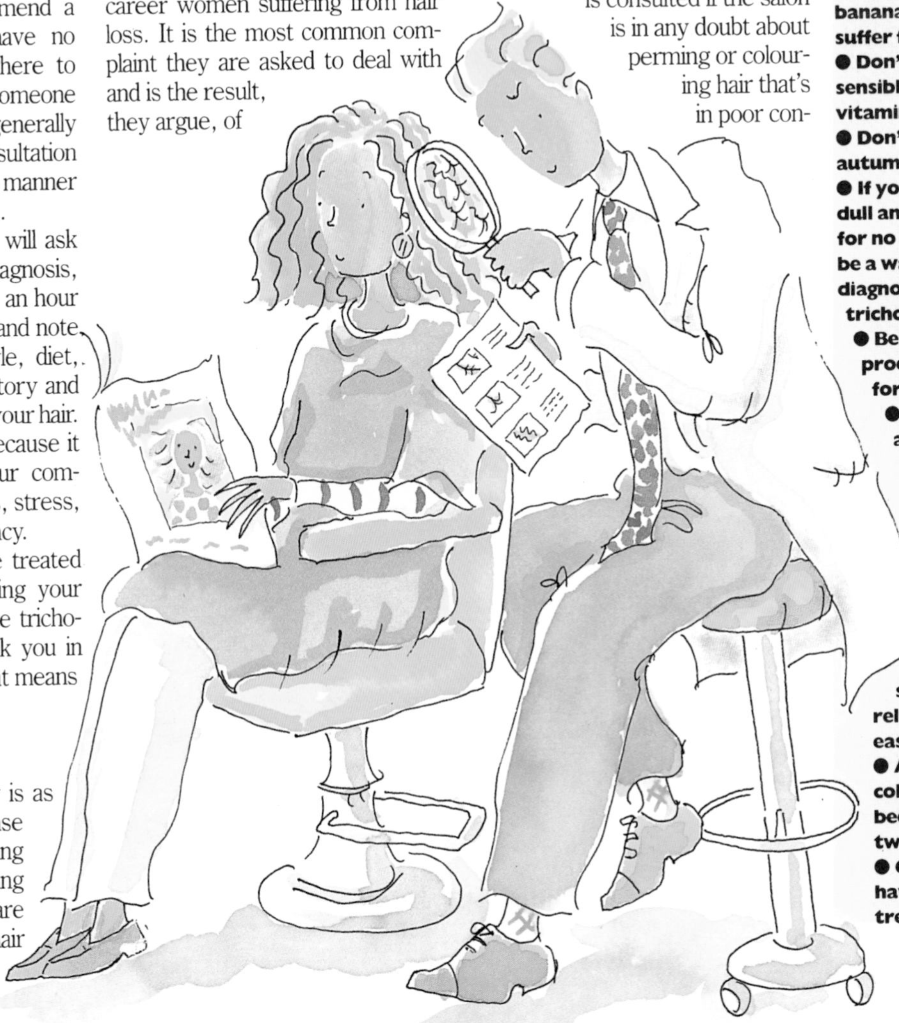

KEEP A CLEAR HEAD

There's a lot you can do to keep your hair and scalp in good condition and prevent disorders:

- **Eat a well-balanced diet.**
- **Avoid dairy produce, nuts, bananas and fatty foods if you suffer from a scaly scalp or dandruff.**
- **Don't go on crash diets. Plan sensible low-calorie menus and take vitamin or mineral supplements.**
- **Don't worry if you lose hair in autumn, it's a normal seasonal loss.**
- **If your hair suddenly becomes dull and dry, or excessively greasy for no apparent reason, this could be a warning. Get an accurate diagnosis from an expert – a trichologist or GP.**
- **Be gentle with your hair. Buy products that are formulated for your hair type.**
- **Don't use heated styling appliances too often. They dry out hair and make it brittle and look dull.**
- **Don't use metal or fine-toothed combs.**
- **Always protect your hair in the sun. Wear a hat or scarf and use products with sunscreens.**
- **Regularly massage your scalp gently to stimulate and relax it (this can also be good for easing headaches).**
- **Avoid having your hair coloured if it feels dry and has been permed during the last two weeks.**
- **Get your hair trimmed and have a deep conditioning treatment regularly.**

With thanks to GLENN LYONS at the PHILIP KINGSLEY TRICHOLOGY CLINIC, London/Illustration: BILL PIGGINS

STEP-BY-STEP

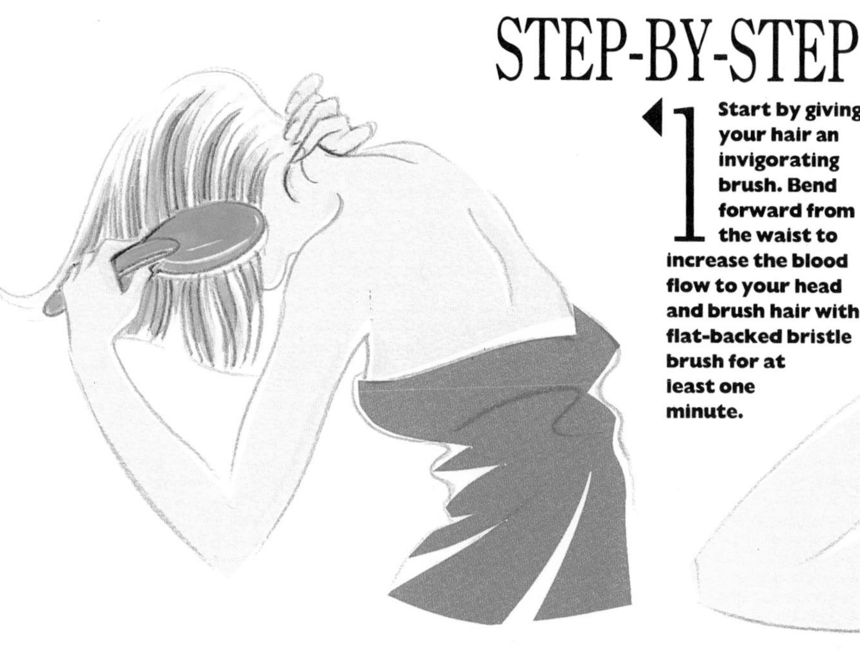

1 Start by giving your hair an invigorating brush. Bend forward from the waist to increase the blood flow to your head and brush hair with a flat-backed bristle brush for at least one minute.

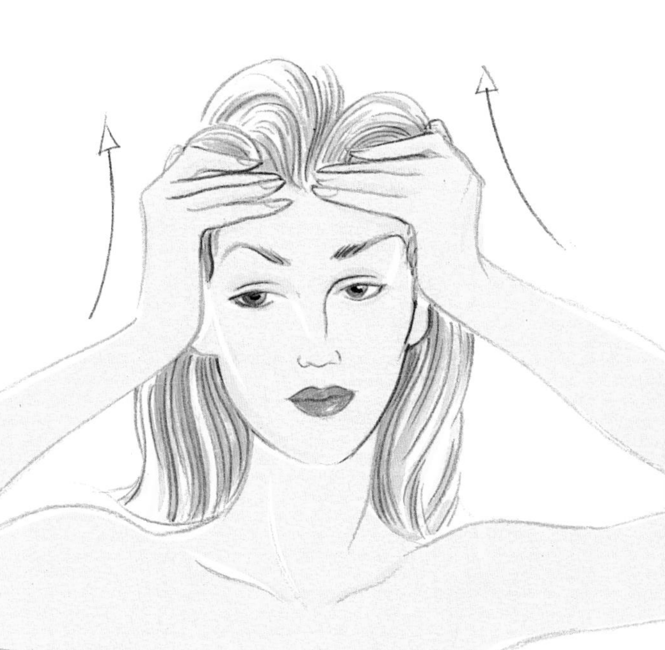

2 Keep your head lowered and run your fingers through your hair from the roots to the ends as quickly as you can. Repeat several times. Your scalp should start to tingle gently.

3 Return to an upright position. Stroke your scalp upwards by placing the fingertips on either side of the head just in front of the ears. Push up to the top of your head until your fingers touch. Repeat this movement all around your head.

GET THE MASSAGE!

Get to grips with your scalp and put your hair through its paces with this easy-to-do massage. Give it a glow!

If your hair's looking dull and lifeless, what it probably needs is a bit of exercise! After all you probably keep your body in trim but how often do you think about giving your hair a work-out?

The best way to exercise your scalp is by massage. Just a few minutes once a week will make a noticeable difference to the look of your hair since massage increases the circulation to your scalp bringing nutrients, oxygen and beneficial hormones to the hair follicles. It can even make it grow faster. But don't expect the results to show on your hair as it is – it will only affect the new growth.

An added bonus is that you'll stroke away the tension that can cause headaches. Include the back of your neck and forehead too and you'll feel the full benefits.

HEAD START

If you've got dry hair you can combine the massage with a nourishing oil treatment. Work a teaspoon of warm olive or almond oil through your hair before you start to massage. The warmth from the massage will help the oil to penetrate the cuticle (outer layer) of the hair. Shampoo your hair afterwards to remove the oil. If your hair's normal then try the massage alone just before you shampoo.

Watchpoint

Oily hair can be made worse by massage. To counteract this, massage while you shampoo and keep your movements light.

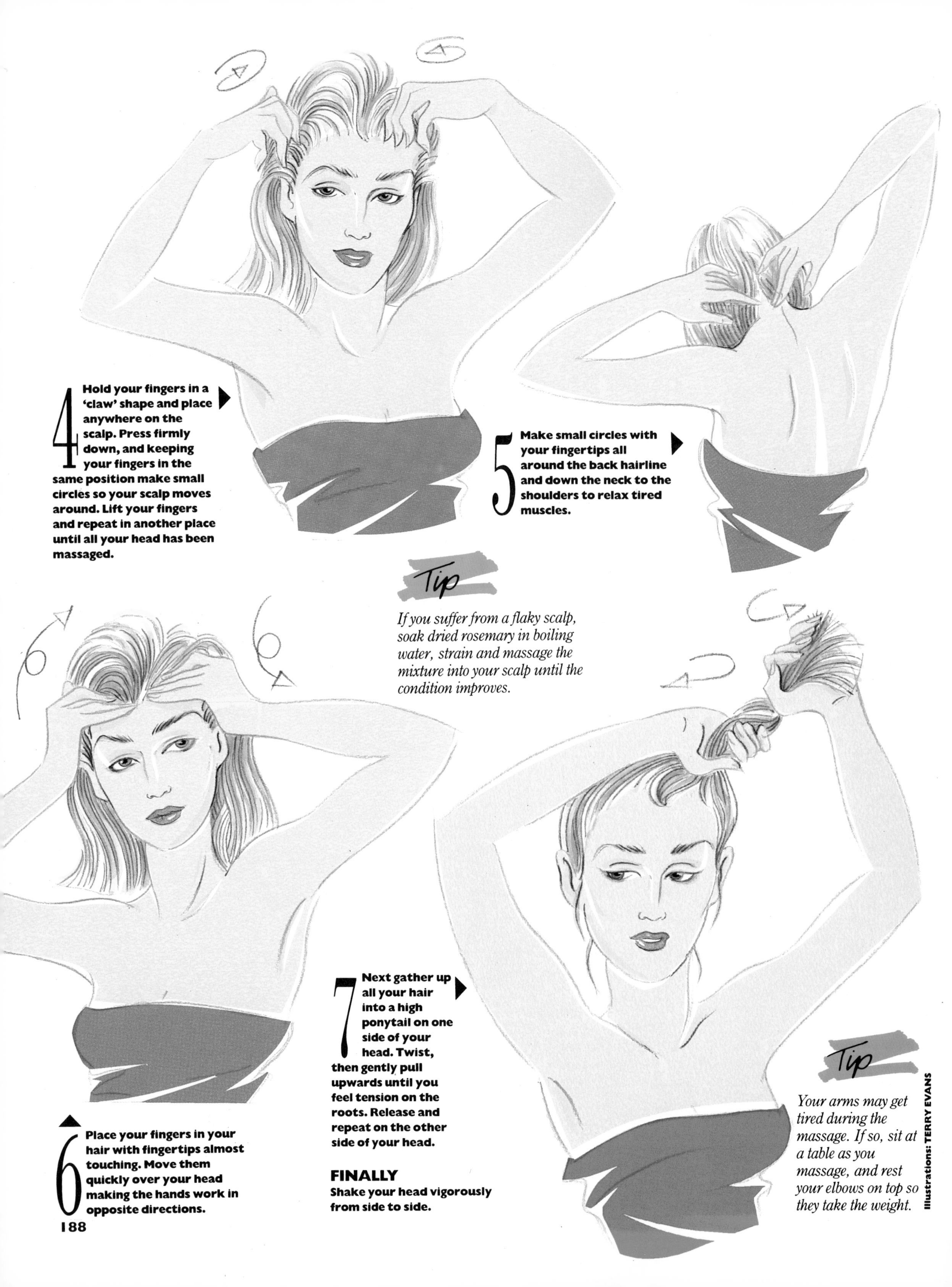

4 Hold your fingers in a 'claw' shape and place anywhere on the scalp. Press firmly down, and keeping your fingers in the same position make small circles so your scalp moves around. Lift your fingers and repeat in another place until all your head has been massaged.

5 Make small circles with your fingertips all around the back hairline and down the neck to the shoulders to relax tired muscles.

Tip

If you suffer from a flaky scalp, soak dried rosemary in boiling water, strain and massage the mixture into your scalp until the condition improves.

6 Place your fingers in your hair with fingertips almost touching. Move them quickly over your head making the hands work in opposite directions.

7 Next gather up all your hair into a high ponytail on one side of your head. Twist, then gently pull upwards until you feel tension on the roots. Release and repeat on the other side of your head.

FINALLY
Shake your head vigorously from side to side.

Tip

Your arms may get tired during the massage. If so, sit at a table as you massage, and rest your elbows on top so they take the weight.

Illustrations: TERRY EVANS

KEEP YOUR HAIR ON!

If your hair's coming out in handfuls and you're starting to look more like your balding uncle than a bouncy-haired beauty then read on and get right to the root of the problem

First of all – don't panic! Worrying about losing your hair will only make things worse and since 90 per cent of all women's hair loss is only temporary, it's probably not as serious as you think. Every hair has a life cycle of its own which ends with it falling out to make room for a new one. At any one time only about 80 per cent of your hairs are growing. The growing phase lasts for two-six years, and the length of time your hair takes to grow will determine the length you can grow your hair. This explains why some people can grow very long hair while others can't get their hair past their shoulders. The other 20 per cent of your hairs have stopped growing and go into an inactive period of around three months before finally falling out.

HOW MUCH HAIR LOSS IS NORMAL?

It's perfectly normal to lose 50-100 hairs every day. This sounds like a lot until you realise that we have a total of between 90,000-150,000 hairs on our heads. Normally we don't even notice losing the odd 100 if we shampoo and brush our hair daily, but if you've got an easy-to-wear hairstyle and style your hair less often you may be taken by surprise at just how many hairs are left behind in the bristles. The longer your hair is, the more you'll notice the loss because the length makes it look more in the brush. But this is only normal. If you are seriously losing your hair you will notice a loss of over 10-50 per cent of the hairs on any one area of your head.

QUICK CHECK

Make a quick diagnosis of the possible cause of your hair loss by looking closely at the roots of the hairs where it's thinnest:

- If the ends are blunt – your hair is breaking off rather than falling out and you need to look at the general condition of your hair. For instance have you had a perm recently? Over-processed hair is more susceptible to breakage.
- If the ends are tapered – your hair has been falling out from the roots.

LOSS CAUSES

There are several common causes of hair loss. Dieticians believe that lack of vitamins B and C and the minerals zinc, iron and sulphur may be prime causes, and so it follows that crash diets can often result in more hair loss than weight loss.

Severe shock is another common cause of hair loss, with the fall occurring about two weeks after the traumatic event. Stress, too, can cause hair to fall, but worrying about it will only make the condition worse.

Menstruation, the Pill and pregnancy also have their contribution to make. A temporary loss of hair can happen around the time of your period, due to hormonal imbalances. If you begin taking the Pill and notice that you're losing your hair, check with your doctor or clinic. It can affect hair growth in some people. But pregnancy causes the most noticeable hair fall of all. During the whole period of pregnancy your levels of the hormone progesterone are very high and this prevents the normal cycle of hair loss. After the birth when your levels drop back to normal all the hairs that should have fallen out during the pregnancy fall out all at once. You can lose up to 30,000 in the course of a few weeks.

Long or short-term illness almost always has an adverse effect on hair, as do some drugs and medical treatments. Check with your doctor if you notice any loss. Alopecia is a disease that results in complete hair loss either in round patches or all over. This is a specific medical condition and must only be treated by a doctor or trichologist.

WHAT YOU CAN DO

- Massage – can help to stimulate the blood supply to the scalp – in fact, it's usually the massaging rather than lotions that gets the hair growing again. Keep your fingers in a claw-like position and press with the pads of your fingertips in small circular movements.
- High frequency treatments, using an electric current to promote hair growth, can be helpful as they will help to stimulate blood supply to the scalp. Check at your local registered hairdressing salons or trichology clinics.
- Step up your mineral and vitamin intakes. Take some extra vitamin E, brewers' yeast and wheatgerm, for example.
- Use gels, setting lotions and mousses as a temporary way of getting your hair to look thicker. Special hair thickeners are also available which work by slightly swelling the hair at the shaft.
- Keep your hair in as good condition as possible to avoid any further complications. Keep away from perms and colouring and do your best to prevent your hair from drying out.
- Keep your hair in a short layered style until it gets thicker. If your hair is long, remember that the weight will pull it flatter on top making it look even thinner.
- Check your combs and brushes aren't doing any further damage. Avoid combs that are too fine and always comb your hair very gently.
- If you're feeling very self-conscious about excessive hair loss, try adding a fake hairpiece, like a ponytail or bun, to give the impression that you've got more than you have. But do be extremely careful when attaching hairpieces as the grips and pins can pull out fragile hair.

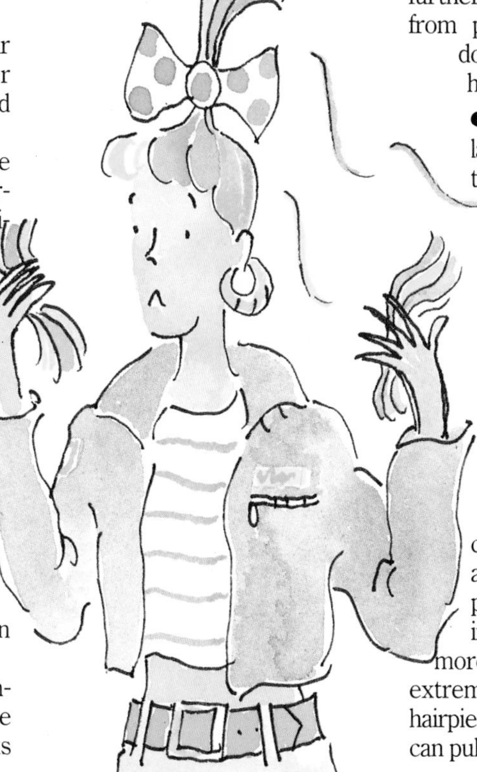

Illustration: BILL PIGGINS

HAIR HELP CLINIC

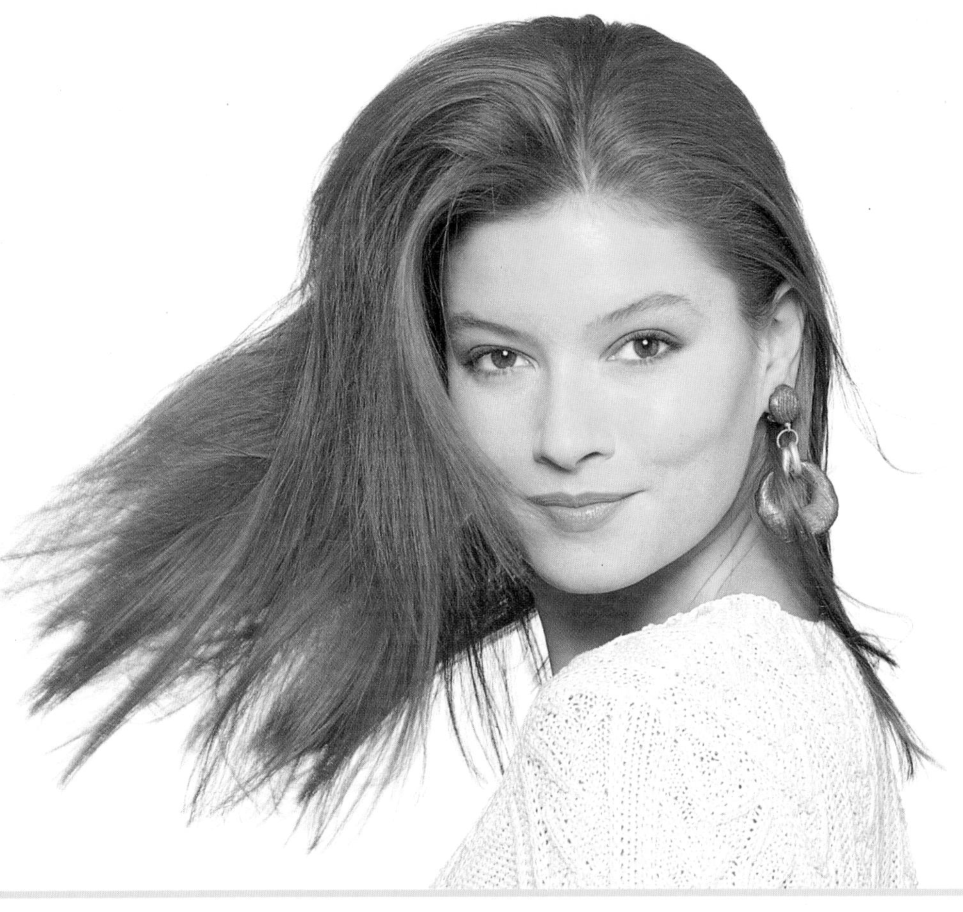

SUNSILK

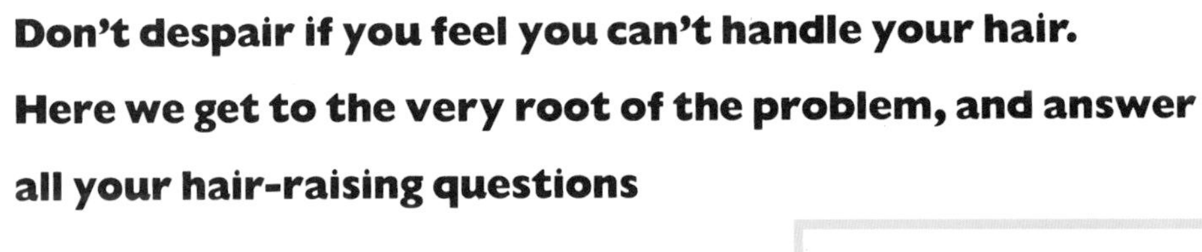

Don't despair if you feel you can't handle your hair. Here we get to the very root of the problem, and answer all your hair-raising questions

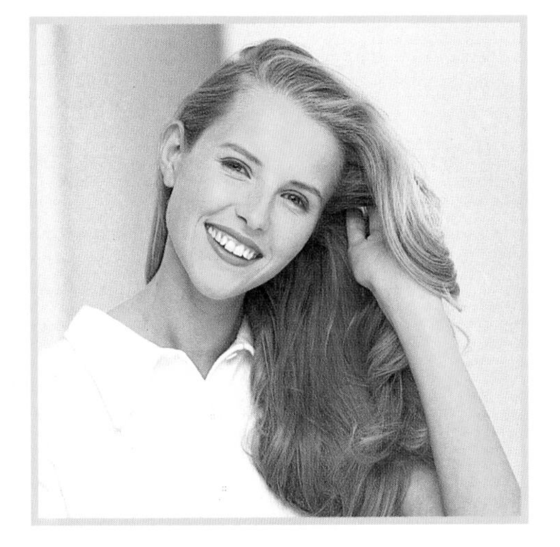

Q I've tried endlessly to grow my hair long, but it always seems to stop when it reaches a certain length. Why is this?

A On average, hair grows about 12 mm/½ in each month, slowing down to about 6 mm/¼ in per month when the hair reaches a length of about 25 cm/10 in. Some will find their hair grows faster than this, others may have a slower growth rate. But the growing phase of your hair varies too. For some people, hair grows for a minimum of two years before it falls out. For others, the growing phase lasts up to seven years.

So the combination of a slow growth rate and short life span means you may never be able to grow your hair very long. You can't extend these factors although it's important to keep healthy if you want a head of hair that will grow to its potential. So make sure you eat a balanced diet. Also condition your hair regularly. Even though it doesn't grow very quickly, don't miss out on going to the hairdresser. Regular trims will stop it looking straggly.

Q I noticed something called panthenol was one of the ingredients in a conditioner I bought. What is it and what does it do?

A Panthenol is a derivative of vitamin B5. It is often added to hair-styling products such as gels, spray gels and mousses as well as conditioners because it helps maintain moisture in your hair, leaving your locks stronger.

Q Mum often asks me to wash my little sister's hair. It always ends in tears. What can I do?

A You can buy a shampoo shield which is like the brim of a hat. Just pop this on her head and lather up without the water and shampoo running onto her face.

You'll find them in shops selling baby care products. But children's hair doesn't get very greasy so you only need a mild baby shampoo. This shouldn't sting as much as adult shampoos.

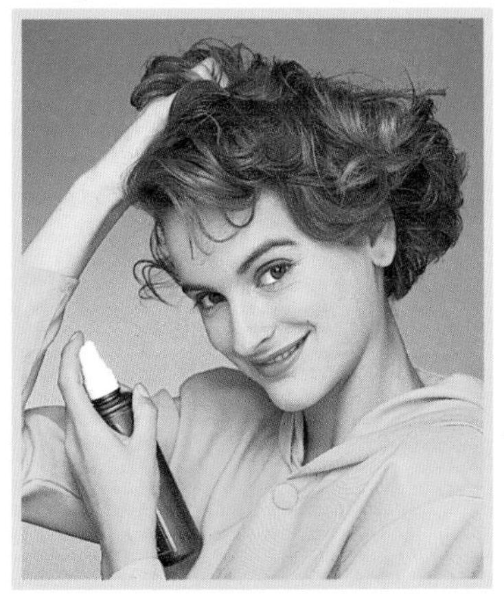

Q I'm pregnant – I was thinking about having my hair permed. Is it okay to do this?

A Yes, it's perfectly safe to have a perm when you're pregnant but the results can be unpredictable and the perm may not take. Although the hair you can see is dead, the growing part is under the scalp and can be affected by your hormones.

My boyfriend's hair is beginning to thin already. Can he do anything about it at all?

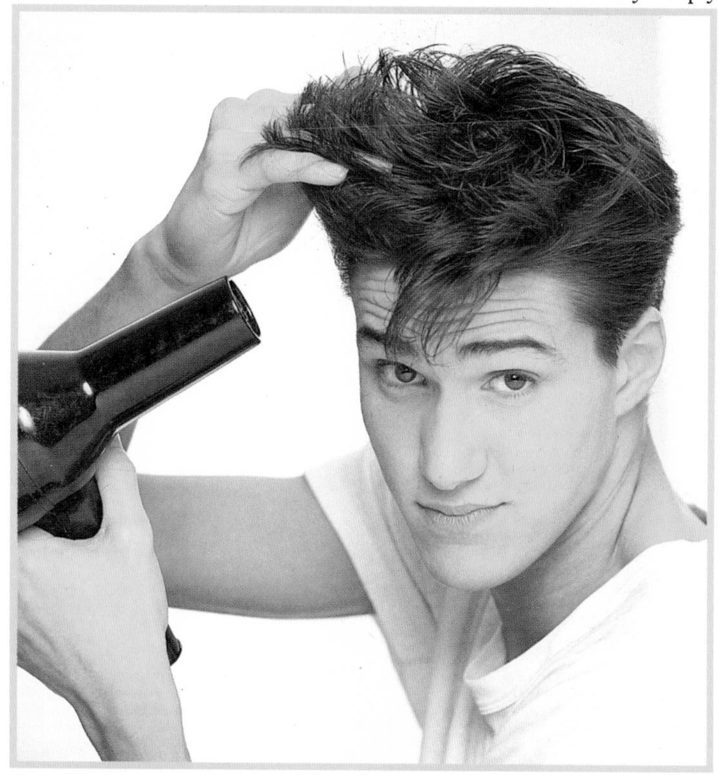

This is a problem men have worried about for centuries and in the past treatments have been bizarre, such as rubbing in bear grease and bird droppings. And still in this age of scientific advancement, there is no real cure. The pattern of baldness is usually inherited and the best advice you can give your boyfriend is to get a good haircut and to ring the changes with mousse, gel and blow-drying.

So many men make the mistake of trying to grow what little hair they have and then trying to use this to disguise the bald patches, usually unsuccessfully. Persuade him against a toupee or hair piece as they can look unnatural and can even have an ageing effect. Hair transplants tend not to be a good idea either, as many men who go through these operations are unhappy with the results. Your boyfriend may also be tempted by the many products on the market claiming to slow down hair loss. Some of these work on the principle that they stimulate the blood supply to the scalp providing essential nourishment to the growing hair follicles, but he can do this for free by simply massaging his scalp with his fingers for a few minutes each day. Other products contain ingredients which plump up the hair shaft so that thin hair looks thicker. Those formulated especially for men tend to be pricey and a straightforward inexpensive body-building shampoo and conditioner can do the job just as well.

Finally, he may have heard of a drug called Minoxidil. A small percentage of men have achieved a degree of hair growth using this but it's only available on prescription and is very expensive. You have to use it all the time – and it doesn't help in every case.

I was looking at a new shampoo which said it conditioned as well. How can it do this?

It's all highly technical but basically the product contains negatively and positively charged molecules. The shampoo molecules detach dirt and grease and are then washed away when you rinse your hair, while conditioning molecules have the opposite effect, and attach themselves to the hair which improves the shine and helps protect it. The conditioning molecules in a two-in-one type shampoo are larger than usual so that the shampoo can't 'attack' them and cancel them out.

These all-in-one products are designed to save time and take up less space. However, some people find they get a build-up of conditioner on the hair after prolonged use which eventually can dull the hair and leave it lank and lifeless. Try keeping two-in-one products for occasional use only such as when you're in a hurry or for holidays. And the rest of the time stick to a separate shampoo and conditioner.

My friend said that if I keep my hair in a ponytail it will start to fall out. Is this true?

Your friend has probably heard of traction alopecia which is a type of hair loss caused by mistreatment that weakens the hair so it falls out or breaks. Causes for this include over-rigorous brushing or hairstyles where the hair is pulled taut at the roots and forced against the natural direction of growth. You can, however, wear your hair in ponytails and plaits if they're not tight and your scalp doesn't feel uncomfortable.

My scalp itches and flakes. Is it dandruff and what can I do to prevent it?

Many people who suffer from an itchy, dry scalp presume that they've got dandruff when in fact the condition is likely to have been caused by other factors. One of the most common culprits is insufficient rinsing of shampoo. Make sure you use a mild shampoo and use a shower attachment afterwards to get your hair and scalp squeaky clean. Similarly, avoid harsh chemical treatments, such as perming and colouring. If the problem doesn't clear up, book an appointment with a trichologist who can analyse your scalp to check for real dandruff and carry out tests to see if you are allergic to anything. A poor diet, lacking in B group vitamins (found in green and yellow veget-

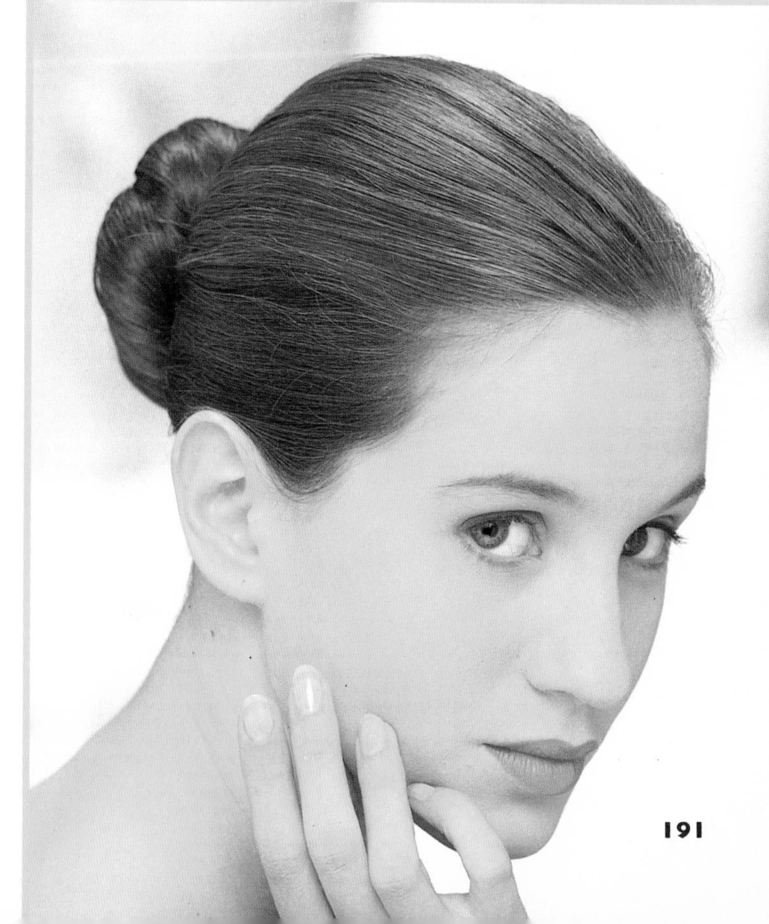

ables, yoghurt, nuts, yeast and wholegrains) is another possible cause. Boost your intake for a healthy scalp and also try a gentle massage to stimulate the hair's blood supply. Insufficient brushing and a sunburnt scalp can also cause itchiness and flakiness.

Q I'd really like to have my Afro hair straightened permanently. Can this be done easily?

A Yes, but only if your hair is healthy. And it's not advisable if your hair is in poor condition. Strong chemicals are used and the hair is pulled straight so the treatment makes hair weaker and very fragile.

Tip

Don't forget to ask your hairdresser's advice on hair care when you go along for an appointment. It's all part of the service and you can pick up some expert tips for free.

Q I dyed my hair and the new colour just doesn't suit me. Is there anything I can do?

A Your best bet is to ask for help from your hairdresser who may be able to sort out the problem using products only available in the salon. Or, you could try disguising or toning down the colour yourself by putting semi-permanent colourant on top. Go for a shade close to the one you have already to avoid an even worse colouring calamity. Semi-permanents simply coat the hair with colour and wash out after about six to ten washes so have less drastic results than permanent colourants which actually penetrate the hair and last until the hair grows out. Read the instructions first to check that the semi-permanent can be used on hair that's already been coloured.

In future, when tinting or lightening do a strand test first to ensure that you're going to be happy with your new hair colour. And always leave the product on for the specified time.

ELIDA GIBBS

Q My perm is starting to fall out and I only had it done a few days ago. What should I do?

A You should go back to your hairdresser and demand the problem is put right. This may mean reperming, if your hair is in good enough condition, but you shouldn't be charged for it. Meanwhile, if it's not possible to have your hair repermed you'll have to make the most of it. If you've long hair, it's best to wear it in a ponytail, French pleat or chignon. Alternatively, you could set it on heated or bendy rollers – at least the small amount of perm in your hair will give the curls more holding power and body than if your hair was dead straight.

Q Since having my baby, my hair seems to be falling out. I'm worried I might end up bald!

A There's a very simple explanation for this and you can rest assured it's highly unlikely you'll end up bald! Basically, each hair goes through three phases. The growing phase, the resting phase, then the fall-out phase. When you're pregnant, hair tends to remain in the growing and resting phases for longer, which is why many expectant mums say their hair is thicker and more luxuriant than usual. Then it goes through the falling-out phase two to six months after the baby is born. So the hair you're losing is only what you would normally have lost over a period of months rather than weeks had you not been pregnant. Because it is falling out rapidly now, it may seem like an extraordinarily large amount, but really your hair is just getting back to normal.

Tip

If you're unsure about choosing and using any hair care product, colourant or perm at home, then don't hesitate to write to the manufacturers for advice and any useful fact sheets.

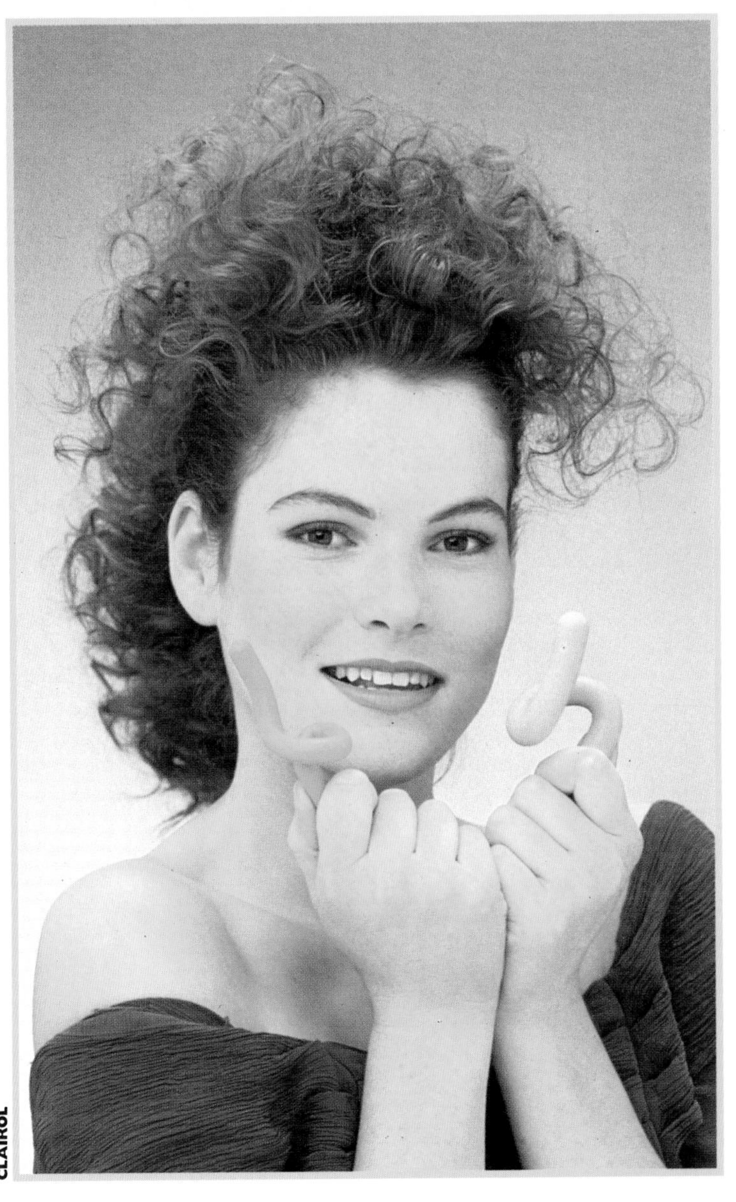

CLAIROL

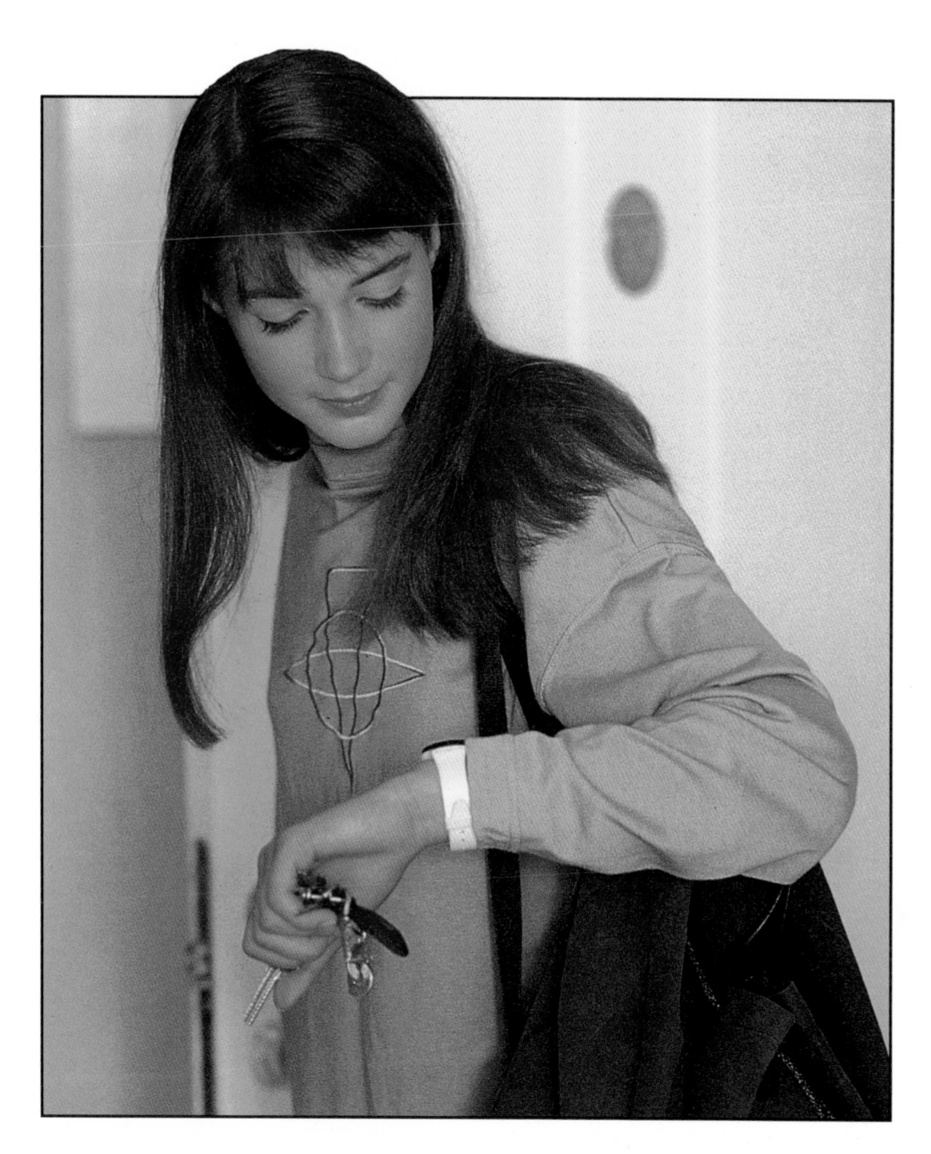

CHAPTER SEVEN

The Lifestyle File

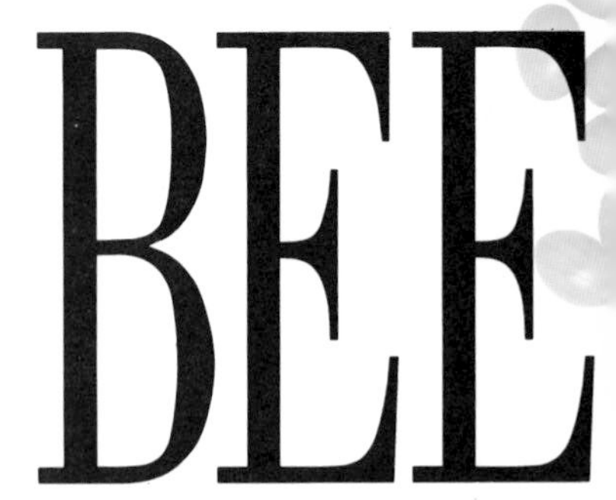

The humble bumble bee provides all sorts of products which can give your looks a boost.

Check out these natural goodies and get buzzing with health and vitality

Royal jelly is the substance worker bees feed to the queen to make her fat and fertile. Many people believe it can work wonders for the human body too, alleviating a wide variety of ailments ranging from acne and abnormal blood pressure to varicose veins, although many take royal jelly supplements simply as a general tonic. They say it helps them fight stress and fatigue and ward off illness. It's even got a reputation as an aphrodisiac!

Unfortunately, there's little scientific evidence to back these claims. However, we do know that royal jelly is rich in nutrients, particularly amino acids which make up the proteins which are essential for maintaining a healthy body, B vitamins important for healthy skin and many minerals including iron.

There's also a mysterious four per cent of the composition of royal jelly that defies analysis, so this could hold the secret to its supposed health-giving and healing properties.

You'll find face creams containing royal jelly and it is possible that its cocktail of nutrients has a beneficial effect when applied directly to your skin, but don't expect it to be any more magical than other moisturisers.

POP A POLLEN PILL

Pollen hasn't had as much publicity as royal jelly, yet it also contains a good balance of nutrients. It's been claimed that pollen supplements can strengthen your immune system, help alleviate flu and hay fever symptoms, rheumatism and arthritis and have a general rejuvenating effect. Athletes often take it believing it keeps them super fit, so if you've been feeling under the weather lately it may be worth trying pollen supplements. Fans have reported improvements in their hair, nails and skin, and even bigger, firmer boobs!

HONEY – GET STUCK IN

In some parts of the world there are communities where the inhabitants live well into their nineties and beyond and their long life has been attributed to the fact that they consume large quantities of honey.

But before you start dipping into the honey pot, remember that most of the honey we buy from the supermarket has been heat-treated and filtered, so much of the essential pollen and precious nutrients are lost.

What you're left with is hardly even a healthy alternative to white sugar. The only difference is that honey is made of more easily digested sugars which are absorbed more quickly by the body so you get a quicker boost of energy. Honey also contains small amounts of B vitamins and minerals such as iron, copper, manganese, sodium, potassium, calcium and phosphorous, required for healthy growth, maintenance and repair of tissues and bones. It has 20 calories per level teaspoon, slightly more than sugar which has 17 calories per level teaspoon.

If there are any health benefits to be gained, you need to buy a honey containing small amounts of pollen. This may be difficult to find, but as a general guideline a pure honey should be better than one which states it's a blend from several different countries.

Make a beeline for farm shops or hunt down a local beekeeper. You'll also find some health food shops sell honeycomb which is a good way to get honey in its most natural form – although the bits of beeswax are rather chewy and not very appetising. Because bees make honey from the nectar they gather from flowers, flavours vary depending on the plants they feed on.

PRECIOUS PROPOLIS

Propolis is the resin bees make from the buds and barks of trees which they then use to seal their hives and protect themselves against invaders such as mice or germs. It serves as their all-purpose disinfectant and if an intruder such as a mouse does get in, they sting it to death then embalm it with propolis! The ancient Greeks and Romans used propolis as a healing ointment and it's also reported to have been used in the Boer War.

Propolis appears to improve our immune system, helping us ward off illnesses and kill infectious organisms. You can buy propolis tablets and capsules or try these:

- Propolis tincture: useful for dabbing on spots to help them clear up.
- Propolis salve: rub it on stiff, swollen or painful joints and muscles for a pain-killing effect.
- Toothpastes with propolis: its antibacterial action is said to help prevent mouth infections and tooth decay.

However, about one person in every 2,000 is sensitive to propolis. To test yourself, rub a little on the inside of your wrist. If the skin becomes red and puffy, don't use propolis products.

THE HEALING POWER OF HONEY

For thousands of years, honey has been valued not just for its taste but because it also has remarkable medicinal and cosmetic properties.

- **It has antiseptic and antibacterial qualities. The Egyptians used it as a preservative when embalming dead bodies.**
- **It's moisturising and extremely soothing.**
- **When applied to the skin, honey has a 'drawing' action so helps deep-cleanse impurities and unplug blackheads.**
- **Burns and wounds heal faster when treated with honey.**

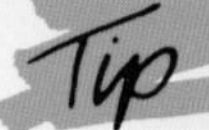

A teaspoon each of honey and lemon juice in a cup of hot water soothes a tickly, sore throat. Or, if you're suffering with a cough and cold, just crush about four fresh cloves of garlic and soak them in ½ lb of honey for a day or two. Take a teaspoon every three or four hours.

A RIGHT ROYAL CURE

Some people swear that regularly taking royal jelly has improved or completely cured:

- **Acne – the B group vitamins and C found in royal jelly capsules can improve the condition of the skin and when combined with vitamin E in cream-form, royal jelly is known to help clear up acne.**
- **Cystitis – vitamins B and C both help to ward off this bladder infection.**
- **PMT – take a royal jelly and Oil of Evening Primrose capsule for 10 days before your period to beat the blues.**

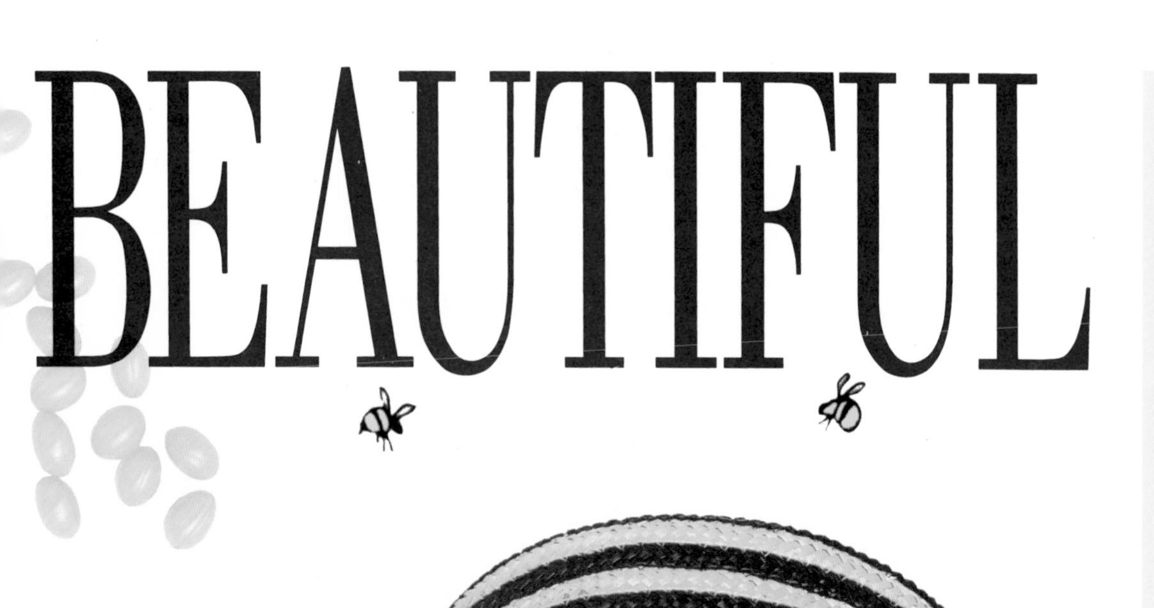

SWEET TREATS

You'll find plenty of toiletries, from moisturisers to cleansers to bubble baths and soaps, made with honey. Combinations such as milk and honey baths, or oat and honey scrubs look tempting but there's no legislation to ensure that these products contain any significant quantity of honey. The alternative is to make your own cosmetics. Here are some simple recipes:

FAST FACIAL

This deep cleanses and nourishes. Mix 2 tbls honey with ½ tsp lemon juice or cider vinegar if you have oily skin, or 1 tsp vegetable oil such as almond if you have dry skin. Apply to cleansed skin, leave for 15 minutes before rinsing off with tepid water.

WHEATGERM SCRUB

This removes dead skin and softens blackheads. Mix 2 tbls clear, runny honey with 1 tbls wheatgerm. Rub this mixture over cleansed skin, then rinse off with plenty of tepid water. Pat face dry gently.

CLEANSE-ALL

For oily skin. Mix 3 tbls runny honey with 2 tsp lemon juice, 2 tsp cider vinegar and half a whisked egg white. Massage into skin, then rinse off with tepid water.

CUTICLE CONDITIONER

Blend 2 tsp beaten egg yolk with 2 tsp almond or olive oil and 2 tsp honey. Massage into nails and cuticles. Leave on overnight.

HAIR CONDITIONER

Mix ½ cup olive oil with 1 cup runny honey. Massage into your hair. Wrap head in a warm towel and leave for an hour before shampooing out.

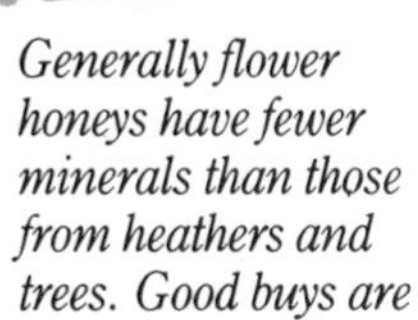

Generally flower honeys have fewer minerals than those from heathers and trees. Good buys are heather honey from Scotland, British willowherb honey, Australian and Hungarian honeys.

Photographs: JAMES HOBSLEY/Still-life: STEVE CABALLERO/Hair: PAULA MANN/ Make-up: KIZZY HARRISON/Hat: THE HAT SHOP/Top: PINEAPPLE/Earrings: REX INTERNATIONAL/Bees: TRIDIAS

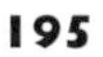

SUPPLEMENTARY BENEFITS

Put a spring in your step and a sparkle in your eyes with the right vitamins and minerals

Did you know that biting into a juicy tomato can help keep wrinkles at bay? Or that polishing off a glass of milk promotes shiny hair? It's all down to the power of vitamins and minerals, a collection of substances you just can't live without.

Despite the fact that you need only tiny amounts of them – in powdered form, the recommended daily allowance of each vitamin would only just cover your thumbnail – vitamins and minerals play an important part in almost every bodily function, governing how your body is built, the way you use food for energy and even your state of mind.

VITAL VITAMINS

Each of the vitamins we need has a specific role to play – here's what they do and where to find them:

Vitamin A looks after your eyes, fights infections, and helps keep skin young-looking and smooth. Good sources: red and green vegetables, eggs and apricots.

Vitamin B which is actually a group of substances usually found together, promotes healthy skin and hair, fights fatigue and helps you deal with stress. It can be found in meat, bread, eggs and cheese.

Vitamin C maintains young-looking skin and helps the body heal itself. Oranges, grapefruits, blackcurrants, tomatoes and leafy green vegetables are some of the best sources.

Vitamin D helps build bones and teeth. The body produces this vitamin when it's exposed to sunlight, but it's also found in dairy products and oily fish.

Vitamin E keeps the blood system healthy, and helps the body to build new cells. It's also thought to help prevent skin ageing. Good sources are vegetable oils, milk, eggs and nuts.

Vitamin K takes care of your liver, and helps blood to clot. It's found in yoghurt, eggs and green vegetables.

MINERAL CURES

The body needs more than a dozen different minerals – these are a few of the most significant:

Calcium is used to build bones and teeth, but it also helps premenstrual problems and acts as a natural tranquiliser. It's found in milk, cheese and leafy green vegetables.

Chromium helps prevent tiredness by regulating blood sugar levels, so it's especially necessary if you're always on the go. Meat, fruit and vegetables all contain useful amounts.

Selenium works with vitamin E to keep skin young-looking, helps digestion, and is even said to cure dandruff! It's found in broccoli, eggs, onions and tuna.

Zinc is something of a wonder-mineral, essential for all kinds of things from healing wounds and rebuilding cells to strengthening hair and preventing stretch marks. Some experts claim it helps beat colds and prevents acne, but this hasn't been proved conclusively. Zinc is available in seafood, nuts and meat.

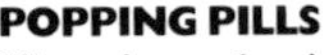

POPPING PILLS

Vitamin and mineral pills are big business. But do we really need them? For certain groups, the answer is often yes. Dieters, elderly people living alone and not bothering to cook or eat properly, strict vegetarians, young babies and pregnant women are all likely to lack a range of nutrients, or to need extra, so for them a multivitamin and mineral supplement may be a good idea. Smokers need extra vitamin C, teenagers just starting their periods may require more iron, women on the pill can always use additional vitamins B, C and E.

Usually though, a balanced, healthy diet supplies all the vitamins and minerals the body needs. Supplements can help when your health is temporarily below par, but in the long term, taking a vitamin pill won't make up for eating badly. And you *can* actually overdose on vitamins and minerals, making yourself just as ill as if you didn't have enough of them. This is much less likely to happen if you get your nutrients from food rather than pills – you'd have to eat an enormous number of carrots before you got too much vitamin A, for example!

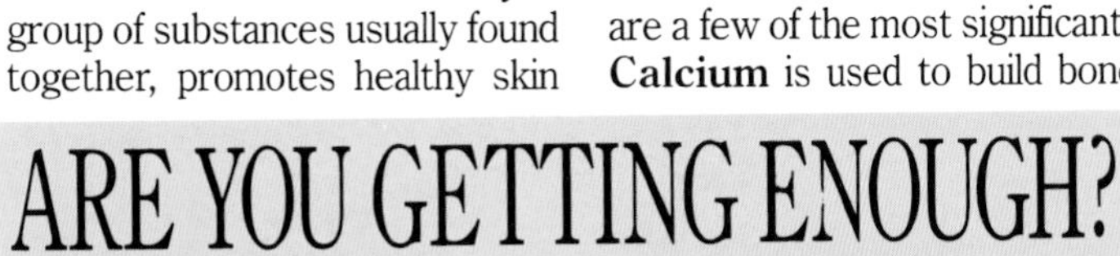

ARE YOU GETTING ENOUGH?

Though severe vitamin deficiency is rare in the Western world, our bodies are so finely balanced that even a slight lack causes tell-tale symptoms – watch out for these:

Puffy eyes: You may be lacking vitamins A and C – eat citrus fruits or fresh vegetables.

Dry hair: Could be you need extra vitamin B – tuck into brown bread, green vegetables and nuts.

White flecks on nails: May mean a lack of zinc – eat lots of shellfish, nuts or whole grains.

Dry skin: Can be a sign of insufficient vitamin A – crunch on yellow and green vegetables, or go to work on an egg.

Dark circles under eyes: Could be a sign of anaemia – get extra iron from liver or spinach.

Always check with your doctor if you get unusual symptoms.

NUTRIENT NOTES

- Women need and take more food supplements than men.
- Shops were stripped bare of certain supplements when scientists claimed they raised a child's IQ. Doctors still argue about whether it's true.
- Scientists can find out whether you're deficient in minerals by analysing your hair.
- Vitamin C is the best-selling single vitamin supplement. Multivitamins sell best overall.

WALK TALL

Don't be a slouch! We all get backache from time to time, but taking some simple steps to improve your posture and avoid strain can put your back together again

Illustrations: DICKY HOWETT/Photographs: JUTTA KLEE/Hair: KARIM MITHA/Make-up: VIRGINIA NICHOLS/Catsuit and headbands: MARY QUANT

Backache can make life a misery because almost every movement you make involves your back.

Most back problems can be blamed on evolution: when humans started walking on two legs, the back had to adapt itself to a less natural, upright stance.

Sadly, eight out of 10 of you will suffer from back pain at some stage, and it's the most common reason for taking time off work.

The usual cause of back problems is bad posture, although the way you do everyday tasks such as lifting and carrying can make things worse. Sometimes, the result of the strain can be pinpointed exactly, for instance, a slipped disc or a crack in a vertebra. Menstrual and labour pains can also cause backaches. But there's a lot you can do to help yourself. Take preventative action now and you'll reduce risks to your back in the future.

POSTURE POINTERS

- Posture is the backbone of beauty and health, but its importance is often forgotten. Being fit doesn't necessarily mean that your posture is good, although it may make your back stronger.
- Poor circulation, tension, stiffness and shallow breathing are also all related to bad posture. Walk tall and you'll not only feel better but look a lot better and have a prettier profile too.
- Good posture is *not,* however, about standing like a sergeant-major or walking around with an imaginary book on your head. It's about aligning the natural curves of the back so that back strain is kept to a minimum. Look around and see how many hunched shoulders, bowed heads and rounded backs there are, then have a critical look at your own posture in a full-length mirror and see how you stand up!

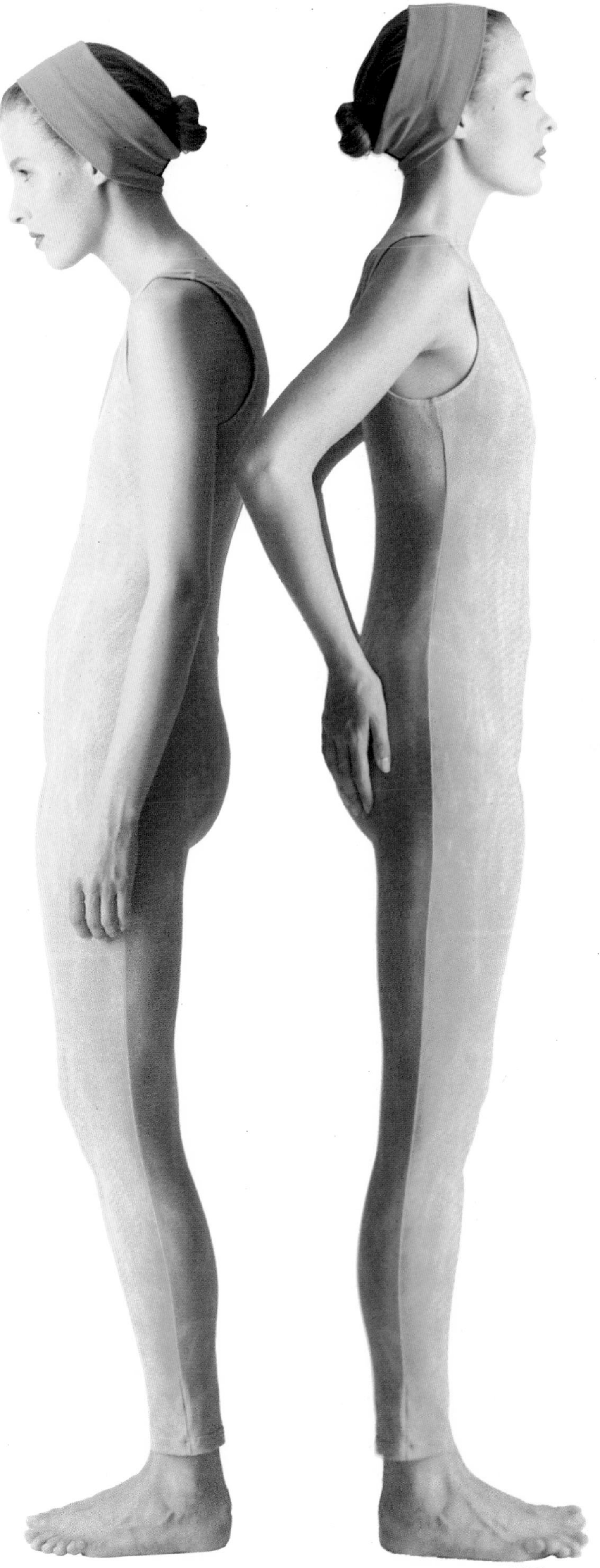

STAND POINTS

Stand sideways and take a good look at yourself in the mirror. Be honest! If you seem to be slouching, try these simple steps to correct your posture:

- Start by positioning your feet 25 cm/10 in apart and balancing your weight evenly.
- Place a finger on the crown of your head and imagine pulling up a string from here so that your spine stretches upwards.
- Keep your neck and chin tucked in and your shoulders relaxed. Tilt your pelvis slightly forwards so your stomach and bottom tuck in.
- Flop forwards gently and then pull yourself up again, relax, and stand normally.

Make an effort to use these measures regularly. With luck, walking tall will become a habit!

SITTING PRETTY

Even when you're sitting, there is a great deal of pressure on your spine. Don't just slouch in front of the telly, but pad out your sofa with cushions to support your lower back.

Also, if your job involves spending hours at a desk, it's vital that your chair is giving your back the support it needs. Ideally it should have:

- Good lower back support.
- The seat of the chair should slope down slightly at the front to reduce pressure on the back of the knees.
- Adjustable height so that your feet rest on the ground.

Make sure you're sitting properly, too. Don't cross your legs (it will reduce circulation) and take regular exercise during the day – even if it's only going to the photocopier and back!

DID YOU KNOW?

There's a greater risk of injuring your back three days before your period as progesterone levels drop, causing muscles and ligaments to soften.

TAKING THE STRAIN

Take care! Follow our tips to stop unnecessary back trouble.

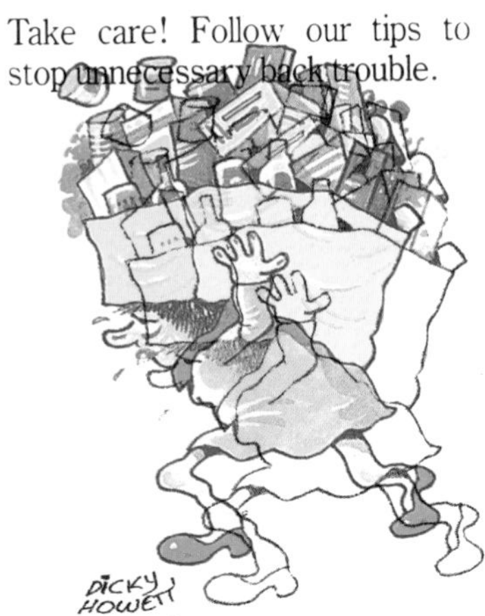

IN THE BAG

Backpacks are the best sort of bag, since the weight is evenly distributed. But if they're not your style, try wearing your shoulder bag diagonally across your body or swap it from shoulder to shoulder occasionally. If you're carrying shopping bags, split the weight evenly between both hands and don't carry too much at once – you can always ask someone to help!

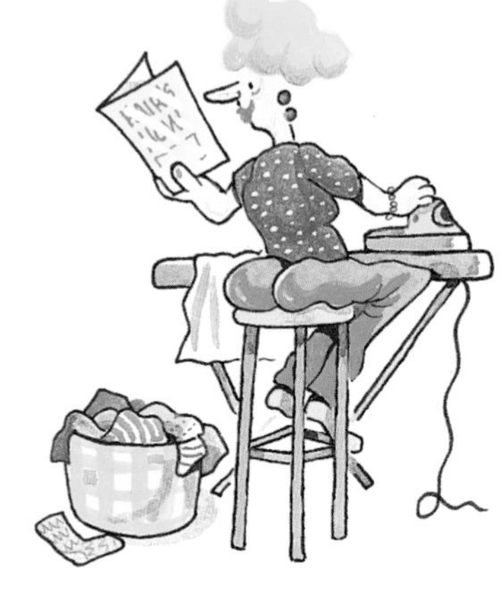

AT HOME

Warning: housework can be bad for your back! Most tasks around the house involve a lot of bending. Sit down when doing the ironing and use an upright vacuum cleaner, if possible.

Take care when gardening. Don't try to dig the whole garden on the first day of spring, take it in easy stages. Kneel when weeding, or use long-handled tools which are specially designed to save you from bending.

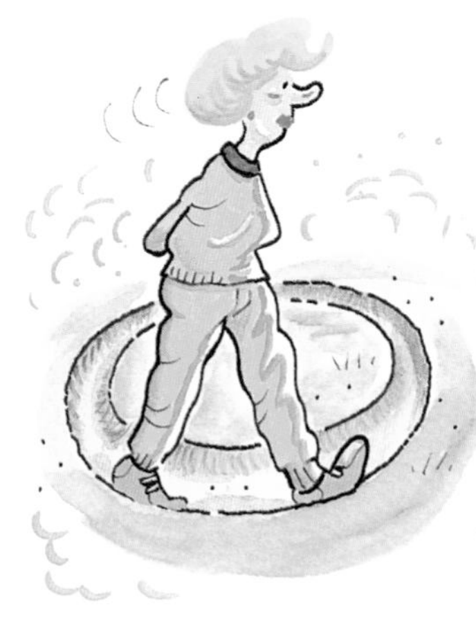

ON THE MOVE

Don't stand when you can walk! Standing in one spot for a long time causes the muscles to tire, so walk around.

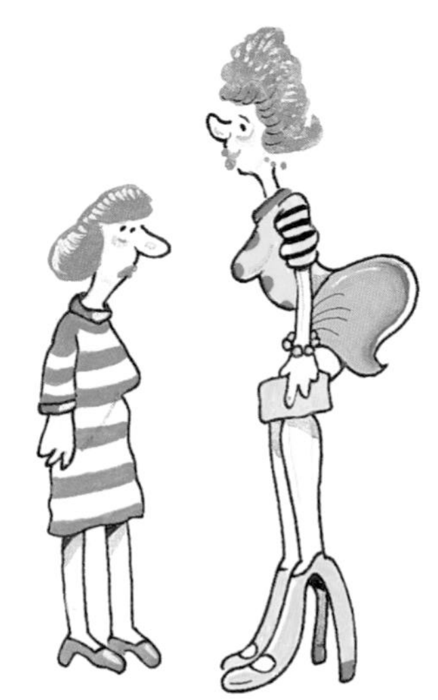

SHOE SOLUTION

High heels throw you off balance, so stick to heels no higher than 5 cm/2 in for everyday use. Thick soles also help to prevent jarring the spine.

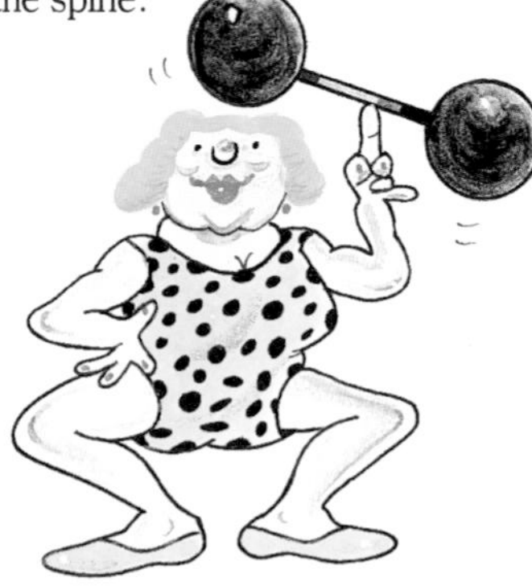

LIFT OFF!

More back injuries are caused by lifting than by almost anything else. To lift properly, bend from your knees so your legs do the work, rather than your back. Stand close to the object you're lifting and try not to twist as you straighten up.

BACK UP

Spine: made up of 24 vertebrae, that stack on top of each and nine lower vertebrae that are fused together.
Spinal cord: a column of nerves that runs through each vertebra, connecting the brain and lower body.
Discs: spongy cushions of cartilage between each vertebra.
Ligaments: tough elastic tissue which holds the bones in place.
Joints: each vertebra has two. They control movement and provide stability.
Muscles: there are 140 which give support and balance.

BACK DOWN

Lying down is the most restful position for your back so long as the surface gives enough support. It's important that your bed is right for you. A bed that's too soft or too hard is not good for your back. Try this simple test:

Lie down on the bed and slip your hand between the small of your back and the mattress. If you can't get your hand in-between, then the mattress is too soft and if there's a big gap, the mattress is too hard. You need a snug fit.

BACK ATTACK

If you injure your back suddenly and are in pain, here's an emergency checklist to help:

- Stop doing whatever caused the backache. Telephone the doctor if you think you need to.
- Lie down on a firm surface, using pillows for support and rest for at least 24 hours. Try a foetal position with your knees bent up if this is more comfortable.
- Hold a hot water bottle on the painful area for 15 minutes, three times a day.
- When the worst of the pain is over, start moving your back very gently to prevent it stiffening up.
- Try soaking in a warm bath.
- Take heart – 75 percent of sudden back injuries get better within a week and 90 percent within a month.

HIGH ENERGY

If your get up and go has got up and gone, then follow our energy-boosting action plan and go all out to get your mind and body back into top gear

There's nothing worse than feeling tired and having no drive. But the good news is that the causes can often be attributed to lifestyle or eating habits. And with a little time and a bit of effort, you can boost flagging energy levels – naturally.

Energy is needed for all the work the body carries out to maintain itself – from blinking and thinking to exercising. So it's important to make energy and then use it positively, if you want to feel fighting-fit every day. If you don't, you'll soon get run down and may start to feel tired, depressed and listless or even find it hard to concentrate.

If it's a real effort to get out of bed in the morning then take a close look at your lifestyle. Are you eating the right foods, getting enough exercise and taking time to relax? Are you on the birth-control pill or any other form of medication? All these factors can affect how lively you feel.

FUELLING UP WITH FOOD

Beat off lethargy with the food that you eat:

- **Avoid sugary foods and drinks and stimulants such as tea and coffee which give you a quick energy burst but then leave you feeling tired.**
- **Eat a well-balanced diet with plenty of high-energy value foods like chicken, fish, fruit, pulses and vegetables.**
- **Start the day with a wholesome breakfast to wake up your digestive system and get your body working.**
- **Drink lots of water, herbal teas, coffee substitutes or mix up a delicious fruit cocktail.**
- **Avoid very low-calorie diets or fasting as you'll feel sluggish and tired even if you do lose those few extra pounds in weight. And never skip meals. Aim to eat little and often.**

FIT FOR ANYTHING

If you're unfit, your body will use more energy to do simple tasks like walking up the stairs. And when you *are* fit you actually *feel* more energetic, so exercising has a twofold effect. Take a brisk walk, go swimming or cycling with your friends and you'll soon begin to feel brilliant. Then aim to do three 30-minute sessions of your favourite exercise a week.

LEARN TO RELAX!

Remember, too, that energy needs to be replenished so it is vital that you allow yourself enough resting time when you have been working out or working hard at home or the office.

Stress is probably one of the major energy-zappers and whereas 'living off your nerves' can sometimes have a positive effect it can also use up a lot of energy. So try not to worry if you've got masses of work on, just plan your time carefully and aim to do the more difficult tasks when you're feeling at your best. Make sure you gradually wind down at the end of the day rather than working flat out all the time.

And always take a short break when you feel you need to.

HEAVY BREATHING

Try and get out into the fresh air as often as possible. If it means walking instead of taking the bus or exercising someone else's dog, give it a go and really get your lungs working. Practice deep breathing by inhaling through your nostrils for a count of ten and then exhaling from your mouth for a count of ten. Also, sit up, rather than hunching over a desk as this will help to ensure that a good supply of oxygen circulates around your body all the time.

HEALTH DRIVE

Fighting an illness, taking the pill or medication over a long period of time can deplete your energy reserves too. If you take the pill you'll probably have lighter periods and there is less chance of you being deficient in energy-producing iron, but there are negative side effects. One of these, and this happens when you take antibiotics too, is to upset the delicate balance of the gut by stripping it of healthy bacteria and allowing harmful bacteria to multiply. This can lead to a condition called *candida albicans*, which in its advanced stage robs the body of vital vitamins and minerals, making you feel very tired. You can help to keep this yeast-like fungus at bay by eating lots of live yoghurt and cutting out sugary foods which the *candida* feeds on.

Finally, bear in mind that you can actually be your own worst energy enemy and think yourself tired out because it's the natural response to a hard day's work. Try putting variety into your life, changing dull routines and thinking yourself full of energy and you probably will be!

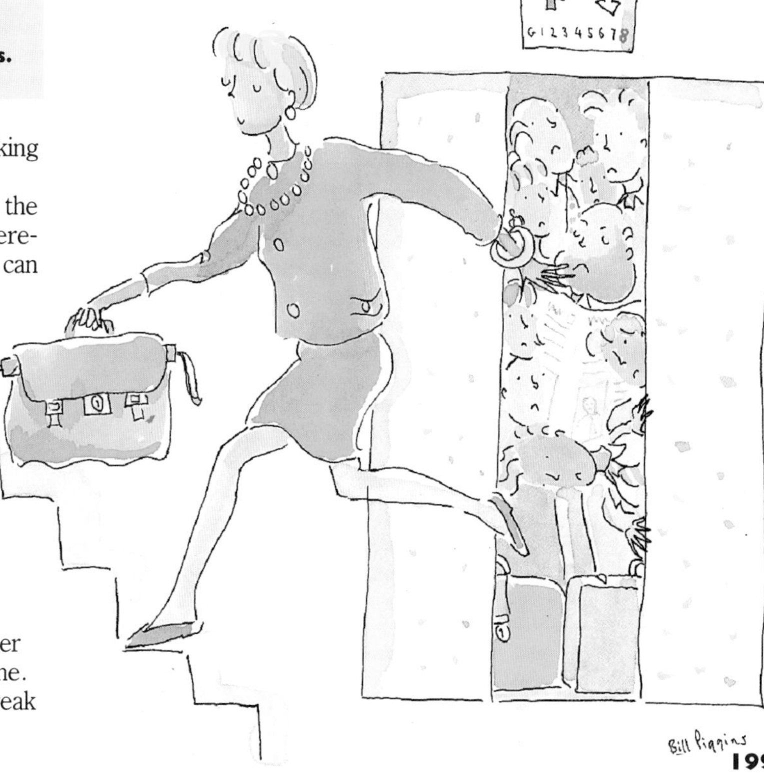

Illustration: BILL PIGGINS

GET UNSTRESSED!

Feeling tetchy and unable to cope? Then your stress levels could be too high. Wind down with our action plan and learn to take stress in your stride

Stress may have become the buzzword of the Nineties, but if you are genuinely suffering, it can spoil your looks and your health. It may be your friends who notice the changes in you first, how you're becoming short-tempered, snappy and tired. Before it gets a grip, act like an accountant and take a stress stocktake (see next column). If your stress levels are too high it's vital that you get them down before they get you down!

HEALTH WARNINGS

Stress can seriously damage your health – and that's official! Acne, ulcers, allergies and even heart attacks are all believed to be related to stress. It's claimed that as much as 70 percent of disease is stress-related, so getting your levels down to a minimum will keep you much healthier and help you live longer.

STRESS STOCKTAKE

Do any of the following symptoms sound familiar? Are you:

- **Irritable**
- **Anxious**
- **Overeating or undereating**
- **Constantly tired**
- **Disinterested in sex**
- **Nail biting**
- **Bursting into tears for no good reason**
- **Finding it difficult to sleep at night**
- **Losing your sense of humour**

STAGGERING CHANGES

Most changes happen without you having any control over them. But if you've got major decisions looming, try to stagger them so you don't get overloaded. If you've just started a new job, don't choose this as a time to go on a diet or give up smoking. Let yourself adjust to one change before moving onto the next, and your stress level will be lower.

HELP YOURSELF

Take one, or more, of these tips to ease your stress load.

● DON'T BE LIST-LESS!

Lists can help cut out stress. Write down everything that's worrying you, then work through them jotting down possible solutions. Also, a list can help you plan a busy work schedule more efficiently. Put down the tasks in order of priority and tick them off when the job is done. Don't set yourself unrealistic targets though – you won't be able to cure everything in a day! And since some of your stress is bound to be in areas that you can't change, you'll need to be flexible enough to compromise.

● ATTITUDE PROBLEMS

It's not so much the amount of stress you're under but how you deal with it that's generally the problem. One person may reach the same level of stress from the break-up of a marriage as another does from missing a train! Changing your attitude can be the most powerful antidote. If something happens that seems like the end of the world, try to see the silver lining in the clouds! Look on it as an experience that'll make you wiser in the future and whatever you do, don't dwell on it and don't blame yourself.

● SMILE PLEASE!

Try – however hard it may be – to smile. Spend a day when you consciously smile at everyone you meet. You'll be amazed at how other people react. They smile back, are more helpful and you'll end up feeling a lot less stressed. Laughter is a great stress breaker too. Why not hire a video of your favourite comedy and invite a few friends round for a bit of a giggle.

● TAKE YOUR TIME

Make sure that you set time aside for yourself. If you're always busy then actually schedule some leisure time into your diary or set aside a regular period each day – maybe when you get home – to relax. Take up a hobby if you don't have one already. Make a list of things you like doing and make sure you do at least one of them once a week.

FULL SCALE ALERT!

Every change in your life requires readjustment and the more drastic it is, the more stress it can cause. The chart below shows a few typical stress ratings. Add up your score for the last year.

EVENTS	RATING		
Death of spouse	**100**	**Death of close friend**	**37**
Divorce	**73**	**Change of job**	**36**
Death of family member	**63**	**Change in duties at work**	**29**
Illness or injury	**53**	**Child leaving home**	**29**
Marriage	**50**	**Begin or end schooling**	**26**
Fired from job	**47**	**Change in residence**	**20**
Retirement	**45**	**Change in sleeping habits**	**16**
Pregnancy	**40**	**Change in eating habits**	**15**
Gain of new family member	**39**	**Holidays**	**13**
Change in financial state	**38**	**Christmas**	**12**

It has been found in various stress tests that the majority of people who scored over 200 in a single year suffered health problems the following year and those scoring over 300 became ill. Although their bodies coped with the stress at the time, their natural resistance to disease was lowered. Such resistance can also be weakened by a relatively simple change in life style. For instance, if you're struggling to cope with the demands of a new job you'll probably find you eat more snack foods, get less sleep and take less exercise. But as long as you're aware of all these pressures and take sensible precautions, your health needn't suffer.

STRESS ZAPPERS!

- **Walking along the beach at sunset**
- **Curl up with a good book**
- **Singing in the bath**
- **Looking through old photos**
- **Watching a favourite film again**
- **Feeding the ducks in the park**
- **Giving yourself a manicure and pedicure**
- **Stroking your pets**
- **Having a body massage**

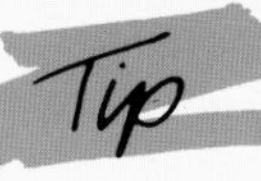

Stress eats up vitamin C – so step up your intake and boost your resistance to infections.

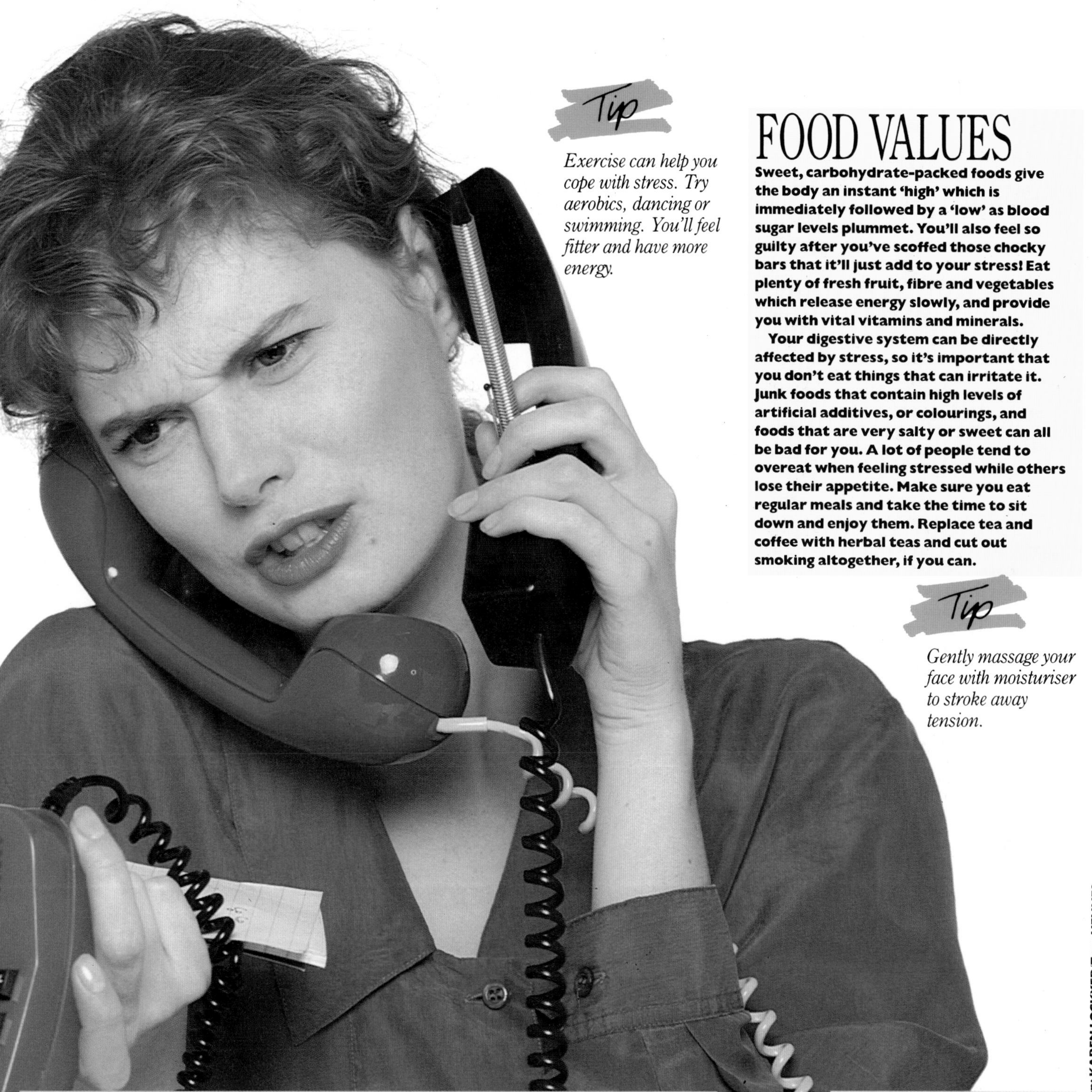

Tip

Exercise can help you cope with stress. Try aerobics, dancing or swimming. You'll feel fitter and have more energy.

FOOD VALUES

Sweet, carbohydrate-packed foods give the body an instant 'high' which is immediately followed by a 'low' as blood sugar levels plummet. You'll also feel so guilty after you've scoffed those chocky bars that it'll just add to your stress! Eat plenty of fresh fruit, fibre and vegetables which release energy slowly, and provide you with vital vitamins and minerals.

Your digestive system can be directly affected by stress, so it's important that you don't eat things that can irritate it. Junk foods that contain high levels of artificial additives, or colourings, and foods that are very salty or sweet can all be bad for you. A lot of people tend to overeat when feeling stressed while others lose their appetite. Make sure you eat regular meals and take the time to sit down and enjoy them. Replace tea and coffee with herbal teas and cut out smoking altogether, if you can.

Tip

Gently massage your face with moisturiser to stroke away tension.

WORK IT OUT

If your work causes you stress you'll need to organise yourself to deal with it.

- **Always take your full lunch hour to go out and walk around. Don't feel guilty about giving yourself time to relax as you'll be much more productive in the time that you are working.**
- **Have the courage to say 'no' if you're asked to do more when you're already overloaded.**
- **Don't put things off. Once you get started you'll find it's much easier than you thought.**
- **Do all your most difficult tasks in the morning when you're most fresh.**
- **After work, allow at least ten minutes to wind down before you face the journey home. This will give you the chance to forget about your work worries.**

Tip

Instead of getting impatient while standing in a queue or sitting in a traffic jam, use the time to plan a special treat for yourself and you won't notice the wait – even if it turns out to be a long one.

WISHFUL THINKING!

Got five minutes to spare? Then you've got just enough time to get to paradise and back! Wherever you're sitting, get comfortable and close your eyes. Try to imagine that you are in the most perfect place in the world. Wherever your idea of bliss is, try to imagine yourself there feeling the warmth, hearing the sounds and smelling the scents. After a few minutes, slowly open your eyes and stretch.

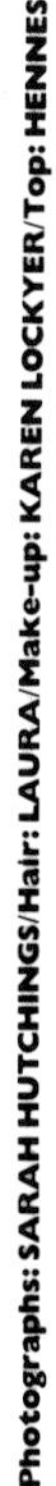

STRESS TEST

Feeling harassed and rushed off your feet? A certain amount of stress can be good for you but too much can have a bad effect on your mental and physical well-being. Test yourself and wise-up to the danger signs

WORK

1 If you have a deadline to meet at work or an exam to study for, do you:
- ○ **Set yourself a schedule and try to keep to it**
- △ **Set yourself schedules but never seem able to keep to them**
- □ **Put off the work until the last minute then try to cram it all in**
- ○ **Don't feel you need to make any special effort and just keep working at your normal pace**

2 During an assessment of your work, your boss/teacher generally praises your achievements but is critical of a few minor things. Do you feel:
- ○ **Pleased and resolve to correct your bad points**
- □ **Upset – you don't feel the things said about you were justified**

3 At your workplace do you feel your work is:
- □ **Not up to scratch – you need to work harder than everyone else to get the same results**
- △ **Better than anyone else**
- ○ **As good as you can do**

4 When you have a bad day at work do you feel:
- ○ **"It's just one of those days" and don't let it worry you**
- △ **Frustrated that you couldn't do what you wanted to but maybe you'll succeed tomorrow**
- □ **It must have been your fault**
- □ **It wasn't your fault and blame other people**

5 How punctual are you?
- ○ **Never more than 5 minutes late**
- △ **Always on time**
- □ **Almost always late – but with an excuse**

6 If you've got behind on your work do you:
- △ **Stay late and work harder to make it up**
- ○ **Ask for some help**
- □ **Worry that you'll never be able to do it**
- ○ **Try to work through it steadily**

7 If there's work that needs to be done as a team and you're put in charge do you find you:
- □ **Want to do it all – "if you want something done well you have to do it yourself"**
- ○ **Try and allocate the work and trust that person to do it well**
- △ **Distribute the work evenly but then check over everyone else's work and change it**

8 There's a new project at work but although it's something you feel you'd be good at it's given to someone else. Do you:
- □ **Feel hurt but don't say anything**
- △ **Ask if you can help out on it**
- ○ **Shrug it off – you're busy enough at the moment anyway**

9 Do you do any of the following (tick as many as you like):
- □ **Bite your nails**
- △ **Use your hands a lot when you talk**
- □ **Talk too fast or loud**
- △ **Fiddle with your hair**
- □ **Touch your face when talking**
- △ **Chew gum**
- □ **Clench your teeth**
- □ **Feel weepy all the time**

HEALTH

10 Do you exercise:
- ○ **Regularly – 2 or 3 times a week**
- △ **Sometimes – 2 or 3 times a month**
- □ **Rarely – you never seem to get time**

11 Do you feel that you drink too much alcohol:
- □ **Yes** ○ **No**

12 Do you feel you smoke too much:
- □ **Yes** ○ **No**

13 Do you suffer from frequent (tick as many as you like):
- □ **Headaches**
- □ **Stomach upsets**
- □ **Constipation/diarrhoea**
- □ **Bouts of short breath when you haven't been exercising**
- □ **Colds and Flu**

14 Do you sleep badly:
- □ **Often**
- ○ **Sometimes**
- ○ **Rarely**

15 Do you have nightmares:
- □ **Often**
- ○ **Sometimes**
- ○ **Rarely**

16 Do you feel tired:
- □ **Most of the time**
- ○ **Only if you've been busy**
- △ **During the week only**

EATING

17 Do you (tick as many as you like):
- ○ **Eat meals at regular times**
- △ **Eat three meals a day but the times vary**
- △ **Skip the occasional meal**
- □ **Never eat breakfast/lunch**
- □ **Grab a sandwich and eat on the run**
- ○ **Always sit down to eat**
- □ **Have no appetite when you're busy**

Drink more than four cups of tea or coffee in a day:
- □ **Yes** ○ **No**
- △ **Sometimes**

18 Do you eat junk food/snacks/chocolate:
- ○ **Rarely**
- △ **Sometimes**
- □ **Frequently**

19 How do you feel about diets:
- △ **As soon as you lose weight you put it all back on again**
- □ **You like to keep in shape so you diet often**
- △ **You only bother after Christmas or before you go on holiday**
- ○ **You're quite happy with your size and rarely diet**

TIME OFF

20 How much free time do you have for yourself:
- △ **Too much**
- □ **Never enough**
- ○ **You get around to doing most things that you want to do**

21 How long is it since you went away on holiday:
- ○ **Up to six months**
- △ **Over six months**
- □ **Over a year**

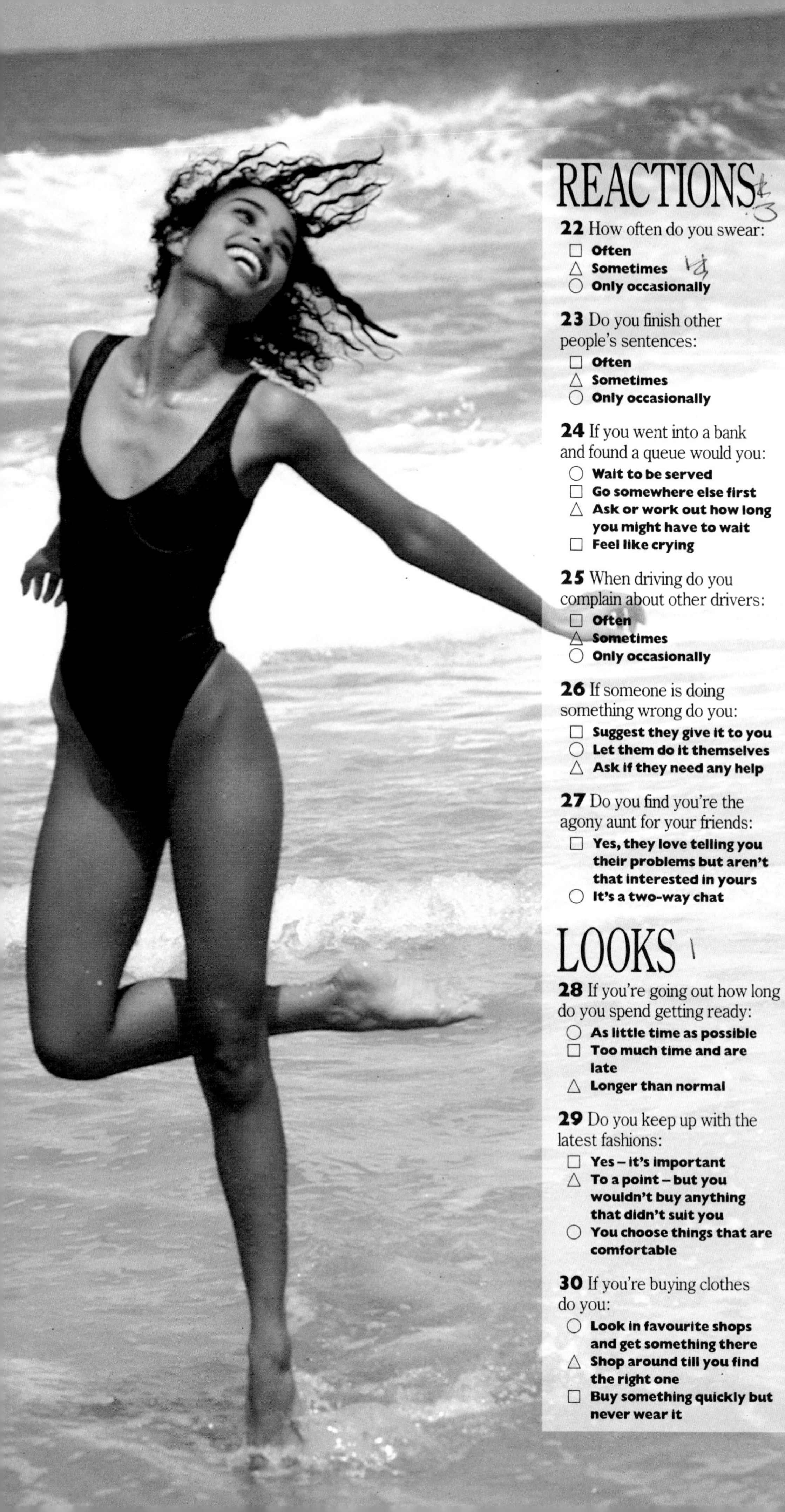

REACTIONS

22 How often do you swear:
- □ **Often**
- △ **Sometimes**
- ○ **Only occasionally**

23 Do you finish other people's sentences:
- □ **Often**
- △ **Sometimes**
- ○ **Only occasionally**

24 If you went into a bank and found a queue would you:
- ○ **Wait to be served**
- □ **Go somewhere else first**
- △ **Ask or work out how long you might have to wait**
- □ **Feel like crying**

25 When driving do you complain about other drivers:
- □ **Often**
- △ **Sometimes**
- ○ **Only occasionally**

26 If someone is doing something wrong do you:
- □ **Suggest they give it to you**
- ○ **Let them do it themselves**
- △ **Ask if they need any help**

27 Do you find you're the agony aunt for your friends:
- □ **Yes, they love telling you their problems but aren't that interested in yours**
- ○ **It's a two-way chat**

LOOKS

28 If you're going out how long do you spend getting ready:
- ○ **As little time as possible**
- □ **Too much time and are late**
- △ **Longer than normal**

29 Do you keep up with the latest fashions:
- □ **Yes – it's important**
- △ **To a point – but you wouldn't buy anything that didn't suit you**
- ○ **You choose things that are comfortable**

30 If you're buying clothes do you:
- ○ **Look in favourite shops and get something there**
- △ **Shop around till you find the right one**
- □ **Buy something quickly but never wear it**

WHAT'S YOUR STRESS SCORE

Total up your points and see which category you're in.

2 points for every □ answer
1 point for every △ answer
0 points for every ○ answer

OVER 55 POINTS

Watch out! Your stress level is reaching overload. If you blow your top at the smallest thing then it's high time you took a break. Stress at this level will be affecting your health both mentally and physically. Take a holiday and try to relax. Make a list – but not an unrealistic one – and sort out your priorities so you're not trying to do everything at once. Next time you start to boil, take a tip and count to ten. Get a new hobby and make sure you set aside more time for yourself. You're probably a perfectionist. Ask yourself, if it's not quite right – does it really matter? Remember it's not the amount of stress that you're under, but how you react to it.

25-55 POINTS

Your stress levels are quite high but if you've got the right attitude you'll be able to enjoy all the action. Check through the quiz again to see which section you've got the most □ points in – these are the areas of greatest stress. If they are all in one section then being aware of it will help you. So long as all the other areas in your life are relatively stress-free this can be fine. If the stress is in different sections take care not to let any one get out of control.

UNDER 25 POINTS

Your life is fairly stress-free. Either you've learnt to handle stress very well or your life is a bit unchallenging. If it's hectic you probably see changes as fun rather than as setbacks and enjoy working them out – with this attitude you'll be able to sail through. A low stress rating could also mean that you're simply not being pushed enough. We all need a certain level of stress to motivate us to do things. Try being a bit more adventurous – you'll find life a lot more fun!

Photograph: DIDIER de FEYS

ALLERGIC REACTION

If your skin breaks out at the very sight of cosmetics and you don't know what to do next, check out our guide and find out the reason for your rashes and the solution to your scratching

There is no simple answer to why your skin is sensitive to one product and perfectly happy with another. But there are many reasons – you can have an allergic reaction to almost anything – food, make-up, or even the air you breathe can cause your skin to erupt. If you do have an allergic reaction don't automatically assume that it is something new that's causing it. Sometimes your skin can be perfectly happy with something for years and then suddenly become vulnerable for seemingly no reason at all.

WHAT IS AN ALLERGY?

Allergy literally means 'altered reaction'. An allergic reaction can show up as a rash, dry scaly skin, blisters, redness or in more severe cases as cracking and oozing skin. An allergic reaction can be temporary, or it can mean that your skin is permanently sensitive to the cause of the allergy. Don't imagine that because a friend who has sensitive skin reacts well to a certain product it will work in the same way for you – it's important to realise that allergic reactions are quite individual.

Your skin exists to protect your internal organs from potential damage through things such as ultra-violet rays in everyday sunlight; weather changes; extremes like wind, cold or sun; any form of shock or stress, or pollution. When you stop to think about everything your skin has to put up with it's not surprising that it doesn't always behave in quite the way you want it to.

PROTECT YOURSELF

Of course if you know what you are allergic or sensitive to, then the remedy can be relatively simple and you should make sure that you avoid the substance creating the allergy. But if you can't work out what is causing the problem there are steps you can take to prevent severe reactions and help you realise why you are at risk. Follow our Protection Plan and your suffering could soon be a thing of the past!

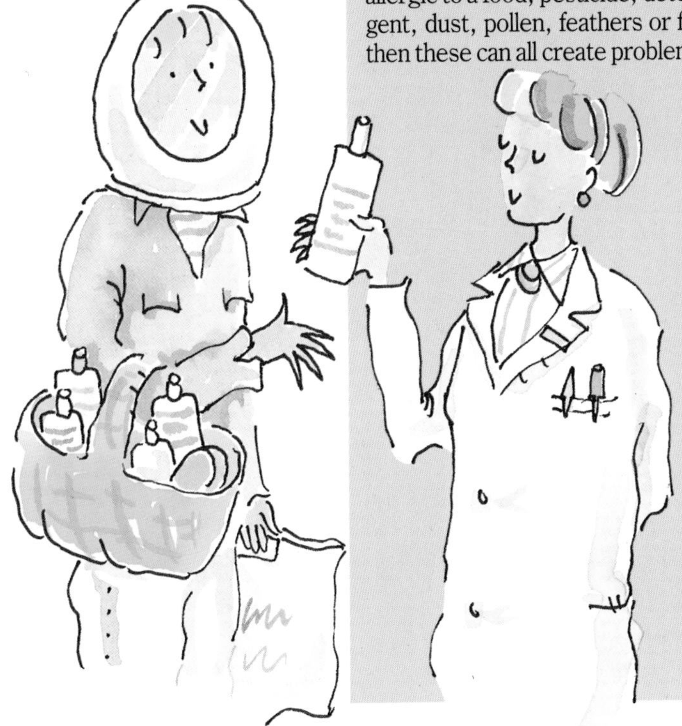

SENSITIVITY SAFEGUARDS: THE PROTECTION PLAN

- Look out for products that are allergy screened, dermatologically or allergy tested or are hypo-allergenic. All these descriptions mean that the contents of the product have been carefully studied by dermatologists and any substance likely to cause an allergic reaction will not have been used. The products will then be tested on humans who are known to have sensitive skin and if a reaction occurs then the product will not be marketed.
- Always wash your hands, brushes or sponges with a mild soap before applying any cream, lotion or make-up product. Then you will avoid any bacteria coming into contact with and growing on the product or coming into contact with your skin. It's important to remember that it is often what is on your hands, make-up brushes or sponges and not what is contained in the product that can cause problems. If you are allergic to a food, pesticide, detergent, dust, pollen, feathers or fur then these can all create problems if they are not removed before you apply a product.
- Use products that are as natural and uncomplicated as possible. Ingredients to look out for because they're kind to skin are allantoin, arnica, benzoin, bisalobol, calendula, camomile, cornflower, harpagophytum, lavender, liquorice, mint, mallow, marjoram, soya and avocado oils. If your skin is sensitive and has shown an allergic reaction soothe and calm it. A good moisturiser will protect your skin from airborne hazards and reduce its vulnerability.
- Remember that your skin is acid and its natural pH value is 5.5 so that if you regularly use a soap, which is alkaline, you are removing your skin's natural protection factor. This doesn't mean you can't use soap or liquid cleanser on your face – just make sure you use something that is unperfumed and as simple as possible. Rinse with lukewarm water.
- If you want to try a new product and are worried that it might cause an allergic reaction, do a patch-test on the inside of your upper arm using a very small dab of the product. Leave for 24 hours and you will know from your skin's reaction whether or not your skin is sensitive to that product. If it is, discontinue use.

BEWARE!

There are certain products that are known to create allergic reactions on sensitive skin:

Nail varnish – avoid anything containing formaldehyde.

Hand cream – avoid anything containing lanolin.

Mascara – avoid mascara with fibres.

Lipstick – avoid lipsticks containing eosin and lanolin.

Deodorant – avoid deodorants containing ammonium sulphide and anti-perspirants that contain aluminium salts.

Illustration: BILL PIGGINS

SEE YOURSELF RIGHT

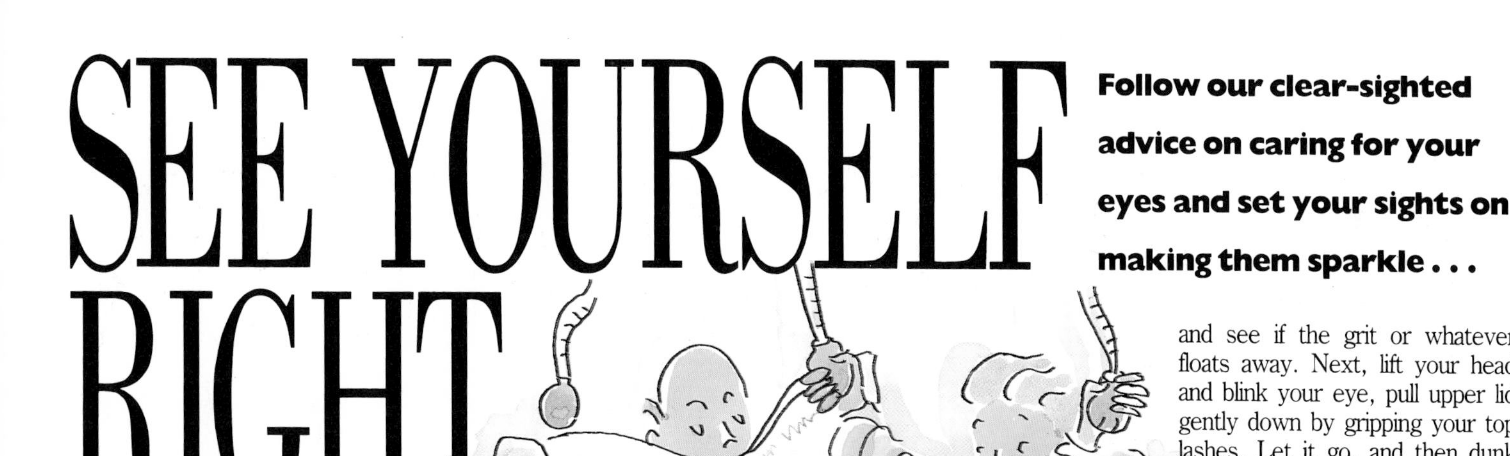

Follow our clear-sighted advice on caring for your eyes and set your sights on making them sparkle . . .

One of the first things people notice about you is your eyes, so the last thing you want is a pair of pink or puffy peepers. But in order to possess a real set of sparklers you need to be healthy (when you're poorly your eyes are generally dull or yellowy), well rested (lack of sleep leaves your eyes bloodshot and gives you under-eye shadows). And, ideally, you should make caring for your eyes a part of your routine in everyday life.

DON'T SHARE . . .

Most of us use eye make-up to make our eyes look bigger and better. But if you don't take basic hygiene precautions when applying it – you may well end up making your eyes look awful. Epidemics of an eye infection called trachoma have occurred amongst schoolgirls and were spread because they used each other's eyeliner pencils. So it isn't a good idea to share eye make-up or eye make-up brushes with your friends, or even family, because it can lead to one person infecting another.

Eye cosmetics *do* contain preservatives and these reduce the risk of you getting a nasty infection – but these don't work for ever so try not to keep things for years.

Take care when you're putting on eye make-up. First of all, make sure you're standing still! Don't put it on in the bus, train, car, or when you're in a hurry. Many serious eye inflammations are caused when the cornea (the delicate protective covering over the front of the eye) is scratched by an eye make-up brush or pencil hitting it.

GENTLY DOES IT

Take care when you remove your eye make-up as well. Eyes are sensitive things and need gentle treatment. For best results, remove your eye make-up before you cleanse your face. The most hygienic method of doing this is to use a light remover (nothing too oily or astringent) and two cotton wool pads – one for each eye. Never pull or drag the delicate skin around the eyes and don't use facial cleansing products such as toners on your eyes, or face packs close to them. They're too harsh.

Similarly, don't even use your usual moisturiser (unless it's a very light formulation). Instead, use special eye creams or gels and pat them on gently.

EYESORES

Even if you are scrupulous about eye care, there are quite a few eye complaints over which you have little control. If you suffer from dark shadows under your eyes and you get plenty of sleep, this may be a hereditary trait.

If you have puffy eyes this may be caused by fluid retention just before your period. But if these symptoms persist and can't be put down to your period or a night on the tiles, then you should get your doctor to check them.

STYES IN THEIR EYES

If you have problems, don't try and treat yourself. Seek specialised help quickly. For instance, if a lump of grit gets into your eye, don't prod around with unwashed fingers. Let your eyes water – this is your body's defence mechanism and often the offending object floats out on your tear fluid. If you can't get the object out this way, then dunk your head in a basin of water and see if the grit or whatever floats away. Next, lift your head and blink your eye, pull upper lid gently down by gripping your top lashes. Let it go, and then dunk your head again. If it's still hurting, go to a doctor, eye hospital or optician where you'll find experts in eye care who will use specialised equipment to deal with these sort of problems.

The eye problem, conjunctivitis, is actually a viral infection, and like styes (small red itchy boils in one of the skin's eyelid glands which are often found in the inner or outer corners of the eyes) some people are just more susceptible to developing them than others. However, anyone can become infected through dust, not removing make-up properly which blocks the glands, and even by the chlorine in swimming pools. If you do get conjunctivitis, you should see your doctor.

VISION ON

Your eyesight is precious, so check it regularly. Go for a test once a year and if you work with a VDU go every six months. VDU users have been found to experience twice the normal incidence of eye problems – so be careful and take regular 10-minute breaks to avoid eye strain.

BRIGHT EYES

Put a twinkle in your eyes by:

- **Eating a well-balanced diet that's rich in vitamin A foods.**
- **Getting enough sleep.**
- **Making your own eye masks. Keep used tea-bags in the fridge, or use chilled cucumber or potato slices and place on your eyelids for about 20 minutes to give you clear, sparkling eyes.**
- **Using a couple of ice cubes in a hanky to reduce puffy eyes.**
- **Keeping all your eye make-up brushes clean. Wash every week.**
- **Throwing away eye make-up that you've had for a year.**
- **Using special eye gels or creams containing ingredients such as elderflower, marigold, camomile and witch-hazel.**
- **Exercising your eyes! A few simple movements, like opening your eyes wide and looking to one side and then the other will keep them healthy, too.**

Illustration: BILL PIGGINS

BOSOM PALS

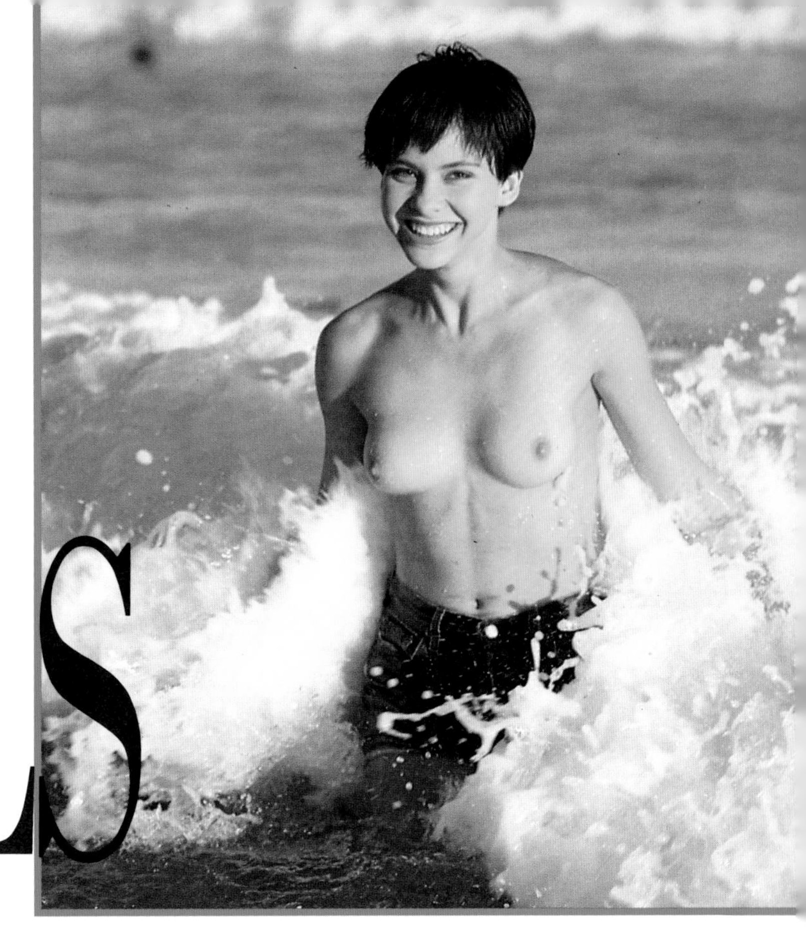

Never mind if you're big up front or your bust just amounts to a couple of bumps! Make the most of your natural assets and start shaping up now

NATURAL ASSETS

The size and shape of your breasts is hereditary but big or small, with proper care you can keep them firm and well-toned. In fact, the sooner you start looking after them the better.

Apart from a small amount of glandular tissue, breasts are made up of fat and have no muscles to help fight the forces of gravity and defy the dreaded droop. A good bra will provide the necessary support and you can also exercise the muscles around your breasts which form a sort of supportive platform. It's a good idea to make sure the skin stays supple, firm and well-toned too.

THE BEST BRA

But it's not good to go bra-less, even if you're quite small, and it's just as bad to wear one that doesn't fit properly. If your bra is too tight it will restrict circulation, causing the skin to slacken. Too big, and it won't provide enough support. So do yourself a favour and throw away that old, over-washed, worn-out bra.

But before getting a new one, make sure you know exactly which size to buy. If you don't know how to measure up properly and are confused about cup sizes, you'll find it's actually quite simple. Here's how to discover your vital statistics:

First measure under your bust. If this is an even figure add four inches; if it's uneven, add five. This gives you your bra size, for example, 30 + 4 = 34, or 31 + 5 = 36.

To work out your cup size, measure around the fullest part of your bust. Take the first total from the second measurement and if it comes to the same figure, you're an A cup; one inch difference is a B cup, two inches C, three inches D, four inches DD and five inches E.

BARING ALL

Your bust can be one of the most neglected areas when it comes to skin care. While your beauty routine may include rubbing lotions into your hands, and creams into your hips, when was the last time you massaged body lotion over your breasts? It's especially important to do this in summer when wearing more revealing clothes as your bust is more exposed to the elements. Apart from keeping the skin soft, moisturising with a massaging action stimulates blood flow which in turn helps to improve skin texture generally.

Instead of your usual body lotion, you could invest in a special bust cream. These won't add extra inches, but will leave a slight film over your skin which has a gentle tightening action so your boobs look and feel slightly firmer.

Always use upward strokes when massaging in bust care cream but avoid using perfumed products near your nipples as they can cause irritation.

BEING UPLIFTED

Points to look for before you buy:

- ***Underwired bras* give a little more support and tend to push up your bust, but make sure the wire doesn't cut into your skin.**
- **Make sure the straps don't cut into your shoulders. Bras like this, worn over the years, can leave small ridges in your skin!**
- ***Cotton bras* are cooler and more comfortable in hot weather than those made from synthetic fibres. The latter can make you perspire more.**
- **There should be no flesh spilling over the top of your bra or bulging out from the sides.**
- ***Seamless bras* are best worn under sweaters and T-shirts.**
- ***Sports bras* are essential for exercise. You want to stop your boobs from bouncing about and so putting too much strain on them. Sports bras are specially designed with features such as straps that won't slip off, extra wide under-the-bust-bands to ensure the bra won't ride up and some have net inserts to allow perspiration to evaporate.**
- ***Invisible support* You may have seen small pads which you stick beneath your bust for support. They're not suitable for large busts but are the answer if you're wearing a revealing top.**

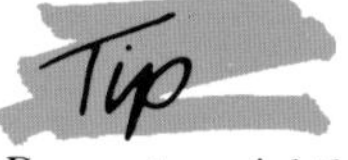

Prevent unsightly spots on your upper chest by washing with a medicated soap.

GOING TOPLESS

As your breasts rarely see the light of day, they can burn more quickly than other parts of your body. Make sure you use a high protection sun cream with a total sun block over your nipples.

Photograph: DIDIER de FEYS/Illustrations: SARAH GARDNER

BREAST BADDIES

HOT BATHS These encourage your skin to soften and slacken over time so try to make sure the water is warm rather than hot.

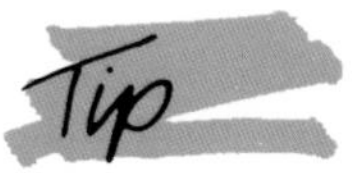

Cold water helps tone up and tighten skin – a quick, cold splash before you get out of the bath will help to keep your boobs perky. If this is too much to bear, wring out a flannel in cold water, and use it like a cold compress, holding it against each breast in turn for a few seconds.

POOR POSTURE Slouch and your boobs will sag. Stand up straight and you'll see an instant improvement. Rounding your shoulders may be a sign you're self-conscious about a big bust, but why try to hide it? If you've got it, flaunt it!

CRASH DIETING Sudden weight loss usually results in sudden weight gain a few weeks later. These fluctuations do nothing for your figure or your bust. You're likely to become flabby as your skin can't spring back into shape easily and stretch marks will start to appear.

It's better to lose weight slowly, gradually learning to improve your eating habits, so that when you reach your target weight, you won't immediately revert to your old ways and pile on the pounds.

HEALTH CHECK Start examining your boobs regularly to ensure you notice any unusual lumps as soon as possible. Your bust naturally has an irregular feel but with frequent checks, you'll become familiar with this and will be able to spot any changes. Don't panic if you do find a lump – very few turn out to be cancerous. They're often just harmless cysts, but do go and see your doctor as soon as you can.

ANY QUESTIONS?

Q Should I have surgery to alter the size of my bust?

A Plastic surgery can give you bigger or smaller breasts but there are risks and complications. Breast implants, for example, can harden while breast reduction can result in scarring. The breast is virtually dismantled which means the nipples need to be moved and sometimes restructured. It's costly too – about the price of an around the world air ticket. If you're seriously considering such an operation, ask your doctor to refer you to a reputable surgeon.

Q What's the best way to get rid of hairs growing around my nipples?

A Just snip the hairs, cutting them close to the skin. Or have them permanently removed with electrolysis, but make sure you go to a qualified electrolysis operator. What you mustn't do is use hair-removing creams or pluck out the hairs – nipples are too sensitive.

Q How can stretch marks and saggy boobs be avoided in pregnancy?

A Some women say they have avoided stretch marks by rubbing oils into their bust every day. But there's no guarantee this will work as stretch marks occur deep down in your skin when fibres overstretch. Stretch marks do eventually fade but your best bet is not to gain too much weight and to wear a good maternity bra, even at night if it's not too uncomfortable.

I MUST, I MUST . . .

. . . improve my bust. Remember reciting these lines at school? Unfortunately, exercise can't increase bust size but will improve shape. Although the breasts themselves contain no muscles, there is a supporting network which runs above your chest to your jaw – grimace or smile broadly and you'll see these tense up – and around the sides from under your armpit. When these are strong and well-toned, they help to keep your boobs pert. These exercises will also help with toning:

SWIMMING is an excellent boob booster, especially breast stroke but also back stroke and crawl.

WEIGHT TRAINING works wonders too. At many gyms you'll find a machine called a pec deck which exercises the pectoral muscles around your breasts. Opening and closing your arms, pushing against the resistance of the weights on the machine will show results in a matter of weeks.

But if you can't get to a gym, use weights at home. And they don't have to be dumb bells – heavy books, cans of baked beans or bags of flour will do the trick. Just lie on your back, on the floor, with knees bent up. Arms should be out to your sides with a weight held in each hand. Now with arms just slightly bent at the elbows, slowly bring them straight up and touch the weights together above your chest. Slowly lower again, and repeat 10 times.

PALM PUSHING is a good one to do when you're watching television. Easy but effective, just put the palms of your hands together, elbows out to the sides, in a praying position. Now push palms together as hard as you can for a count of three. Relax for a count of three. Repeat five times.

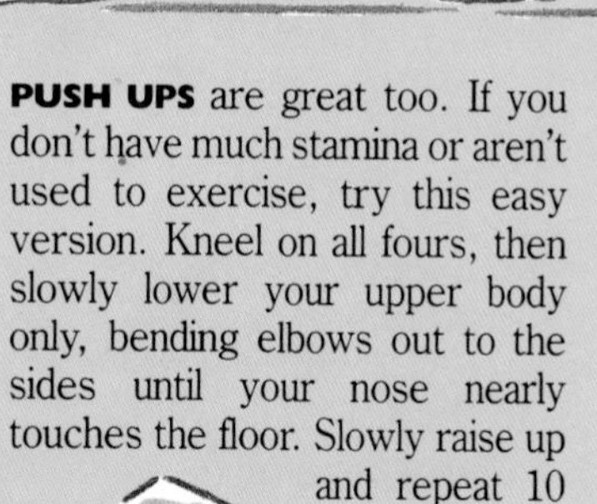

PUSH UPS are great too. If you don't have much stamina or aren't used to exercise, try this easy version. Kneel on all fours, then slowly lower your upper body only, bending elbows out to the sides until your nose nearly touches the floor. Slowly raise up and repeat 10 times.

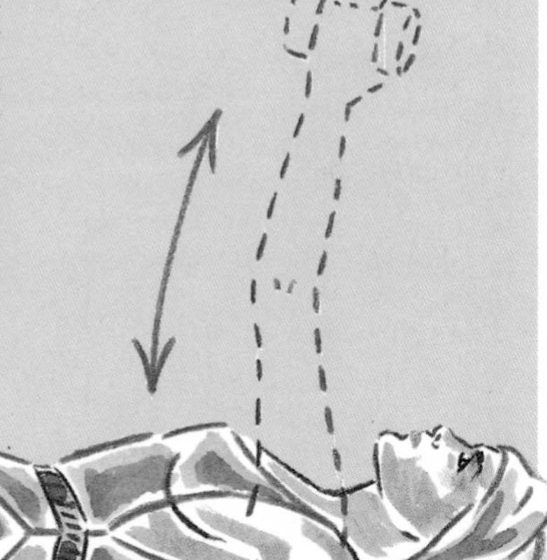

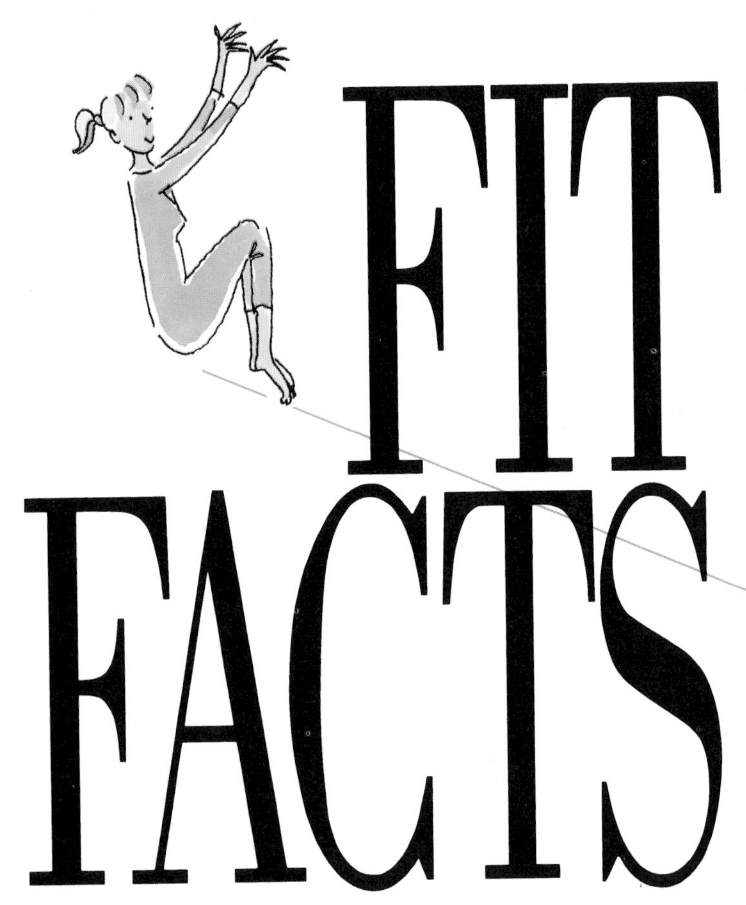

FIT FACTS

If the very thought of exercise makes you sweat, find out how easily you can get fit for life – fast!

Everyone looks and feels better when they're fit. And your body needs to exercise regularly to keep the heart and lungs healthy, your joints loose, and your spine supple and strong. Exercise also helps you to shake off tiredness and lethargy by boosting your circulation and increasing energy and stamina. Regular activity also helps you to cope with stress, sleep better and generally produces a much fitter, healthier looking you. Flab becomes firmer, your skin starts to glow, muscles become stronger and your posture improves.

GYM 'N' TONIC

The most important factor is to find a form of exercise that suits you and your lifestyle. Bear in mind whether you prefer solitary activities such as weight-training or team sports. Will you need to buy special, and often very expensive, equipment or clothing or can you hire what you need? Are there extra costs like membership or class fees? And, of course, do the times of classes fit in with your schedule?

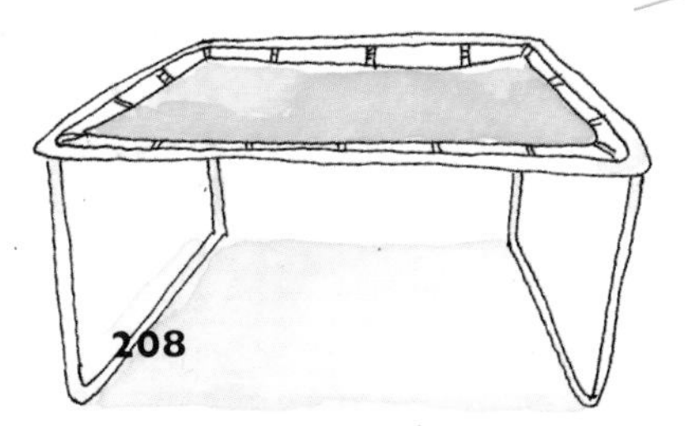

BE A SPORT

Here's a rundown of some of the most popular ways to get fit:

- **Walking** – brisk walking is great for the heart, lungs and lower leg muscles.
- **Swimming** – improves your stamina and suppleness by toning up the whole body. For best results vary the strokes.
- **Dancing** – great for improving the condition of your heart and lungs, building up your leg muscles, burning up calories and improving your social life!
- **Jogging** – works out the heart, lungs and tones up your legs, thighs and bottom. It's essential to wear the right running shoes.
- **Cycling** – helps to improve the condition of the heart, lungs, legs and lower body. Fast or uphill cycling is best.
- **Tennis** – the running, bending and stretching involved gives your whole body a work-out.
- **Weight-training** – builds up the strength and tone of specific muscle groups and particular problem areas.

WARM UPS

Whatever exercise you choose to do, always warm up first. Limbering up in this way means that you're less likely to pull a muscle or injure yourself. Try a few simple stretching movements, run or skip on the spot or even try a short stint of light trampolining.

Wind down slowly after vigorous activity. If you suddenly stop dead you are quite liable to feel faint and dizzy.

GENTLY DOES IT

If you can't bear the thought of exercise, just making a few minor changes in your lifestyle can make you fitter. Walk to work instead of catching the bus and climb the stairs instead of taking the lift. If you sit at a desk all day, get up regularly and walk around to keep your circulation moving. Have a good stretch too – it'll do you the world of good. Make exercise part of your social life and it won't feel such an effort. Go out dancing or organise cycling outings. At home, dance to your favourite record. Even bouncing on your bed is better than no exercise at all!

WORK-OUT WORDS

Here's a quick jog through some popular types of exercise:

Aerobic means 'with air'. This type of activity pumps more oxygen-rich blood around the body.

Anaerobic means 'without air'. You do this exercise in short bursts, like sprinting or gymnastics.

Callanetics is a new exercise system that uses controlled movements to tone up the body.

Cardio-vascular activity gives your heart and circulation system a work-out. Most forms of exercise are cardio-vascular.

Isometrics are resistive muscle exercises – for example pushing or pulling against an immovable object (like a wall). Great for toning up specific areas of your body.

GOOD TRAINING

Get into good exercise habits early and you'll feel and see the benefits in no time:

- Choose a type of exercise that you enjoy, otherwise you'll soon get bored and won't keep it up.
- Join a sports centre with a friend – you'll be much more likely to keep going.
- Stick to your chosen sport for at least 20 minutes three times a week.
- If you start to feel dizzy or faint, stop immediately.
- Don't go on a low-calorie diet and do vigorous exercise at the same time. You'll feel faint.
- Be careful not to push yourself too soon. It's much better to build up slowly, rather than over-exerting yourself in the first five minutes.

One final word of warning – if you have a history of back or respiratory problems, chest pains or you suffer from frequent dizzy spells or diabetes – do go to your doctor for a check-up before you start any new exercise programme. If you're pregnant, check with your doctor about exercising at home or joining antenatal classes.

ROW FOR IT

If you're thinking of investing in home exercise equipment, a rowing machine is probably your best buy. Rowing tones, firms and generally fine tunes the whole of your body. Unlike cycling or running it uses all major, and most minor, muscle groups – not just the legs.

Watchpoint

Choose safe and sensible sports gear. Invest in a good sports bra and buy the right footwear to cushion your legs if you're exercising on concrete roads. Avoid clothing made of synthetic materials and go for natural fibres instead.

Illustration: BILL PIGGINS

If you've been feeling the squeeze around your waistband lately, you know you could probably do with losing a few pounds. So at the same time as embarking on our exercise programme here, start a diet. Get a good, healthy regime from your doctor or join a slimming club and be a winning loser!

Most dieticians now agree that to lose weight you need to cut down on your fat intake which means less butter, fatty red meat, fry-ups and fewer foods with hidden fat such as cakes, biscuits and pastry. You can, however, eat fish and poultry as well as a controlled amount of bread, rice and pasta. These are nutritious sources of energy but make sure you opt for wholemeal varieties. Most of your diet should be fruit and vegetables which are high in fibre, an important ingredient when slimming since being constipated can make you bloated!

BULGE BEATERS

Even if you're not overweight, you can still have a bulging tummy caused by slack stomach muscles and poor posture. There's a whole network of muscles around your midriff that need exercising. These include:

- The straight abdominals – they run down the centre of your midriff from your chest to your lower tummy and allow you to bend your body forwards.
- The oblique muscles – you'll find these on either side of your midriff. They enable your trunk to turn to each side.
- The transverse abdominals – situated low down on either side of your tummy, by your hips. Just another part of the network that holds your organs in place!

Once you have got all these muscles toned up, they'll act like a natural corset, holding your tummy and waist in as well as supporting your back. Try our routine and you'll soon see a difference. But remember, although you need to put some effort into the exercises to make them effective, never overdo it. Also, if you have any back problems, are seriously overweight or pregnant, check with your doctor first.

Note: each exercise, except where specified should be repeated five times. After a few days, make it six times and after a few weeks, you should be able to manage 20 repeats with ease.

ALWAYS warm up first.

NEVER arch your back, jerk your body, strain your neck or shoulders, or hold your breath.

WAIST DISPOSAL

A fat tummy and spare tyre are unsightly when you're in your undies and they also spoil the look and feel of your clothes. So if you can pinch a wodge around your middle, banish the bulge with our waist-whittling tips

WARM UP

March on the spot for a minute, lifting your knees up high and pumping your arms vigorously. Now stand with feet slightly apart, hands resting on shoulders. Then bend your left knee over your left foot and stretch your left hand up high. Repeat on other side, 20 times in all.

ABDOMINAL STRENGTHENER

Lie on your back, knees bent up, stomach pulled in, back pushed into floor. Now slightly raise your head and shoulders and stretch hands either side of knees. Slowly lower, breathing out.

TWIST AND TRIM

Lie flat on your back, hands behind your head. Lift your legs up vertically, crossing them over at the ankles and with knees bent slightly. Now reach up and try to touch your right knee with your left elbow. Then without lowering your shoulders too much, reach your right elbow over to your left knee.

SPIN AND SLIM

Stand with feet apart, knees slightly bent. Hold a long brush handle at either end behind your neck and shoulders. Fixing your eyes on a point straight ahead twist from the waist to the left then slowly to the right. DON'T twist your hips or head, only your waist.

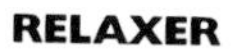

RELAXER

After each exercise you should repeat this movement so that your muscles don't tense up. Just lie flat on your back, hugging your knees to your chest. Now turn head slowly to left and slowly to right.

Tip

While sitting in front of the TV, clench and relax your tummy muscles – it'll firm them up.

Photograph: WILL WHITE/Illustrations: GILLIAN SAUNDERS/Hair: SHIRALEE LAW/Make-up: VIRGINIA NICHOLS

CLEVER CLOTHING

Until your waist's in shape, you can disguise the bulges by opting for flattering outfits.
DO go for long, loose tops.
DO buy belts that are on the wide side and fasten them on a loose notch so that they skim over your body or even dip slightly below your waist.
DO opt for tailored, well-cut clothes like coat dresses.
DO go for comfortable draped fabrics.
DO fit small, padded shoulders to balance your outine and help give the illusion of a narrower waist.
DO think about your underwear. Lycra high cut panties give a slimmer, smoother look and avoid that visible panty line.
DON'T wear midriff skimming jackets and tops.
DON'T wear very tight narrow waistbands or belts that force flab to bulge over the top.
DON'T even think about coats or dresses with tie belts.
DON'T wear ultra tight and clingy Lycra, velour or knitted outfits.
DON'T buy gathered or dirndl skirts that may make your waist look small but will make your hips and tummy look huge.

Watchpoint

Avoid swimming costumes with detail around the middle, or low-cut tops and high-cut bottoms – they'll accentuate your tum!

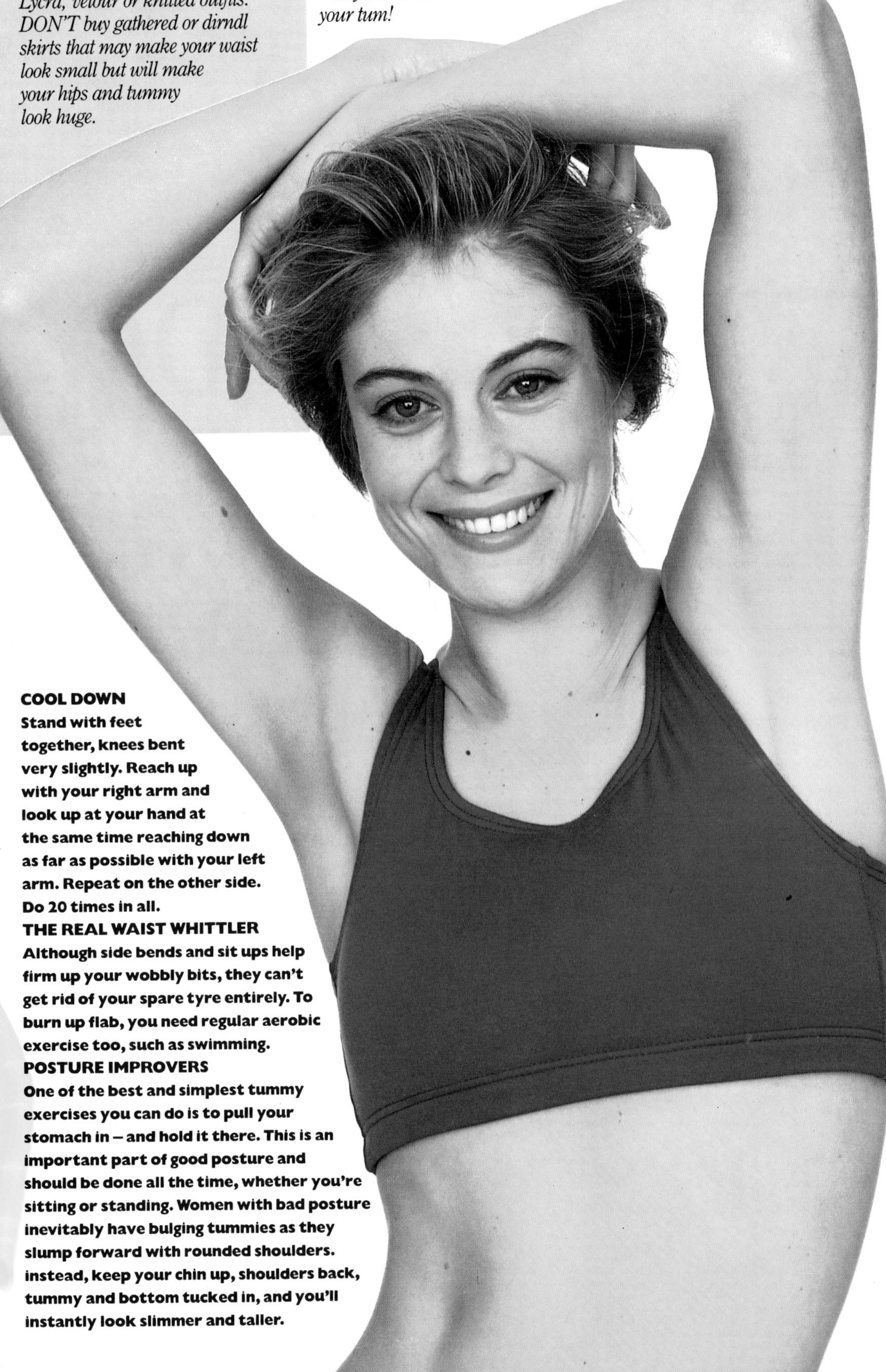

SIDE STRETCH
Stand with feet shoulder-width apart, knees slightly bent. Bend elbows and cross hands in front of waist. Then as you lift one elbow up to the side stretch the other arm out to the other side at shoulder level and lean towards it slightly. Return to starting position and repeat on the other side.

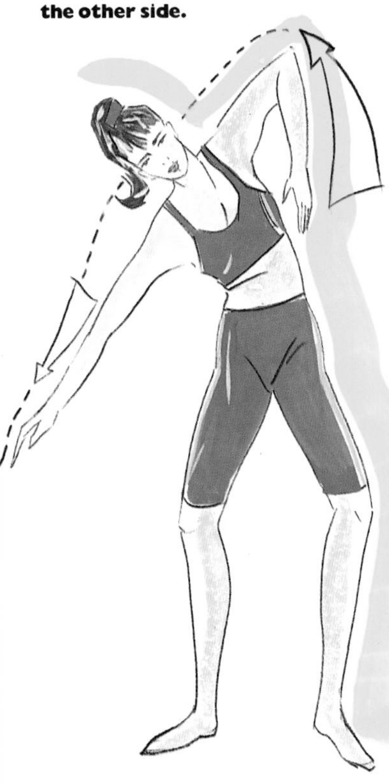

COOL DOWN
Stand with feet together, knees bent very slightly. Reach up with your right arm and look up at your hand at the same time reaching down as far as possible with your left arm. Repeat on the other side. Do 20 times in all.

THE REAL WAIST WHITTLER
Although side bends and sit ups help firm up your wobbly bits, they can't get rid of your spare tyre entirely. To burn up flab, you need regular aerobic exercise too, such as swimming.

POSTURE IMPROVERS
One of the best and simplest tummy exercises you can do is to pull your stomach in – and hold it there. This is an important part of good posture and should be done all the time, whether you're sitting or standing. Women with bad posture inevitably have bulging tummies as they slump forward with rounded shoulders. instead, keep your chin up, shoulders back, tummy and bottom tucked in, and you'll instantly look slimmer and taller.

LIGHTWEIGHT MATTERS

Are you constantly the butt of jokes about twigs and pipe cleaners? Then help's at hand if you're seriously skinny with our plan to help you shape up your thin body

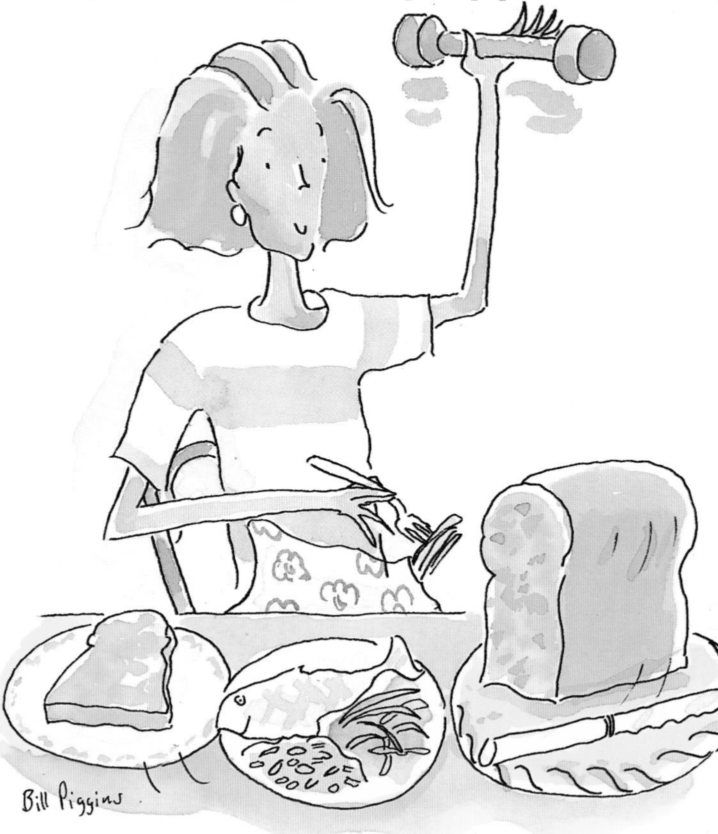

If your clothes hang off you, your bikini looks baggy and people are always calling you names like chicken legs or tin ribs – then you just may be underweight.

Being too skinny can be a temporary condition – the result of illness, injury or a period of stress – when your food intake hasn't been able to keep up with your body's energy levels and causes it to draw on its natural stores of fat. But don't think that all you have to do is eat masses of chips and cakes to fill out in all the right places. Some people stay skinny (more than 10 percent below the ideal weight for their height) all through their lives whatever they eat.

Being underweight is not like being anorexic. It's not a disease and most underweight people have excellent health. However, women that are skinny generally feel that they look bony and not curvy enough. Needless to say it doesn't really do a lot for self-esteem. But even if being too thin is due to hereditary factors there are things you can do to give yourself a better body shape. In the meantime try not to feel bad about being thin. After all, ideal weight charts are worked out statistically and aren't necessarily right for you.

WHY ME?

Why are some of us too thin? There are six important possibilities to consider:

FAMILY HISTORY

Recent studies have suggested that if your biological mum and dad are knobbly-kneed skinnies with mammoth appetites, then you are quite likely to be too. Your metabolism – the rate at which the body converts food to energy or stores it as fat – may be hereditary too.

AGE

If you're under 21, you could still be using all your energy to grow upwards. When you finally reach your adult height that energy will be used to fill you out!

DIET

Maybe you're not eating enough or you're eating too many low-calorie foods. Alternatively, you could be eating the right foods to gain weight, but your metabolism is very high and you just 'burn off' excess food energy before any of it is stored as fat in your body.

EXERCISE

You may be scared to exercise in case you lose even more weight. But exercising doesn't just burn up calories – it gets all parts of your body working more efficiently. It also stimulates the digestive tract – making you feel hungrier – so that you'll want to eat more – and often. Regular exercise like weight-training can also help to build up specific parts of your body.

HEALTH

A bout of illness or suffering an injury can cause temporary appetite loss, so it's quite normal to lose a bit of weight then. If you're constantly feeling tired and listless or look pale and spotty and have no interest in eating – then you should go to your doctor for a check-up. It could be something serious that is causing your weight to drop.

STRESS

Anxious or nervous people often tend to be thin. This is because all their energy is taken up keeping their nervous systems in one piece! A certain amount of stress is good for you, but you can have far too much and this can keep your weight down. So learn to relax (try yoga or deep breathing exercises) if you're trying to fatten up!

FILLING OUT!

The younger you are, the more likely it is that time and nature will sort out your problem. But there's no harm in helping them along a little – follow our hints:

DIET

- **To get your digestion working and give your body the best chance to build you up, eat fresh energy-giving foods like fish, fruit, raw vegetables, bean sprouts, brown rice, muesli and brown bread. Always eat when you're hungry but try to avoid eating after 9pm.**
- **Don't let yourself binge on fast food, fry-ups, cakes, sweets or milkshakes; they'll just make you feel sluggish. And don't be tempted by products that claim to increase body weight. There's no evidence that they work.**

EXERCISE

- **Make it regular – at least three half-hour sessions a week. Exercise, like swimming or dancing, improves the absorption of essential nutrients in the body – and helps you relax.**

RELAXATION

- **Stress could be the biggest single cause of being underweight, so learn to relax! Imagine you're floating in a warm bath or on a cloud – whatever you choose, do it *every* day!**
- **Get to the bottom of your problems. Worrying about them can make you lose weight so take the time to sort them out.**

HEALTH

- **It's always a good idea to see your doctor about any health matter, including being underweight, just to make sure there isn't a serious problem. If you get a clean bill of health it could be a deep-seated psychological problem that's making you lose weight – so it might be worth going to a counsellor.**

Illustration: BILL PIGGINS

TRIM THOSE

For these, or any other exercises, to have a real effect they must be repeated regularly. Make and take time to do the ones which tackle *your* trouble spots every day or every other day. Warm up with a gentle jog on the spot and a few stretches first, and cool down afterwards with a repeat of the warm-up sequence, but in reverse order.

THE WORRY: A double chin
THE WORKOUT: (No joke!) Stick your tongue out as far as you can, then try to touch it to the tip of your nose. Repeat 10 times. Next, tilt your head back, making your neck long. Push your jaw forward and lift the lower lip over the top lip. Repeat 10 times. Once a day, pat the skin under and around your jaw and chin, using your fingertips.

THE WORRY: Wobbly thighs.
THE WORKOUT: Kneel upright and stretch both arms straight out in front at shoulder level. Now lean back, as far as is comfortable, and at the same time press your thighs together. Straighten up, relax, then repeat nine times.

Sit upright but cross-legged on the floor. Lightly, rest hands on knees, then press the knees down and out towards the floor. Relax, then repeat nine times.

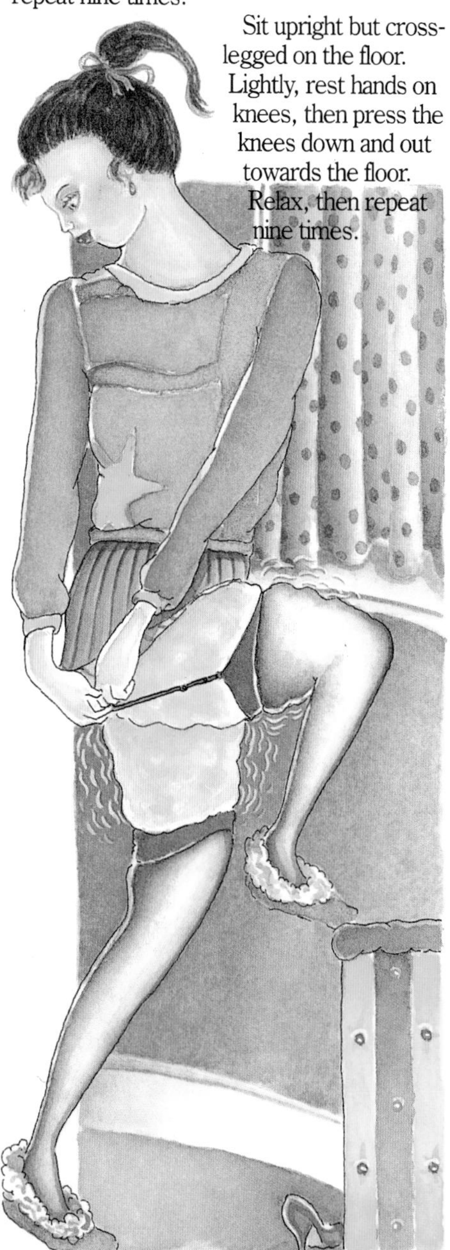

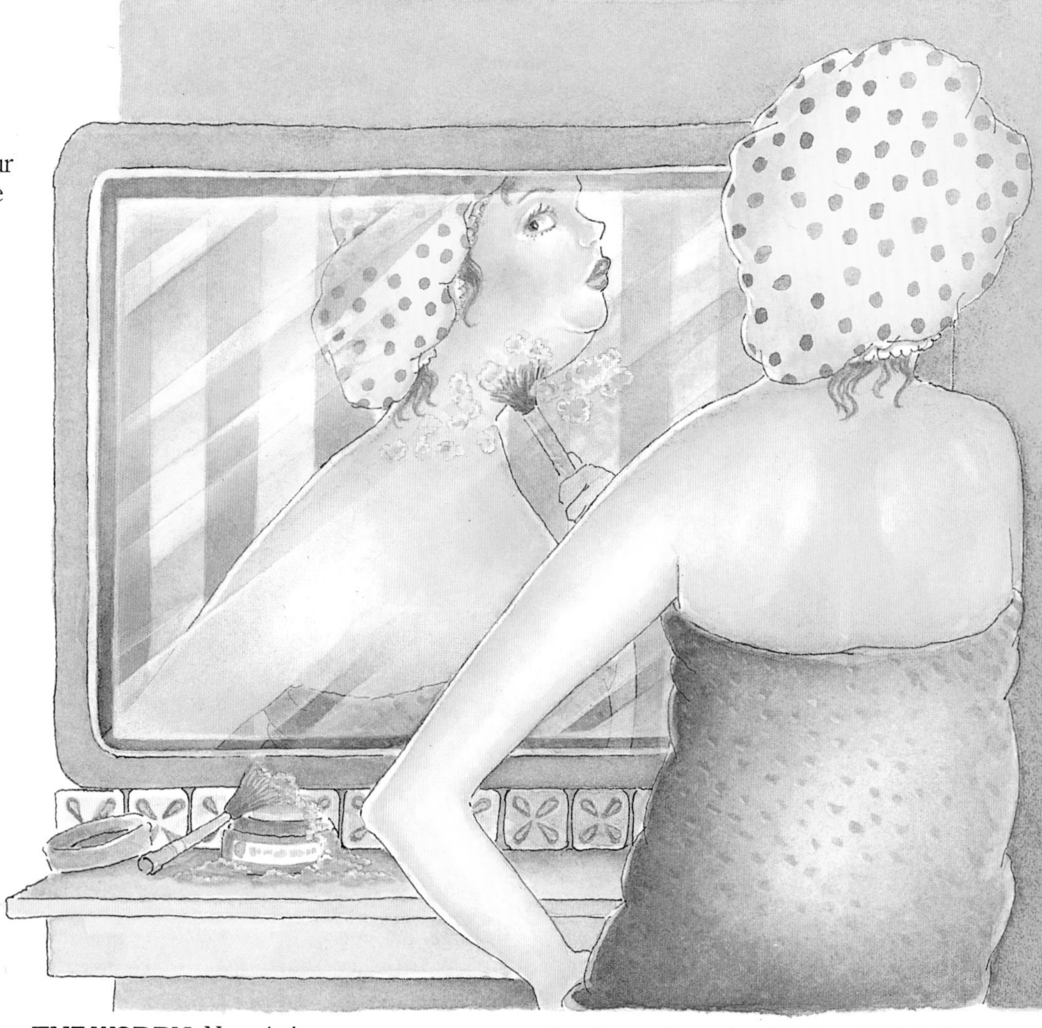

THE WORRY: No waist!
THE WORKOUT: Stand tall, right hand on hip, left arm at side. Bend from the waist, to the left, letting left arm slide down leg as far as is comfortable. Take care to keep your body in a straight line, without leaning backwards or forwards as you bend to the side. Repeat nine times, then change sides and repeat 10 times.

Then, with right hand on right hip, stretch left arm out to the side at shoulder level. Keeping hips facing to the front, twist the top of your body to the left, swinging left arm to the right. Straighten out, and repeat nine times. Then change sides and repeat 10 times.

THE WORRY: Flabby hips
THE WORKOUT: Kneel on the floor with arms outstretched (holding on to a support if you need to). With knee still bent, raise right leg out to the side, then unbend knee and stretch leg out fully. Bend knee again and return leg to starting position. Repeat sequence with left leg. Repeat nine times, alternating right leg with left. Lie flat on your back on the floor and pull both knees tight in to chest, clasp your hands around them. Roll to the right then to the left, touching knees to floor on each side as you do so. Aim to repeat this exercise about another 19 times.

THE WORRY: A pot belly!
THE WORKOUT: Do sit-ups in reverse – sit up with knees bent and feet flat on the floor. Rest palms on knees, pull stomach in and lower your torso backwards as far as is comfortable. Then turn hands over and sit up again as smoothly as possible. Repeat nine times.

Now sit on the floor with legs stretched out in front, hands flat on the floor at either side for support. Bend one knee, keeping the foot flat on the floor. Then raise the other outstretched leg just a short way off the floor, keeping the toes pointed. Lower and raise leg four times more. Then work on your other leg and repeat five times in all.

TROUBLE SPOTS

Do you wobble when you walk and sag when you sit, despite the fact you've lost weight? Then what you need is a workout to shape you up

THE WORRY: A seat that sags!
THE WORKOUT: Simply stand tall, pull seat up and in, then press buttocks tightly together and hold for a count of five. Release, and repeat nine times. Next lie face down on the floor. Put arms at sides, palms down, and stretch chin forward, but keep it touching the floor. With knee locked, lift right leg off floor – just a little way – keeping the pelvis pressed hard into the floor. Repeat nine times, then change legs and repeat 10 times.

Watchpoint

If you have joint or back problems, are pregnant or overweight, have recently had a baby or have any other doubts about your fitness, consult your doctor before you try these exercises.

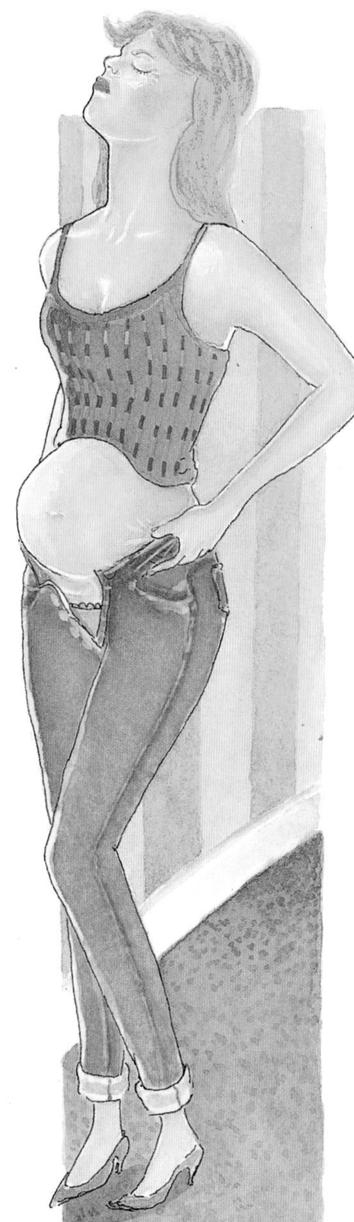

THE WORRY: Fat across the back of your shoulders.
THE WORKOUT: Stretch your arms out to the sides and bend back from elbows so that fingertips are resting on your shoulders. Make circular movements for 15 seconds in a clockwise direction and then repeat in an anti-clockwise direction for 15 seconds. Alternatively, stand upright with your arms relaxed at sides. Shrug shoulders six times, then hold the next one for a count of four. Repeat sequence eight times.

THE WORRY: Flabby upper arms.
THE WORKOUT: Stand upright with your legs shoulder-width apart, arms stretched straight out at either side of you. Clench your fists and, with elbows locked, make small circles for 15 seconds. Repeat in other direction for 15 seconds.

THE WORRY: A sagging bust.
THE WORKOUT: To tone up the muscles which help to support the bust, fold arms across chest, each hand gripping the opposite forearm. Lift your arms up to shoulder level, then push arms upwards. Relax and repeat nine times more.

Finish off by pressing the palms of your hands together in front of you, at bust level, as if in prayer. Push hard, then relax, 10 times in all.

Tip

Use exercise (and massage) to help prevent cellulite forming on your thighs and upper arms.

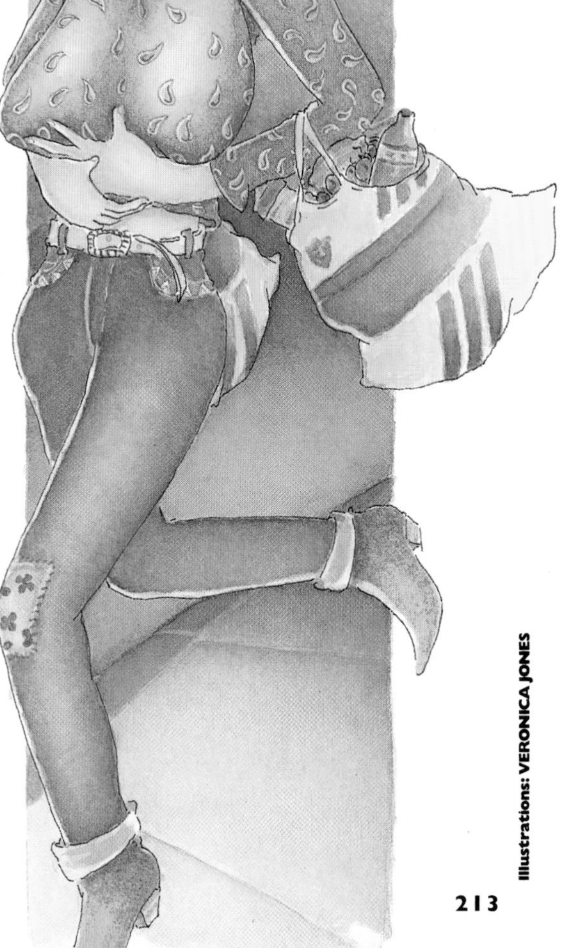

Illustrations: VERONICA JONES

A DOSE OF YOUR OWN MEDICINE . . .

Feeling poorly? Nothing the doctor gives you seems help? Try homoeopathy and find out how natural remedies can work

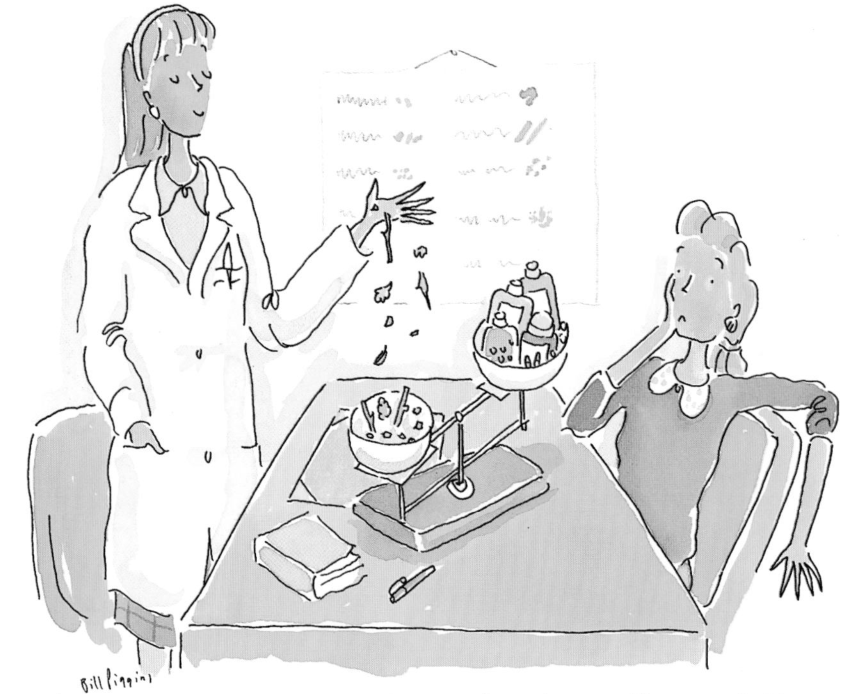

Like lots of the great scientific advances, homoeopathy (pronounced home-ee-op-pathy) was discovered by accident. Two hundred years ago, a German doctor Samuel Hahnemann was experimenting on himself by taking quinine (a drug used to treat malaria). To his amazement, he started to develop the symptoms of malaria, even though he'd never been near a mosquito! He went on to test other drugs and discovered that a drug could cause the symptoms of a disease in a healthy person and could cure them in a person with the actual disease. He called this way of treating illness homoeopathy, which means treating 'like with like', and he went on to discover that the more he diluted his potions, the more potent they became. Even stranger, they seemed to cause fewer and fewer side effects. So whether the remedy was made from silver, thorn-apple, or snake venom, it couldn't poison him or give him the kind of side effects which would usually be expected from other drugs.

It's not just the medicines that are different with homoeopathy: it aims to turn your ideas about illness upside down too. For instance, if you went to your doctor with spots or a cold you'd expect to get something to zap the spots or stop your nose running. But a homoeopath will leave those minor symptoms alone; they're a sign your body is cleaning itself out and getting your system back in balance. Just getting rid of the symptoms can be dangerous. It forces your body to choose another route to heal you, which could mean a more serious illness.

Instead, homoeopathy works on the same vital energy sources as acupuncture; once that energy's flowing again, your symptoms will disappear since your immune system is gently kick-started into operation. Homoeopathy helps you build up your resistance to diseases for life, not just for the present.

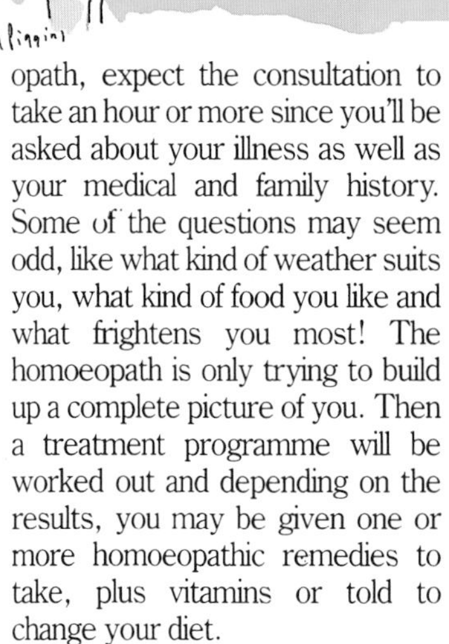

HOME HELP

It's a brilliant first-aid medicine as well; you can easily learn to use it at home for cuts and bruises, stings, shock, burns and tummy upsets. You can buy homoeopathic remedies at most good health food shops, but always receive a professional diagnosis before treating yourself at home.

When you go to see a homoeopath, expect the consultation to take an hour or more since you'll be asked about your illness as well as your medical and family history. Some of the questions may seem odd, like what kind of weather suits you, what kind of food you like and what frightens you most! The homoeopath is only trying to build up a complete picture of you. Then a treatment programme will be worked out and depending on the results, you may be given one or more homoeopathic remedies to take, plus vitamins or told to change your diet.

You may need to pay the homoeopath several visits and if you suffer from certain allergies you'll need to keep up the diet recommended for life.

WORKING TIME

The idea of homoeopathy is to heal as gently and quickly as possible. Sometimes you'll start to feel better immediately after you take the recommended remedy. But more often the remedy works by 'spring-cleaning' your system, which might mean the symptoms get worse for a few days, or new ones such as a runny nose, a sore throat or a rash may develop, before you get any improvement. Don't worry – you'll soon feel better! Homoeopathy works 'from the inside out' – which means that serious problems will clear up first whereas the spots you originally complained about may take months to disappear! And as you get better, you'll be more in touch with the way your body works naturally.

So instead of automatically rushing for the painkillers or the antibiotics, start to see illness as signals to slow down, take a look at how you're living your life and make changes for the better.

WHAT CAN HOMOEOPATHY TREAT?

Like any treatment, there is no guaranteed cure, but it is claimed that homoeopathy can help all sorts of problems from migraine to cancer.

Here are a few of the well-known ones:

- **period pains, heavy and irregular periods**
- **sports injuries**
- **depression**
- **spots and acne**
- **eating problems**
- **phobias**
- **eczema and asthma**
- **hay fever**
- **constipation and flatulence**
- **allergies**
- **anaemia**
- **headaches**

Illustration: BILL PIGGINS

THE GENTLE TOUCH

Nothing beats a massage for stroking away the stresses of the day. We show you how to put the magic in your fingertips or – better still – get a friend to do one for you . . .

WORK OUT ON THE JOB

Feeling tense and grouchy at work? Instead of reaching for another cup of coffee or bar of chocolate, try our mini massages.

NECKS & SHOULDERS

Press fingertips lightly on either side of your neck, just below the nape (see above). Work around neck to the front, then back again. Knead each shoulder. Squeeze and release flesh on shoulders and the tops of your arms. Clench your fist and pummel each shoulder 20 times (see right).

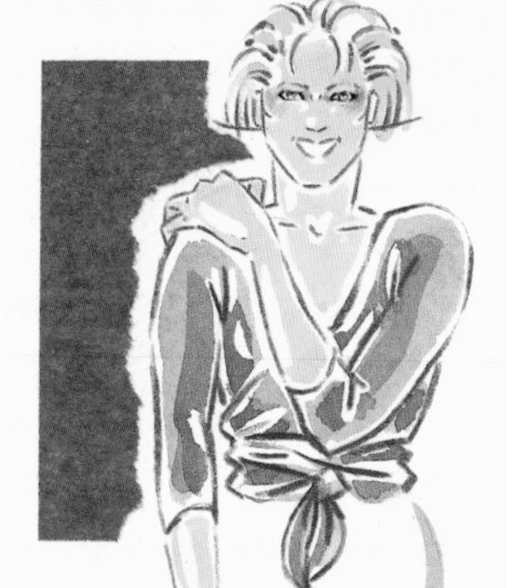

SHOULDERS & ARMS

Stroke your right shoulder (see above left). Move down to the elbow. Glide back to your neck, repeat three times. Do the other side. Start at your right shoulder, knead the skin down to the elbow and up to the top of the spine (above right). Do the other side.

Photograph: PAUL MITCHELL/Masseur: ALDO at FOGAZZA/Illustrations: JACQUELINE BISSETT

If you've ever had a massage you'll know how wonderfully relaxing it is. Whether it was an hour of professional pampering or a friend gently rubbing your tired shoulders, it probably left you feeling on top of the world. In a way, it's something you do instinctively when you give someone a cuddle or a pat on the back, and with massage, you're merely taking the power of touch a step further . . .

For centuries, massage has been used to relieve aches and pains and relax both body and mind. The back is the best place to start on – that's where the benefit of massage is really felt and, since backache is one of the most common complaints, it's worth knowing ways to prevent it or relieve the symptoms. You can then massage all over or move on to your neck and shoulders for a really relaxing treat.

There's no need for years of training before you start – all you need do is to perfect a few basic massage techniques. It won't cost you much either – just the price of some baby oil or a wonderfully scented essential oil like lavender. So get together with a friend and you're guaranteed to be in top form – mentally and physically – in no time at all.

MASSAGE IS GOOD FOR:
- **improving circulation**
- **giving body functions a gentle boost**
- **all-over total relaxation**
- **keeping skin supple**
- **reducing insomnia**

GET THE MASSAGE?

A good massage isn't necessarily one that has lots of complicated techniques. It's more important that you get the atmosphere and general feel right so the person who's being massaged can unwind. So don't worry if your technique isn't perfect – stick to one or two movements. For instance, begin with long, light, rhythmic, stroking movements that relax the muscles, rather like warming up before exercise. The strokes can then get gradually stronger, as you move on to smaller movements concentrating on areas of tense muscles.

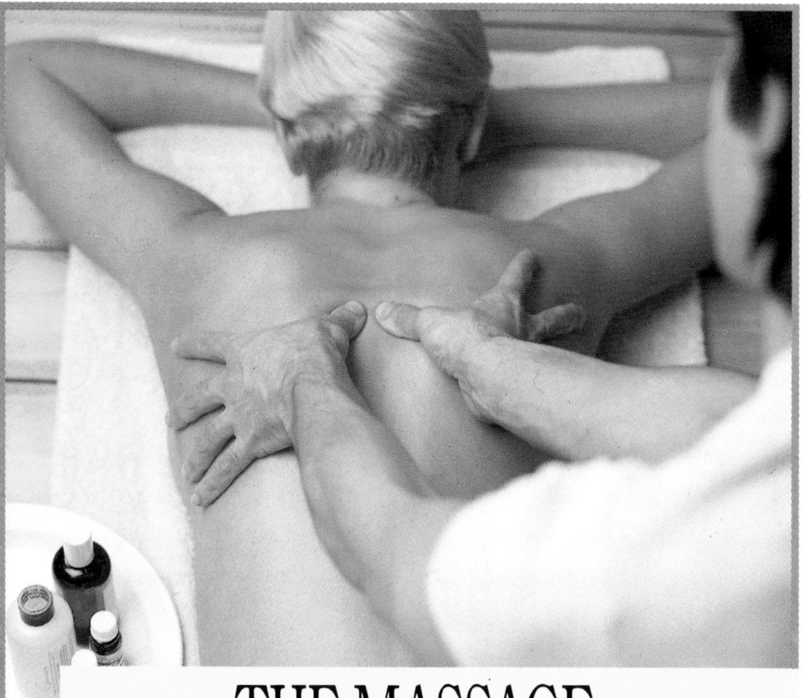

THE MASSAGE

For a proper all-over massage, it's worthwhile knowing a few of the basic strokes and their benefits:

MOVEMENT	BENEFITS
Stroking	As the name implies, stroking is good for relaxing at the start of the massage. Use long, light movements or firmer strokes to boost the circulation.
Kneading	This is called petrissage – and it's just like kneading dough. You literally pick up the flesh and squeeze it, then, using the whole hand, with fingers loosely together, press the flesh against the palm. Good for tense and 'knotty' shoulders and backache.
Pinching	Similar technique, with the same effects as kneading, but use only the thumbs and forefingers.
Wringing	Work with both hands, and imagine you're wringing out a cloth. Pick up the flesh, squeeze and twist it – but be careful not to bruise it! Good for relaxing and toning.
Clapping/ slapping	Slap skin with two fingers held loosely, or use the side or back of hands and even fists. Boosts a sluggish system – an instant reviver.
Caterpillar walking	Press left hand flat against the skin, fingers together. Cover with right hand. Lift up left palm so only fingers are in contact with the skin. Apply slight pressure to the bottom hand with right hand then relax. Continue this movement up the skin and repeat. Good for a 'knotty', stiff back.

Finish off with deep strokes again, this time getting lighter and lighter until the fingers can hardly be felt on the skin.

The whole massage should last somewhere between five and 20 minutes, with each movement being repeated at least 10 times before moving on to the next..

Surprisingly, you don't need to be strong or muscular to give a good massage. The secret lies in using your own body weight and leaning into the movements to give them pressure. After a few massages, you'll know just how much pressure is needed. Remember, it's almost impossible to hurt a healthy body by massaging it – always using light, gentle strokes won't do any good at all.

BARE ESSENTIALS

You don't have to spend a fortune on oils – grapeseed or baby oil are as good as anything else.

For an extra special massage, try adding a few drops of essential or aromatherapy oils. The smells from these are believed to affect your mood and so enhance the effects of the massage. For one massage, pour about a teaspoon of a base oil, such as almond or wheatgerm, on to a saucer and add just two or three drops of the essential oil. Try one, or a combination, of the following mood enhancers:

RELAXING: lavender, rose, jasmine and geranium
INVIGORATING: rosemary, cinnamon, thyme, sage
WARMING: eucalyptus, ginger, bay, cypress
SENSUAL: ylang ylang, patchouli, clove, sandalwood
HEALING: tea tree, lavender, camomile, ylang ylang

BODY TALK

- Choose a warm, quiet room to work in. Draw the curtains and turn down the lights.
- Arrange a massage for when you've got plenty of time and won't be distracted.
- Put on your favourite relaxing music. Use a tape rather than an LP so you don't have to keep changing it.
- Have everything you need to hand before you begin.
- Spread a large soft towel on the floor for your friend to lie on and keep another handy for covering up. If you want to use a table it must be steady and large enough so the person who's being massaged doesn't hang off the ends!
- Make your friend as comfortable as possible. (A warm shower beforehand will help to relax muscles).
- The fewer clothes worn the better – you don't want them to get in the way while you massage. Cover parts of the body not being massaged with towels to keep them warm. The masseuse should also wear loose, comfortable clothing so she can move more freely.
- Both of you should tie long hair out of the way and take off rings and dangly jewellery.
- Try not to talk too much during the massage! The quieter it is the more relaxing the massage will be.

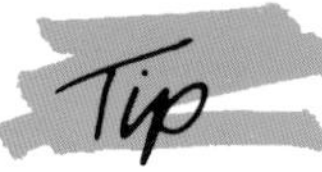

Always start by pouring about a teaspoonful of oil into your hand to warm it up. Cold oil poured directly onto someone's body will wake rather than relax them!

DO'S AND DON'TS

DO

Use talc instead of oil if a greasy or spotty back is a problem.
Make sure nails are short and snag-free to prevent scratching.

DON'T

Use too much oil as hands will just slip over the skin and not get a proper grip.
Worry if the skin goes a bit red – it's due to an increase in the blood circulation, and means that a good job is being done.
Be massaged or massage someone with serious back, skin or health problems.
Use an undiluted essential oil on the skin as this can cause irritation, always use a base oil.
Massage or be massaged on a bed – it doesn't provide enough support for the body, and it will sink away from the pressure rather than absorbing it.

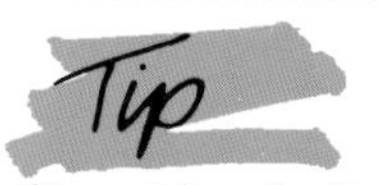

Spread the oil all over the skin before you start the massage movements. Then, for a really professional massage, try to keep your hands in contact with the skin all the time.

MOODY BLUES

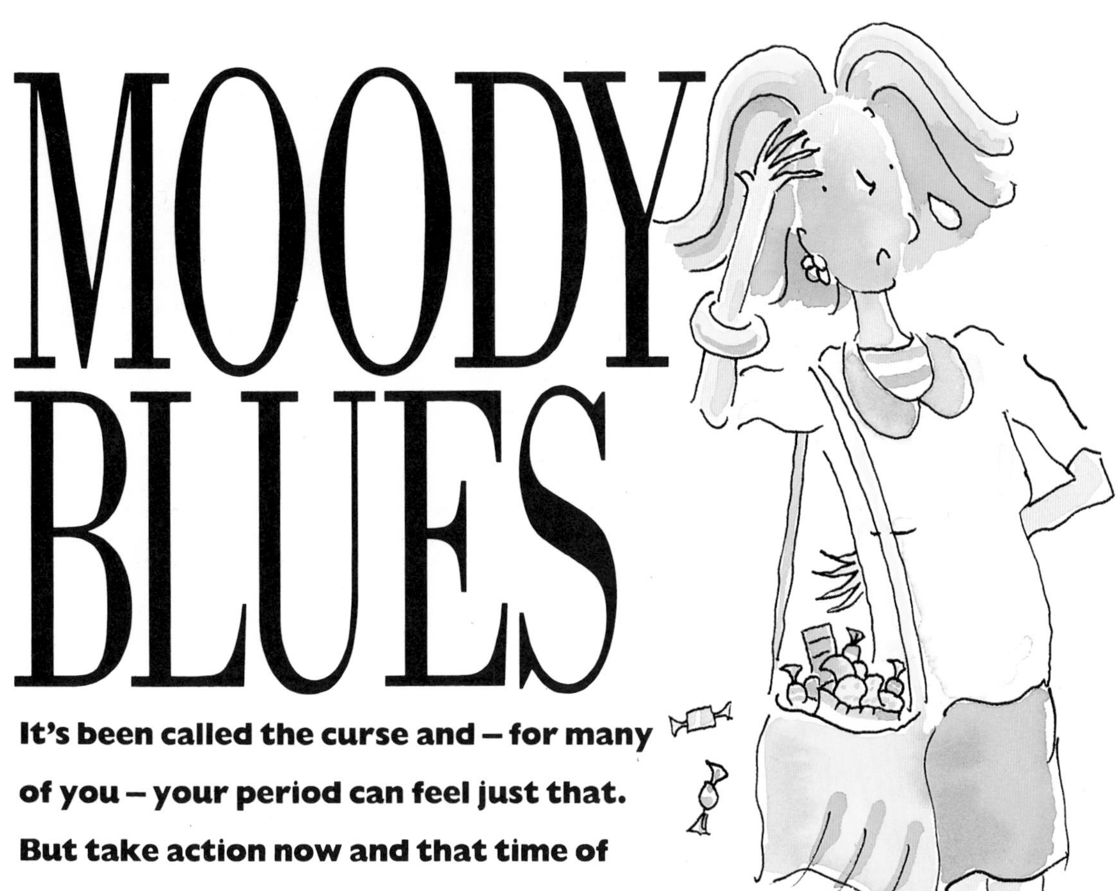

It's been called the curse and – for many of you – your period can feel just that. But take action now and that time of the month could look a lot rosier!

You know how it is: you get out the diary to pencil in an important event – maybe it's a first date, a big exam, or a long-awaited holiday – and, just your luck, it coincides with *that* 'time of the month': the week when you can't help snapping at your family, throwing weepy wobblies all over the place for no reason and feeling tense and tired.

It just doesn't seem fair that your body can ruin your life like this month after month, but it's a frustrating fact of life that nine out of ten of you will suffer from Pre-Menstrual Syndrome (or PMS for short) at some time or another.

AT RISK?

PMS can start at any time of life, but events that cause big changes in your hormone levels put you more at risk, like: going on or coming off the pill; having a baby, a miscarriage or an abortion; having two or more children close together; and if your mother has suffered from Pre-Menstrual Syndrome.

So, what exactly is PMS and, more importantly, what can you do about it?

WHAT IS PMS?

Pre-Menstrual Syndrome is the name for a collection of symptoms many women experience during about ten days before their period starts each month. It's not an illness, but it can make you behave totally out of character. There are over 150 recognised symptoms of PMS, although most women are only likely to experience some of the following:

- Mood swings.
- Cravings for sweet food.
- Irritability, tension, anxiety.
- Depression or sadness.
- Outbursts of anger.
- Overwhelming tiredness.
- Water retention.
- Swollen breasts, feet or hands.
- Migraine.
- Backache.
- Spotty skin.
- Weepiness.
- Lank hair.

If you suffer three or four of these symptoms every month you could be suffering from PMS.

Doctors disagree about the causes of PMS. Some think that it's due to diet, lifestyle, or stress; others that it's hereditary, hormonal or to do with your attitude to menstruation. All may play a part.

WHAT CAN I DO ABOUT IT?

Start by looking at how you feel about menstruation. Is it 'the curse', unclean and embarrassing? Or is it a special time to pamper yourself and feel proud to be a woman? Feeling resentful or disgusted with yourself will make the discomfort, swelling, or bad temper seem much worse, so try to welcome your periods and don't treat them like an embarrassing secret. After all, how can people be nice to you if they don't have a clue why you're feeling moody?

THE WRITE WAY

It can also help to keep a diary, making a note of things you feel bad about, people you're angry with, or problems worrying you. Talking it all through with a friend when the PMS has passed means there's less reason for an outburst next month! Yoga, or any kind of dance, will make you feel more positive and teach you to relax so you'll be less moody.

YOU ARE WHAT YOU EAT

It helps to eat a fresh, wholefood diet. Include wheatgerm, eggs, nuts, green leafy vegetables, avocados, bananas and liver to give you the Vitamin B6 (pyridoxine) and other essential minerals such as magnesium, zinc and iron that it is claimed help ward off PMS.

And it goes without saying that lots of fresh air, exercise and regular sleep can work wonders!

HELP YOURSELF

Here are a few simple guidelines to help you cope when the next bout of PMS is upon you:

- DO accept that you get PMS, and plan to take it easy for a few days before your period.
- DO try to avoid heavy housework, important appointments, special dates or confrontrations at work.
- DO keep evenings free for warm baths, chatting to friends or pottering about.
- DO try Evening Primrose Oil – available in capsule form – as it is thought to help the body produce GLA, an essential fatty acid, which can help relieve common PMS symptoms.
- DON'T skip meals. Eat a regular, healthy diet, with plenty of green vegetables and fruit to ensure you get the necessary vitamins and minerals.
- DON'T binge on sweets, fatty foods, or drink too much alcohol, tea or coffee. All of these can prevent the body from properly absorbing essential minerals.
- DON'T suffer in silence – ask for understanding and support.
- DON'T sprinkle salt on your food as it can contribute to water retention.

Illustration: BILL PIGGINS

Never mind if your legs aren't as long as you'd like – they can still look lovely if you give them some attention

PERFECT PINS

Don't neglect your legs so they let you down – just follow our advice to keep them in tip-top condition.

Exfoliate – skin on the legs has a tendency to be dry so scrub away dead cells regularly. Try using a loofah and lather up with soap in the bath, or invest in a body scrub. Work up from ankles to thighs, concentrating on dry shins, goose-pimply flesh and cellulite.

Moisturise – after your daily bath or shower, lavish lots of body lotion on your legs. This soothes dry skin and prevents flaking. On thicker skin, over your knees for instance, you may need a richer cream to keep the skin soft.

Defuzz – legs look and feel better when they're silky smooth and waxing is the best way to achieve this. Do it yourself at home or have the treatment done at a salon. You will need to let the hairs grow until they're at least 6 mm/¼ in long so the wax has something to grip on to. But in time, the hairs will grow back sparser and finer. Depilatory creams only need to be used about once a fortnight, if that, and are fairly effective but in the long term, waxing may work out cheaper and be less time consuming. Shaving is a last resort. It may be quick, cheap and convenient but you'll probably find your legs feel stubbly again within a matter of days so only use this method in emergencies.

FLATTER AND FLAUNT

Even the plumpest pins look more attractive when they're tanned, so if you're going bare-legged, touch them up with a little fake tan. A body lotion with a hint of shimmer applied along your shins will also enhance them for a special evening.

A spot of bother? Fake tan also helps to disguise blemishes, and is especially helpful for hiding stretch marks. But if you're really self-conscious about scars, bruises or birth marks, try a concealer – the sort you'd use on your face, or look for specialised concealing creams with concentrated pigmentation to provide even greater coverage.

Broken veins? Tiny spidery thin veins may appear on your legs if you have sensitive skin. To prevent them, avoid hot baths which can encourage blood vessels to break and avoid exposure to sudden extremes of temperature – putting your legs too near the fire when you've just come in from the cold can make your skin red and blotchy, or give you chilblains.

If you want to do more than simply disguise these veins, you could have them treated at a beauty salon. One of the most popular methods is electrolysis which uses heat to cauterise the blood vessel so it's no longer visible.

Another less common type of treatment uses a chemical which is injected into the vein to shrink it. It's very important, however, to ensure you visit a qualified therapist for these treatments – try a beauty salon in a reputable department store.

SUPPORT ACT

If you thought support tights were thick, ugly passion killers, you're wrong. Now they're available in sheer and fashionable colours. They're a bonus for women who are on their feet all day or if you're pregnant – we all need a little support sometimes to help us stand up for ourselves! So how do they help? Basically they're tighter at the ankle than at the top so they help to fight the pull of gravity and pump and squeeze the blood up your legs, thus helping to prevent varicose veins, swollen feet and ankles, and that tired, lead-weight feeling in your legs. You can get light, medium or strong support tights.

FIGHT CELLULITE

This is a common complaint which mars many women's thighs. But whether you're suffering from cellulite already or trying to avoid it, tackling the problem with a daily routine rather than occasional and expensive salon treatments is your best bet. If you're overweight, slim down and aim to stimulate your blood circulation to help your body pump out the fluid and toxins which seem to be the main cause.

Boost circulation with daily massages in the bath using a friction sponge or mitt and afterwards use an anti-cellulite cream. Finally, splash problem areas with cold water and remember to exercise. Try our exercises as well as regular cycling, swimming and brisk walking.

LEG WORK

There's little you can do to alter the underlying shape of your legs but don't be disheartened. Regular exercise will fight flab and help to avoid problems in later life such as varicose veins and brittle bones. Stair climbing is excellent exercise, so skip lifts and escalators. You can even buy stair-

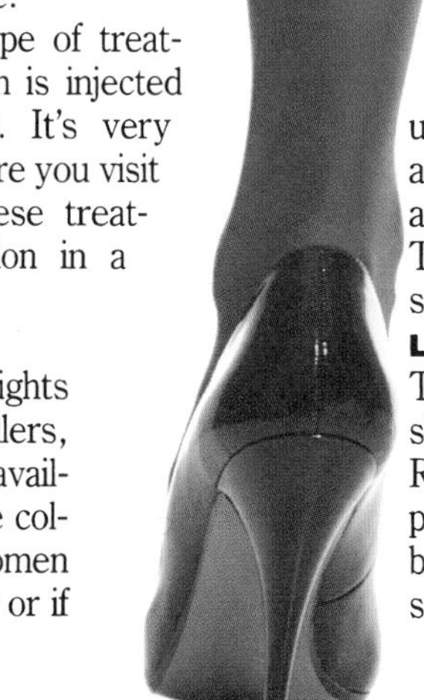

climbing machines now for use at home – a worthwhile investment, great for shaping legs and bottoms.

Most doctors recommend a brisk 20-minute walk, cycle ride, ride, swim or aerobics lesson at least three times a week. But in addition, slot in this routine whenever possible to keep leg muscles stretched, flexible and toned.

WARM UP: stretch, then jog gently on the spot for about a minute.

COMPLETE LEG TONER: lie on your side supporting your head with your hand, the other hand placed in front of your chest. Now slowly raise your upper leg – not too high, it's more difficult to hold it just a few inches up. Then slowly lower. Repeat 10 times on each side. Then repeat a further 10 times on each side, but this time lift the bottom leg to meet the top leg.

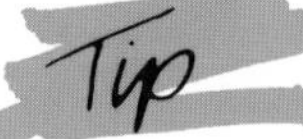

Feeling weary? Look out for the revitalising leg lotions and gels on the market. These usually contain refreshing ingredients such as cooling peppermint oil and invigorating seaweed extracts to leave you tingling instead of tired. Rub in with strong, sweeping upward movements.

CALF STRETCH: this is good for girls who like to wear high heels. Stand about 30 cm/12 in away from a wall with palms flat against the wall. Now without raising your heels, lean your upper body slowly towards the wall, bending your elbows out, and you'll feel the stretch in the back of your legs. Don't bounce. Hold for a count of three and repeat 10 times. ▶

SIMPLE STRENGTHENER: knees and ankles take a lot of strain and need to be strong if you're going to avoid injuries, so try this exercise. Sit on a chair and grip a round wastepaper bin between your ankles. Now slowly lift the bin up until your legs are horizontal. Hold for a count of three, then lower. Repeat 10 times. ▶

COOL DOWN: finish with this stretch to avoid pulled muscles. Lie on your back with one leg bent, the knee pointing towards the ceiling. Now gently stretch your other leg up and gripping it around the calf, very carefully pull it towards your chest, trying not to bend your knee, but don't force it. Flex and point your ankle three times. Slowly lower and repeat with other leg. ▶

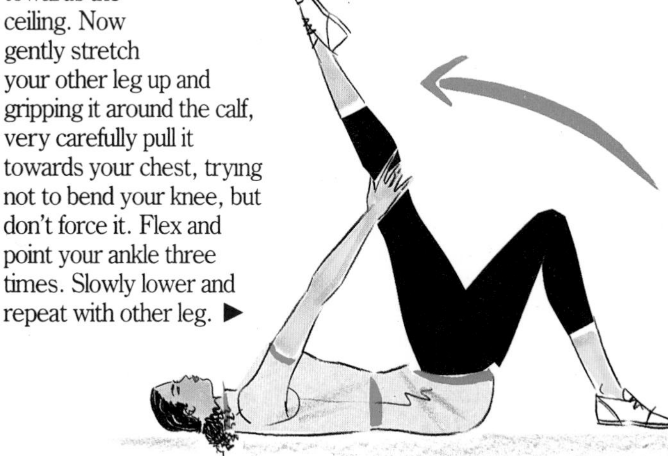

Tip

Legs look slimmer in dark tights. Also match tights to the colour of your shoes as this gives the illusion of longer legs. And steer clear of skirts that fall at mid calf as these will draw attention to the fattest part of your legs and make them look larger. If, however, you feel your legs are too spindly, opt for pale coloured tights.

ANY QUESTIONS?

Q My mum has varicose veins. Will I get them too?

A Varicose veins do tend to run in families but with a little care you may be able to avoid them. They occur when valves in the veins of your leg fail and instead of being pumped around, the blood pools and makes your vein stretch and bulge. So obviously it's important to keep the blood moving. Therefore, you must avoid tight restrictive clothing and underwear; don't allow yourself to become overweight and eat plenty of fibre to prevent constipation as both these things can put a strain on leg veins. Try to avoid long periods of standing and if you have a a job where you're on your feet all day, invest in some support tights. Exercise stimulates circulation and strong leg muscles help the veins to do their job properly. Also when you're resting, lie with your feet propped up in a higher position than your head so the blood doesn't have to fight the pull of gravity and can flow up easily. Serious varicose veins should be treated – ask your doctor for advice.

Q What can I do about my thick ankles?

A If they are just temporarily puffy, you could be suffering from water retention. The above advice for varicose veins also applies to you – follow those tips and you should find the puffiness disappears. Perhaps, however, you have simply inherited thick ankles in which case no amount of ankle circling exercises will slim them down. You can disguise them by wearing dark tights, and court shoes which are low at the front to draw the attention from your ankles.

Illustrations: JACQUELINE BISSETT/Photograph: ADRIAN BRADBURY

HEALTH WARNINGS!

Are you fit for anything or do you live dangerously? Wise up to every day hazards – some may surprise you!

You may feel virtuous starting your day with a jog round the block, but if you live in a city a half-hour run in congested traffic means you may be breathing in as much carbon monoxide as a heavy smoker. You could also be picking up airborne dust particles which can clog your pores and lead to blackheads and spots. If that's the case, try another form of exercise, like swimming, or visit a gym for a work-out.

If you do jog, always wear a good sports bra and proper training shoes. And jog in the evening or after it has rained when the air is fresher.

BYE GUM

Do you chew gum to help keep trim? Think again – it really gets your digestive juices flowing, leaving you with too

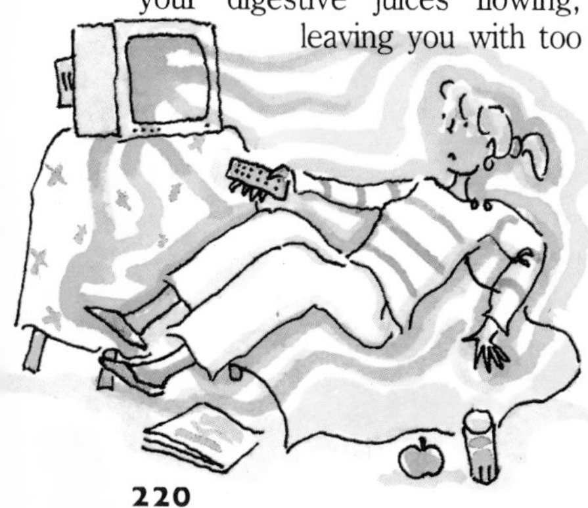

much stomach acid. This can cause tummy pain and wind. If you need to nibble, snack on fruit.

EAU YES

A simple way to a clear skin is to drink lots of water to flush out toxins. However, tap water can often have a metallic taste and there have been reports that it is not as pure as it looks. High levels of nitrates in particular are a cause for concern, so it may be a good idea to invest in a water filter.

ANYONE FOR A CUPPA?

Tea and coffee are strong in caffeine – so watch how much you drink. If you feel anxious, irritable and have trouble sleeping it could be because you're drinking too much tea or coffee. Try decaffeinated coffee or switch to herbal teas.

WORK IT OUT

Modern offices look smart and hygienic. But studies have shown that a number of office workers can suffer from 'sick building syndrome.' Symptoms include lethargy, headaches and itchy eyes. Too-hot central heating dries the skin, while air conditioning may simply spread a host of bugs. You can bring your office back to health by filling it with indoor plants. They give off oxygen essential for a healthy, moist atmosphere, or you could try an ioniser which puts out negative ions. They cling on to positively charged particles of pollen, dust and smoke, weighing them down so they fall as dust and can be vacuumed away.

Working under fluorescent lights can be tiring. Work in daylight or use a desk lamp and go for a walk at lunch time.

Even the photocopier can be a bit of a hazard – if it's poorly ventilated it may leak ozone. Ozone, vital to the earth's upper atmosphere, can cause depression and appetite loss in concentrated doses. Check that the copier is well-maintained and in a separate, ventilated room.

Use a VDU? There has been much controversy about side effects such as eyesight deterioration and itchy skin, so always take regular breaks, turn off the computer when you're not using it and get a special shield for the screen to filter the rays. If you're pregnant, or thinking of starting a family, use a VDU as

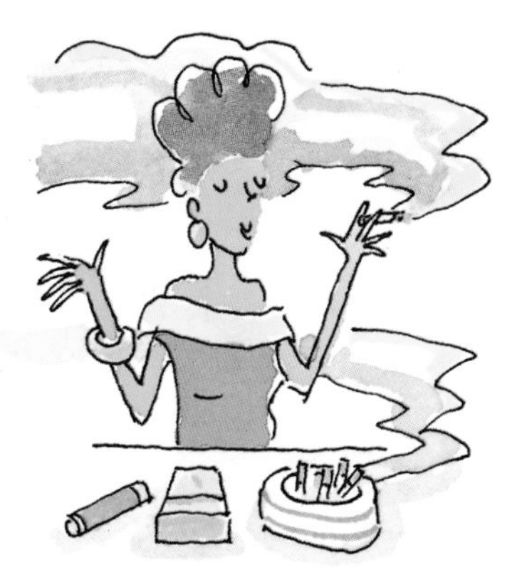

little as possible – recent studies have linked them with foetal abnormalities.

EVENINGS IN

There's nothing like curling up in front of the telly after a stressful day, but if you sit closer than 3 m/10 ft, you can be exposing yourself to small doses of harmful X-rays which leak from the set.

WILD NIGHTS OUT

While a glass of wine now and then can be relaxing, too much booze is self destructive. If you're drinking more than two glasses each night – that's too much! It can give you broken veins and serious liver problems. It also hinders the absorption of vitamins such as the B group, which keeps your nerves calm and your skin glowing. Don't ever feel you have to drink just because your friends do.

Smoking also has serious side-effects. As well as running the risk of lung cancer, smoking will give you poor circulation, greyish skin, bad breath, wrinkles, and you'll be more likely to get spots. Give up the habit by cutting down gradually and make sure you're getting enough vitamin C – smoking uses it up! Burning the midnight oil will also take its toll on your looks so plan a quiet weekend from time to time. Turn your home into a health farm – no fags, booze or junk food – just relax and recharge your batteries.

TALKING SCENTS

When you buy an anti-perspirant deodorant, choose a natural herbal or fragrance-free hypo-allergenic brand. Other deodorants may contain aluminium salts to absorb sweat but this also constricts pores and sometimes causes an itchy rash.

THE GOOD NEWS

If all this sounds as if life's not worth living, don't despair! Make a few changes and you'll still keep the fun in your life.

Illustrations: BILL PIGGINS

CRISIS POINTS

Trying to deal with disaster or shake off severe shock isn't easy. So be prepared and learn how to fight back and start living again

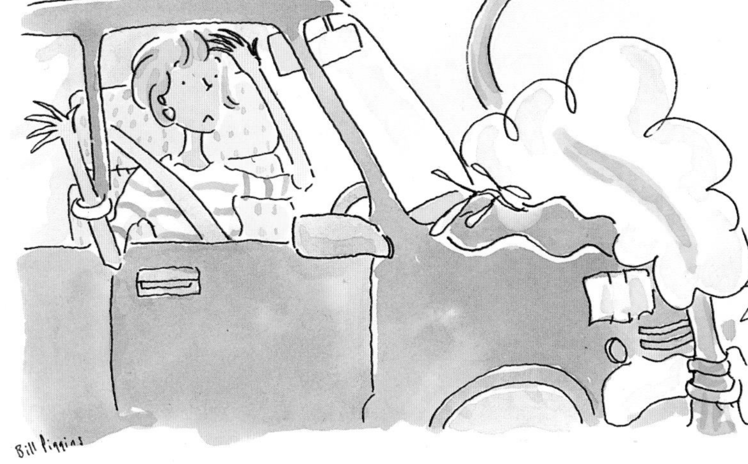

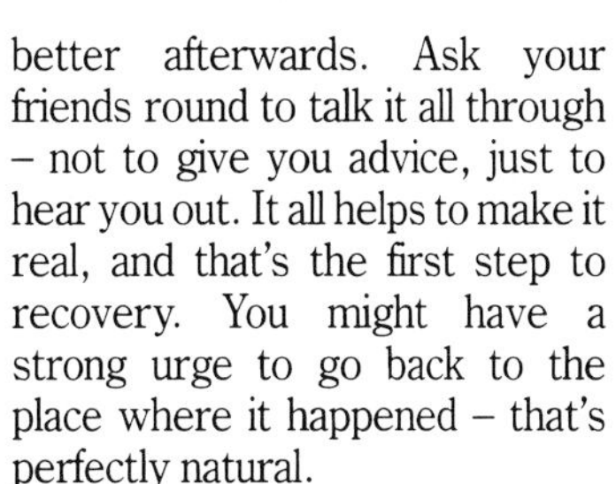

Life's full of everyday knocks: failing a driving test or not getting the job that you'd pinned your hopes on are unpleasant, and a blow. They're often called minor traumas and most of us take them in our stride, or after a few tantrums and tears we are able to put them in perspective – or vow to do better next time!

Real medical trauma is a shock so bad it knocks you sideways and changes your way of life for days, months, or even years. It can be caused by many things and usually happens when you least expect it, which makes the after-effects even more unbearable. For instance, a car accident, a brush with death, being burgled, the end of a long-term relationship, the death of a loved one, divorce in the family or being raped. The kind of things that you read about or think they only happen to others – not you or your family.

FUTURE SHOCK

The first effects of trauma are physical: trembling, turning pale, fainting, even being sick. If you've been in an accident you may have physical injuries that bring their own problems, or even permanent disability.

However, your emotional reaction to trauma is deeper and can be more serious, and without proper after-care you can be left mentally scarred for life. The usual symptoms are a loss of a sense of reality. You'll probably start off by refusing to believe what's happened, or feeling totally numb and distant from the event, unable even to cry.

It's common to feel yourself pretending to be okay. But of course, everyone reacts differently. Some of your feelings may take you by surprise, but it's quite normal to feel the exact opposite of what you expect: strong anger, bitterness, fear and 'why me?' syndrome after a trauma, as well as disbelief and sorrow. If you've had a brush with death at a young age, you may dwell on the fact that you're not immortal after all.

Similarly, you may try to make the trauma 'unhappen' by bargaining, along the lines of 'please God turn the clock back to before and I'll promise never to be horrible to anyone again'. But it has happened, and all you can do is to work towards accepting it, and learning what you can from the experience. The healing process will be slow, but there are many positive ways that you can start to rebuild your life – now!

HOW TO COPE

So how do you start coping? Well, trying to pretend it hasn't happened simply doesn't work. So give yourself time for reality to sink in. Cancel appointments and take as much time as you need to rest away from the hubbub. If you live away from the family home, go back. It can give you great comfort and security to be surrounded by familiar things.

If you've been in a car accident or fallen off a horse, get a friend to help you back into a car or on to a horse as soon as you can; it'll help to conquer the fear. When you've split up with a boyfriend, lost a member of the family or a friend, forget the stiff upper lip – bottling things up just creates trouble for the future. It's true, some of your feelings may be very uncomfortable, but let them come to the surface all the same. If that means howling in rage or sobbing into the night, go ahead – you'll feel a lot better afterwards. Ask your friends round to talk it all through – not to give you advice, just to hear you out. It all helps to make it real, and that's the first step to recovery. You might have a strong urge to go back to the place where it happened – that's perfectly natural.

The shock of a trauma can often make you rush around trying to fill the gap or stop yourself feeling and thinking. This can be a mistake. Make time to listen to music, meditate, walk or whatever helps you to feel still and in touch with yourself. Think about what you've been through, what or who you've lost, the sadness and the disappointment. It can help to write it all down – when you look back in a month or two you'll be surprised how much you've healed. On the positive side, begin to understand what you've learned about yourself and other people from the trauma. If it happened again, would you – or could you – have acted differently? What might you have done to avoid it or make it less hurtful? Trauma is painful – accept that you need to feel the pain in order to recover. At the same time, use all the help you can get from family, friends, helplines, problem pages, or local self-help groups. Sharing your feelings with other people who've had the same experience is also very useful – it helps reconnect you to the real world, understand your own feelings and see that there is life after what's happened.

COMING TO TERMS

In the long term, you may find that counselling, psychotherapy, natural or spiritual healing are necessary for you to come to terms with what's happened and integrate it into your life. More and more people these days are taking advantage of these services, whether it's specialist counselling for rape, trauma or bereavement, or more general talking sessions.

Recovery means not only accepting it really did happen and acknowledging the effects that it's had – and going to have – on your life, but also realising that every trauma is an opportunity to grow up a little. That may sound rather hard to believe,but how many times have you heard people saying 'It was awful, but it was the spur I needed!'?

You'll know you're on the road to recovery when you can remember without it hurting, and when you understand that although trauma is horrible, it can show you where you may be wasting your time, and what's really important in your life.

Illustration: BILL PIGGINS

SLEEP EASY

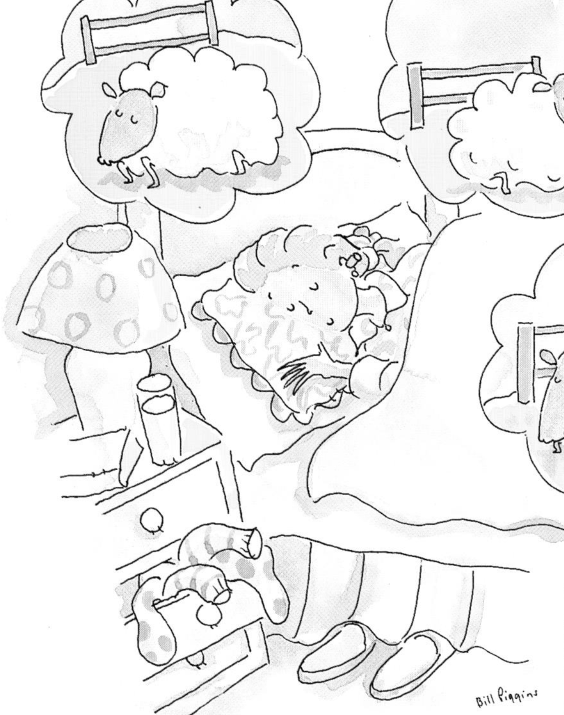

TEN TIPS TO IMPROVE YOUR KIP

1 *Have a warm, relaxing bath.*
2 *Camomile and peppermint are natural soporifics – so try them as tea. They're available from most health foodshops. Drink a cup of one of them about 30 minutes before you go to bed.*
3 *Or have a glass of milk. It contains an amino acid called tryptophan which helps encourage restful sleep.*
4 *Is your bed comfortable? A sagging mattress causes backache and tension. Your mattress should be firm and support your spine.*
5 *Use soothing scented herb pillows, they smell delicious.*
6 *Avoid alcohol. It may seem to relax you, but it can stimulate the brain and wake you early.*
7 *If noise is a problem, use a pair of ear-plugs.*
8 *Avoid tight nightwear.*
9 *Try a pair of socks for cold feet.*
10 *Check that your bedroom is well-ventilated.*

Do you drop off with ease or toss and turn all night? Sleep is a vital natural process, so wake up to the facts and help yourself to sweet dreams

How much sleep did you have last night? Eight hours may be the average, but individual needs vary. Some people need 10 to 12 hours a night, while others sparkle after only three to four. Your need for sleep tends to decrease with age which is why babies need the most (14-16 hours) and the elderly need least (six hours or less).

A refreshing night's sleep alternates both slow-wave (dreamless) sleep to rest the body, and REM (dreaming) sleep to refresh the mind. Sleep progresses through several stages which occur in 60-90 minute cycles.

Stage One. A light sleep in which the muscles relax, pupils contract, and temperature, breathing and heart rate lower. Brainwaves get smaller, slower and more uneven.

Stage Two. Sleep deepens. Your metabolic rate drops further, while the brain shows occasional bursts of activity.

Stage Three. Sleep is quite deep now, with brainwaves becoming larger and slower. Metabolic rate is still dropping. The eyes may roll slowly from side to side.

Stage Four. (Delta Sleep). This occurs within an hour, and is a deep level of sleep from which you are hard to rouse. Temperature, blood pressure and heart rate are at their lowest, breathing is at its slowest and most even, brainwaves are largest.

Stage Five. (REM Sleep). This is when dreaming occurs and REM (Rapid Eye Movement) takes place under your lids. Blood pressure, pulse and breathing rates increase.

Not being able to sleep bothers all of us at one time or another. Common causes of occasional sleeplessness include jet-lag, stress, a change of routine, a different bed, hunger, pain, cold, noise, over-tiredness and some kinds of drugs. Missing out on the odd night's sleep won't do you any harm, it only becomes a problem when you go for weeks or months without any deep sleep.

It's common sense to avoid any kind of stimulus before bed. Avoid vigorous exercise, and don't overload your stomach with food since your digestive system slows down during the night. Avoid sugar, salt and caffeine. The effects of caffeine may last up to six hours.

If you can't nod off, relax. Fear of not being able to sleep, often makes matters worse. It's better to just rest quietly than to spend the night tossing, turning and worrying. Counting sheep may seem an old trick, but monotonous mind games can help induce drowsiness. Add up a list of figures in your mind or try counting backwards from 500! Yoga, meditation and massage are all aids to relaxation. Also, try breathing exercises such as inhaling to a count of four, then exhaling very gently to a count of 12. Or sleep with your ear on the pillow, so you can hear your heartbeat.

Sedatives are a last resort and only a short-term solution since your body eventually builds up a tolerance. If necessary, try alternative remedies like hypnosis, homoeopathy or acupuncture.

However, prolonged insomnia can be a symptom of depression or chronic anxiety. See your doctor if you're concerned.

BEDTIME BEAUTY

- *A cleansing beauty ritual before bedtime will keep skin clear, as well as helping you to relax.*
- *Brush your teeth and floss them.*
- *Cleanse, tone and moisturise your skin, using slow, rhythmic movements.*
- *Tie your hair into a topknot so you don't add grease to your pillow.*
- *Morning puffiness under the eyes may be caused by your sleeping position. Keep your head slightly raised with a firm pillow.*

Illustration: BILL PIGGINS

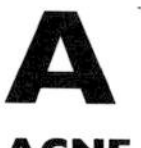

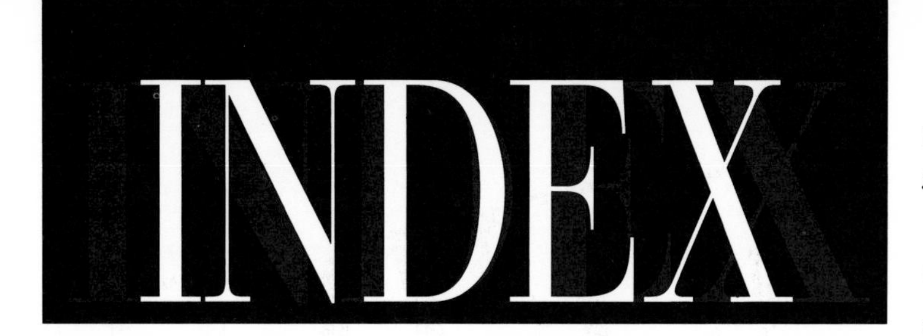

IJ

L

M

N

OPQ

S

T

UV

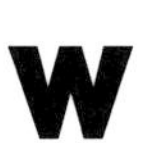